SECOND CANADIAN EDITION

Nursing Research in Canada

Methods and Critical Appraisal for Evidence-Based Practice

Geri LoBiondo-Wood, RN, PhD, FAAN
Associate Professor
University of Texas Health Sciences
    Center
School of Nursing
Nursing Systems and Technology
Houston, Texas

Judith Haber, APRN, BC, PhD, FAAN
Professor and Associate Dean for
    Graduate Programs
Master's Program and Post-Master's
    Advanced Certificate Program
College of Nursing
New York University
New York, New York

CANADIAN EDITORS

Cherylyn Cameron, RN, PhD
Associate Vice-President
University Partnership Centre,
    Research and Scholarship
Georgian College
Barrie, Ontario

Mina D. Singh, RN, PhD
Assistant Professor
School of Nursing
York University
Toronto, Ontario

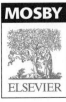

MOSBY

ELSEVIER

NOTICE
Neither the Publisher nor the Authors assume any responsibility for any loss or injury and/or damage to persons or property arising out of or related to any use of the material contained in this book. It is the responsibility of the treating practitioner, relying on independent expertise and knowledge of the client, to determine the best treatment and method of application for the client.

The Publisher

Library and Archives Canada Cataloguing in Publication
LoBiondo-Wood, Geri
    Nursing research in Canada : methods and critical appraisal for evidence-based practice /
Geri LoBiondo-Wood, Judith Haber. — 2nd
Canadian ed. / Canadian editors, Cherylyn Cameron, Mina D. Singh

Includes index.
Has supplement: Study guide to accompany Nursing research in Canada.
ISBN 978-0-7796-9995-7

    1. Nursing—Research—Canada—Textbooks. I. Haber, Judith II. Cameron, Cherylyn, 1958–
III. Singh, Mina D. IV. Title.

RT81.5.N8724 2008   610.73072'071   C2007-907298-4

ISBN-13: 978-0-7796-9995-7
ISBN-10: 0-7796-9995-5

Publisher, Education: Ann Millar
Developmental Editor: Dawn du Quesnay
Managing Developmental Editor: Martina van de Velde
Managing Production Editor: Lise Dupont
Copy Editor: Holly Dickinson
Proofreader: Mariko Obokata
Cover, Interior Design: Monica Kompter
Typesetting and Assembly: Jansom
Printing and Binding: Transcontinental

Elsevier Canada
905 King Street West, 4th Floor
Toronto, ON, Canada M6K 3G9
Phone: 1-866-896-3331
Fax: 1-866-359-9534

Printed in Canada

2 3 4 5   13 12 11 10 09

TABLE OF CONTENTS

CONTRIBUTORS

Cherylyn Cameron, RN, PhD
Associate Vice-President
University Partnership Centre, Research and
    Scholarship
Georgian College
Barrie, Ontario
The Role of Research in Nursing
Theoretical Framework
Critical Reading Strategies: Overview of the
    Research Process
Developing Research Questions and Hypotheses
Literature Review
Introduction to Qualitative Research
Qualitative Approaches to Research
Qualitative Data Analysis
Critiquing Qualitative Research
Use of Research in Practice

Marlene Z. Cohen, RN, PhD, FAAN
John S. Dunn, Sr., Distinguished Professor in
    Oncology Nursing
Interim Chair
Department of Target Populations
School of Nursing
The University of Texas Health Science Center
Houston, Texas
Professor
Department of Symptom Research
The University of Texas M.D. Anderson Cancer
    Center
Houston. Texas
Nurse Researcher
Lyndon B. Johnson General Hospital
Houston, Texas
Introduction to Qualitative Research

Betty J. Craft, RN, PhD, CS
Retired, Faculty Emeritus
College of Nursing
University of Nebraska
Omaha, Nebraska
Critiquing Quantitative Research

Barbara Davies, RN, PhD
Associate Professor, Nursing
University of Ottawa
Ottawa, Ontario
Premiers Research Excellence Award
Co-Director Nursing Best Practice Research Unit
Research Vignette: Nursing Best Practice

Nancy C. Edwards, RN, BScN, MSc, PhD
Full Professor
School of Nursing
Department of Epidemiology and Community
    Medicine
University of Ottawa
Ottawa, Ontario
CHSRF/CIHR Nursing Chair
Director, Community Health Research Unit
Research Vignette: Tackling the Prevention of
    Falls Among Seniors

Julie Gaudet, RN, MN (Admin.)
Professor
Ryerson, Centennial, George Brown
    Collaborative Nursing Degree Program
School of Nursing
Centre for Health Sciences
George Brown College
Toronto, Ontario
Research Vignette: Interprofessional Learning:
    Impetus for Collaborative Nursing Practice

Margaret Grey, RN, DrPH, FAAN
Dean and Annie Goodrich Professor of Nursing
Yale School of Nursing
Yale University
New Haven, Connecticut
Experimental and Quasiexperimental Designs
Data Collection Methods
Quantitative Data Analysis

Judith Haber, APRN, PhD, CS, FAAN
Professor and Director
Master's Program and Post-Master's Advanced
    Certificate Program
Division of Nursing
New York University
New York, New York
The Role of Research in Nursing
Critical Reading Strategies: Overview of the
    Research Process
Developing Research Questions and Hypotheses
Legal and Ethical Issues
Nonexperimental Designs
Sampling
Rigour in Research

Judith A. Heermann, RN, PhD
Associate Professor
College of Nursing
University of Nebraska
Clinical Nurse Researcher
University of Nebraska Medical Center
Omaha, Nebraska
Critiquing Quantitative Research

Carl Kirton, RN, APRN BC, MA,
Adjunct Faculty
College of Nursing
New York University
Director, Ambulatory Care and Nurse Practitioner
AIDS Clinic
Mount Sinai Hospital
New York, New York
Quantitative Data Analysis

Barbara Krainovich-Miller, APRN BC, EdD,
Clinical Professor
College of Nursing
New York University
New York, New York
Critical Reading Strategies: Overview of the
    Research Process
Literature Review
Critical Thinking Challenges

Patricia R. Liehr, RN, PhD
Professor, Associate Dean for Nursing Research
    and Scholarship
Christine E. Lynn College of Nursing
Florida Atlantic University
Boca Raton, Florida
Theoretical Framework
Qualitative Approaches to Research

Geri LoBiondo-Wood, RN, PhD, FAAN
Associate Professor
University of Texas Health Science Center—
    Houston
School of Nursing
Nursing Systems and Technology
Houston, Texas
The Role of Research in Nursing
Critical Reading Strategies: Overview of the
    Research Process
Qualitative Approaches to Research
Introduction to Quantitative Research
Nonexperimental Designs
Rigour in Research
Presenting the Findings

Janice M. Morse, RN, PhD
Professor, Faculty of Nursing
Director, International Institute for Qualitative
    Methodology
Faculty of Nursing
University of Alberta
Edmonton, Alberta
Research Vignette: Creating Qualitatively
    Derived Theory

Barbara Paterson, RN, Med, PhD
Professor and Tier 1 Canada Research Chair
Faculty of Nursing
University of New Brunswick
Fredericton, New Brunswick
Research Vignette: How Nurses Use and
    Respond to Research

ix

Mina D. Singh, RN, PhD
Assistant Professor
School of Nursing
York University
Toronto, Ontario
The Role of Research in Nursing
Legal and Ethical Issues
Introduction to Quantitative Research
Experimental and Quasiexperimental Designs
Nonexperimental Designs
Sampling
Data Collection Methods
Rigour in Research
Quantitative Data Analysis
Presenting the Findings
Critiquing Quantitative Research

Glenda L. Smith, RNC, NNP, APRN BC,
    PNP DSN
Associate Professor of Nursing
Department of Nursing
Tuskegee University
Tuskegee, Alabama
Critical Thinking Challenges

Mary Jane Smith, RN, PhD
Professor and Associate Dean for Graduate
    Academic Affairs
School of Nursing
Robert C. Byrd Health Sciences Center
West Virginia University
Morgantown, West Virginia
Theoretical Framework

Helen J. Streubert Speziale, RN, EdD
Professor
Nursing Department
College Misercordia
Dallas, Pennsylvania
Critiquing Qualitative Research

Marita G. Titler, RN, PhD, FAAN
Director, Research, Quality, and Outcomes
    Management
Department of Nursing Services and Patient
    Care
University of Iowa Hospitals and Clinics
Iowa City, Iowa
Use of Research in Practice

Judith Wuest, RN, BScN, MN, PhD
Professor and Canadian Institutes of Health
    Research/UNB Investigator
Faculty of Nursing
University of New Brunswick
Fredericton, New Brunswick
Research Vignette: Evolution in a Program
*   of Research Focusing on Family Violence,*
*   Caregiving, and Women's Health*

Robin Whittemore, APRN, PhD
Associate Research Scientist, Lecturer
School of Nursing
Yale University
New Haven, Connecticut
Experimental and Quasiexperimental Designs
Data Collection Methods
Quantitative Data Analysis

REVIEWERS

Dr. Pat H. Bailey, RN, PhD
Professor
School of Nursing
Laurentian University
Sudbury, Ontario

Janet Bryanton, RN, MN, PhD (Cand.)
Associate Professor
School of Nursing
University of Prince Edward Island
Charlottetown, Prince Edward Island

Donna Bulman, RN, MEd, PhD
Assistant Professor
School of Nursing
Memorial University
St. John's, Newfoundland

Tam Donnelly, RN, PhD
Assistant Professor
Faculty of Nursing
University of Calgary
Calgary, Alberta

Sherry Espin, RN, PhD
Associate Professor
School of Nursing
Ryerson University
Toronto, Ontario

Angela Gillis, RN, PhD
Professor
School of Nursing
St. Francis Xavier University
Antigonish, Nova Scotia

Brad Hagen, RN, PhD
Associate Professor
School of Health Sciences
University of Lethbridge
Lethbridge, Alberta

June Kaminski, MSN, PhD(c)
Faculty of Nursing
Kwantlen Polytechnic University
Surrey, British Columbia

Judith C. Kulig, RN, DNSc
Professor
School of Health Sciences
University of Lethbridge
Lethbridge, Alberta

Colleen Norris, RN, PhD
Assistant Professor
Faculty of Nursing
University of Alberta
Edmonton, Alberta

Karin Olson, RN, PhD
Associate Professor
Faculty of Nursing
University of Alberta
Edmonton, Alberta

Maryse Pelletier-Hibbert, BN, MN, PhD
Professor
Faculty of Nursing
University of New Brunswick
Fredericton, New Brunswick

Barbara Pesut, RN, PhD
Assistant Professor
School of Nursing
University of British Columbia—Okanagan
Kelowna, British Columbia

Louise Racine, RN, BScN, MScN, PhD
Assistant Professor
College of Nursing
University of Saskatchewan
Saskatoon, Saskatchewan

Anne Sales, RN, PhD
Associate Professor
Faculty of Nursing
University of Alberta
Edmonton, Alberta

Richard Sawatzky, PhD
Assistant Professor
Department of Nursing
Trinity Western University
Langley, British Columbia

Jasna K. Schwind, RN, PhD
Associate Professor
School of Nursing
Ryerson University
Toronto, Ontario

Veryl Margaret Tipliski, RN, PhD, CPMHN(c)
Instructor
Nursing Department
Langara College
Vancouver, British Columbia

PREFACE

The foundation of the second Canadian edition of *Nursing Research in Canada: Methods and Critical Appraisal for Evidence-Based Practice* is the belief that nursing research is integral to all levels of nursing education and practice. Over the past three years (since the first Canadian edition of this textbook), we have seen the depth and breadth of nursing research in Canada grow, with more nurses conducting and using research to shape clinical practice, education, administration, and public policy. Nurses use research data to influence the nature and direction of health care delivery and to document outcomes related to the quality and cost-effectiveness of client care. As nurses continue to develop a unique body of nursing knowledge through research, decisions about clinical nursing practice are becoming increasingly both research based and evidence based.

Nurses need not only to understand the research process but also how to read, evaluate, and apply research findings critically in practice. Understanding research is a challenge for many students, but we believe the negative perception of research as "complex" and difficult to understand can be overcome provided that students have stimulating, lively, and learner-friendly learning opportunities.

Consistent with the perspective that all nurses need to understand both the research process and how to apply research findings in practice is the belief that nursing research must be an integral aspect of nursing education, evident not only in specific research courses but also throughout the curriculum. The research role of nursing graduates calls for the skills of critical appraisal; in other words, nurses must be competent research consumers.

Preparing students to be active consumers of research involves developing their critical thinking and reading skills, thus enhancing their understanding of the research process, their appreciation of the role of the critiquer, and their ability to critique research. An undergraduate course in nursing research is designed to develop this basic level of competence, which is an essential requirement if students are to participate in evidence-based clinical decision making and practice. This approach is in contrast to a graduate-level research course in which the emphasis is on conducting research, as well as understanding and appraising it.

This book was written primarily to introduce undergraduate students to the steps of the research process, the critique of published research literature, and the use of research findings to support evidence-based clinical practice; however, others will also find this book an excellent resource. Students at the master's and doctoral levels will benefit from a concise review of the basic steps of the research and critiquing process. Practising nurses can refer to this book when using research findings (rather than tradition, authority, or trial and error) as the basis for clinical decision making and in their development of evidence-based policies, protocols, and standards. Those who collaborate with nurse scientists to conduct clinical research will also find this book a valuable resource.

Building on the success of the first Canadian edition of *Nursing Research in Canada*, this edition was strengthened with input from Canadian educators from across the country. The text was revised to reflect equally the paradigms of qualitative research and quantitative research. An important addition is a new chapter dedicated to the methods of qualitative research analysis. The section on quantitative methods was augmented with current statistical trends. This second Canadian edition prepares nursing students and practising nurses to become knowledgeable nursing research consumers by focusing on the following:

- Addressing the role of the nurse as a research consumer
- Demystifying research, which is sometimes viewed as a complex process
- Using an evidence-based approach to teaching the fundamentals of the research process

- Introducing the fundamentals of the research process and presenting the critical appraisal process in a user-friendly, logical, and systematic progression
- Promoting a lively spirit of inquiry to develop critical thinking and critical reading skills, facilitating a mastery of the critiquing process
- Developing information literacy and research consumer competencies to prepare students and nurses to effectively locate and manage research information
- Elevating the critiquing process and research consumership to a position of importance comparable to that of producing research (before students become researchers themselves, they must become knowledgeable research consumers)
- Emphasizing the role of evidence-based practice as the basis for clinical decision making and nursing interventions that support nursing practice, demonstrating quality and cost-effective outcomes of nursing care delivery
- Presenting numerous examples of recently published Canadian research studies to provide students with a Canadian viewpoint, to demonstrate the diversity of nursing research across Canada, and to reinforce the research and critiquing process
- Showcasing **Research Vignettes** by renowned Canadian nurse researchers whose careers exemplify the links between research, education, and practice
- Providing numerous pedagogical chapter features, including **Key Terms, Learning Outcomes, Helpful Hints, Evidence-Based Practice Tips, Critical Thinking Decision Paths, Critiquing Criteria, Critical Thinking Challenges, Key Points,** and numerous tables, boxes, and figures
- Providing a study guide that promotes active learning and assimilation of nursing research content

The second Canadian edition of *Nursing Research in Canada: Methods and Critical Appraisal for Evidence-Based Practice* is organized into the following six parts, each of which is preceded by a provocative "Research Vignette" (i.e., a "real" and interesting research story) told by a well-known Canadian nurse researcher:

- PART ONE, RESEARCH OVERVIEW, contains six chapters. Chapter 1, "The Role of Research in Nursing," provides an overview of contemporary research roles, approaches to research, and issues in nursing research. The chapter introduces the importance of the nurse's role as a research consumer and provides a futuristic perspective on the research and evidence-based practice principles that will shape clinical practice in this new millennium. An in-depth examination of the role of research and the history of nursing research in Canada is also included. Chapter 2, "Theoretical Framework," addresses the importance of theoretical foundations to the design and evaluation of research studies. Chapter 3, "Critical Reading Strategies: Overview of the Research Process," speaks directly to students by highlighting critical thinking and critical reading concepts and strategies that facilitate students' understanding of the research process and its relationship to the critiquing process. The style and content of this chapter are designed to make subsequent chapters easier to understand for students. The next three chapters address components of the research process. Chapter 4, "Developing Research Questions and Hypotheses," focuses on how research questions and hypotheses are derived, operationalized in research studies, and critically appraised. Numerous clinical examples illustrate different types of research questions and hypotheses to maximize students' understanding. Chapter 5, "Literature Review," showcases cutting-edge information related to research consumer competencies that prepare students and nurses to effectively locate, manage, and evaluate research studies and their findings. Chapter 6, "Legal and Ethical Issues," provides an overview of the increased emphasis on the legal and ethical issues facing researchers in Canada.
- PART TWO, QUALITATIVE RESEARCH, contains two interrelated qualitative research chapters. Chapter 7, "Introduction to Qualitative Research," provides an expanded framework for understanding qualitative research designs and literature. Chapter 8, "Qualitative Approaches to

Research," presents and illustrates major qualitative designs and methods using examples from the literature. Taking into account feedback from the reviewers of the first edition, the authors have included in this chapter more information on qualitative methods, thus balancing the qualitative content with quantitative methods.

- PART THREE, QUANTITATIVE RESEARCH, contains Chapters 9 to 11, which delineate the essential steps of the quantitative research process, using published clinical research studies to illustrate each step. Links between the steps and their relationship to the total research process are examined and then synthesized in Chapter 19.
- PART FOUR, PROCESSES RELATED TO RESEARCH, contains Chapters 12 to 17. These six chapters on the process related to research, from sampling to analysis, were renamed and reorganized to meet both students' interests and the demand to balance qualitative and quantitative information. For example, Chapter 14 was restructured to incorporate both qualitative and quantitative rigour in research.
- PART FIVE, CRITIQUING RESEARCH, contains Chapters 18 and 19, which synthesize the essential components and criteria for critiquing qualitative and quantitative research reports and include four studies with accompanying critiques.
- PART SIX, APPLICATION OF RESEARCH: EVIDENCE-BASED PRACTICE, contains Chapter 20, "Use of Research in Practice," which provides a dynamic conclusion to this text through its vibrant presentation of how to apply the best available evidence in clinical practice using an evidence-based practice framework.

Throughout this textbook, critical thinking is reinforced through the presentation of the potential strengths and weaknesses of each step of the research process. Critical thinking is also enhanced by innovative chapter features, such as Critical Thinking Decision Paths, Helpful Hints, and Critical Thinking Challenges, which promote development of research consumer decision-making skills. Each chapter includes both a section describing the critiquing process related to the focus of the chapter and lists of critiquing criteria designed to stimulate a systematic and evaluative approach to reading and understanding qualitative and quantitative research literature. Extensive Internet resources are provided on the accompanying Evolve Web site and can be used to develop evidence-based knowledge and skills.

The **study guide** that accompanies the second Canadian edition has been designed to enhance student learning outcomes through interesting learning activities that enhance students' mastery of research consumer competencies. Students will also be required to use the Internet to locate research articles for review and evaluation. In addition, crossword puzzles, word searches, and critical thinking exercises are presented to challenge students.

The Evolve Web site that accompanies this edition provides interactive learning activities designed to develop the critical thinking, critical reading, and information literacy skills required of informed consumers of nursing research. Student resources include Critiquing Exercises, which consist of research articles and corresponding multiple-choice questions that review cross-chapter content to challenge students and a comprehensive list of nursing research Weblinks and important content updates. A bonus chapter, Chapter 21, "Tools for Applying Evidence to Practice," is also provided on the accompanying Evolve Web site.

Instructor resources include a passcode-protected **faculty Web site** where faculty can access all instructor materials online, including content outlines, lecture guides, coordinating classroom activities, transparencies, and a Microsoft Word–based or Rich Text–based test bank from which instructors can export test bank questions into their own online software. Also available to instructors via the password-protected Web site are an instructor's resource manual, an image collection, lecture slides, and a test bank that allows instructors to create examinations using the Exam-View test generator program.

The development and refinement of a scientific foundation for clinical nursing practice remain essential priorities for the future of professional nursing practice. The second Canadian edition of *Nursing Research in Canada: Methods and Critical Appraisal for Evidence-Based Practice* will help students understand the steps of the research process, critically analyze research studies, judge their merit, and judiciously apply research findings in clinical practice. To the extent that this goal is accomplished, the nursing profession will have a cadre of clinicians who derive their practice from theory and research evidence specific to nursing.

ACKNOWLEDGEMENTS

This major undertaking was accomplished with the help of a many of people, some of whom made direct contributions to the new edition and some of whom contributed indirectly. We acknowledge with deep appreciation and our warmest thanks the following people who made this second Canadian edition possible:

- Nursing educators across Canada who provided valuable and insightful comments that help to direct the revisions featured in this edition
- Our students, particularly the nursing students of the Georgian College, Seneca College, and York University Collaborative Nursing programs and the York University Second-Entry programs, who inspired us with their feedback and willingness to use the information in this text by becoming research assistants
- Ann Millar, Publisher, Elsevier Canada, who had faith in us and provided much needed guidance and direction
- Dawn du Quesnay, Developmental Editor, who patiently guided us and kept us on track

- Lise Dupont, Managing Production Editor, Elsevier Canada, who shepherded the manuscript through the publication process
- Our vignette contributors, whose willingness to share their wisdom and evidence of their innovative research made a unique contribution to this edition
- All of the reviewers, who provided thoughtful feedback not only on the first Canadian edition but also on the second Canadian edition manuscript
- Our families, who supported us and picked up the "loose ends" while we wrote and revised
  - John and Don Cameron, thanks for all of your love, support, and encouragement. Thanks to Jennie Cameron for giving feedback on the text during your nursing studies and for providing research assistance and office management.
  - Neranjan and Sandhya Singh and Ram and Betty Laljie, thanks for your ongoing love, patience, support, and encouragement toward making this endeavour a reality.

Cherylyn Cameron
Mina D. Singh

STUDENT PREFACE

We invite you to join us on an exciting nursing research adventure that begins as you turn the first page of the second Canadian edition of *Nursing Research in Canada: Methods and Critical Appraisal for Evidence-Based Practice*. The adventure is one of discovery! You will discover that the nursing research literature sparkles with pride in, dedication to, and excitement about the research dimension of professional nursing practice. Whether you are a student or a practising nurse whose goal is to use research as the foundation of your practice, you will discover that nursing research and a commitment to evidence-based practice position is integral to meeting the challenge of providing quality health care in partnership both with clients and their families or significant others and with the communities in which they live. Finally, you will discover the richness in the "who, what, where, when, why, and how" of nursing research and evidence-based practice, developing a foundation of knowledge and skills that will equip you for clinical practice today and into the future.

We think you will enjoy reading this text. The six-part organization and special features of this text are designed to help you to develop your critical thinking, critical reading, information literacy, and clinical decision-making skills, while providing a user-friendly approach to learning that expands your competence to deal with these new and challenging experiences. The study guide that accompanies this text provides a self-paced learning tool to reinforce the content of the text, chapter by chapter.

Research consumer skills are used in every clinical setting and can be applied to every client population and every clinical practice issue. Whether your present or future clinical practice involves primary care or specialty care, and whether it provides in-patient or outpatient treatment in a hospital, clinic, or home, you will be challenged to apply your research consumer skills in practice settings and to use nursing research as the foundation for your evidence-based practice. The second Canadian edition of *Nursing Research in Canada: Methods and Critical Appraisal for Evidence-Based Practice* will guide you through this new adventure, in which you will discover your ability to play a vital role in building an evidence-based professional nursing practice.

Cherylyn Cameron
ccameron@georgianc.on.ca

Mina D. Singh
minsingh@yorku.ca

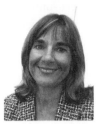

GERI LoBIONDO-WOOD, RN, PHD, FAAN, is an Associate Professor at the University of Texas Health Science Center at Houston (UTHSC-Houston), School of Nursing. She received her diploma in nursing at St. Mary's Hospital School of Nursing in Rochester, New York, her bachelor's and master's degrees from the University of Rochester, and a Ph.D. in nursing theory and research from New York University. Dr. LoBiondo-Wood currently teaches research and theory to undergraduate, graduate, and doctoral students at UTHSC-Houston, School of Nursing. She also holds a joint appointment for the development of evidence-based practice at the M.D. Anderson Cancer Center in Houston. She has extensive experience guiding nurses and other health care professionals in the development and utilization of research in clinical practice. Dr. LoBiondo-Wood is currently a member of the Editorial Board of *Progress in Transplantation* and a reviewer for *Nursing Research*, the *Journal of Advanced Nursing*, and *Nephrology Nursing Journal*. Her research and publications focus on chronic illness and the impact of solid organ transplantation on child and adult recipients and their families throughout the transplantation process.

Dr. LoBiondo-Wood has been active locally and nationally in many professional organizations, including the Southern Nursing Research Society, the Midwest Nursing Research Society, and the North American Transplant Coordinators Organization. She has received local and national awards for her teaching and contributions to nursing. In 1997, she received the Distinguished Alumnus Award from New York University, Division of Nursing Alumni Association. In 2001, she was inducted as a Fellow of the American Academy of Nursing.

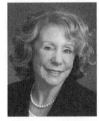

JUDITH HABER, APRN, PHD, CS, FAAN, is Professor and Associate Dean for Graduate Programs in the College of Nursing at New York University. She received her undergraduate nursing education at Adelphi University in New York and holds a master's degree in adult psychiatric –mental health nursing and a Ph.D. in nursing theory and research from New York University. Judith Haber is internationally recognized as a clinician and educator in psychiatric–mental health nursing. She has extensive clinical experience in psychiatric nursing, having been an advanced practice psychiatric nurse in private practice for over 30 years, specializing in treatment of families coping with the psychosocial sequelae of acute and chronic catastrophic illness. Dr. Haber is currently on the Editorial Board of the *Journal of the American Psychiatric Nurses Association (JAPNA)* and, as a contributing editor, writes a column on policy and politics for this journal. Her areas of research involvement include tool development, particularly in the area of family functioning. She is internationally known for developing the Haber Level of Differentiation of Self Scale. Another program of research addresses physical and psychosocial adjustment to illness, focusing specifically on women with breast cancer and their partners. Based on this research, she and Dr. Carol Hoskins have written and produced an award-winning series of psychoeducational videotapes, *Journey to Recovery: For Women with Breast Cancer and Their Partners*, which they are currently testing in a randomized clinical trial funded by the National Cancer Institute.

Dr. Haber has been active locally and nationally in many professional organizations, including the American Nurses Association, the American Psychiatric Nurses Association (APNA), and the American Academy of Nursing. She has received numerous local, state, and national awards for public policy, clinical practice, and research, including the APNA Psychiatric Nurse of the Year Award in 1998. In 1993, she was inducted as a Fellow of the American Academy of Nursing.

CANADIAN EDITORS

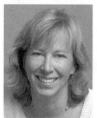

CHERYLYN CAMERON, RN, PHD, is the Associate Vice-President of the University Partnership Centre, Research and Scholarship, Georgian College. She received her bachelor of science in nursing degree from the University of Alberta and a master of arts degree from Central Michigan University. She received her Ph.D. from the Ontario Institute for Studies in Education (OISE)/ University of Toronto in theory and policy studies in education. Her dissertation "The Lived Experience of Transfer Students from a Baccalaureate Nursing Program" won the Best Dissertation award from the Council for Study of Community Colleges in the United States. Dr. Cameron currently teaches courses as an adjunct professor for Central Michigan University in the master of arts degree in education with a community college specialization. At Georgian College, she works with university partners to provide degree-level studies for college students and is responsible for research and scholarship at the college. Her research interests include college–university relations, student experiences, transfer from college to university, and the implementation of best practice guidelines.

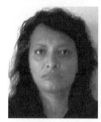

MINA D. SINGH, RN, PHD, is an Assistant Professor at York University School of Nursing. She received her bachelor of science in nursing from the University of Toronto and started her clinical nursing in neurosurgery but spent most of her career in mental health and public health nursing. Her interests in program evaluation encouraged her to pursue her education in quantitative research. She earned her doctorate in measurement and evaluation from the University of Toronto. Her current interests, as a specialist in quantitative methods, relate to program evaluation in health care and nursing education. She also conducts research in chronic disease prevention and cultural diversity in health care.

PART ONE

Research Overview

How Nurses Use and Respond to Research

A few years ago, I was fortunate to work as a nurse scholar on an acute care medical unit in a large urban hospital. This experience gave me a unique opportunity to observe at first hand how nurses use and respond to research. During that time, one of the staff nurses on the unit made a comment that I believe captures many Canadian nurses' attitudes toward research. She said, "I used to think that nursing research was bunk. Just something we had to learn in school that I could put away with my textbooks when I graduated. I thought that we learned research in school because the professors were hoping to convince some of us to go on to graduate school. I really didn't see it as having anything to do with the real world of bedside nursing." She added that because of our regular research discussions on the unit and our continual efforts to use research findings in the care of clients, her attitude about research had changed. She said, "When I saw research as relevant to what I did and not just some pie-in-the-sky idea from school, I began to use research as a tool—something that helped me do my job better."

Practising nurses' positive attitudes toward research are not unique. During the three years I worked on the unit, I observed nurses searching for research evidence to answer their practice questions, chatting with each other about research articles, and quoting research findings to clients and other health care professionals. Put simply, these nurses used research to "do the job" of nursing more effectively. For example, they consulted research articles to find solutions to several practice issues on the unit, such as how to help an anxious client cope with invasive procedures; how to help nurses deal with their feelings about clients who use injection drugs and leave the hospital in compromised medical conditions, against medical advice; and how best to structure nursing assignments so that clients receive the care they need.

Sometimes, when nurses discovered that little research existed about the issues that arose, they were forced to imagine how other research might apply. For example, when the nurses became concerned that some clients were not eating enough and not eating nutritionally sound foods, they consulted the research about the nutritional status of hospitalized clients. As it turned out, the existing research had been conducted in long-term care facilities and, to a lesser extent, in surgical units. Therefore, the existing research did not address the particular concerns that the nurses expressed pertaining to the nutritional status of clients with exceptionally high metabolisms who also use injection drugs, late-night admissions of homeless clients who might not have eaten prior to admission, and clients with neurological deficits who experienced difficulty handling cutlery and cups.

Nevertheless, the nurses were able to apply some of the research conducted in long-term care facilities to their unit. For example, the nurses learned that if clients are fed by nursing staff who are hurried, those clients' nutritional status was often poor. Many of the unit's clients required feeding, and the research conducted in long-term care facilities caused the nurses to reflect on the staff who fed the clients and how long the feeding took. This consideration, in turn, caused the nurses to change the feeding directions they gave to support staff (e.g., unit assistants) and to reinforce that it is the nurse's responsibility to make sure that the client has eaten enough.

The nurses also initiated research on the unit. For example, they were continually frustrated with the behaviour of many clients who use injection drugs. The nurses reported these clients were often hostile, manipulative, and noncompliant. Hospital statistics demonstrated that this particular client population accounted for most of the nurses' security calls. Several nurses said they dreaded working with this type of client. Initially, they suggested strategies that were inadequate or unrealistic (e.g., building a seclusion room in the unit for clients who use injection drugs). Ultimately, the nurses decided to seek advice from the hospital's chemical dependency experts. After consulting with the nurses, the chemical dependency team developed a program of workshops and conducted weekly rounds over the course of a year to help nurses better understand and care for clients who use injection drugs.

Because other units had similar issues with the same client population, the nurses decided to report the results of the program to others in a tangible way, as research findings. The nurses set to work formally evaluating the program that had been created by the chemical dependency experts. For example, the nurses administered questionnaires and participated in group interviews. The research revealed that most nurses now enjoyed caring for clients who use injection drugs. The nurses better understood the behaviour of these clients and what could be done to help them. Following a presentation of the research findings, the nurses celebrated their accomplishments of the program with a cake and coffee party on the unit.

Another example of nurses initiating research involved investigating whether nurses' medication errors could be decreased by using personal digital assistants (PDAs), such as PalmPilot devices. The idea for the research project arose when the nurses discovered that many of the medication errors were related to nurses not recognizing that a new order had been provided, misreading the order, or forgetting that a medication had not been administered. The nurses submitted a proposal for the research project and received funding for it from the University of British Columbia (UBC). The first component of this research consisted of observing the nurses administering medication and writing documentation. Based on their observations, the nurses then developed a program for PDAs that told nurses which medications should be given and which had not yet been administered. This program included the ability to link to other information about clients and their medications. In the end, the research confirmed that the use of PDAs did reduce medication errors. Subsequently, the research findings were submitted to a publishing company that is hoping to incorporate them into new PDA software for nurses.

Nurses' commitment to research does not occur overnight, and some nurses will be more excited by research than others. In three years, however, the nurses I observed began to see research in a new light: as something they *need* to care for clients effectively. When I told the nurses mentioned in this vignette that I was writing this piece, one nurse said, "They will read it and think that our stories do not represent the real world. They will think it can't happen in most hospitals or for most nurses. They will think that research took place in our case only because you were here with us and you understood research." If that nurse is correct and that is what you are thinking, I invite you to consider the following: What if all we need to inspire nurses to use research as a method of helping them do their jobs more effectively is someone who believes that research can do just that? What if that someone is you? Are you prepared to be the nurse who says to colleagues, "Let's see what research has been done about that. I bet someone has studied it and that the results will be helpful to us." After reading this chapter and this book, I hope that you will use research as the foundation of your nursing practices. I have seen how much research influences practising nurses, and I'm here to tell you that it works.

Barbara Paterson
RN, MEd, PhD
Professor and Tier 1 Canada
  Research Chair
Faculty of Nursing
University of New Brunswick
Fredericton, New Brunswick

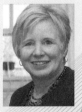

CHAPTER 1

Geri LoBiondo-Wood

Judith Haber

Cherylyn Cameron

Mina D. Singh

The Role of Research in Nursing

LEARNING OUTCOMES

*After reading this chapter, the student should
be able to do the following:*

- State the significance of research to the
  practice of nursing.
- Identify the role of the consumer of
  nursing research.
- Discuss the differences in trends within
  nursing research in Canada.
- Describe how research, education, and
  practice relate to each other.
- Evaluate the nurse's role in the research
  process as it relates to the nurse's level of
  education.
- Identify future trends in nursing research.
- Formulate the priorities for nursing
  research in the twenty-first century.

KEY TERMS

consumer 8

critique 6

data 7

evidence-based practice 5

generalizability 17

research utilization 5

Depth 16

STUDY RESOURCES

evolve Go to Evolve at
http://evolve.elsevier.com/Canada/LoBiondo/Research/
for Weblinks, content updates, and additional
research articles for practice in reviewing
and critiquing.

W e invite you to join us on an exciting nursing research adventure that begins as you read the first page of this chapter. The adventure is one of discovery! You will discover that the nursing research literature sparkles with pride in, dedication to, and excitement about this dimension of professional nursing practice. Whether you are a student or a practising nurse whose goal is to use research as the foundation of your professional practice, you will also discover that nursing research is integral to meeting the challenge of providing quality health care in partnership with clients, their families and significant others, and the communities in which they live. Finally, you will discover the "who, what, where, when, why, and how" of nursing research and develop a foundation of knowledge, evidence-based practice, and competencies that will equip you for twenty-first-century nursing practice.

Your nursing research adventure will be filled with new and challenging learning experiences that will develop your skills as a research consumer. Your critical reading, critical thinking, and clinical decision-making skills will grow as you read and review the research literature and raise questions about your practice. For example, you will be encouraged to ask adventurous questions, such as the following:

- What makes an intervention effective with one group of clients who are diagnosed with congestive heart failure but not with another group?
- What is the effect of using computer learning modules to educate children about self-management of asthma?
- What is the experience of men who undergo prostate surgery and therapy?
- What is the quality of therapeutic touch studies that have been conducted in recent years?
- Is research conducted on pain management ready for use in practice?

This chapter begins your nursing research adventure by developing your appreciation of the significance of nursing research and of the nurse's role in the research process, both in the future and in the past.

SIGNIFICANCE OF RESEARCH IN THE FIELD OF NURSING

The health care environment is changing at an unprecedented pace. Hinshaw's portrait of twenty-first-century nursing stated that "an unprecedented explosion of nursing knowledge guided practice and advanced the health and well-being of individual clients, families, and communities" (Hinshaw, 2000, p. 117). Carper (1978) described four fundamental patterns of knowing in nursing: (1) empirics, the science of nursing; (2) aesthetics, the art of nursing; (3) the component of personal knowing; and (4) ethics, the component of moral knowledge of nursing. Empirical (empirics) knowledge based on research findings represents "one source of knowledge within a larger body of knowledge" (Tarlier, 2005, p. 131). The challenges associated with nursing's rapid pace of growth can best be met by integrating evidence-based knowledge about biological, behavioural, and environmental influences on health care into nursing practice. Nursing research provides specialized scientific knowledge that empowers nurses to anticipate and meet these constantly shifting challenges and maintain the profession's societal relevance.

Evidence-based practice is the conscious and judicious use of the current "best" evidence relating to the care of clients and the delivery of health care services (Titler, Mentes, Rakel, Abbott, & Baumler, 1999). The Canadian Nurses Association (CNA) states that "evidence-based nursing refers to the incorporation of evidence from research, clinical expertise, client preferences and other available resources to make decisions about patients" (CNA, 1998, p. 1). Through **research utilization** efforts, knowledge obtained from research is transformed into clinical practice, culminating in nursing practice that is evidence based.

For example, to understand the importance of evidence-based practice, consider the study by Tourangeau, Giovannetti, Tu, and Wood (2002), which sought to examine the effects of nursing-related hospital variables on mortality rates for hospitalized clients while testing a proposed 30-day mortality model. The findings of this retrospective design revealed that lower 30-day mortality is related to richer mix of Registered Nurse (RN) skills, nurses' years of experience on the clinical unit, and the number of shifts a nurse missed. On average, teaching hospitals had the lowest risk-adjusted mortality rate, whereas nonurban community hospitals had the highest rate. Of significance to nursing staffing issues, the study revealed that a 10% increase in the proportion of RNs across all hospital types was associated with five fewer client deaths for every 1000 discharged clients. These findings have implications for the organization of nursing in acute care hospitals and for the mix of nursing skill required on each unit. Such data provide evidence to support staffing models, but changes should not be advocated based on the results of only one study. Replication of this study is necessary to build more empirical evidence to support staffing changes.

Nurses must also be accountable for the quality of client care they deliver. In an era of consumerism when the quality of health care and high health care costs are being questioned, consumers and employers—the purchasers of health insurance—are asking health care professionals to document the effectiveness of their services (DiCenso, Guyatt, & Ciliska, 2005; Hinshaw, 2000; Melnyk & Fineout-Overholt, 2002). Essentially, nurses are being asked, "How do nursing services make a difference?" The message can hardly be clearer: how consumers and employers perceive the value of nurses' contributions will determine the profession's role in any future delivery system (Dykes, 2003; Naylor, 2003; Titler, Cullen, & Ardery, 2002). Public- and private-sector reimbursement groups (i.e., provincial health plans and private health insurance companies) also require accountability for services provided. For example, the standards of the Canadian Council on Health Services Accreditation require health care institutions to complete a self-assessment and to follow up on promises to improve health care and safety (Canadian Council on Health Services Accreditation, 2006). With this information

in hand, short- and long-term plans can be developed to demonstrate the link between quality care and cost-effective client outcomes.

Just as nursing research is critically important to members of the public, who are primary health care consumers, research is also important to many national and provincial or territorial nursing organizations. Advancing the importance of nursing research with respect to quality of care, client safety, and health promotion, among others, requires a coordinated national effort. In 2002, the Office of Nursing Policy (ONP) at Health Canada laid the groundwork for the development of the Canadian Consortium for Nursing Research and Innovation. After an initial think-tank session with leaders of nursing research from across Canada, the ONP contracted the Canadian Nurses Foundation to provide leadership for the consortium. Now, four key nursing organizations (CNA, the Canadian Association of Schools of Nursing [CASN], the Canadian Association for Nursing Research, and the Academy of Canadian Executive Nurses), together with the ONP and Canada's nursing research chairs, are working to develop a strategic plan to support research funding and infrastructure (ONP, 2007).

For nationally coordinated nursing research to be effective, all professional nurses must possess and use basic research skills. All nurses should share a commitment to the advancement of nursing science by conducting research and using research findings in practice. Also, baccalaureate graduate nurses should have the critical appraisal skills to inform and validate practice. In other words, nurses must be knowledgeable consumers of research who can **critique** research and use existing standards to determine the merit and readiness of research for use in clinical practice (CASN, 2006; CNA, 2002; College of Nurses of Ontario [CNO], 2002).

Pringle (1999) captured the importance of research intertwining with practice in her double helix analogy. In the following extract, she redefined Fawcett's 1978 double helix to incorporate practice as one helix

. . . spiralling from an individual's demands for care or need for health education, through nurses' responses to those demands or needs, to the nurses' evaluation of the effectiveness of the responses. Research is the second helix, spiralling from questions that arise about the nature of the demands or needs, through tests of a series of responses for effectiveness, to determination of the most effective response and generalizing from it. (p. 166)

The remainder of this book is devoted to helping you develop the consumer expertise required to understand and use research.

RESEARCH: The Element That Links Theory, Education, and Practice

Research links theory, education, and practice. Theoretical formulations supported by research findings may become the foundations of theory-based practice in nursing. Your educational setting, whether a nursing program or the health care organization where you are employed, provides an environment in which you, as a student or an employee, can learn about the research process. In the setting of a nursing program or a health care organization, you can also explore different theories and begin to evaluate them in light of research findings.

Consider the program of research that focused on building knowledge about improving the health and health care of women who experience intimate partner abuse. This program extended over a decade and focused on the experiences of women who left abusive partners, the health of the women after leaving the relationships, and the degree of health care improvement for women after they left their abusive partners (Ford-Gilbe, Wuest, Varcoe, & Merritt-Gray, 2006). The knowledge gained from this body of interrelated research led to the development of comprehensive interventions to support the health and quality of life of women who leave abusive partners.

The findings of the 2006 study on the health and heath care of women who experience intimate partner abuse have had enormous implications for both nurses and other health care professionals, which comprise the interdisciplinary health care team that works with women who experience intimate partner violence (IPV). Meaningful intervention is critical for these women because health problems persist after they leave their partners. Many of these women report continued abuse and harassment from their ex-partners and experience financial hardships. Although health care workers have an interest in improving health care for these women, most health care workers do not have the knowledge required to address their clients' needs in a meaningful and effective way. As the researchers noted, ". . . the vast majority of health practitioners [are] unprepared to recognize and respond to IPV in ways that are sensitive to the complexity of women's experiences and respectful of women's safety and choices" (Ford-Gilbe, Wuest, Varcoe, & Merritt-Gray, 2006, p. 148).

One of the foundational studies leading to the development of an evidence-based program of study is the exploration of the health promotion processes of families headed by a lone parent during the aftermath of IPV (Ford-Gilbe, Wuest, & Merritt-Gray, 2005). The researchers discovered that a central social problem for these families is intrusion, defined as "unwanted interference in everyday life, arising from abuse and its fallout, that demands attention, diverts attention away from family priorities, and limits choices for moving on" (p. 478). Families learned to limit intrusion through subprocesses described as regenerating family, renewing self, and rebuilding security. The theory generated in this study provides a framework for nurses and other health care professionals to organize health assessments and interventions to support families who are trying to minimize intrusion.

The preceding examples attempt to answer a question that may have presented itself to you before taking this course: How will the theory and research content of this course relate to my nursing practice? The **data** from each study discussed thus far have clearly demonstrated societal and practice implications. In an era of continuing concern about health care costs, empirically supported programs that are cost-effective without compromising quality are essential. Many studies directly evaluate the cost-effectiveness of treatment models, including the study by Forchuk, Martin, Chan, and Jensen (2005), which found that a transition discharge model of care for clients experiencing chronic mental illness resulted in their early discharge from a psychiatric hospital by an average of 116 days, resulting in considerable cost savings (see Appendix A).

Bear in mind, however, that research is of little value unless it is used in practice to improve the health care of clients. Several studies have demonstrated that the use of research-based interventions is more likely to result in better outcomes than traditional or ritual-based nursing care (Heater, Becker, & Olson, 1988; Titler, Goode, & Mathis, 1992). In its efforts to develop the nursing discipline, the CASN identified the dissemination of scholarship and research as one of the mandates directing the future activities of the association (CASN, 2006). In addition, the Canadian Health Services Research Foundation (CHSRF) supports research dissemination by hosting workshops and other communication initiatives.

At this point in your nursing research adventure, you may be wondering how education in nursing research links theory and practice. The answer is two-fold. First, learning about nursing research will provide you with an appreciation and understanding of the research process so that you can more easily become a participant in research activities. Second, learning the value of nursing research helps you to become an intelligent *consumer* of research. A **consumer** of research actively uses and applies research. To be a knowledgeable consumer, a nurse must have knowledge about the relevant subject matter, the ability to discriminate and to evaluate information logically, and the ability to apply the knowledge gained. Note that you need not conduct research to be able to appreciate and use research findings in practice. Rather, to be intelligent consumers, nurses must understand the research process and develop the critical evaluation

skills needed to judge the merit and relevance of evidence before applying it to practice. The success of evidence-based practice depends on your ability, as a consumer of research, to understand the research process and to evaluate the evidence.

ROLES OF THE NURSE IN THE RESEARCH PROCESS

Every nurse practising in the twenty-first century has a role to play in the research process. The CASN states that it "strongly supports nursing research and the training of nurse researchers across Canada [and] works to encourage and improve the quality of nursing research, as well as to promote research findings and support Canada's current and upcoming nursing research leaders" (CASN, 2006). More specifically, the Research and Scholarship Committee stated in its 2004/05 strategic plan that, in collaboration with other nursing bodies, it would advocate for funding to support the training of nurse researchers and to develop policy, position statements, and guidelines on issues related to research and scholarship, including the training of nurse researchers (CASN, 2004).

On a provincial level, each province in Canada has its own standards for entry into nursing practice, and many of these standards have specific related research competencies. For, example, the CNO has outlined, in the standard relating to knowledge, the following competencies that incorporate research (CNO, 2002):

- Reviewing research in nursing, health sciences, and related disciplines

- Using research to inform practice and professional service

- Critically evaluating research related to outcomes and advocating for its application to practice

The Alberta Association of Registered Nurses (2005) also clearly states in its Entry-to-Practice Competencies document that "the registered nurse supports decisions with evidence-based rationale"

(Section 2.1) and "supports, facilitates or participates in research relevant to nursing" (Section 2.7).

The CNA states that "nurses are expected to know how to locate and use results of research findings to inform and build an evidence-based practice" (CNA, 2002). The Canadian Registered Nurse Examination (CNRE) outlines competencies related to research on which examination questions for licensing to practice are based. The following sections from the RN examination competencies explicitly highlight the importance of research for practice (CNA, 2002):

Professional Practice	provides rationale for nursing care actions and decisions based on theoretical and evidence-based knowledge from nursing, health sciences, and related disciplines (Competency: PP-38) reads and participates in critiquing evidence-based literature in nursing, health sciences, and related disciplines (i.e., research articles and reports) (Competency: PP-40)
Nursing Practice: Health and Wellness	provides evidence-based health-related information to the person (Competency: HW-18)
Nursing Practice: Alterations in Health	uses evidence-based information to assist the person to understand interventions and their relationship to expected outcomes (e.g., possible risks and benefits, discomforts, inconveniences, costs) (Competency: AH-22)

Graduates of nursing programs from across Canada must demonstrate an awareness of the value or relevance of research in nursing. The College of Nurses of Ontario specifically states that nurses may help identify problem areas in nursing practice, assist in data collection activities, and—in conjunction with the professional nurse—appropriately integrate research findings into clinical practice and thus engage in evidence-based practice (CNO, 1999). In other words, RNs must participate as team members in evidence-based practice activities, including development and revision or implementation of clinical standards, protocols, and critical paths (see Chapter 20).

Nurses must also be intelligent consumers of research; that is, they must understand all steps of the research process and their interrelationships. A professional nurse interprets, evaluates, and determines the credibility of research findings. The nurse discriminates between interesting findings that require further investigation and those that are sufficiently supported by evidence before applying findings to practice. Nurses should then use these competencies to advance the nursing or interdisciplinary evidence-based practice projects (e.g., developing clinical standards, tracking quality improvement data, or coordinating implementation of a pilot project to test the efficacy of a new wound care protocol) of the workplace committees to which they belong.

RNs are also responsible for generating clinical questions to identify nursing issues that require investigation and for participating in the implementation of scientific studies. Clinicians often generate research ideas or questions from hunches, gut-level feelings, intuition, or observations of clients or nursing care. These ideas then often become the seeds of research investigations.

Paterson (2002) related the story of Vini and Suzanne, two nurses working in an intensive care unit. They observed that the blood pressure of a certain client dropped each time he received acetaminophen for a fever. He would then need to receive additional treatment for the corresponding low blood pressure. This situation raised several questions for Vini and Suzanne, and they wondered whether treating the fever was truly beneficial and what would be the effects of leaving the fever untreated. They spoke to other health care professionals, conducted a literature review, and concluded that treatment with antipyretics, such as acetylsalicylic acid, should be immediately applied and that, in some clients, leaving the fever untreated had clear benefits. Vini and Suzanne subsequently disseminated their research findings to their colleagues and other health care professionals at a critical care conference. These two nurses exemplify the circularity between practice generating research and research improving practice. Systematic collection of data about a clinical problem, such as the one identified by Vini and Suzanne, contributes to the refinement and extension of nursing practice.

RNs may also participate in research projects as members of interdisciplinary or intradisciplinary research teams in one or more phases of a project. For example, a staff nurse may work on a clinical research unit where a particular type of nursing care is part of an established research protocol (e.g., for pain management, prevention of falls, or treatment of urinary incontinence). In situations such as these, the nurse administers care according to the format described in the protocol. The nurse may also be involved in collecting and recording data relevant to the administration of, and the client response to, nursing care.

As important as the generation of research is the sharing of research findings with colleagues. Examples include developing an article or presentation for a research or clinical conference on the findings of a study or sharing the findings of a research report that was critiqued and found to have merit and the potential for application to practice. In a more formal way, it may involve joining a health care agency's research committee or its quality assurance or quality improvement committee, where research articles, integrative reviews of the literature, and clinical practice guidelines are evaluated for evidence-based clinical decision making.

Nurses who have graduate degrees must also be sophisticated consumers of research and additionally are specially prepared to conduct research as co-investigators or primary investigators. At the master's level, nurses are prepared to be active members of research teams. Nurses with master's-level training can assume the role of clinical expert, collaborating with an experienced researcher in

proposal development, data collection, data analysis, and interpretation. Nurses with master's degrees enhance the quality and relevance of nursing research by providing not only clinical expertise but also evidence-based knowledge about the way clinical services are delivered. Nurses with master's-level training also facilitate the investigation of clinical problems by providing a climate that is open to nursing research and by engaging in evidence-based practice projects. In the capacity of "change champions" (see Chapter 20), nurses collaborate with others in investigations, promote the competency of staff nurses as research consumers, and expand implementation of evidence-based practice projects. At the master's level, nurses conduct research investigations to monitor the quality of nursing in clinical settings and help others to apply scientific knowledge to nursing practice.

To achieve the greatest expertise in appraising, designing, and conducting research, nurses must complete doctorates. Nurses with Ph.D. degrees develop theoretical explanations for phenomena relevant to nursing, develop methods of scientific inquiry, and use qualitative and empirical methods to modify or extend existing knowledge so that it is relevant to nursing (or to other areas of health care). In addition to their role as researchers, nurses with doctoral-level training act as role models and mentors to guide, stimulate, and encourage other nurses who are developing their research skills. Nurses with doctoral degrees also collaborate and consult with social, educational, and health care institutions or governmental agencies in their respective research endeavours. These nurses then disseminate their research findings to the scientific community, clinicians, and—as appropriate—the general public through scientific journal articles and presentations for nursing research conferences. Seminars and newsletters are also viable mechanisms for research dissemination (Fitzpatrick, 2000).

Another essential responsibility of nurses, regardless of the level of education they receive, is that they pay special regard to the ethical principles of research, especially the protection of human subjects. For example, nurses caring for clients who are participating in antinausea chemotherapy research must ensure that the clients have signed the informed consent form and have had all questions answered by the research team before beginning the research. Furthermore, nurses who see clients having an adverse reaction to the medication must not administer more doses until they have notified an appropriate member of the research team (see Chapter 6). Not all nurses must or should conduct research, but all nurses must play some part in the research process. Nurses at all educational levels—whether they are consumers, researchers, or both—need to view the research process as integral to the growing professionalism in nursing.

As professionals, nurses must take time to read research studies and evaluate them, using the standards congruent with scientific research. Also, nurses should use the critiquing process to identify the strengths and weaknesses of each study. Bearing in mind that each study has its limitations, nurses should consider whether sound and relevant evidence from one particular study can be used in other settings as well.

HISTORICAL PERSPECTIVE[1]

Nursing research has undergone many changes and developments over the last few decades. In addition, the groundwork for the research that exists today was laid in the late nineteenth century and throughout the twentieth century. To capture the specifics of nursing research and the works of many excellent researchers, especially in the 1980s and 1990s, is beyond the scope of this chapter. Box 1–1 shows the major milestones in the development of nursing research.

Nineteenth Century

In the mid-nineteenth century, nursing as a formal discipline began to take root with the ideas and practices of Florence Nightingale. Her concepts have

[1]This section (i.e., from page 11 to page 15) is adapted with permission from Potter, P., Perry, A. G., Ross-Kerr, J., & Wood. M. (2006). *Canadian fundamentals of nursing* (3rd ed., pp. 82–84). Toronto: Elsevier Canada.

contributed to, and are congruent with, the present priorities of nursing research. Promotion of health, prevention of disease, and care of the sick were central ideas of her practice and publications. Nightingale believed that systematic collection and exploration of data were necessary for nursing. Her collection and analysis of data on the health status of British soldiers during the Crimean War led to a variety of reforms in health care. Nightingale also noted the need for measuring the outcomes of nursing and medical care (Nightingale, 1863) and had expertise in statistics and epidemiology. She stated, "Statistics are history in repose, history is statistics in motion" (Keith, 1988, p. 5). Other than Nightingale's work, little research was conducted during the early years of nursing's development. Schools of nursing had just begun to be established and were unequal in their ability to educate, whereas nursing leadership had just started to develop.

Twentieth Century

In the twentieth century, research focused mainly on nursing education, but some client- and technique-oriented research was also evident (see Box 1–1). In 1923, in the United States, the Committee for the Study of Nursing Education studied the preparation of educators, administrators, and public health nurses and the clinical experiences of nursing students, publishing the results in the Goldmark report (Committee for the Study of Nursing Education, 1923). This report identified gaps in the educational background of nurses. As a result of the Goldmark report, the method for educating nurses changed, producing more university-based nursing curricula. A decade later in Canada, a similar comprehensive study of nursing and nursing education was carried out by Dr. George Weir, sponsored jointly by the CNA and the Canadian Medical Association. The Weir report, published in 1932, documented serious problems in nursing education and drew attention to the need for changes to improve standards in education and practice. The Weir report's recommendation that authority and responsibility for schools of nursing be vested within provincial

BOX 1–1	Historical Milestones in the Development of Nursing Research

1858	Florence Nightingale publishes *Notes on Matters Affecting the Health, Efficiency and Hospital Administration of the British Army* and *Notes on Hospitals*
1920	Public health courses are offered at the universities of British Columbia (UBC), Alberta, Toronto, McGill, Dalhousie, and Western Ontario (UWO)
1923	The Goldmark report on US nursing education identifies deficiencies in the system
1932	The Weir report, sponsored by the Canadian Nurses Association and the Canadian Medical Association, calls for better nursing education and service
1952	The American Nurses Association first publishes *Nursing Research*
1959	The first Canadian nursing master's degree program is launched at UWO
1964–1965	The first nursing research project is funded by a Canadian federal granting agency; *International Journal of Nursing Studies* and *International Nursing Index* are launched
1969–1970	*Nursing Papers*, the forerunner of the *Canadian Journal of Nursing Research*, is published at McGill; the Lysaught report, *An Abstract for Action*, is published
1971	McGill launches the Centre for Nursing Research; the first national Canadian conference is held on nursing research; both are financed by the Department of National Health and Welfare
1978	Heads of university nursing schools and deans of graduate studies attend the Kellogg National Seminar on Doctoral Education in Nursing
1982	The Alberta Foundation for Nursing Research, the first funding agency for nursing research, is established; the Working Group on Nursing Research is established by the Medical Research Council of Canada (MRC)
1985	The report of the Working Group on Nursing Research is released by MRC
1988	The MRC and the National Health Research and Development Program establish a joint initiative to structure nursing research grants
1991	The first fully funded Canadian nursing Ph.D. programs are launched first at University of Alberta, followed by University of British Columbia, McGill University, and University of Toronto
1994	McMaster University launches its nursing Ph.D.; MRC's mandate includes health research
1999	The Nursing Research Fund is launched with a $25 million grant over 10 years; the Canadian Health Services Research Foundation (CHSRF) administers the funds; the Ph.D. nursing program is launched at the University of Calgary
2000	Five CHSRF/Canadian Institutes of Health Research (CIHR) Chairs Awards are granted to nursing
2002	The Office of Nursing Policy organizes a think tank called, "Pathfinding for Nursing Science in the 21st Century," which advocates for a coordinated voice for nursing science
2004	The Ph.D. in nursing program is initiated at Dalhousie University
	A forum on doctoral education is held in Toronto under the auspices of the Canadian Association of Schools of Nursing to develop a national position paper on the Ph.D. in nursing for Canada; the Canadian Consortium for Nursing Research and Innovation is established to develop a strategic plan, build partnerships, and advocate for funding to support research programs and infrastructure

Adapted from Potter, P., Perry, A. G., Ross-Kerr, J., & Wood, M. (Eds.). (2006). *Canadian fundamentals of nursing* (3rd ed., p. 82). Toronto: Elsevier Canada.

systems of education was revolutionary at the time and took more than half a century to be fully implemented across the country.

Changes in the educational system for nurses were crucial for the development of nursing research. In Canada, the establishment of university nursing courses in the 1920s, followed by master's degree programs in the 1950s and 1960s, was key to the development of nursing research. The first master's degree program, established at the University of Western Ontario (UWO) in 1959, highlighted the need for Canadian research in nursing.

The first nursing research journal, *Nursing Research*, was established in the United States in

1952. The first nursing research journal published in Canada, *Nursing Papers* (later called the *Canadian Journal of Nursing Research*), was established at McGill University in 1969. Other journals slowly followed. Today, nurses publish their research in a variety of journals, including those for nursing (see Chapter 5, Box 5–3) and those for other disciplines.

In 1971, McGill University established the Centre for Nursing Research. In the same year, the first National Conference on Nursing Research in Canada was held in Ottawa. These conferences were held annually or biennially for several years. Papers of the early conferences were published as monographs. Nursing research conferences increased and began to be sponsored by professional, research, and academic organizations. As well, nurses began to participate in the research conferences of interdisciplinary groups, such as the Canadian Association on Gerontology.

Throughout the 1970s and 1980s, university faculties and schools of nursing built their research resources so that they could mount doctoral programs. The first provincially approved doctoral nursing program was established at the University of Alberta Faculty of Nursing in 1991. The UBC School of Nursing followed later that year, with programs at McGill University and the University of Toronto following in 1993. In the late 1990s and early 2000s, other programs were launched, bringing the total to 15. The growing number of nursing doctoral programs in Canada (15), the United States (88), and outside North America (over 130), in addition to new programs currently being developed, will prepare a record number of nurse researchers worldwide for the challenge of applying research methods that are diverse enough to address the compelling needs of clients around the world (Hegyvary, 1999; L. Berlin, personal communication, August 12, 2000; Ross-Kerr & Wood, 2006). A critical mass of new nursing scholars is increasing as evidenced by the 171 nurses who completed their Ph.D.s in nursing from a Canadian university in a five-year period from 2001 to 2006 (CNA and CASN, 2007).

Growing awareness of the importance of nursing research gradually led to research funds becoming available. The year 1964 marked the first time that a federal granting agency funded nursing research in Canada (Good, 1969). For the next few decades, the National Health Research and Development Program was the primary source of federal funds for nursing research. In 1982, the Alberta government responded to requests for funding and established the Alberta Foundation for Nursing Research, with $1 million to be distributed over the first five years. This was the first research granting agency in Canada to fund nursing research exclusively. The Foundation did excellent work for 12 years before tight budgets and downsizing led to the government's decision not to award it further funds.

Also in 1982, the Medical Research Council of Canada (MRC) instituted the Working Group on Nursing Research, which recommended the establishment of doctoral nursing programs and the mandatory funding of nursing research by the MRC (1985). In 1988, the MRC and the National Health Research and Development Program launched a joint initiative to provide support for nursing researchers. Several key Canadian researchers received funding under this venture. In 1994, the MRC broadened its mandate from exclusively biomedical research to health research. Under the new guidelines, most nursing research was now eligible for funding.

Meanwhile, in the United States, a study of nursing by the Institute of Medicine (IOM, 1983, p. 19) recommended that the federal government increase funds for scientific research in nursing and that a national organization be established to place nursing research "in the mainstream of scientific investigation." Acting on this recommendation, the US Congress established the National Center for Nursing Research (NCNR) in 1985 and the National Institute of Nursing Research (NINR) in 1993. The NINR's mission is "to promote and improve the health of individuals, families, communities, and populations. [It] supports and conducts clinical and basic research and research training on health and illness across the lifespan" (NINR, 2007).

In Canada, insufficient and inconsistent funding for nursing research indicated a need for a national funding body similar to the NINR. Nurses had long been asking for such assistance. Adequate numbers of nursing researchers with doctoral degrees now existed, and their research priorities were clear (see Box 1–2). In 1999, in response to intensive lobbying by the CNA, the federal government established the Nursing Research Fund, budgeting $25 million for nursing research (i.e., $2.5 million over each of the following 10 years), with the CHSRF to administer the funds. The research areas targeted for support included nursing policies, management, human resources, and nursing care. Each year, $500,000 is designated for the Open Grants Competition, $500,000 for the Canadian Nurses Foundation for research on nursing care, $500,000 for nursing chairs, $750,000 for training (postdoctoral fellowships and student grants), and $250,000 for knowledge networks and dissemination activities. To date, five chairs in nursing research have been funded by this initiative, representing excellence in nursing research across Canada (CHSRF, n.d.). The incumbents are charged with developing research capacity in one particular area of nursing, as is illustrated in the list below:

- Dr. Lesley Degner, University of Manitoba: Development of Innovative Nursing Interventions to Influence Practice and Policy in Cancer Care, Palliative Care, and Cancer Prevention
- Dr. Alba DiCenso, McMaster University: Evaluation of Nurse Practitioner/Advanced Practice Nurse Roles and Interventions
- Dr. Nancy Edwards, University of Ottawa: Multiple Interventions in Community Health Nursing Care
- Dr. Janice Lander, University of Alberta: Evaluating Innovative Approaches to Nursing Care
- Dr. Linda O'Brien-Pallas, University of Toronto: Nursing Human Resources for the New Millennium

During the developmental period of nursing research, nursing studies tended to focus on the roles and characteristics of nurses rather than on delivering professional care to clients. The Lysaught (1970) report on nursing in the United States recommended

---

BOX 1–2   Canadian Nursing Research Priorities

PRIORITY 1: NURSING PRACTICE

- Context (including determinants of health, health reform, and ethical issues)
- Populations (vulnerable groups and specific clinical populations)
- Interventions (wide range, from health promotion to comfort measures)

PRIORITY 2: OUTCOMES

- Development of valid measures for multiple dimensions
- Links with clinical judgement

PRIORITY 3: ENHANCED LINKS BETWEEN RESEARCH AND PRACTICE

- Development of a body of nursing knowledge

Adapted from Potter, P., Perry, A. G., Ross-Kerr, J., & Wood, M. (2006). *Canadian fundamentals of nursing* (3rd ed., p. 84). Toronto: Elsevier Canada.

---

increased research in nursing practice and education. Terms such as *conceptual framework, conceptual model, nursing process*, and *theoretical base of nursing practice* began to appear in the nursing literature. From the 1970s on, more nurses received doctoral preparation and initiated their own research, in both the United States and Canada. In the report of the Commission on Canadian Studies, Professor Thomas Symons commented as follows:

> *The slowness in developing graduate schools of nursing in Canada has, in turn, adversely affected the amount of research undertaken in this field. Little support has been available for publication, or for investigating problems in nursing health care of particular interest to Canadians. Little has been written about the history and achievements of the profession in Canada. There have been almost no biographical studies of outstanding members of the profession. It is regrettable that some of the leaders in Canadian nursing seem to have received more recognition in the United States, and in Britain and Western Europe, than in their own country. (1975, p. 212)*

Nursing research has focused progressively on evidence-based practice in response to demands to justify care practices and systems by improving client outcomes and controlling costs. The scope of nursing research has also broadened to include historical and philosophical inquiry. The establishment of the Centre for Philosophical Nursing Research at the University of Alberta exemplifies this new direction.

The following four training centres funded by the CHSRF are mandated to increase research capacity in nursing and related disciplines:

- The Atlantic Regional Training Centre increases health services research capacity throughout Atlantic Canada and is a collaborative initiative among four Atlantic Canada universities: Dalhousie University in Nova Scotia, Memorial University of Newfoundland, the University of New Brunswick, and the University of Prince Edward Island (http://www.artc-hsr.ca/).

- The FERASI Centre in Quebec (FERASI stands for "Formation et expertise en recherche et administration des services infirmiers"; in English, "Training and Expertise in Nursing Administration Research") is a joint initiative among l'Université de Montréal, McGill University, and l'Université Laval to build research capacity in the administration of nursing services (http://www.ferasi.umontreal.ca).

- The Ontario Training Centre in Health Services and Policy Research comprises six Ontario universities for the purpose of enhancing health services and policy research. The centre is located at McMaster University and involves collaboration with Toronto, York, Ottawa, Laurentian, and Lakehead universities (http://www.otc-hsr.ca).

- The Western Regional Training Centre for Health Services Research based at the UBC's Department of Health Care and Epidemiology and the University of Manitoba's Department of Community Health Sciences is designed to support graduate training of applied health services researchers, equipping them to address the research needs of a wide range of health care policymakers (http://www.wrtc-hsr.ca).

Throughout the 1990s and to the present, some of the original nursing research pathfinders and many new ones have conducted research on a wide range of clinical topics, describing phenomena and testing interventions. A review of the many nursing journals shows the growth in the variety, quality, and depth of research available for potential use in practice. Tracing nursing's research roots shows that nursing has made significant contributions to health care. Naturally, nurses are far from finished with their quest for knowledge and research, but the nursing leaders of the twentieth century have—by example—paved the way for those who will emerge in this new millennium.

FUTURE DIRECTIONS

In the twenty-first century, the continuing expansion of nursing research provides numerous opportunities for nurses to study important research questions, promote health care, and ameliorate the side effects of illness and the consequences of treatment while also optimizing the health outcomes of clients and their families (Jennings & McClure, 2004). *Toward 2020: Visions for Nursing,* includes a prediction that

> *nurse researchers in 2020 [will] conduct studies that place less emphasis on nurses and nursing processes than was the case 20 years ago, focusing instead on health, the needs of patients and communities, and providing sound evidence to guide policy and practice. Research conducted by nurses [will be] interdisciplinary. Research to determine more cost-effective ways to provide safe, high-quality health and illness services [will be] led by nurse researchers. (Villeneuve & MacDonald, 2006, p. 99)*

Major shifts in the delivery of health care include the following:

- An emphasis on community-based care
- An emphasis on reducing health care disparities
- A focus on health promotion and risk reduction
- An increased severity of illness in inpatient settings
- An increased incidence of chronic illness
- An expanding population of elderly people
- An emphasis on provider accountability through a focus on quality and cost outcomes
- The use of technology to serve human needs

Consistent with these trends, nurse researchers are beginning to focus on the development of quantitative and qualitative research programs and clinically based outcome studies. Strategies that enhance nurses' focus on outcomes management through evidence-based quality improvement activities and the use of research findings for effective clinical decision making also are being refined and identified as priorities (see Chapter 20). Evidence-based practice guidelines, standards, protocols, and critical pathways will become benchmarks for cost-effective, high-quality clinical practice (O'Neill & Dluhy, 2000; Titler et al., 2002). Also, nurse researchers and nurse leaders will continue to be increasingly visible at the national level, functioning in policymaking roles, representing nursing on expert panels, and lobbying for more funding dollars. The extent of growth in nursing research is evidenced by the establishment of the Nursing Research Fund, which will provide financial support for research opportunities identified by the community of nurse researchers.

Promoting Depth in Nursing Research

Depth in nursing science becomes evident when research is replicated. Research programs that include a series of studies in a similar area, each of which builds on a prior investigation, promote *depth* in nursing science (Whittemore and Grey, 2002). Moreover, to maximize use of resources and to prevent duplication, researchers must develop intradisciplinary and interdisciplinary networks in similar areas of study (Larson, 2003; O'Neill & Dluhy, 2000). Researchers from a variety of professions can come together to delineate common and unique aspects of client care (i.e., medicine, nursing, and respiratory therapy). Cluster studies, multiple-site investigations, and programs of research facilitate the accumulation of evidence supporting or negating a theory. Furthermore, the increasing emphasis on health services research promotes scientific inquiry that produces a better understanding of health care delivery and issues that cross disciplines, such as resource utilization and policymaking (Aiken, Clarke, Cheung, Sloane, & Silber, 2003; Buerhaus, Staiger, & Auerbach, 2000).

The work of Dr. Nancy Edwards, the director of the Community Health Research Unit (CHRU), provides an excellent example of depth in nursing research. Working in partnership with Public Health and Long-Term Care–City of Ottawa, the University of Ottawa, and a large team of co-researchers, Dr. Edwards is enhancing the scientific and evidence-based practice in public health. One of her areas of study is the incidence, causes, and prevention of falls among the elderly. For example, one study collected qualitative data on seniors' beliefs about falls and prevention behaviour; the key findings guided further study on the use of fall prevention devices, such as grab bars in the bathroom. A more recent research study by Dr. Edwards built on the existing body of knowledge about falls and focused on fall prevention by engaging First Nations elders in community action (CHRU, 2005).

Dr. Edwards's work illustrates the value of building replication studies into research programs. Stone, Curran, and Bakken (2002) proposed that the adoption of research findings in practice, with their potential risks and benefits (including the cost of implementation), should be based on a series of replicated studies that provide a body of evidence, thereby increasing the degree to which the findings can be applied and generalized. A greater focus on **generalizability** is important if the evolving science is to be considered reliable and usable in health care settings and in health care policies. As such, in the future, replication studies will be more credible and will play a crucial role in developing depth in nursing science (Fahs, Stewart, & Kalman, 2003).

Dr. Edwards's work also highlights why research training is likely to increasingly become an essential component of a research career plan. A larger cadre of nurse researchers who begin their research careers at a young age is important to the development of research programs like Edwards's. The goal is to increase the longevity of research careers, enhance the discipline's science development, promote mentoring opportunities, prepare the next generation of researchers, and provide leadership in health care for interdisciplinary health care debates.

Nurse researchers should also be committed to developing publicly and privately funded research programs and to subscribing to a life of periodic education and retraining supported by awards, grants, and fellowships. Research programs facilitate growth in the depth and breadth of research expertise and recognize that some researchers must be retrained as they develop or shift the emphasis of their research, seek to broaden their scientific background, and acquire new research capabilities.

An International Perspective

The continuing development of a national and international research environment is essential to the nursing profession's mission to establish a global research community (Chang, 2000; Hegyvary, 2004). The opportunities for cross-cultural and cross-national studies on subjects of common interest are consistent with the priority for global research (Hegyvary, 2004; Hinshaw, 2000). Challenges associated with developing a global research community include establishing international networks, Web sites, and databases; understanding different cultural perspectives and adapting research accordingly; and obtaining funding for international projects (Evers, 2003; Hinshaw, 2000; Messias, 2001).

Because of nursing's emphasis on the cultural aspects of care and the influence of such factors on practice, increasing international research is likely to emerge as a future trend. Access to multiple populations as a function of globalization allows the testing of nursing science from various perspectives. Interaction with colleagues from other countries provides a rich context for the generation and dissemination of research (Dickenson-Hazard, 2004; Ward, 2003). Evidence supporting the need for global nursing research is provided by the number of measurement tools that have been, and are being, translated and validated in the language of the nurse researcher's country of origin (Nahcivan, 2004).

Alliances with international organizations committed to the goal of health for all will create natural research partnerships. For example, the World Health Organization (WHO), through the Pan-American Health Organization (PAHO), has designated that four WHO Collaborating Centres for Research and Clinical Training in Nursing be located in American schools and colleges of nursing. In Canada, the WHO and the PAHO have designated three locations as collaborating centres for the development of nursing and midwifery (http://www.bireme.br/whocc/). These centres will provide research and clinical training to nurses worldwide. The International Council of Nurses and research conferences in general are just two examples of international nursing research forums designed to educate nurses about the global nature of health- and health care–related topics. Forums for global research dissemination will continue to increase, challenging nurse researchers in various regions of the world to form collaborative research relationships in which research expertise, educational opportunities, and the ability to conduct research projects of mutual interest can be shared and in which international research agendas can be created (Evers, 2003; Hinshaw, 2000).

Research Priorities

As the number of nurses with doctoral degrees increased, and as nursing chairs were created, and funding was expanded, a distinct set of Canadian nursing research priorities emerged (see Box 1–2 on page 14). Often, funding agencies determine research priorities based on their particular needs and interests. In 2007, the CHSRF's priority research themes included (1) managing the delivery of high-quality services in the health care workplace; (2) managing the safe delivery of high-quality services in the health care workplace; (3) providing primary health care; and (4) providing nursing leadership, organization, and policy. These themes were established after consultation with health sector administrators and policymakers and researchers across Canada. For example, under the rubric of primary health care, policymakers were particularly interested in research dedicated to exploring which models of primary health care work best in specific contexts (CHSRF, 2007).

The CIHR's nursing grants funded $11.6 million for 105 research projects in 2005. Although the availability of funding contributes to interest in nursing research, only 15% of nurses' submissions to the CIHR are successful.

In 2006, 50 Canadian nursing leaders identified additional priorities for nurses during a Nursing Leadership, Organization, and Policy Network Day sponsored by the CHSRF. Over the course of the day, several research themes were identified as requiring further research, including "human resources planning and management, nursing roles and scopes of practice, education, worklife, staffing, leadership, and use of research through knowledge transfer and exchange" (CHSRF, 2006, p. 7).

The National Research Institute developed a set of nursing research priorities relating to the study of gender and health. The Institute identified the following five major themes pertaining to female versus male health status, health behaviour, and use of health services across the lifespan:

1. Access and equity for vulnerable groups
2. Promoting health in the context of chronic conditions
3. Gender and health across the lifespan
4. Promoting positive health behaviours
5. Gender and the environment

Vis-à-vis the theme of promoting health in the context of chronic conditions, one of the priority issues is the relationship between gender and cardiovascular disease. Further investigation is required to understand gender differences in symptom reporting, access to health services, and change in role status (Stewart, Kushner, & Spitzer, 2001).

Reducing health disparities in poor communities and vulnerable populations is another topic that will shape the focus of future nursing- and interdisciplinary-related research agendas. By 2010, the North American population will include a higher proportion of children and elderly who are chronically ill or disabled (Dochterman et al., 2005). The health concerns of mothers and infants will continue to spur research that deals effectively with the maternal–infant mortality rate. Individuals of all ages who have sustained life-threatening illnesses will live by means of new life-sustaining technology that will create new demands for self-care and family support. Cancer, heart disease, arthritis, asthma, chronic pulmonary disease, diabetes, and Alzheimer's disease are prevalent during middle age and later life and will command large proportions of the available health care resources. Human immunodeficiency virus/acquired immune deficiency syndrome (HIV/AIDS), a chronic illness that affects men, women, and children, will continue to have a significant impact on health care delivery. As a wave of national initiatives are launched to improve end-of-life care, the shortage of nurses—as clinicians and investigators—will become a major problem worldwide (WHO, 2001). A better understanding of mental disorders will emerge as a result of advancements in psychobiological knowledge and research initiatives. Mental health illnesses will continue to be a major public health issue. Depression has been cited as the number one mental illness worldwide (WHO, 2001). Alcohol and drug abuse will continue to be responsible for significant health care expenses. Investigations that address quality-of-care outcomes related to nursing are a top priority for psychiatric nurses in the twenty-first century (President's New Freedom Commission on Mental Health, 2003), as well as nursing contributions to end-of-life research (Matzo & Sherman, 2001).

Undoubtedly, one of the most exciting research opportunities for nurses in the future relates to genetics and the human genome, where study prospects range from basic biological topics to clinical decision making and behavioural interventions (Williams, Tripp-Reimer, Schutte, & Barnette, 2004). Grady (2003) proposed that nurse researchers can make significant contributions to the following areas:

- Understanding the gene–environment–behaviour interface
- Developing and using biological, psychosocial, and neuroimmunological markers
- Participating in biological–psychosocial intervention
- Providing counselling related to genetic health
- Developing and testing cognitive models for decision making regarding genetic factors and genetic therapies
- Investigating new delivery models for health care given the evolving genetic knowledge
- Addressing related ethical issues and dilemmas

Hinshaw (2000) suggested that nurses must play a major role in the field of genetics research so that the evolving knowledge is structured within a "holistic" understanding of the client.

Over the next 10 years, many hard questions relating to cost containment and access to care will need to be addressed through interdisciplinary studies, and the research will also need to address the related ethical dilemmas. An important emphasis of research studies will be related to improvement of client outcomes by addressing clinical and systems' issues and problems (Kohn, Corrigan, & Donaldson, 1999; Stone, Curran, & Bakken, 2002). The pre-eminent goal of nursing research will be the ongoing development of knowledge for use in the practice of nursing, particularly client care initiatives related to the organization and delivery of nursing care. This type of research, sometimes referred to as health services research, includes studies that predict the future supply and demand

for nursing care (Aiken et al., 2003; Rogers, Hwang, Scott, Aike, & Dinges, 2004).

In light of the priority given to clinical research issues, the funding of investigations increasingly emphasizes populations of interest. For example, the historical exclusion of women as subjects in clinical research is well documented. Minority women as subjects have been even more likely to be excluded from research studies; as a result, research data on the health of minority women are extremely scarce.

Along with national nursing research initiatives, specific nursing interest groups frequently establish their own research priorities specific to their specialty. For example, one of the objectives of the Aboriginal Nurses Association of Canada is "to conduct research on cross-cultural medicine and develop and assemble material on Aboriginal health" (2005). Some associations provide funds to support research initiatives. The Canadian Association of Critical Care Nurses, for example, established a small research grant to support specific research activities. The grant will be awarded to a researcher whose work directly relates to the clinical practice of critical care nurses (Canadian Association of Critical Care Nurses, 2007).

Other types of research investigations (e.g., those using historical, feminist, or case study methods) embody the rich diversity of nursing research methods. The nursing profession must continue to value and promote creativity and diversity in research endeavours at all educational levels as a way of empowering nurses for the future. As opportunities are recognized and gaps in science are observed, nurses will conduct, critique, and use nursing research in ways that publicly demonstrate how nursing care makes a difference.

Nurse researchers will have an increasingly strong voice in shaping public policy relating to health care. Shaver (2004) stated that disciplines such as nursing—because of its focus on treatment of chronic illness, health promotion, independence in health, and care of the acutely ill, all of which are heavily emphasized values for the future—will be central to the shape of health care policy in the future. Research data providing evidence that supports or refutes the merit of health care needs and programs focusing on these issues will be timely and relevant. Thus, nursing and its science base will be strategically placed to shape health policy decisions (Fitzpatrick, 2004).

info

Because we will continue to live in the "information age," dissemination of nursing research becomes increasingly important. Research findings will continue to be disseminated in professional arenas (e.g., international, national, regional, and local electronic and print publications and conferences) and in consultations and staff development programs that are implemented on-site, through Web-based programs, or via satellite. Dissemination of research findings in the public sector, however, is an exciting new trend that has already begun.

Nurse researchers are increasingly asked to testify at governmental hearings and to serve on commissions and task forces related to health care. Nurses are increasingly quoted in the media when health care topics are addressed, and their visibility has expanded significantly. Today, nurses and nurse researchers participate in teleconferences, develop their own home pages on the Internet, star in DVDs, and appear in interviews on television and radio and in printed and electronic media (e.g., the Internet, newspapers, and magazines). Nurses have their own radio shows and are beginning to host their own television shows. Consider Sue Johanson, RN, host of the *Sunday Night Sex Show*, who brings over 25 years of experience in sexual education to the public discourse on sex. In addition to addressing all aspects of sex in a nonjudgemental manner on her show, Johanson has written several books and writes a weekly column on health for the *Toronto Star*. Dissemination of research through the public media provides excellent exposure to thousands of potential viewers, listeners, and readers.

Tech

Practising nurses also use technological innovations (e.g., computerized documentation systems and electronic access to databases and literature searches, interactive telecommunication educational offerings, online journals, and research-based

practice guidelines) to make research-related clinical practice activities come alive (Carty, 2001; Jenkins & Dunn, 2004).

Nurses have a research heritage to be proud of and a challenging and exciting future ahead of them. Both researchers and consumers of research will engage in a united effort to acknowledge research findings that make a difference in the care that is provided and the lives that are touched by our commitment to evidence-based nursing practice.

Critical Thinking Challenges

- How will expanding your computer technology "comfort zone" generate evidence-based practice information that can affect health care?
- What assumption underlies the recommendation that the role of the nursing graduate in the research process is primarily that of a knowledgeable consumer?
- What effects will evidence-based client outcome studies have on the practice of nursing?
- Discuss how research will contribute to the development of intradisciplinary and interdisciplinary networks.

KEY POINTS

- Nursing research expands the unique body of scientific knowledge that forms the foundation of evidence-based nursing practice. Research is the component that links education, theory, and practice.

- Nurses become knowledgeable consumers of research through educational processes and practical experience. As consumers of research, nurses must have a basic understanding of the research process and must demonstrate critical appraisal skills to evaluate the strengths and weaknesses of research before applying the research to clinical practice.

- Nursing research blossomed in the second half of the twentieth century: graduate programs in nursing expanded, research journals began to emerge, and funding for graduate education and nursing research increased dramatically.

- All nurses, whether they possess baccalaureate, master's, or doctoral degrees, have a responsibility to participate in the research process.

- The role of the baccalaureate graduate is to be a knowledgeable consumer of research. Nurses with master's and doctoral degrees are obliged to be researchers and sophisticated consumers of research studies.

- A collaborative research relationship within the nursing profession will extend and refine the scientific body of knowledge that provides the grounding for theory-based practice.

- The future of nursing research will focus on the extension of scientific knowledge Collaborative research relationships between education and practice will multiply. Cluster research studies and replication of studies will have increased value.

- Research studies will emphasize clinical issues, problems, and outcomes. Priority will be given to research studies that focus on health promotion, care for the health needs of vulnerable groups, and the development of cost-effective health care systems.

- Both consumers of research and nurse researchers will engage in a collaborative effort to further the growth of nursing research and accomplish the profession's research objectives.

REFERENCES

Aboriginal Nurses Association of Canada. (2005). *Our objectives.* Retrieved August 13, 2007, from http://www.anac.on.ca/objectives.html

Aiken L., Clarke S. P., Cheung R. B., Sloane D. M., & Silber J. H. (2003). Education levels of hospital nurses and patient mortality. *Journal of American Medical Association, 290,* 1617–1623.

Alberta Association of Registered Nurses. (2005). *Entry-to-practice competencies.* Retrieved July 6, 2007, from http://www.nurses.ab.ca/profconduct/npa.html

Buerhaus, P., Staiger, D., & Auerbach, D. (2000). Implications of a rapidly aging nursing workforce. *Journal of American Medical Association, 283*(22), 2948–2954.

Canadian Association of Critical Care Nurses. (2007). *CACCN research grant.* Retrieved August 13, 2007, from http://www.caccn.ca/new/index.php?fuseaction=view.content&item=64

Canadian Association of Schools of Nursing. (2004). *CASN Research and Scholarship Committee strategic plan for 2004/05.* Retrieved September 6, 2007, from http://www.casn.ca/media.php?mid=166

Canadian Association of Schools of Nursing. (2006). *CASN research and scholarship.* Retrieved September 6, 2007, from http://www.casn.ca/content.php?sec=7

Canadian Council on Health Services Accreditation. (2006). *About us.* Retrieved September 6, 2007, from http://www.cchsa.ca/

Canadian Health Services Research Foundation. (n.d.). *Nursing research fund: CHSRF/CIHR chair awards—Nursing.* Retrieved January 16, 2008, from http://www.chsrf.ca/nursing_research_fund/chairs_e.php

Canadian Health Services Research Foundation. (2006). *Looking forward, working together: Priorities for nursing leadership in Canada.* Retrieved August 7, 2007, from http://www.chsrf.ca/research_themes/pdf/NLOP_e.pdf

Canadian Health Services Research Foundation. (2007). *Primary research themes.* Retrieved August 13, 2007, from http://www.chsrf.ca/research_themes/ph_e.php

Canadian Nurses Association. (1998). *Evidence-based decision-making and nursing practice.* Retrieved September 28, 2003, from http://www.cna-nurses.ca

Canadian Nurses Association. (2002). *RN exam competencies.* Retrieved July 3, 2007, from http://cna-aiic.ca/CNA/nursing/rnexam/competencies/default_e.aspx

Canadian Nurses Association and Canadian Association of Schools of Nursing. (2007). *Nursing education in Canada statistics: 2005–2006.* Ottawa: Canadian Nurses Association.

Carper, B. A. (1978). Fundamental patterns of nursing. *Advanced Nursing Science, 1*(1), 13–24.

Carty, B. (Ed.). (2001). *Nursing informatics: Education for practice.* New York: Springer.

Chang, W. Y. (2000). Priority setting for nursing research. *Western Journal of Nursing Research, 22,* 119–121.

College of Nurses of Ontario. (1999). *Entry to practice competencies for Ontario Registered Nurses as of January 1, 2005.* Toronto: College of Nurses of Ontario.

College of Nurses of Ontario. (2002). *Professional standards* (revised 2002). Toronto: CNO.

Committee for the Study of Nursing Education. (1923). *Nursing and nursing education in the United States. Report of the committee and report of a survey by Josephine Goldmark.* New York: Macmillan.

Community Health Research Unit. (2005). *Research projects funded in 2005.* Retrieved August 13, 2007, from http://aix1.uottawa.ca/~nedwards/chru/english/research2005.html

DiCenso, A., Guyatt, G., & Ciliska, D. (2005). *Evidence-based nursing.* Toronto: Elsevier.

Dickenson-Hazard, N. (2004). Global health issues and challenges. *Journal of Nursing Scholarship, 36*(1), 6–10.

Dochterman, J., Titler, M., Wong, J., Reed, D., Pettit, D., Mattlew-Watson, M., et al. (2005). Describing use of nursing interventions in three groups of patients. *Journal of Nursing Scholarship, 37*(1), 57–66.

Dykes, P. C. (2003). Practice guidelines and measurement: State of the science. *Nursing Outlook, 51,* 65–69.

Evers, G. (2003). Developing nursing science in Europe. *Journal of Nursing Scholarship, 35*(1), 9–13.

Fahs, P. S., Stewart, L. L., & Kalman, M. (2003). A call for replication. *Journal of Nursing Scholarship, 35*(1), 67–72.

Fitzpatrick, J. J. (2000). A decade of applied nursing research: A new millennium and beyond. *Applied Nursing Research, 13*(1), 1.

Fitzpatrick, J. J. (2004). Translating clinical research into research policy. *Applied Nursing Research, 17*(2), 71.

Forchuk, C., Martin, M. L., Chan, Y. L., & Jensen, E. (2005). Therapeutic relationships: From psychiatric hospital to community. *Journal of Psychiatric and Mental Health Nursing, 12*, 556–564.

Ford-Gilboe, M., Wuest, J., & Merrit-Gray, M. (2005). Strengthening capacity to limit intrusion: Theorizing family health promotion in the aftermath of woman abuse. *Qualitative Health Research, 15*, 477–501.

Ford-Gilboe, M., Wuest, J., Varcoe, C., & Merrit-Gray, M. (2006). Developing an evidence-based health advocacy intervention for women who have left an abusive partner. *Canadian Journal of Nursing Research, 38*, 147–167.

Good, S. R. (1969). *Submission to the study of support of research in universities for the Science Secretariat of the Privy Council.* Ottawa: Canadian Nurses Association and Canadian Nurses Foundation.

Grady, P. A. (2003). A NINR initiative to address health disparities. *Nursing Outlook, 51*(1), 5.

Heater, B. S., Becker, A. M., & Olson, R. K. (1988). Nursing interventions and patient outcomes: A meta-analysis of studies. *Nursing Research, 37*, 303–307.

Hegyvary, S. T. (1999). An open letter from the new editor. *Image, 31*, 203.

Hegyvary, S. T. (2004). Working paper on grand challenges in improving global health. *Journal of Nursing Scholarship, 36*, 96–101.

Hinshaw, A. S. (2000). Nursing knowledge for the 21st century: Opportunities and challenges. *Journal of Nursing Scholarship, 32*, 117–123.

Institute of Medicine. (1983). *Nursing and nursing education: Public policies and private actions* (p. 19). Washington, DC: National Academy Press.

Jenkins, M. L., Dunn, D. (2004). Enhancing web-based health information for consumer education. *Applied Nursing Research, 17*(1), 68–70.

Jennings, B. M., & McClure, M. L. (2004). Strategies to advance health quality. *Nursing Outlook, 52*, 17–22.

Keith, J. M. (1988). Florence Nightingale: Statistician and consultant epidemiologist. *International Nursing Review, 35*(5), 147–149.

Kohn, L., Corrigan, J., & Donaldson, M. (Eds.). (1999). *To err is human: Building a safer health system.* Washington, DC: National Academy Press.

Larson, E. (2003). Minimizing disincentives for collaborative research. *Nursing Outlook, 51*, 267–271.

Lysaught, J. P. (1970). *An abstract for action.* New York: McGraw-Hill.

Matzo, M., & Sherman, D. W. (Eds.). (2001). *Pallliative care nursing: Quality care to the end of life.* New York: Springer.

Medical Research Council of Canada. (1985). *Report to the Medical Research Council of Canada by the Working Group on Nursing Research.* Ottawa: Medical Research Council.

Melnyk, B. M., & Fineout-Overholt, E. (2002). Putting research into practice. *Reflective Nursing Leadership, 28*(2): 22–25.

Messias, D. K. H. (2001). Globalization, nursing, and health for all. *Journal of Nursing Scholarship, 33*(1), 9–11.

Nahcivan, N. O. (2004). Turkish language equivalence of the exercies of self-care agency scale. *Western Journal of Nursing Research, 26*(7), 813–824.

National Institute of Nursing Research. (2007). *About NINR.* Retrieved January 13, 2008, from http://www.ninr.nih.gov/

Naylor, M. (2003). Nursing intervention research and quality of care. *Nursing Research, 52*, 380–385.

Nightingale, F. (1863). *Notes on hospitals.* London: Longman Group.

Office of Nursing Policy. (2007). *Nursing issues: Research.* Retrieved July 3, 2007, from http://www.hc-sc.gc.ca/hcs-sss/alt_formats/hpb-dgps/pdf/nurs-infirm/2006-res_e.pdf

O'Neill, E. S., & Dluly, N. M. (2000). Utility of structured care approaches in education and clinical practice. *Nursing Outlook, 48*, 132–135.

Paterson, B. (2002). An answer for Sandra. *Canadian Nurse, 98*(4), 14.

Potter, P., Perry, A. G., Ross-Kerr, J., & Wood, M. (Eds.). (2006). *Canadian fundamentals of nursing* (3rd ed.). Toronto: Elsevier Canada.

President's New Freedom Commission on Mental Health. (2003). Achieving the promise: Transforming mental health care in America: Final report. DHHS Pub No. SMA-03-3832. Rockville, MD.

Pringle, D. (1999). Another twist on the double helix: Research and practice. *Canadian Journal of Nursing Research, 30*, 165–179.

Rogers, A. A. E., Hwang, W., Scott, L., Aike, L. H., & Dinges, D. F. (2004). The working hours of hospital staff nurses and patient safety. *Health Affairs, 23*, 202–212.

Ross-Kerr, J., & Wood, M. (2006). Research as a basis for practice. In P. Potter, A. G. Perry, J. Ross-Kerr, & M. Wood (Eds.), *Canadian fundamentals of nursing* (3rd ed., pp. 81–94). Toronto: Elsevier Canada.

Shaver, J. (2004). Improving the health of communities: The position. *Nursing Outlook, 52,* 116–117.

Stewart, M., Kushner, K., & Spitzer, D. (2001). Research priorities in gender and health. *Canadian Journal of Nursing Research, 33,* 5–15.

Stone, P. W., Curran, C. R., & Bakken, S. (2002). Economic evidence for evidence-based practice. *Journal of Nursing Scholarship, 34*(3), 277–282.

Symons, T. H. B. (1975). *To know ourselves: The report of the Commission of Canadian Studies.* Ottawa: Associations of Universities and Colleges of Canada.

Tarlier, D. (2005). Mediating the meaning of evidence through epistemological diversity. *Nursing Inquiry, 12,* 126–134.

Titler, M. G., Cullen, L., & Ardery, G. (2002). Evidence-based practice: an administrative perspective. *Reflective Nursing Leadership, 28*(2), 26–27, 46.

Titler, M. G., Goode, C., & Mathis, S. (1992). Nursing research in times of economic cutbacks: Implications for nurse administrators. *Series on Nursing Administration, 4,* 167–182.

Titler, M. G., Mentes, J. C., Rakel, B. A., Abbott, L., & Baumler, S. (1999). From book to bedside: Putting evidence to use in the care of the elderly. *The Joint Commission Journal on Quality Improvement, 25*(10), 545–556.

Tourangeau, A., Giovannetti, P., Tu, J., & Wood, M. (2002). Nursing-related determinants of 30-day mortality for hospitalized patients. *Canadian Journal of Nursing Research, 33,* 71–88.

Villeneuve, M., & MacDonald, J. (2006). *Toward 2020: Visions for nursing,* p. 99. Ottawa: Canadian Nurses Association.

Ward, L. S. (2003). Race as a cross-variable in research. *Nursing Outlook, 51*(3), 120–125.

Weir, G. M. (1932). *Survey of nursing education in Canada.* Toronto: MacMillan. Note that this publication is often referred to as the Weir Report or the Weir Survey.

Whittemore, R., & Grey, M. (2002). The systematic development of nursing interventions. *Journal of Nursing Scholarships, 34*(2), 115–120.

Williams, J. K., Tripp-Reimer, T., Schutte, D., & Barnette, J. (2004).Advancing genetic nursing knowledge. *Nursing Outlook, 52*(3), 73–79.

World Health Organization (2001). *The world health report 2001—Mental health: new understanding, new hope.* Geneva: WHO.

Patricia R. Liehr
Mary Jane Smith
Cherylyn Cameron

CHAPTER 2

Theoretical Framework

LEARNING OUTCOMES

After reading this chapter, the student should be able to do the following:

- Define key concepts in the philosophy of science.
- Identify assumptions underlying the positivist or postpositivist view (positivism) and the constructivist view (constructivism) of research.
- Compare inductive and deductive reasoning.
- Differentiate between conceptual and theoretical frameworks.
- Identify the purpose and nature of conceptual and theoretical frameworks.
- Describe how a framework guides research.
- Differentiate between conceptual and operational definitions.
- Describe the relationships among theory, research, and practice.
- Discuss levels of abstraction related to frameworks guiding research.
- Differentiate among grand, midrange, and microrange theories in nursing.
- Describe the points of critical appraisal used to evaluate the appropriateness, cohesiveness, and consistency of a framework guiding research.

KEY TERMS

aims of inquiry 26
35 concept
34 conceptual definition
38 conceptual framework
constructivist paradigm 26
constructivism 26
context 26 27
deductive reasoning 33
empirical analytical 28
34 empirical factors
epistemology 26
36 grand theory
38 hypothesis
inductive reasoning 33
34 metaparadigm
37 microrange theory
36 midrange theory
30 mixed methods research
33 model
ontology 26
35 operational definition
25 paradigm
25 philosophical beliefs
25 positivism
qualitative research 28
quantitative research 28
text 28
38 theoretical framework
32 31 theory
triangulation 30
25 worldview

STUDY RESOURCES

evolve Go to Evolve at
http://evolve.elsevier.com/Canada/LoBiondo/research/
for Weblinks, content updates, and additional
38 research articles for practice in reviewing
and critiquing.

THE NATURE OF KNOWLEDGE

When nurses have clinical questions, Carper's (1978) ways of knowing provide answers to consider in guiding their practice (empirical, aesthetic, personal, and moral patterns of knowledge). Nurses also learn from experts who have experience and wisdom to share and from other disciplines, which is why nursing students take courses in chemistry, philosophy, psychology, and other fields. Nurses also learn from, and act on, their intuition and sometimes know what to do from trial and error, although solving problems through trial and error is not very efficient. Nurses also learn from scientific problem solving.

The knowledge gained from scientific research can be used to guide nursing practice. Knowledge acquired through scientific reasoning or research is less vulnerable than that acquired through individual experience. What nurses do naturally and by "instinct" may be effective, but if nurses are tired or upset, their performance may be adversely affected.

Nurses learn from conducted research that what they believe is helpful, but what they have learned from outside experts may not, in fact, be helpful to a specific group of clients. For example, for many years, medical experts taught nurses that clients should not be provided with information about their conditions and care. However, early nursing research clearly showed that providing clients with this information did improve their health (Johnson, Fieler, Jones, Wlasowicz, & Mitchell, 1997).

Philosophers deal with the following questions: What is truth? How do we know what we know? What is real? What counts as evidence? What is good (of value)? What is ethical or right conduct? The answers to these questions are important guides to nursing practice as they shape how nurses see the world and their roles in it. How nurses provide care and how they conduct research differ depending on how they answer these philosophical questions.

PHILOSOPHIES OF RESEARCH

Every specialty has characteristic terminology for communicating important features of the work of that specialty that are not as relevant to others. Learning new terminology is part of what nursing students do when they learn research methods and skills. Each research method and all philosophies of science have specialized language that nursing students will encounter in the **literature**. Thus, to help you comprehend the research you will read, it is important to clarify a few terms.

The word *science* comes from a word meaning "knowledge," and the word *philosophy* comes from a word that means "wisdom" (Oxford University Press, 2004). All research is based on **philosophical beliefs** about the world; these beliefs are also known as a **worldview** or **paradigm**. *Paradigm* is from a Greek word meaning "pattern." Thomas Kuhn (1962) first applied the word paradigm to science to describe the way people in a particular society think about the world. According to Olson (2006), "Paradigms are sets of beliefs and practices, shared by communities of researchers, which regulate inquiry within disciplines" (p. 459).

All research is based on philosophical beliefs and assumptions. Although those who conduct qualitative research are more likely to describe their philosophical beliefs and assumptions explicitly when discussing their findings, all research is based on these beliefs. Therefore, knowing and comprehending these beliefs is important to understanding and using research findings. These beliefs are not right or wrong; rather, they represent different views of the world and their utilization is dependent upon the goals of the research.

The paradigms of positivism and constructivism are the basis of research. **Positivism** and, more recently, postpositivism, is the basis of *empirical analytical* (quantitative) research. The notion of positivism first emerged from the work and thoughts of the nineteenth-century philosopher Auguste Comte. The main assumption underlying positivism is that a reality exists that can be observed, measured, and known as fact. Related to this paradigm is the notion of determinism, the view that every phenomenon is brought about by an antecedent event. For example, the events leading to the development of heart disease can be determined. Postpositivists are still interested in reality and seek to understand it, but their views are tempered by the belief that no absolute truth exists. **Constructivism** is the basis for *naturalistic* (qualitative) research and developed from writers such as Immanuel Kant, who sought alternative ways of thinking about the world. Constructivists believe that reality is not fixed but is a construction of the people perceiving it and that many constructions are possible; thus, no ultimate truth exists. The paradigms of positivism and constructivism can be thought of as extremes at either end of a continuum of research approaches.

Helpful Hint

All research is based on a paradigm, however it is seldomly identified in a research report.

Table 2-1 compares these two paradigms; however, the philosophical language in the table needs to be clarified. **Epistemology** deals with what we know, that is, "truth." The origins, nature, and limits of knowledge are included. Epistemology deals with why and how we know some things and what constitutes our knowing. **Ontology** (from the Greek *onto*, meaning "to be") is the science or study of being or existence and its relationship to nonexistence.

Existentialists and phenomenologists discuss being and nonbeing or nothingness as categories. Ontology deals with what is real (versus fiction or appearance) and the nature of reality (or matter). There are two views of reality: in the received or positivist view, one reality exists and humankind seeks to learn the laws of nature, whereas in the perceived or constructivist view, reality is constructed differently by different people. For example, what the client perceives as real and important may go unnoticed by nurses. **Context** refers to the environment where something occurs. The context of research studies can include physical settings, such as the hospital or home, or less concrete "environments," such as the context that cultural understandings and beliefs bring to an experience. The **aims of inquiry**, or the goals of the research, also vary with the paradigm. How the researchers' *values* are viewed, the researchers' role or *voice*, and the *methodology* they use also vary with different paradigms.

The **constructivist paradigm** is the basis of most qualitative research, and the positivist or contemporary empiricist paradigm is the basis of most empirical analytical or quantitative research. An example from oncology research may clarify that some types of research are more congruent with the positivist paradigm than with the constructivist paradigm, and vice versa. Consider the example of

TABLE 2-1	**Basic Beliefs of Research Paradigms**	
	Constructivist Paradigm	**Positivist or Postpositivist Paradigm**
Epistemology	"Truth" is determined by the individual or cultural group Subjectivism is valued	Truth is sought via replicable observation Objectivism is valued
Ontology	Multiple realities exist, influenced by culture and environment	"Real reality" exists "out there" Driven by natural laws
Context	Emphasized; value is placed on rich details of context in which the phenomenon occurs Time and place are important	Minimized; value is placed on generalizability across contexts
Aims of inquiry	Description (narrative), understanding, transformation, reconstruction	Description (statistical), explanation, prediction, and control
Values	Included; they add to understanding of the phenomenon	Excluded; they detract from the inquiry aim
Researcher's voice	Active participant	Neutral observer
Methodology	Dialogic, transformative	Experimental, controlled

Adapted from Lincoln, Y., & Guba, E. (2000). Paradigmatic controversies, contradictions, and emerging confluences. In N. K. Denzin. & Y. S. Lincoln (Eds.), *Handbook of qualitative research* (2nd ed.). Thousand Oaks, CA: Sage.

chemotherapy for cancer. When studying the efficacy of a drug for the treatment of cancer, logic suggests that experimental research should be used. This approach, based on the positivist paradigm, is guided by the ontological view of one reality; in other words, all clients will respond in the same way to this chemotherapy drug. Of course, responses to drugs may vary according to clients' age, gender, ethnicity, and so on, but those features can be considered by research that includes persons of diverse ethnicity and both genders and by looking at the effects of the drugs according to these groups.

Epistemology leads to seeking truth in an objective, replicable way. Continuing with the previous example, the way the chemotherapy drug is prepared and provided to people will be the same for each person, and other researchers in other parts of the world would do the research in the same way. In this paradigm, the emphasis is on studying parts, so the focus might be on the responses of tumour cells rather than the effect on the whole person. Because the context is not central to this research, researchers would expect to find the same response to drugs in different parts of the world because the researchers are focused only on the tumour itself, not on the effect on the person and their experiences.

With respect to the previous example, the goal of oncology research is guided by the received or positivist view to statistically describe, explain, and predict the outcome, and, finally, to eliminate or, at least, control the cancer. In this view, which is the basis of most quantitative research, researchers are neutral observers, meaning, for example, that they do not have a vested interest in showing that one drug is better than another. Quantitative researchers believe that values detract from the inquiry. Of course, values are always a part of what we do—we would not study something we did not value or believe was important. For researchers who subscribe to the positivist view, the goal is to keep the values as separate from their work as possible.

However, when we are interested in what it means to people to have cancer or cancer treatment, a qualitative study is more appropriate. Qualitative studies, based on the constructivist paradigm, are guided by the ontological view that multiple realities exist. As Olson (2006) stated, "Phenomena are studied through the eyes of people in their lived situations" (p. 461). For example, the meaning of cancer will likely be different for a young mother than for a grandmother. The meaning of cancer also may be different in Canada than in Japan. Epistemology includes the view that truth varies and is subjective. Context is important, and description of the experience(s) is vital. When seeking to understand clients' experiences of a treatment, we would expect that what is important and "true" for one person may not be so for another. Some of the differences may result from context. The experience may well vary according to where the client is treated and the client's characteristics, such as age, gender, and ethnicity. The experience of having cancer may be different for a client whose parent died a painful death from cancer than for a client who knew people whose cancer was cured. The values of all involved are acknowledged in qualitative research.

Researchers work to ensure that their values do not cloud their attitudes and behaviours toward research or prevent them from understanding how others view experiences. What is valued by and important to participants in the research also helps researchers understand experiences. Qualitative research is conducted in dialogues or interviews with "participants," a word that recognizes their active role in the research, whereas quantitative research is conducted with "subjects" (i.e., passive participants), in keeping with the constructionist paradigm. The results from qualitative research would be useful in describing experiences, leading to a better understanding of others' experiences, and through this understanding lead to practices that can transform or improve peoples' health or their experiences of illness.

Helpful Hint

Values are involved in all research. It is vital, however, that values do not influence the results of the research.

Another way of thinking about the positivist and constructivist paradigms and linking them to research is illustrated in the Critical Thinking Decision Path. This algorithm illustrates that beliefs lead to different questions, which in turn lead to the selection of different research approaches. Qualitative and quantitative research methods are associated with different assumptions that are consistent with each method and are more specific than these global worldviews (i.e., positivism and constructivism). These beliefs and approaches lead to different research activities, as illustrated in the decision path.

TYPES OF RESEARCH:
Qualitative and Quantitative

As you can see from the critical thinking pathway, research processes are divided into two major categories: qualitative and quantitative. Researchers choose between these categories based primarily on the questions they are asking. In other words, a researcher may wish to test a cause-and-effect situation or to assess whether variables are related, or a researcher may wish to discover and understand the meaning of an experience or process.

A researcher would choose to conduct a **qualitative research** study if the question to be answered concerns understanding the meaning of a human experience, such as grief, hope, or loss. The meaning of an experience is based on the view that meaning varies and is subjective. The context of the experience also plays a role in qualitative research. For example, the experience of loss as a result of a miscarriage would be different from the experience of the loss of a parent. Qualitative research is generally conducted in natural settings and uses data that are words or **text** rather than numbers to describe the experiences being studied. Data are collected from a small number of subjects, allowing an in-depth study of a particular phenomenon. For example, Smith, Edwards, Varcoe, Martens, and Davies (2006) (see Appendix B) studied the in-depth the experience of 16 key informants who worked in policy, leadership, and

provider positions within the "maternal/child" health care system. Although qualitative research is systematic in its approach, it uses a subjective approach. Data from qualitative studies help nurses understand experiences or phenomena that affect clients; these data also assist in generating theories that lead clinicians to develop improved care and further research. Table 3–2 (see p. 47) outlines the general steps of qualitative studies and the journal format for a qualitative article. Chapters 7 and 8 provide an in-depth view of the underpinnings, designs, and methods of qualitative research.

Whereas qualitative research seeks to interpret meaning and phenomena, **quantitative research** encompasses the study of research questions or hypotheses (or both) that describe phenomena, test relationships, assess differences, and seek to explain cause-and-effect interactions between variables and tests for intervention effectiveness. The numerical data in quantitative studies are summarized and analyzed using statistics. Quantitative research techniques are systematic, and the methodology is controlled. Appendices A and C illustrate different quantitative approaches to answering research questions. Table 3–1 (p. 46) indicates where the steps in the research process can usually be located in a quantitative research article and where they are discussed in this text. When reading research articles, remember that a researcher may vary the steps slightly, depending on the nature of the research problem, but all of the steps should be addressed systematically.

Empirical analytical is a general label for quantitative research approaches that test hypotheses. These methods are discussed in detail in Part 3. Note that although all research is based on philosophy, researchers who use quantitative approaches are less aware of, or, at least, often make less explicit, the philosophy underlying their research. Positivism or postpositivism is the basis of research focused on testing hypotheses that are derived from theories or conceptual frameworks. The goal is to support the research hypothesis with the data from the study. In addition to the positivist view beliefs already discussed, other

Critical Thinking Decision Path. Selecting a Research Process

If your beliefs are

Researcher beliefs	Humans are biopsychosocial beings, known by their biological, psychological, and social characteristics.	or	Humans are complex beings who attribute unique meaning to their life situations. They are known by their personal expressions.
	Truth is objective reality that can be experienced with the senses and measured by the researcher.		Truth is the subjective expression of reality as perceived by the participant and shared with the researcher. Truth is context laden.

then you will ask questions, such as

Example questions	What is the difference in blood pressure and heart rate for adolescents who are angry compared with those who are not angry?	or	What is the structure of the lived experience of anger for adolescents?

and select approaches

Approaches	**Quantitative/deductive**	or	**Qualitative/inductive**

leading to research activities:

Research activities	Researcher selects a representative (of population) sample and determines size before collecting data.	or	Researcher selects participants who are experiencing the phenome non of interest and collects data until saturation is reached.
	Researcher uses an extensive approach to collect data.		Researcher uses an intensive approach to collect data.
	Questionnaires and measurement devices are preferably administered in one setting by an unbiased individual to control for extraneous variables.		Researcher conducts interviews and participant or nonparticipant observation in environments where participants usually spend their time. Researcher bias is acknowledged and set aside.
	Primarily deductive analysis is used, generating a numerical summary that allows the researcher to reject or accept the null hypothesis.		Primarily inductive analysis is used, leading to a narrative summary, which synthesizes participant information, creating a description of human experience.

assumptions underlie contemporary empiricism in nursing (Im & Meleis, 1999); these are outlined in Box 2–1.

Matching Research Goals with Research Philosophy

Some researchers write about qualitative research and quantitative research as incompatible approaches. The value of one approach over the other has been argued. However, other researchers have recognized that different research methods accomplish different goals and have advocated using the method appropriate to the research question and combining methods when this approach is compatible with the research goals. Understanding the philosophy underlying each method can help researchers use the method that best meets the intended purpose and can guide the reader to use the research findings in appropriate ways.

Combining research methods is known as **mixed methods research**, which is used more extensively in the social sciences to solve practical research problems (Teddlie & Tashakkori, 2003). Tashakkori and Creswell (2007) defined mixed methods "as research in which the investigator collects and analyzes data, integrates the findings, and draws inferences using both qualitative and quantitative approaches or methods in a single study or a program of inquiry" (p. 4). Consider the earlier example regarding chemotherapy. When studying the effectiveness of a drug for cancer, not measuring changes in tumour size would be foolish. Equally foolish would be ignoring what clients say is important to them when they take this drug, if researchers want to understand what it means to the clients. Because the meanings clients make of their experiences may well determine the needs that can be met with nursing interventions, such as the need for information or the need to talk about the fear of death, this information is vital to guide effective nursing practice. Thus, according to the above example, both qualitative and quantitative methods are necessary.

Interest in combining qualitative and quantitative research methods has increased as researchers recognize that although each paradigm has inherent strengths and weaknesses, a combination of methods maximizes the strengths of each (Cameron, 2003). Locke, Spirduso, & Silverman (1993) maintained that research combining qualitative and quantitative designs had contributed to program evaluation, organizational studies, and policy development. Mixed methods research has now evolved to the point where researchers are developing a separate methodological orientation with its own vocabulary, techniques, and design (Teddlie & Tashakkori, 2003). Mixed method studies are one form of **triangulation** in which the researcher uses more than one research strategy in a single study (Speziale & Carpenter, 2007).

However, nursing researchers debate whether mixed methods research is, in fact, a hidden way of promoting one paradigm—positivism—over another (Giddings & Grant, 2007). To ensure that researchers do not fall into this trap (of promoting one paradigm over another), researchers must recognize the epistemological differences between the two approaches, including the philosophical and methodological features. According to Ford-Gilboe, Campbell, and Berman, "in both post-positivist and interpretative paradigms, it is possible to justify the use of quantitative and qualitative methods to meet the purposes of the research without violating paradigm assumptions" (1995, p. 22). Teddlie and Tashakkori (2003) argued that the results from mixed methods research are greater

---

BOX 2–1   Assumptions of Contemporary Empiricism

1. The world is, to some extent, predictable. Although nothing is absolute, reasonable predictions about health and illness are possible.
2. Human responses to health and illness can be identified, measured, and understood.
3. The notion of explanation results from linking observable processes to unobservable processes.
4. Careful scientific research provides results that can be corroborated.

than the sum of the contributions from the qualitative and quantitative components and that mixed methods designs will become the most dominant methodological tool in the twenty-first century.

FRAMEWORKS FOR RESEARCH

As an introduction to frameworks for research, put yourself in the shoes of Kate. Read her story and consider its message for the practising nurse who wishes to critique, understand, and conduct research.

Kate has worked in a coronary care unit (CCU) for nearly three years since graduating from nursing. She has grown more comfortable over time and now believes that she can readily manage the complexities of client care in the CCU. Recently, she has observed the pattern of blood pressure (BP) change when health care providers enter a client's room. This observation began when Kate noticed that one of her clients, a 62-year-old woman who had continuous arterial monitoring, showed dramatic increases in BP, as much as 100%, each time the health care team made rounds in the CCU. Furthermore, this elevated BP persisted after the team left the client's room and then slowly decreased to preround levels within the following hour. Conversely, when the nurse manager visited the same client on her usual daily rounds, the client engaged calmly in conversation and was often left with lower BP when the nurse manager moved on to the next client. Kate thought about what was happening and adjusted her work so that she could closely observe the details of this phenomenon over several days.

Team rounds were led by the attending cardiologist and included nurses, pharmacists, social workers, medical students, and nursing students. The team discussed the client, and, occasionally, she was asked to respond to a question about her history of heart disease or her current experience of chest discomfort. Participants took turns listening to her heart, and the students responded to questions related to her case. In contrast, the nurse manager's visit occurred one-on-one, giving the client the nurse's full attention. Kate noticed that the nurse manager was especially attentive to the client's experience. In fact, the nurse manager usually sat and spent time talking to the client about how her day was going, what she was thinking about while lying in bed, and what feelings were surfacing as she began to consider how life would be when she returned home.

Kate decided to talk to the nurse manager about her observations. The nurse manager, Alison, was pleased that Kate had noticed these BP changes associated with interaction with health care professionals. She told Kate that she, too, noticed these changes during her eight-year experience of working in the CCU. Her observation led her to the theory of *attentively embracing story* (Liehr & Smith, 2000; Smith & Liehr, 2003), which seemed applicable to the observation. Alison had learned the theory as a first-year master's degree student and now was applying it in practice and beginning plans to use the theory to guide her thesis research. The theory of attentively embracing story proposes that intentional nurse–client dialogue, which engages the human story, enables connecting with self-in-relation to create ease (see Figure 2–1). As depicted by the theory model, the central concept of the theory is intentional dialogue, which is what Kate first observed when she noticed Alison interacting with the client.

Alison was fully attentive to the client, following her lead and pursuing what mattered most to the client. Alison seemed to obtain a lot of information in a short time, and the client seemed willing to share things she was not sharing with other people.

According to the theory of attentively embracing story, the three concepts of intentional dialogue, connecting with self-in-relation, and creating ease are intricately connected. So, when Kate observed intentional dialogue, she also observed connecting with self-in-relation as the client reflected on her experience in the moment and creating ease when she saw the client's BP decrease after the nurse manager's visit.

Alison and Kate shared an understanding that a relationship existed between client–health care provider interaction and BP. They discussed several possible issues

Figure 2–1 Attentively embracing story

Connecting with Self-in-Relation
Personal history
Reflective awareness

Intentional Dialogue
True presence
Querying emergence

Nurse Client

Creating Ease
Remembering disjointed story moments
Flow in the midst of anchoring

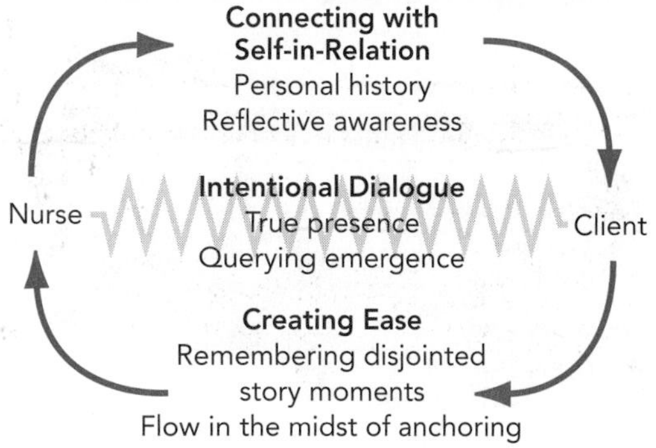

TABLE 2–2 Issues Affecting Blood Pressure Change and Related Research Question

Issues	Research Questions
Number of people in the client's room	Is there a difference in BP for clients in the CCU when interacting with one person compared with interacting with two people or a group of three or more people?
Involvement of the client	For the client in the CCU, what is the relationship between BP and the amount of time spent listening to the health care team's discussion of personal qualities during routine rounds? What is the effect of nurse–client intentional dialogue on BP within the hour after the dialogue?
Continuing effect of experience on BP over the next hour	What is the BP pattern of clients in the CCU from the beginning of routine health care rounds until one hour after the completion of rounds?
Content of dialogue	What is the relationship between issues discussed during intentional dialogue and BP?
Meaning of experience for the client	What is the client's experience of being the object of routine health care rounds? What is the client's experience of sharing personal matters with a nurse while in the CCU?

BP: blood pressure; CCU: coronary care unit.

that might be affecting this relationship and made a list of research questions related to each issue (see Table 2–2). Their list serves only as a reflection of the complexity of the relationship; other issues could generate a research question contributing to understanding of the relationship between client–health care provider interaction and BP. The list developed by Kate and Alison highlights the fact that the relationship cannot be understood with one study; rather, a series of studies may enhance understanding and offer suggestions for change. For instance, a thorough understanding may lead to testing different approaches for conducting team rounds.

LINKS CONNECTING PRACTICE, THEORY, AND RESEARCH

Several important aspects of frameworks for research are embedded in the story of Kate and Alison. First, it is important for the reader to notice the links connecting practice, theory, and research. Each is intricately connected with the other to create knowledge for the discipline of nursing (see Figure 2–2). A **theory** is a set of interrelated concepts that provides a systematic view of a phenomenon. Theory guides practice and research; practice enables testing of theory and generates questions for research; and research contributes to theory building and establishing practice guidelines. So, what is learned through practice, theory, and research interweaves to create the knowledge fabric of the discipline of nursing. From this perspective, each reader is in the process of contributing to the

knowledge of the discipline. For example, if you are practising, you can use focused observation (Liehr, 1992), just as Kate did, to consider the nuances of situations that matter to client health. Kate noticed the changes in BP occurring with interactions and systematically began to pay close attention to the effect of different interactions. This logical process often generates the questions that make the most sense for enhancing client well-being.

Another major theme in the story of Kate and Alison can be found in each nurse's approach to the phenomenon of the relationship between health care provider–client interaction and BP. Each nurse was using a different approach to look at the situation, but both were systematically evaluating what was observed. This approach is the essence of science—

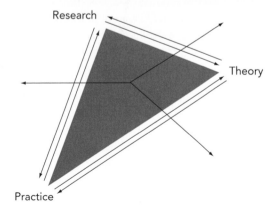

Figure 2–2 Discipline knowledge: the theory–practice–research connection

Research

Theory

Practice

systematic collection, analysis, and interpretation of data. Kate was using **inductive reasoning**, a process of starting with the details of experience and moving to a general picture. Inductive reasoning involves the observation of a particular set of instances that belong to and can be identified as part of a larger set. Alison told Kate that she, too, had begun with inductive reasoning but now was using **deductive reasoning**, a process of starting with the general picture, in this case, the theory of attentively embracing story, and moving to a specific direction for practice and research. Deductive reasoning uses two or more related concepts that, when combined, enable the researcher to suggest relationships between the concepts.

Inductive and deductive reasoning are basic to frameworks for research. Inductive reasoning is the pattern of "figuring out what's there" from the details of the nursing practice experience and is the foundation for most qualitative inquiry. Research questions related to the issue of the meaning of experience for the client (see Table 2–2) can be addressed with the inductive reasoning of qualitative inquiry. Deductive reasoning begins with a structure that guides searching for "what is there." All but the last two research questions listed in Table 2–2 would be addressed with the deductive reasoning of quantitative inquiry.

Given Alison's use of deductive reasoning guided by the theory of attentively embracing story, we can assume that she has read and critiqued the literature on theoretical frameworks and has chosen *attentively embracing story* to guide her master's thesis research. For Kate to move on in her thinking about research to study the way changes in BP are related to health care provider–client interaction, she needs to become well-versed in the importance of theoretical frameworks. As she reads the literature and reviews research studies, she will critique the theoretical frameworks guiding those studies. By critiquing existing frameworks, she will develop the knowledge and understanding needed to choose an appropriate framework for research. As a beginning, Kate is reading this chapter, recognizing that she is critiquing nursing research.

Helpful Hint

Investigators may not always provide a detailed, explicit statement of the observation(s) that led them to their conclusion(s) when using inductive reasoning. Likewise, you will not always find a clear picture of the structure guiding a study that uses deductive reasoning.

FRAMEWORKS AS STRUCTURES FOR RESEARCH

Whether evaluating a qualitative or a quantitative study, look for the framework that guided the study. Generally, when the researcher is using qualitative inquiry and inductive reasoning methods, the critical reader will find the framework at the end of the publication in the discussion section. From the study's findings, the researcher builds a structure for moving forward. For example, in the study on women and violence in improving pregnancy and parenting care for Aboriginal families (Smith et al., 2006) (see Appendix B), the researchers investigated experiences from community members. These stories were analyzed, and the findings were synthesized at the theoretical level. The researchers moved from the particulars of the experiences of pregnancy and parenting care to a general structure of concepts that included pregnancy as an opportunity for change, safe health care places and relationships, responsive care, and making interventions safe and responsive. These concepts were described in the context of the subjects' stories and relevant literature, creating a conceptual structure that could be modelled.

A **model** is a symbolic representation of a set of concepts that is created to depict relationships. Figure 2–1 is the model of *attentively embracing story*. It represents the nurse–client connection through the rhythmic symbol labelled intentional dialogue. The model depicts process by connecting the concepts through nurse–client dialogue with linking arrows. This model could be the basis for deductive reasoning. An example of a deductive question that could be derived from the model is as follows:

> *What is the difference in salivary cortisol (an indicator of ease) for cancer clients who engage with participants (connecting with self-in-relation) in a nurse-led (intentional dialogue) cancer support group?*

When the researcher uses quantitative inquiry and deductive reasoning methods, the critical reader will find the framework at the beginning of the article, before a discussion of study methods. For example, in a study seeking to understand the stress and psychological distress in single mothers, Samuels-Dennis (2006) (see Appendix C) used the Stress Process Model as the theoretical framework. The model posits stress as a dynamic and evolving process composed of three core elements: stressors, stress moderators, and stress outcomes (Pearlin, 2002). The model and the related literature led Samuels-Dennis to hypothesize the following:

- Social assistance recipients will report greater stressful events than employed single mothers.
- Social assistance recipients will report greater depressive symptoms than employed single mothers.
- Employment status and stressful events will predict depression among single mothers.

Samuels-Dennis (2006) used deductive reasoning to move from the model, which she substantiated with the literature, to the hypotheses, or best guesses, regarding what she would find. Her model provided a framework to guide her research from theory to hypotheses, or from the abstract to the concrete.

The Ladder of Abstraction

The ladder of abstraction is a way for the reader to gain a perspective when reading and thinking about frameworks for research. When critiquing the framework of a study, imagine a ladder (see Figure 2–3). The highest level on the ladder, the worldview, includes beliefs and assumptions—the **metaparadigm** of the researcher. The metaparadigm of

nursing transcends all specific philosophies, thus providing a frame of reference for thinking about the discipline of nursing. Fawcett (2000) stated that a metaparadigm is "extremely global and provides no specific direction for such activities as research and practice" (p. 4). Instead, a metaparadigm provides a general orientation and helps us focus on what nursing is and what it is not. Fawcett (2000) stated that a metaparadigm for nursing includes the following four concepts: person, environment, health, and nursing. Although these four concepts are not always explicitly stated in a publication, they do exist.

The middle portion of the ladder includes the frameworks, theories, and concepts the researcher uses to articulate the problem, purpose, and structure for the research. For example, as stated by Samuels-Dennis (2006), the purpose of her study was to further understand employment status as a social determinant of psychological distress among single mothers. Using the literature base, a model of stress process was used to identify specific variables to measure, form a hypothesis, and logically structure the study.

Following the "middle of the ladder" position of frameworks, theories, and concepts is a lower rung where empirical factors are located. **Empirical factors** refer to those elements that can be observed through the senses. These factors include the variables measured and described in quantitative research studies and the story that is described in qualitative studies. The key empirical aspects of a study—its concepts and variables—are generally articulated through conceptual and operational definitions.

A **conceptual definition** is much like a dictionary definition, conveying the general meaning of

Figure 2–3 The ladder of abstraction

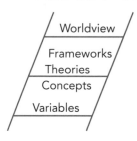

the concept. However, the conceptual definition goes beyond the general meaning found in the dictionary: it defines the concept as it is rooted in the theoretical literature. The **operational definition** specifies how the concept will be measured—that is, what instruments will be used to capture the variable, which comprises the lower rung of the ladder of abstraction (or "closer to the ground").

Helpful 💡 Hint

Some research reports embed conceptual definitions in the literature review. The reader should find the conceptual definitions so that the logical fit between the conceptual and the operational definitions can be determined.

Frameworks, Theories, and Concepts

Consider closely the middle portion of the ladder of abstraction, where frameworks, theories, and concepts are located. Pretend to look at the middle section through a magnifying glass so that the information located there can be distinguished and clarified. Frameworks, theories, and concepts can be compared with each other from the perspective of abstraction, with concepts being the lowest on the middle portion of the ladder and frameworks the highest. However, some concepts are closer to the ground than others. The same is true for theories and frameworks. For example, the concept of pain relief would be closer to the ground than the concept of caring. The idea of varying levels of abstraction within the middle of the ladder is emphasized in the section below on theories, but it has relevance for concepts and frameworks as well.

CONCEPTS

Building from the lower end of the ladder of abstraction, a **concept** is an image or symbolic representation of an abstract idea. Chinn and Kramer (1999, p. 51) defined a concept as a "complex mental formulation of experience." Concepts are the major components of theory and convey the abstract ideas within a theory. In this chapter, the concepts of the theory of attentively embracing story, intentional

dialogue, connecting with self-in-relation, and creating ease have been defined and their relationships have been modelled. Each concept creates a mental image that is explained further through the conceptual definition. For example, the concept of pain creates a mental image based on experience. Its experiential meaning is different for the child who has just fallen off a bike, for the older adult with rheumatoid arthritis, and for the nurse with a doctoral degree who is studying pain mechanisms using an animal model. These definitions and associated images of the concept of pain incorporate different experiential and knowledge components, all with the same label—pain. Therefore, it is important to know the meaning of the concept for the person. For a reader, it is important to know the meaning that the researcher gives to the concepts in a research study.

THEORIES

A theory is a set of interrelated concepts that structure a systematic view of phenomena for the purpose of explaining or predicting. A theory is like a blueprint, a guide for modelling a structure. A blueprint depicts the elements of a structure and the relationship of each element to the other, just as a theory depicts both the concepts that compose it and how they are related. Chinn and Kramer (1999, p. 63) defined a theory as an "expression of knowledge . . . a creative and rigorous structuring of ideas that project a tentative, purposeful, and systematic view of phenomena" (p. 268).

On the ladder of abstraction, theories are located relative to their scope. An often-used label in nursing is "grand theory," which suggests a broad scope, covering major areas of importance to the discipline. Grand theories arose at a time when nursing was addressing its nature, mission, and goals (Im & Meleis, 1999); thus, the development of grand theories are historically important. However, the significance of grand theory extends beyond history to have implications for guiding the discipline of nursing today and in the future. For the purpose of introducing the reader to theory as a framework for nursing research, grand theory is discussed, as well as midrange theory and microrange theory. As is suggested by the names of these theory categories, grand theories are highest and microrange theories are lowest in level of abstraction.

Grand Theory. Theories unique to nursing help to define how this discipline is different from other disciplines. Nursing theories reflect the metaparadigm of nursing with particular views of person, health, environment, and nursing (Fawcett, 2000) that contribute to the development of knowledge specific to nursing's concerns. A **grand theory** is an all-inclusive conceptual structure that tends to include the metaparadigm views on person, health, and environment to create a perspective for nursing. This most abstract level of theory has established knowledge for the discipline and is critical to further knowledge development in the discipline.

The grand theories of several well-known nursing theorists have served as a basis for practice and research. Among these theories are Rogers's science of irreducible human beings (1990, 1992), Orem's theory of self-care deficit (1995), Newman's theory of health as expanding consciousness (1997), Roy's adaptation theory (Roy & Andrews, 1991), Leininger's culture care diversity and universality theory (1996), King's goal attainment theory (1997), and Parse's theory of human becoming (1997). Each of these grand theories addresses phenomena of concern to nursing from a different perspective. For example, Rogers viewed the person and the environment as energy fields coextensive with the universe. As a result, she recognized person–environment unity as a mutual process. In contrast, King distinguished the personal system from the interpersonal and social systems, focusing on the interaction among systems and the interaction of the systems with the environment. For King, person and environment interact as separate entities, which is different from the person–environment mutual process described by Rogers.

If a researcher uses Rogers's theory to guide plans for a study, the research question will reflect values different from those if the researcher had used King's theory. The researcher using Rogers's theory might study the relationship of therapeutic touch to other phenomena that reflect the importance of energy fields and pattern appreciation, whereas the researcher using King's theory might study outcomes related to the shared goals of nurses and clients or other phenomena related to interacting systems. Note that one grand theory is not necessarily better than another. Rather, these varying perspectives allow the nurse researcher to select a framework for research that facilitates movement of concepts of interest down the ladder of abstraction to the empirical level, where they can be measured as study variables. What is most important about the use of theoretical frameworks for research is the logical connection of the theory to the research question and the study design.

Midrange Theory. **Midrange theory** is a focused conceptual structure that synthesizes practice–research (i.e., the link between practice and research) into ideas central to the discipline of nursing. According to Merton (1968), the original source for much of the description of midrange theory, midrange theories lie between everyday working hypotheses and all-inclusive grand theories. Merton's view of the "middle" allows for a great deal of space between grand theories and hypotheses. Efforts have been made to more clearly articulate the middle and to distinguish the characteristics of midrange theory. For example, in a 10-year review of nursing literature using specific criteria, Liehr and Smith (1999) identified 22 midrange theories. Following the suggestion of Lenz (1996), they considered the scope of the 22 midrange theories and grouped them into high-middle, middle-middle, and low-middle categories using the theory names (see Table 2–3). The groupings move from a higher to a lower level of abstraction. Because midrange theories are lower in level of abstraction than grand theories, they offer a more direct application to research and practice. In other words, as the level of abstraction decreases, translation into practice and research simplifies.

In their conclusion, Liehr and Smith recommended that nurses thoughtfully construct midrange theory, weaving practice and research threads to create a fabric that is meaningful for the discipline. In the text on advanced nursing practice by Hamric, Spross, and Hansen, Brown (2005) stated the following:

> Middle-range theories typically address a particular patient experience (e.g., living with rheumatoid arthritis) or problem (e.g., managing chronic pain); thus their range of applicability is relatively narrow. However, this narrow range of applicability allows them to be developed to address specific issues encountered in clinical practice. (p. 163)

Midrange theory can be developed in a number of ways, including the following (Peterson & Bredow, 2004):

1. Inductive theory, building theory through research
2. Deductive theory, building from grand nursing theories
3. Combining existing nursing and non-nursing theories
4. Synthesizing theories from published research findings
5. Developing theories from clinical practice guidelines

The theory of attentively embracing story, introduced on page 31, is a midrange theory. Generated from nursing practice and research experience (Smith & Liehr, 1999), the theory provides a structure for engaging clients to share what is important to them about a health challenge they are facing. Many of the midrange theories have evolved from inductive or qualitative research, such as the work of Ford-Gilboe, Wuest, and Merritt-Gray (2005), on how families limit intrusion via four subprocesses. You may also wish to consider Falk-Rafael's (2005) research combining theories from power, empowerment, and caring science, which led to the development of a midrange theory of critical theory for public health nursing practice. Midrange theories, such as those described above or in Table 2–3, can help nurses practice as these theories can provide the nurse with an understanding of a client's behaviour and recommend interventions to guide nursing practice.

Microrange Theory. **Microrange theory** (also known as microtheory or situation-specific theory) links concrete concepts into a statement that can be examined in practice and research. According to Meleis (2005), microrange theories "focus on specific nursing phenomena that reflect clinical practice and are limited to specific populations or to a particular field of practice" (p. 18). Narrow in scope, microrange theories produce specific directions for practice. Higgins and Moore (2000) distinguished two levels of microrange theory, one at a higher level of abstraction than the other. They suggested that

TABLE 2–3 Midrange Theory by Level of Abstraction		
High-Middle	**Middle-Middle**	**Low-Middle**
Caring	Uncertainty in illness	Hazardous secrets and reluctantly taking charge
Facilitating growth and development	Unpleasant symptoms	Affiliated individuation as a mediator of stress
Interpersonal perceptual awareness	Chronic sorrow	Women's anger
Self-transcendence	Peaceful end of life	Nurse–midwife care
Resilience	Negotiating partnerships	Balance between analgesia and side effects
Psychological adaptation	Cultural brokering	Homelessness–helplessness
	Nurse-expressed empathy and client distress	Individualized music intervention for agitation

Adapted from Liehr, P., & Smith, M. J. (1999). Middle range theory: Spinning research and practice to create knowledge for the new millennium. *Advanced Nursing Science, 21*(4), 81–91.

microrange theories at the higher level of abstraction are closely related to midrange theories, composed of a limited number of concepts, and applicable to a narrow issue or event. The low-middle theory in Table 2–3 may fit this category. Hypotheses are an example of low-abstraction microrange theories. Readers will recall that a hypothesis is a best guess or prediction about what one expects to find. Chinn and Kramer (1999) defined a **hypothesis** as a "tentative statement of relationship between two or more variables that can be empirically tested." Higgins and Moore (2000) also emphasized the value of microrange theory allowing researchers to describe, organize, and test their ideas.

As you read this text, you will learn how to articulate a microrange theory at the level of a hypothesis, just as Kate formulated a hypothesis about the relationship between client–health care provider interaction and BP. Although Kate did not label her idea as a hypothesis, it was a best guess based on observation. Take a minute to recall an experience from nursing practice that has provoked confusion, and state it as a hypothesis. A mismatch between what is known or commonly accepted as fact and what we experience creates a hypothesis-generating moment. Every nurse experiences such moments. Cultivating hypothesis-generating moments requires noticing them, focusing one's observation on specific details and the relationships between them, and allowing time for creative thinking and dialogue (Liehr, 1992), leading to possibilities for creating a low-level microrange theory or hypothesis.

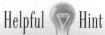

Helpful Hint

The reader of research will find conflicting views regarding levels and placement of theory. Whereas one author will label a particular theory "grand," another author will label the same theory "midrange." The reader can evaluate the theory and assign it a level on the ladder of abstraction. If a theory is at the more concrete level on the ladder, then it falls into microrange theory.

FRAMEWORKS FOR RESEARCH

The Critical Thinking Decision Path on page 39 takes readers through the thinking of a researcher who is about to begin conducting research. Readers can expect to find some, but not all, of the phases of decision making addressed in a research publication. Beginning with the worldview, the highest rung on the ladder of abstraction, the researcher is inclined to approach a research problem from the perspective of inductive or deductive reasoning. Researchers who pursue an inductive reasoning approach generally will not present a framework before beginning the discussion of methods. This is not to say that the literature will not be reviewed prior to introducing the methods. For example, Bottorff, Johnson, Moffat, Grewal, Ratner, and Kalaw (2004) (see Appendix D) were interested in understanding how adolescents view cigarette addiction because an understanding of how adolescents view smoking and addiction can lead to more effective smoking prevention and cessation programs. So, the point of the literature review is to build a case for doing the research. Researchers do not provide a framework for the study because they are planning an inductive approach to study the problem.

Conversely, researchers who use deductive reasoning must choose between a conceptual or a theoretical framework. In the theory literature, these terms are used interchangeably (Chinn & Kramer, 1999). However, in the case presented in the Critical Thinking Decision Path, each term is distinguished from the other on the basis of whether the researcher is creating the structure or whether the structure has already been created by someone else. Generally, each of these terms refers to a structure that will provide guidance for research. A **conceptual framework** is a structure of concepts, theories, or both pulled together as a map for the study. A **theoretical framework** provides structure for concepts that exist in the literature, a ready-made map for the study.

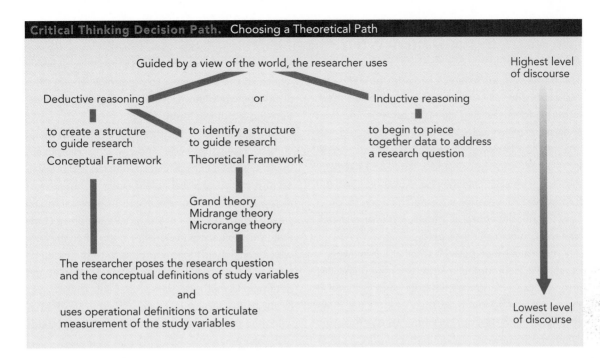

Critical Thinking Decision Path. Choosing a Theoretical Path

Guided by a view of the world, the researcher uses

Highest level of discourse

Deductive reasoning   or   Inductive reasoning

to create a structure to guide research

to identify a structure to guide research

to begin to piece together data to address a research question

Conceptual Framework   Theoretical Framework

Grand theory
Midrange theory
Microrange theory

The researcher poses the research question and the conceptual definitions of study variables

and

uses operational definitions to articulate measurement of the study variables

Lowest level of discourse

To understand these differences, see the study by Forchuk, Martin, Chan, and Jensen (2005) in Appendix A. The authors created a conceptual framework for their study that incorporated a transitional discharge model and identified several variables related to quality of life. In contrast, McCormick, Naimark, and Tate (2002) used a theoretical framework to guide their research: Mishel's Middle-Range Nursing Theory of Uncertainty in Illness, which posits that the appraisal of symptoms may lead to illness uncertainty. The authors examined the symptoms' experience of clients waiting for cardiac bypass surgery. Instead of creating a structure, these authors used a theoretical framework that already existed in the literature.

From the perspective of the Critical Thinking Decision Path, theoretical frameworks can incorporate grand, midrange, or microrange theories. Whether the researcher is using a conceptual or a theoretical framework, conceptual and then operational definitions will emerge from the framework. The decision path moves down the ladder of abstraction from the philosophical to the empirical level, tracking thinking from the most abstract to the least abstract for the purposes of planning a research study and accruing evidence to guide nursing practice and research.

As shown in the Critical Thinking Decision Path, theoretical frameworks can incorporate grand, midrange, or microrange theories. Whether the researcher uses a conceptual or theoretical framework, conceptual and then operational definitions will emerge from the framework. The decision path moves down the ladder of abstraction from the philosophical to the empirical level, tracking thinking from the most abstract to the least abstract for the purpose of planning a research study.

Helpful 💡 Hint

When researchers have used conceptual frameworks to guide their studies, you can expect to find a system of ideas, synthesized for the purpose of organizing thinking and providing study direction.

Critiquing the Framework

The framework for research provides guidance for the researcher as study questions are fine-tuned, methods for measuring variables are selected, and analyses are planned. Once data are collected and analyzed, the framework is used as a basis for comparison. Did the findings coincide with the framework? If discrepancies exist, can they be explained using the framework? The reader of research needs to know how to critically appraise a framework for research (see the Critiquing Criteria box).

The first question posed is whether a framework is presented. Sometimes, a structure may guide the research, but a diagrammed model is not included in the report. The reader must then look for the study structure in the description of the study concepts. When the framework is identified, consider its relevance for nursing. A nurse does not have to create the framework, but the importance of the study's content for nursing should be clear. The question of how the framework depicts a structure congruent with nursing should be addressed. Sometimes, frameworks from very different disciplines, such as physics or art, may be relevant to nursing. The author must clearly articulate the meaning of the framework for the study and link the framework to nursing.

Once the meaning and relationship to nursing are articulated, the reader will be able to determine whether the framework is appropriate to guide the research. For instance, a blatant mismatch occurs if a researcher is studying students' responses to the stress of being in the clinical setting for the first time but presents a framework of stress related to recovery from chronic illness. Such obvious mismatches do not generally arise; however, subtle versions of mismatch do occur. So, the reader needs to look closely at the framework to determine whether it is appropriate and the "best fit" for the research question and proposed study design.

Next, the reader focuses on the concepts being studied. Does the reader know which concepts are being studied and how they are defined and translated into measurable variables? Does literature exist to support the choice of concepts? Concepts should clearly reflect the area of study; for example, a study that uses the general concept of stress when the concept of anxiety is more appropriate to the research focus will lead to difficulties in defining variables and determining methods of measurement. These issues relate to the logical consistency within the framework, the concepts being studied, and the methods of measurement.

Throughout the entire critiquing process, from worldview to operational definitions, the reader is evaluating whether the theoretical framework is appropriate. Finally, the reader will expect to find a discussion of the findings as they relate to the model. This final point enables readers to evaluate the framework for use in further research. The point may suggest necessary changes to enhance the relevance of the framework for continuing study and thus sets future research direction.

Evaluating frameworks for research requires skill that can be acquired only through repeated critique and discussion with others who have critiqued the same publication. The novice reader of research must be patient while these skills are developed. With continuing education and a broader knowledge of potential frameworks, nursing students will build a repertoire of knowledge to enable them to judge the foundation of a research study, the framework for research.

CRITIQUING CRITERIA

1. Is the framework for research clearly identified?

2. Is the framework consistent with a nursing perspective?

3. Is the framework appropriate to guide research on the subject of interest?

4. Are the concepts and variables clearly and appropriately defined?

5. Did the study present sufficient literature to support the selected concepts?

6. Is there a logical, consistent link between the framework, the concepts being studied, and the methods of measurement?

7. Are the study findings examined in relation to the framework?

Critical Thinking Challenges

- Explain the difference between research that uses a constructivist paradigm and research that uses a positivist paradigm as the basis of a study.

- Discuss how a researcher's values could influence the results of a study. Include an example in your answer.

- You are taking an elective course in advanced pathophysiology. The professor compares the knowledge of various disciplines and states that nursing is an example of a nonscientific discipline, declaring in support of this position that nursing's knowledge has been generated with unstructured methods, such as intuition, trial and error, tradition, and authority. What assumptions has this professor made? Would you defend or support this position?

- Nurse researchers claim that a theoretical framework is essential for systematically identifying the relationship among the chosen variables. If this is true, why do non-nursing research studies not identify theoretical frameworks?

- As a consumer of research, how would you use computer databases to verify tools for measuring operational definitions?

- How would you argue against the following statement: "As a beginning consumer of research, it is ridiculous to expect me to determine whether a researcher's study has an appropriate theoretical framework; I've only had Nursing Theory 101."

- Is it possible for a research study's theoretical framework and variables to be the same?

KEY POINTS

- The scientific approaches used to generate nursing knowledge reflect both inductive and deductive reasoning.

- The interaction among theory, practice, and research is central to knowledge development in the discipline of nursing.

- Conceptual frameworks are created by the researcher, whereas theoretical frameworks are identified in the literature.

- The use of a framework for research is important as a guide to systematically identify concepts and to link appropriate study variables with each concept.

- Conceptual and operational definitions are critical to the evolution of a study, whether or not they are explicitly stated.

- In developing or selecting a framework for research, knowledge may be acquired from other disciplines or directly from nursing. In either case, that knowledge is used to answer specific nursing questions.

- Theory is distinguished by its scope. Grand theories are the broadest in scope and at the highest level of abstraction, whereas microrange theories are the most narrow in scope and at the lowest level of abstraction. Midrange theories are in the middle.

- Midrange theories are at a level of abstraction that enhances their usefulness for guiding practice and research.

- When critiquing a framework for research, examine the logical, consistent link between the framework, the concepts for study, and the methods of measurement.

REFERENCES

Bottorff, J. L., Johnson, J. L., Moffat, B., Grewal, J., Ratner, P., & Kalaw, C. (2004). Adolescent constructions of nicotine addiction. *Canadian Journal of Nursing Research, 38*, 22–39.

Brown, S. J. (2005). Direct clinical practice. In A. B. Hamric, J. A. Spross, & C. M. Hansen (Eds.), *Advanced nursing practice* (3rd ed., pp. 143–186). Philadelphia: W.B. Saunders.

Cameron, C. (2003). *The lived experience of transfer students in a collaborative baccalaureate nursing program.* Unpublished doctoral dissertation, University of Toronto.

Carper, B. A. (1978). Fundamental patterns of nursing. *Advanced Nursing Science, 1*, 13–24.

Chinn, P. L., & Kramer, M. K. (1999). *Theory and nursing: A systematic approach* (5th ed.). St. Louis, MO: Mosby.

Falk-Rafael, A. (2005). Advancing nursing theory through theory-guided practice: The emergence of a critical caring perspective. *Advances in Nursing Science, 28*, 38–49.

Fawcett, J. (2000). *Analysis and evaluation of contemporary nursing knowledge: Nursing models and theories.* Philadelphia: Davis.

Forchuk, C., Martin, M. L., Chan, Y. L., & Jensen, E. (2005). Therapeutic relationships: From psychiatric hospital to community. *Journal of Psychiatric and Mental Health Nursing, 12*, 556–564.

Ford-Gilboe, M., Campbell, J., & Berman, H. (1995). Stories and numbers: Coexistence without compromise. *Advances in Nursing Science, 18*, 14–26.

Ford-Gilboe, M., Wuest, J., & Merritt-Gray, M. (2005). Strengthening capacity to limit intrusion: Theorizing family health promotion in the aftermath of woman abuse. *Qualitative Health Research, 15*, 477–501.

Giddings, L. S., & Grant, B. M. (2007). A Trojan horse for positivism? A critique of mixed methods research. *Advances in Nursing Science, 30*, 52–60.

Hamric, A. B., Spross, J. A., & Hanson, C. M. (2005). *Advanced nursing practice* (3rd ed.). Philadelphia: W.B. Saunders.

Higgins, P. A., & Moore, S. M. (2000). Levels of theoretical thinking in nursing. *Nursing Outlook, 48*, 179–183.

Im, E., & Meleis, A. I. (1999). Situation-specific theories: Philosophical roots, properties and approach. *Advances in Nursing Science, 22*, 11–24.

Johnson, J., Fieler, V. K., Jones, L. S., Wlasowicz, G. S., & Mitchell, M. L. (1997). *Self-regulation theory: Applying theory to your practice.* Pittsburgh, PA: Oncology Nursing Press.

King, I. M. (1997). King's theory of goal attainment in practice. *Nursing Science Quarterly, 10*, 180–185.

Kuhn, T. (1962). *The structure of scientific revolutions.* Chicago: University of Chicago Press.

Leininger, M. M. (1996). Culture care theory. *Nursing Science Quarterly, 9*, 71–78.

Lenz, E. (1996). Middle range theory—role in research and practice. In *Proceedings of the Sixth Rosemary Ellis Scholar's Retreat: Nursing science implications for the 21st century.* Cleveland, OH: Frances Payne Bolton School of Nursing, Case Western Reserve University.

Liehr, P. (1992). Prelude to research. *Nursing Science Quarterly, 5*, 102–103.

Liehr, P., & Smith, M. J. (1999). Middle range theory: Spinning research and practice to create knowledge for the new millennium. *Advanced Nursing Science, 21*, 81–91.

Liehr, P., & Smith, M. J. (2000). Using story to guide nursing practice. *International Journal of Human Caring, 4*(2), 13–18.

Lincoln, Y., & Guba, E. (2000). Paradigmatic controversies, contradictions, and emerging confluences. In N. K. Denzin & Y. S. Lincoln (Eds.), *Handbook of qualitative research* (2nd ed., 163–188). Thousand Oaks, CA: Sage.

Locke, L. F., Spirduso, W. W., & Silverman, S. J. (1993). *Proposals that work: A plan for planning dissertations and grant proposals* (3rd ed.). Newbury Park, CA: Sage.

McCormick, K., Naimark, B., & Tate, R. (2002). Symptoms and distress in patients awaiting coronary artery bypass surgery. *Canadian Journal of Nursing Research, 34*, 95–105.

Meleis, A. I. (2005). *Theory: Who needs it . . . What is it?* In A. I. Meleis (Ed.), *Theoretical nursing: Development and progress* (3rd ed., 8–24). Philadelphia: Lippincott, Williams & Wilkins.

Merton, R. K. (1968). *Social theory and social structure.* New York: Free Press.

Newman, M. A. (1997). Evolution of the theory of health as expanding consciousness. *Nursing Science Quarterly, 10*(1), 22–25.

Olson, J. (2006). Understanding paradigms used for nursing research. *Journal of Advanced Nursing, 53*, 459–469.

Orem, D. E. (1995). *Nursing: Concepts of practice* (5th ed.). St. Louis, MO: Mosby.

Oxford University Press. (2004).Oxford English dictionary (online). Retrieved September 3, 2004, from http://dictionary.oed.com

Parse, R. R. (1997). Transforming research and practice with the human becoming theory. *Nursing Science Quarterly, 10*, 171–174.

Pearlin, L. I. (2002). Some conceptual perspectives on the origins and prevention of social stress. In A. Maney & J. Ramos (Eds.), *Socioeconomic conditions, stress and mental disorders: Towards a new synthesis of public policy* (pp. 1–35). Bethesda, MD: NIH Office of Behavioural and Social Research. Retrieved May 2, 2002, from http://www.mhsip.org/pdfs/pearlin.pdf

Peterson, S., & Bredow, T. (2004). *Middle range theories: Application to nursing research.* Philadelphia: Lippincott.

Rogers, M. E. (1990). Nursing: Science of unitary, irreducible human beings: Update 1990. In E. Barrett (Ed.), *Visions of Rogers' science-based nursing.* New York: National League for Nursing.

Rogers, M. E. (1992). Nightingale's notes on nursing: Prelude to the 21st century. In M. E. Rogers (Ed.), *Notes on nursing: What it is and what it is not* (Commemorative ed.). Philadelphia: Lippincott.

Roy, C., & Andrews, H. A. (1991). *The Roy adaptation model: The definitive statement.* Norwalk, CT: Appleton & Lange.

Samuels-Dennis, J. (2006). Relationship among employment status, stressful life events, and depression in single mother. *Canadian Journal of Nursing Research, 38,* 58–80.

Smith, D., Edwards, N., Varcoe, C., Martens, P. J., & Davies, B. (2006). Bringing safety and responsiveness into the forefront of care for pregnant and parenting aboriginal people. *Advances in Nursing Science, 29*(2), E27–E44.

Smith, M. J., & Liehr, P. (1999). Attentively embracing story: A middle range theory with practice and research implications. *Scholarly Inquiry for Nursing Practice, 13*(3), 3–27.

Smith, M. J., & Liehr, P. (2003). *Middle range theory for nursing.* New York: Springer.

Speziale, H., & Carpenter, D. (2007). *Qualitative research in nursing: Advancing the humanistic imperative.* Toronto: Lippincott

Tashakkori, A., & Creswell, J. W. (2007). Editorial: The new era of mixed methods. *Journal of Mixed Methods Research, 1*(1), 3–7.

Teddlie, C., & Tashakkori, A. (2003). Major issues and controversies in the use of mixed methods in the social and behavioral sciences. In A. Tashakkori & C. Teddlie (Eds.), *Handbook of mixed methods in social & behavioral research* (pp. 3–50). Thousand Oaks, CA: Sage.

Geri LoBiondo-Wood

Judith Haber

Barbara Krainovich-Miller

Cherylyn Cameron

CHAPTER 3

Critical Reading Strategies:

Overview of the Research Process

LEARNING OUTCOMES

After reading this chapter, the student should be able to do the following:

- Identify the steps that researchers use to conduct quantitative and qualitative research.
- Identify the importance of critical thinking and critical reading for the reading of research articles.
- Identify the steps associated with critical reading.
- Use the steps of critical reading to review research articles.
- Use identified strategies to critically read research articles.
- Use identified critical thinking and critical reading strategies to synthesize critiqued articles.
- Identify the format and style of research articles.

KEY TERMS

54 abstract

49 analysis

assumptions 47

critical reading 47

critical thinking 45

critique 50

50 critiquing criteria

54 qualitative research

54 quantitative research

STUDY RESOURCES

evolve Go to Evolve at
http://evolve.elsevier.com/Canada/LoBiondo/Research/
for Weblinks, content updates, and additional research articles for practice in reviewing and critiquing.

As you read this text, you will learn how the steps of the research process unfold. The steps are systematic and orderly and relate to the development of nursing knowledge. Understanding the step-by-step process that researchers use will help you to develop the critiquing skills necessary to judge the soundness of research studies. Throughout the chapters, research terms pertinent to each step are identified and illustrated with many examples from the research literature. Four published research studies are featured in the appendices and used as examples to illustrate significant points in each chapter. Judging not only the study's soundness but also a study's applicability to practice is key.

Before you can judge a study, you need to understand the differences between and among studies. As you read the chapters and the appendices, you will encounter many different study designs, as well as standards for critiquing the soundness of each step of a study and for judging both the strength of evidence provided by a study and its application to practice. The steps of the quantitative research process generally proceed in the order outlined in Table 3–1. Table 3–2 outlines the highlights of the general steps associated with qualitative research. Remember that a researcher may vary the steps slightly, depending on the nature of the research problem, but all of the steps should be addressed systematically.

This chapter provides an overview of critical thinking, critical reading, and critiquing skills. The chapter also introduces the overall format of a research article and provides an overview of subsequent chapters in the book. These components of the chapter are designed to help you read research articles more effectively and with greater understanding. You will learn about the research process so that you will be able to practise from a base of evidence to improve client outcomes.

CRITICAL THINKING AND CRITICAL READING SKILLS

As you read a research article, you may be struck by the difference in style or format between a research article and a theoretical or clinical article. With respect to the former, the terms may be new to the reader, and the focus of the content is different. You may also think that the research article is too difficult for you to understand or that it is too technical or boring. You may simultaneously wonder, "How will I possibly learn to evaluate (critique) all of the steps of a research study, as well as all the terminology? I'm only on Chapter 3. This is not easy; research is as hard as everyone says."

Try to reframe these thoughts with a "glass is half full" approach. In other words, tell yourself, "Yes, I can learn how to read and critique research, and this chapter will provide the strategies for me to learn this skill." Remember that learning occurs with time and help. Reading research articles can be difficult and frustrating at first, but the best way to become a knowledgeable consumer of research is to use critical thinking and critical reading skills when you read research articles. As a student, you are not expected to completely understand a research article. It is also understood that you will find it challenging to critique research articles until you gain repeated experience doing so. Nor are you expected to develop critiquing skills on your own. An essential objective of this book is to help you acquire critical thinking and critical reading skills. No perfect critique exists; your interpretation will be based on your current knowledge, experience, and understanding. Remember that becoming a competent critical thinker and consumer of research, like learning the steps of the research process, takes time, patience, and experience.

Critical thinking is the rational examination of ideas, inferences, assumptions, principles, arguments, conclusions, issues, statements, beliefs, and actions (Elder & Paul, 2004). As a critical thinker, you are therefore engaged in the following:

- Disciplined, self-directed thinking that exemplifies the perfection of thinking appropriate to a specific domain of thinking (research)
- Thinking that displays a mastery of intellectual skills and abilities (use of criteria for critiquing research)

TABLE 3–1 Steps of the Research Process and Journal Format—Quantitative Research

Research Process Steps and/or Format Issues	Usual Location in a Journal Heading or Subheading	Text Chapter
Research problem	In the abstract and/or the introduction (not labelled) or in a separate section labelled "Problem"	4
Purpose	In the abstract and/or the introduction or at the end of the literature review or theoretical framework section, or labelled with a separate heading, "Purpose"	4
Literature review	At the end of the heading "Introduction," but not labelled as such, or labelled as a separate heading, "Literature Review," "Review of the Literature," or "Related Literature," or not labelled, but the variables reviewed appear as headings or subheadings	5
Theoretical framework (TF) or conceptual framework (CT)	Combined with "Literature Review" or found in a separate heading. Each concept or definition used in the TF or CF may appear as a separate heading or subheading	2, 5
Hypothesis/research	Can be found as a statement or implied near the end of the introductory section. Sometimes may be labelled or found in a separate heading or subheading, such as "Hypothesis" or "Research Questions," or reported for the first time in the "Results" section	4
Research design	Stated or implied in the abstract or introduction or under the heading "Methods"	2, 7, 8, 9, 10, 11
Sample: size and type	"Size" may be stated in the abstract, in the Methods section, or as a separate subheading under the Methods section as "Sample," "Sample/Subjects," or "Participants" "Type" may be implied or stated in any of the previous headings or described under "Size"	12
Legal–ethical issues	Stated or implied in headings labelled "Methods," "Procedures," "Sample," or "Subjects"	6
Instruments (measurement tools)	Found in headings labelled "Methods," "Instruments," or "Measures"	13
Validity and reliability	Specifically stated or implied in headings labelled "Methods," "Instruments," "Measures," or "Procedures"	14
Data collection	Stated in the Methods section under the subheading "Procedure" or "Data Collection" or under a separate heading, "Procedure"	13
Data analysis	Stated in the Methods section under the subheading "Procedure" or "Data Analysis"	15, 16
Results	Stated in a separate heading, "Results"	15, 16, 17
Discussion of findings	Combined with results or as a separate heading, "Discussion"	17
Implications, limitations, and recommendations	Combined in the Discussion or presented as separate or combined major headings	17
References	At the end of the article	2, 4
Communicating research	Research articles, poster and paper presentation results	1, 2, 20

- The art of thinking about your thinking while thinking, to make your thinking better—more clear, more accurate, or more defensible (clarifying what you do understand and what you do not know)

In other words, being a critical thinker means that you are consciously thinking about your own thoughts and what you say, write, read, or do, as well as what others say, write, or do. Simultaneously, you are questioning the appropriateness of the content, applying standards or criteria, and evaluating the arguments or overall position of the author.

Developing the ability to evaluate research critically requires both critical thinking skills and

TABLE 3–2 Steps of the Research Process and Journal Format—Qualitative Research*

Research Process Steps and/or Format Issues	Usual Location in a Journal Heading or Subheading
Identifying the phenomenon	In the abstract or the introduction, or both
Research question and study purpose	In the abstract or at the beginning or end of the introduction, or both
Literature	In the abstract, introduction, or discussion, or two or all of these sections
Design	In the abstract or the introductory section, or both, or in the method section, entitled "Design"
Sample	In the method section, labelled "Sample" or "Subjects"
Legal–ethical issues	In the data collection, procedures, or sample section
Data collection procedure	In the data collection or procedures section
Data analysis	In the methods section under the subheading "Data Analysis" or "Data Analysis and Interpretation"
Results	Stated in a separate heading: "Results" or "Findings"
Discussion and recommendation	Combined in a separate section: "Discussion" or "Discussion and Implications"
References	At the end of the article

*See Chapters 7 and 8.

critical reading skills. **Critical reading** is "an active, intellectually engaging process in which the reader participates in an inner dialogue with the writer. Most people read uncritically and so miss some part of what is expressed while distorting other parts" (Paul & Elder, 2002). Critical readers enter into a point of view other than their own: the point of view of the writer. To interpret and assess a text accurately, critical readers actively look for **assumptions** or accepted truths, key concepts and ideas, reasons and justifications, supporting examples, parallel experiences, implications and consequences, and any other structural features (Paul & Elder, 2003). Actively looking for assumptions means examining supposedly true or accepted statements that are actually unsupported by research or scientific evidence.

Critical thinking and critical reading skills can be further developed by learning the research process. You will find that critical thinking and critical reading skills used in the nursing process can be transferred to understanding the research process and reading research articles. You will gradually be able to read an entire research article and reflect on it by identifying and challenging assumptions, identifying key concepts, questioning methods, and determining whether the conclusions are based on

the study's findings. Once you have obtained this competency in critiquing research, you will be ready to synthesize the findings of multiple research studies to use in developing evidence-based practice.

PROCESS OF CRITICAL READING

To read a research study critically, you must have reading and writing skills and reasoning ability. A research study commonly requires several readings. A minimum of three or four readings—or even as many as six—is common. Keep your research textbook at your side as you read. Using this book while you read a study may be helpful for you to do the following:

- Identify concepts
- Clarify unfamiliar concepts or terms
- Question assumptions and the study's rationale
- Determine supporting evidence

Critical reading can be viewed as a process that involves various levels or stages of understanding, including the following:

- Preliminary understanding
- Comprehensive understanding
- Analysis understanding
- Synthesis understanding

Preliminary Understanding: Familiarity (Skimming)

Preliminary understanding is gained by scanning or skimming an article to become familiar with its content or to get a general sense of the material. During the preliminary reading, the title and abstract are read closely, but the content is skimmed The title endeavours to signal to readers the main purpose of the study. The **abstract** is a brief overview of a study that outlines the main components of the study. Skimming includes reading the introduction, major headings, one or two sentences under a heading, and the summary or conclusion of the study.

Box 3–1 outlines the reading strategies associated with preliminary reading. Using these strategies will enable you to identify the main theme or idea of the article and bring this knowledge to the second comprehensive reading. Complete each of the strategies for critical reading as you read the articles that appear in the appendices.

BOX 3–1   Highlights of Critical Reading Process Strategies

Make notations directly on the copy (i.e., on a photocopy or an e-copy of the book).

STRATEGIES FOR PRELIMINARY UNDERSTANDING

- Keep a research text and a dictionary by your side.
- Review the chapters in the text on various steps of the research process, critiquing criteria, unfamiliar terms, etc.
- Highlight or underline new terms, unfamiliar vocabulary, and significant sentences.
- Look up the definitions of new terms and write down the definitions.
- Review old and new terms before subsequent readings.
- Highlight or underline identified steps of the research process.

STRATEGIES FOR COMPREHENSIVE UNDERSTANDING

- Before critiquing the article, make sure you understand the main points of each reported step of the research process.
- Identify the main idea or theme of the article; state it in your own words in one or two sentences.
- Continue to clarify terms that may be unclear on subsequent readings.

STRATEGIES FOR ANALYSIS UNDERSTANDING

- Using the critiquing criteria, determine how well the study meets the criteria for each step of the research process.
- Determine which level of evidence fits the study.
- Write down cues (or keywords), relationships of concepts, and questions.
- Ask fellow students to analyze the same study using the same criteria and then compare the results.
- Consult faculty members about your evaluation of the study.

STRATEGIES FOR SYNTHESIS UNDERSTANDING

- Review your notes on the article and determine how each step discussed in the article compares with the critiquing criteria.
- In your own words, write a one-page summary of the reviewed study.
- Cite article references at the top according to American Psychological Association (APA) or another reference style.
- Using the critiquing criteria, briefly summarize each reported research step in your own words.
- Briefly describe the study's strengths and weaknesses in your own words.

Comprehensive Understanding: Content in Relation to Context

The main purpose of reading a research study is to understand the intent of the researcher(s), the methods used, and the findings. Perhaps you have been assigned to read a research article on a topic you were interested in but found it difficult to understand how the researcher conducted the study or the meaning of the findings. This difficulty may have occurred because you could not read at that comprehension level (i.e., you may not have understood the terms the researcher used and therefore could not understand the terms in relation to the study's context or even whether the terms were used appropriately). For example, when reading the qualitative study by Smith, Edwards, Varcoe, Martens, and Davies (2006) (see Appendix B) for comprehension, you must understand that the purpose of participatory research is to acknowledge different value systems and beliefs and to generate knowledge with and for stakeholders. Participatory research is also useful for solving practical problems. So, for the Smith et al. article, rather than merely focusing on the experiences of health care among Aboriginal people, you would also comprehend the impact of colonial and postcolonial practices on the health experiences of pregnant and parenting Aboriginal people.

When reading for comprehension, keep your research text and a dictionary nearby. Although some terms may seem clear during the preliminary reading, they may become unclear upon a second reading. Do not hesitate to write cues or keywords on your copy of the article. If the article still does not make sense after the second reading, ask for assistance from faculty before reading it again. The content that you have highlighted and not highlighted, as well as the comments on the copy, may help a faculty member understand your difficulty. Further reading on the topic may be necessary for you to comprehend the article. For example, if you are unfamiliar with Martha Rogers's *science of unitary human beings* (Rogers, 1990), reading a study and testing a proposition of the model in it may be difficult.

Helpful Hint

If you still have difficulty understanding a research study after using the strategies related to skimming and comprehensive reading, make another copy of your marked-up research article, include your specific questions or area of difficulty, and ask your professor for assistance.

Comprehensive understanding is necessary to analyze and synthesize the material. Understanding the author's perspective for the study reflects critical thinking (Paul & Elder, 2002) and facilitates analysis of the study according to established criteria. Subsequent readings will allow for analysis and synthesis of the study.

Analysis Understanding: Breaking the Content into Parts

The purpose of reading for **analysis** is to break the content into parts to understand each aspect of the study. Some of the questions that you can ask yourself as you begin to analyze the research article are as follows:

- Am I confident that I know the specific type of design so that I apply the appropriate criteria when critiquing the study?
- Did I capture the main idea or theme of the article in one or two sentences?
- How are the major parts of the article organized in relation to the research process?
- What is the purpose of the article?
- How was the study carried out? Can I explain it step by step?
- What are the main conclusions of the author(s)?
- Do I understand the parts of the article, and can I summarize each section in my own words?

In a sense, you are determining how the steps of the research process are presented or organized in the article and the content that is related to each step. At the same time, you are beginning to critique or evaluate the study by asking and answering the questions related to the research process used by the author(s). At this point of critical reading, you are ready to begin the critiquing process that will help determine the study's merit.

Helpful 💡 Hint

Remember that not all research articles include headings related to each step or component of the research process, but each step is presented at some point in the article.

The **critique** involves objectively and critically evaluating the content of a research report for scientific merit and application to practice, theory, and education. Although the reader strives to be as objective as possible, it is understood that all readers have their own perceptions, history, and knowledge. Readers should understand their own biases and acknowledge them as they review the research. Additionally, the critique requires some knowledge of the subject matter and knowledge of how to read critically and use critiquing criteria. Chapters 18 and 19 contain summarized examples of critiquing questions and examples of critiques for qualitative and quantitative studies, respectively.

Critiquing criteria are the standards, evaluation guides, or questions used to judge (critique) a product or behaviour. In analyzing the research report, the reader must evaluate each step of the research process and ask whether each explanation meets the criteria.

As a beginner, you are not expected to write a critique at the same level as an experienced researcher who critiques a colleague's work. Remember that when you write a critique, you should point out strengths and weaknesses. Developing critical reading skills at the comprehension level will enable you to complete a critique successfully. The critiquing strategies that facilitate the understanding gained by reading for analysis are listed in Box 3–1 on page 48.

Synthesis Understanding: Pulling the Parts Together

Synthesis is the pulling together or combining of parts into a whole. The purpose of reading for synthesis is to pull all of the information together to form a new whole, make sense of it, and explain relationships between the bits of information. Although the process of synthesizing the material may take place as the reader analyzes the article, a fourth reading is recommended. During this synthesis reading, the understanding and critique of the whole study are put together. In this final step, the reader decides how well the study meets the critiquing criteria and how useful the research findings are to practice. The reader can also decide how well each step of the research process relates to the previous step.

Synthesis can be thought of as looking at a completed jigsaw puzzle. Does a comprehensive picture form, or is a piece out of place? Reading for synthesis is essential in critiquing research studies. For example, once you have answered the critiquing questions in Box 3–1 after reading for synthesis in relation to the Bottorff, Johnson, Moffat, Grewal, Ratner, and Kalaw (2004) study (see Appendix D), you might add the following to your critique:

The authors clearly indicated that although most smokers start smoking in adolescence, little is known about how teenagers understand nicotine addiction. If this social process is more clearly understood, health promotion interventions may become more effective to address nicotine addiction among adolescents. This qualitative study was designed to gain in-depth accounts of adolescents' experience with tobacco, including personal experiences with smoking, observations of others' smoking behaviour, and adolescents' personal views on addiction. The researchers conducted 80 open-ended interviews with adolescents with a variety of smoking histories, as well as a focus group interview. After transcribing each of the interviews, the researchers entered data into NVivo to search for text that discussed explanations of dependence, addiction, loci of control over smoking, and experiences with quitting smoking. A detailed thematic analysis identified the adolescents' construction of nicotine addiction. Five constructions emerged, with some adolescents drawing from more than one, including nicotine addiction as (1) repeated use, (2) the body and the brain getting used to the nicotine, (3) personal weakness, (4) family influence, and (5) image. Overall, the researchers were struck by the adolescents' minimization of their own role in and the extent of nicotine addiction. The authors made several recommendations, including providing a scientific understanding of addiction.

A summary such as the one above can be the first draft of a final written critique. Writing a summary teaches brevity, facilitates easy retrieval of data to support the critiquing evaluation, and increases your ability to write a scholarly report. In addition, the ability to synthesize one study prepares you for the task of critiquing several studies on a similar topic and comparing the findings.

Helpful Hint

If you are assigned to write a paper on a specific concept or topic that requires you to critique and synthesize the findings from several studies, you might find it useful to create a table of the data. Include the following information: author, date, type of study, design, sample, data analysis, findings, and implications.

Perceived Difficulties and Strategies for Critiquing Research

The best way to become an intelligent consumer of research is to use critical thinking and critical reading skills (see Box 3–1). Read the entire article and reflect on it. Most importantly, draw on previous knowledge, common sense, and the critical thinking skills you already possess.

Another important strategy is to ask questions—remember that questioning is essential to developing critical thinking. Asking faculty members questions and sharing your thoughts about what you are reading are effective ways to develop your reading skills. Do not hesitate to write or call a researcher if you have a question about his or her work. You will be pleasantly surprised by the willingness of researchers to respond to your questions.

Throughout this book, you will find special features that will help refine the critical thinking and critical reading skills essential to developing your competence as a consumer of research. The Critical Thinking Decision Paths related to each step of the research process will sharpen decision-making skills for critiquing research articles. Internet resources (identified by computer icons in the margin) will enhance research consumer activities. Critical Thinking Challenges, which appear at the end of each chapter in this book, are designed to reinforce critical thinking and critical reading skills in relation to the steps of the research process. Helpful Hints, designed to reinforce understanding and critical thinking, appear at various points throughout the chapters, and Evidence-Based Practice Tips will help you apply evidence-based practice strategies to your clinical practice.

When you complete your first critique, congratulate yourself: mastering these skills is not easy at the beginning, but we are confident that you can do it. Once you complete a research critique or two, you will be ready to discuss your critique with your fellow students and professor. Best of all, you can look forward to discussing the points of your critique because it will be based on objective data, not just personal opinion. As you continue to use and perfect critical analysis skills by critiquing studies, remember that these skills are an expected clinical competency for delivering evidence-based nursing care.

LEVELS OF EVIDENCE

Along with gaining comfort while reading and critiquing research studies, a final step must be undertaken. The final step of reading and critiquing the research literature is deciding how, when, and whether to apply a study or studies to your practice so that your practice is evidence based. Evidence-based practice is the careful and judicious use of research literature in making client care decisions (Sackett, Straus, Richardson, Rosenburg, & Hayes, 2000). Evidence-based practice is the systematic use of the best available evidence and the integration of individual clinical expertise and the client's values and preferences into clinical decision making; however, in nursing, the complexities of practice (i.e., the fact that nurses cannot apply evidence without considering the whole) must also be considered. Some nursing scholars have proposed that in addition to research findings, and thus evidence-based practice, client choice and clinical judgement and experience are also important forms of evidence (Estabrooks, 1998; Rycroft-Malone, Seers, Tichen, Harvey, Kitson, & McCormack, 2004).

When using evidence-based practice strategies, the first step is to decide which level of evidence a research article provides. Table 3–3 illustrates a model for determining the levels of evidence (Melnyk & Fineout-Overholt, 2005) that are associated with the design of a study, ranging from systematic reviews of randomized controlled trials to expert opinions. This model represents a hierarchy for judging the strengths of a study's design, which, in turn, influences the confidence in the conclusions the researcher has drawn. Assessing the strength of scientific evidence provides a vehicle to guide nurses in evaluating research studies for their applicability to clinical decision making. Grading the strength of a body of evidence should incorporate three domains: quality, quantity, and consistency (Agency for Healthcare Research and Quality, 2002), which are defined as follows:

- Quality is the extent to which a study's design, implementation, and analysis minimize bias.
- Quantity refers to the number of studies that have evaluated the research question, including the overall sample size across studies and the strength of the findings from the data analyses.
- Consistency is the degree to which studies that have similar and different designs but investigate the same research question and report similar findings.

You will note from Table 3–3 that research evidence is traditionally categorized from weakest to strongest, with an emphasis on support for the effectiveness of interventions. The concept of levels of evidence tends to dominate the evidence-based practice literature rendering unclear the merit of qualitative studies. The previous chapter suggests that different research methods provide different types and levels of evidence, all of which inform practice. Although evidence provided by qualitative studies seems to rank lower in the hierarchy of evidence presented (that is, Levels V and VI), as

TABLE 3–3 **Levels of Evidence: Rating System for the Hierarchy of Evidence**	
Assessing Level of Evidence	**Source of Evidence**
Level I	Evidence from a systematic review or meta-analysis of all relevant randomized controlled trials (RCTs) or evidence-based clinical practice guidelines based on systematic reviews of RCTs
Level II	Evidence obtained from at least one well-designed RCT
Level III	Evidence obtained from well-designed controlled trials without randomization (e.g., quasiexperimental study)
Level IV	Evidence from nonexperimental studies (e.g., case-control and cohort studies)
Level V	Evidence from systematic reviews of descriptive and qualitative studies
Level VI	Evidence from a single descriptive or qualitative study
Level VII	Evidence from the opinion of authorities or reports of expert committees

Adapted from Melnyk, B. M., & Fineout-Overholt, E. (2005). Making the case for evidence-based practice. In B. M. Melnyk & E. Fineout-Overholt (Eds.), *Evidence-based practice in nursing and health care* (pp. 3–25). Philadelphia: Lippincott Williams & Wilkins.

a research consumer, you should consider that qualitative methods are the most effective way to attempt to answer clinical and research questions when little is known or when a new perspective is required.

Sandelowski (2004) noted that the use of hierarchies assumes that randomized clinical trials are the gold standard, thereby devaluing qualitative research. Yet, qualitative research has increased and thrived over the years. Thousands of reports of well-conducted qualitative studies exist on topics such as the following: (a) personal and cultural constructions of disease, prevention, treatment, and risk; (b) living with disease and managing the physical, psychological, and social effects of multiple diseases and their treatment; (c) decision-making experiences with beginning and end of life, as well as assistive and life-extending, technological interventions; and (d) contextual factors favouring and mitigating against quality care, health promotion, prevention of disease, and reduction of health disparities (Sandelowski, 2004). The answers provided by qualitative data reflect important evidence that may provide valuable insights about a particular phenomenon, client population, or clinical situation.

The meaningfulness of levels of evidence will become clearer in the remaining chapters of this text. For example, the Forchuk, Martin, Chan, and Jensen (2005) study in Appendix A falls into Level II because of its experimental design, whereas the Bottorff et al. (2004) study in Appendix D falls into Level VI because of its qualitative design. The **level of evidence** in and of itself does not indicate the full worth of a study but is another tool to help you think about the strengths and weaknesses of a study and the nature of the evidence provided in the findings and conclusions.

However, several nursing scholars are concerned that hierarchical rating of nursing research methodologies is problematic owing to an inherent bias against qualitative research methods. Promotion of one form of research over another can limit the development of multiple and diverse methodologies to explain the human experience and to guide

practice (Tarlier, 2005). Nonetheless, it is important to be familiar with levels of evidence because they are commonly referred to in practice. Although several different types of evidence hierarchy exist, this text refers to the level of evidence hierarchy presented in Table 3–3.

RESEARCH ARTICLES: Format and Style

Before you consider reading research articles, you need to have a sense of their organization and format. Many journals publish research articles, either as the sole type of article in the journal or in addition to clinical or theoretical articles. Although many journals have some common features, they also have unique characteristics. All journals have guidelines for manuscript preparation and submission, which are generally published in the journal or on the journal's Web site, if one is available. A review of these guides will give you an idea of the format of articles that appear in specific journals. Remember that even though each step of the research process is discussed at length in this text, you may find only a short paragraph or a sentence in the research article that gives the details of the step in a specific study. Because of the journal's space limitations or other publishing guidelines, the study published in a journal is a shortened version of the complete work done by the researcher(s). You will also find that some researchers devote more space in an article to the results, whereas others present a longer discussion of the methods and procedures. In recent years, most authors have given more emphasis to the method, results, and discussion of implications than to details of assumptions, hypotheses, or definitions of terms. Decisions about the amount of information to present on each step of the research process within an article are bound by the following:

- A journal's space limitations
- A journal's author guidelines
- The type or nature of the study
- An individual researcher's evaluation of the most important component of the study

The following discussion provides a brief overview of each step of the research process and how it might appear in an article. Refer to Table 3–1, which outlines where the steps can usually be located in a quantitative research article and where they are discussed in this text. Table 3–2 outlines the format of a qualitative research article. Remember that a quantitative research article differs from a qualitative research article. The primary difference is that **qualitative research** seeks to interpret meaning and phenomena, whereas **quantitative research** seeks to test a hypothesis or answer research questions based on a theoretical framework.

Abstract

An **abstract** is a short, comprehensive synopsis or summary of a study that appears at the beginning of an article and focuses the reader on the main points of the study. A well-presented abstract is accurate, self-contained, concise, specific, nonevaluative, coherent, and readable (APA, 2001). Abstracts can vary in length from 50 to 250 words; the journal's style dictates the length. Both quantitative and qualitative research studies feature abstracts. The following example of an abstract can be found at the beginning of the study by Samuels-Dennis (2006) (see Appendix C):

> The purpose of this study was to extend our understanding of employment status as a social determinant of psychological stress among single mothers. A cross-sectional survey assessing stressful life events and depression was completed with 96 single mothers . . . . The findings suggest that women's employment status significantly impacts on their psychological well-being. Implications for nursing practice, policy development, and future research are identified and discussed. (p. 59)

Within the first sentence of this example, the author provides a view of the study variables. The remainder of the abstract provides a synopsis of the methodology, the sample size, and the results. The studies in Appendices A, B, C, and D all feature abstracts. For ease of reading, some journals provide structured abstracts with the headings "Background," "Objectives," "Method," "Results," and "Conclusions."

Helpful Hint

A journal abstract is usually a single paragraph that provides a general reference to the research purpose, research questions, and hypotheses; highlights the methodology and results; and outlines implications for practice or future research.

Identification of a Research Purpose or Problem

Early in a research article, in a section that may or may not be labelled "Introduction," the researcher presents the research purpose or problem. In the study by Forchuk et al. (2005) (see Appendix A), the research problem appears early:

> The transition from hospital to community is complex and can be challenging for individual clients. A recent study of 85 long-term patients showed that 25% met the criterion for relocation trauma when moved from hospital to community. In order to successfully move the focus of care to the community, effective models of care are required. (p. 556)

In other studies, the authors do not state the problem clearly in a few short sentences but instead explain it over a number of paragraphs. The important component of the introduction is the description of the problem and the need for the study, within the context of a brief literature review and, in some cases, a theoretical framework.

Definition of the Purpose

The purpose of the study is defined either at the end of the abstract or initial introduction or at the end of the "Literature Review" or "Conceptual Framework" section. The study's purpose may or may not be labelled as such. For example, Bottoroff et al. (2004) (see Appendix D) clearly stated the purpose in the first sentence of the abstract: "The purpose of this qualitative study was to extend our understanding of how adolescents view nicotine addiction" (p. 22). Forchuk et al. (2005) (see Appendix A) and Samuels-Dennis (2006) (see Appendix C) also stated the purpose early in the abstract. In contrast, Smith et al. (2006) (see Appendix B) stated the purpose clearly in the first sentence of the third paragraph as follows: to "describe community-based stakeholders' perspectives on their experience improving care for pregnancy and parenting Aboriginal women and families" (p. E28).

Literature Review and Theoretical Framework

Authors of studies and journal articles present the literature review and theoretical framework in different ways. Many research articles merge the "Literature Review" and the "Theoretical Framework" into one section. This section includes the main concepts investigated and may be called "Review of the Literature," "Literature Review," "Theoretical Framework," "Related Literature," "Background," or "Conceptual Framework," or the section may not be labelled. In the studies that appear in Appendices B and C, the authors labelled the section on the literature and theoretical framework as "Background" and "Literature Review," respectively, whereas the authors of the studies that appear in Appendices A and D included their review in unlabelled introductory paragraphs. Note that one style is not regarded as better than another; all of the studies in the appendices contain the critical elements but present them differently.

Hypothesis, Research Problem, and Research Question

Authors can also present the study's hypothesis, research problem, and research question in different ways. Research reports in journals often do not feature separate headings for reporting the hypothesis or research problem, which are often embedded in the "Introduction" or "Background" section or not labelled at all (e.g., as in the studies that appear in the appendices). If a study uses hypotheses, the researcher may report whether the hypotheses were or were not supported toward the end of the article in the "Results" or "Findings" section. Quantitative research studies feature research problems, hypotheses, or research questions. For example, Forchuk et al. (2005) (see Appendix A) stated their hypothesis as follows:

> It was hypothesized that in the year following discharge from a psychiatric hospital, individuals participating in the [Transitional Discharge Model] would: (1) have an improved quality of life and (2) incur fewer health and social services costs compared with individuals receiving standard discharge care. (p. 558)

Qualitative research studies do not include hypotheses but instead include research questions and purposes. The articles by Smith et al. (2006) (see Appendix B) and Bottorff et al. (2004) (see Appendix D) have research purposes.

Research Design

The type of research design used in the study can be found in the abstract, in the purpose statement, in the introduction to the "Procedures" or "Methods" section, or not stated at all. For example, Forchuk et al. (2005) (see Appendix A) stated in the abstract that their study was a randomized clinical trial using a cluster design, whereas Smith et al. (2006) (see Appendix B) indicated that a postcolonial stance and participatory research perspectives shaped the study methods.

One of the first objectives when critically reading a study is to determine whether the research is qualitative or quantitative so that the appropriate criteria can be used. Although the rigour of the critiquing criteria addressed does not change substantially, some of the terminology of the questions differs for qualitative and quantitative studies. For example, with regard to Forchuk et al.'s study (2005) (see Appendix A), as a critical reader, you might be asking whether the hypotheses were generated from the theoretical framework or literature review and whether the design chosen was appropriate and consistent with the study's problem and purpose. However, with a qualitative study, such as Smith et al.'s (2006) (see Appendix B), you might be asking whether the researchers conducted the study consistent with the principles of participatory research and therefore focused on valuing all forms of knowledge and the useful practices to improve health care among Aboriginal pregnant and parenting families.

Do not get discouraged if you cannot easily determine the design. More often than not, authors do not state the specific design or, if an advanced design is used, do not spell out the details. One of the best strategies is to review the chapters in this text that address designs and ask your professors for assistance after you have read the chapters. Determining designs is not an easy process. The following tips will help you determine whether the study you are reading uses a quantitative design:

- The research problem demands measurement.
- Hypotheses are stated or implied.
- The terms *control* and *treatment group* appear.
- The term *survey*, *correlational*, or *ex post facto* is used.
- The term *random* or *convenience* is mentioned in relation to the sample.
- Variables are measured by instruments or scales.
- The reliability and validity of instruments are discussed.
- Statistical analysis is used.

In contrast, generally, qualitative studies do not usually focus on numbers; rather, they focus on rich descriptions of people's experiences and explanations of social processes (Miles & Huberman, 1994). Some qualitative studies may use standard quantitative terms (e.g., subjects) rather than qualitative terms (e.g., informants). Deciding on the type of qualitative design that was used can be difficult; one of the best strategies is to review this text's chapters on qualitative design and to critique qualitative studies. Do not hesitate to ask faculty members for assistance after you have read these chapters. Although many studies may not specify the particular design used, all studies inform readers of the specific methodology used, which can help determine the type of design used to guide the study.

Sampling

The population from which the sample was drawn is discussed in the methods section (entitled "Methods" or "Methodology") under the subheadings "Subjects" or "Sample." For example, Forchuk et al. (2005) (see Appendix A) discussed the sampling procedure of their quantitative sample in the "Methods" section under the subheadings "Sample Size Calculation" and "Sample and Data Collection," whereas Samuels-Dennis (2006) (see Appendix C) used the subheading "Participants." Although many researchers do not use subheadings to identify the sample, researchers should reveal both the population from which the sample was chosen and the number of subjects that participated in the study, as well as whether some subjects dropped out of the study. The authors of all of the studies that appear in the appendices discussed their samples in enough detail that it is clear who the subjects were and how they were selected.

Reliability and Validity

The discussion related to instruments used to measure the variables of a study is usually included in a "Methods" section under the subheading "Instruments" or "Measures." The researcher usually describes the particular measure (i.e., the instrument or scale) used by discussing its reliability and validity. Forchuk et al. (2005) (see Appendix A) discussed each of the instruments used in their study in the "Methods" section under the subheading "Instruments." The authors used several instruments, including those they developed. If the instrument was widely used, they included data on the internal consistency and reliability and prior use of each instrument from the literature.

In some cases, researchers do not report commonly used valid and reliable instruments in an article. Seek assistance from your instructor if you are in doubt about the validity or reliability of a study's instruments.

Procedures and Data Collection Methods

The procedures used to collect data or the step-by-step way that the researcher(s) used the measures (instruments or scales) is generally provided under the "Procedures" heading (see Chapter 14). In Samuel-Dennis's (2006) study (see Appendix C), the researcher indicated in detail how she conducted the study under the subheading "Data Collective." Other authors describe the procedure in the "Methods" section without a specific subheading. Generally, researchers also indicate that the studies were approved by a research ethics board, thereby ensuring that each study met ethical standards. Some researchers use this opportunity to describe in great detail the type of methodology used, particularly if it is under development, complex, or relatively new to research. For example, Smith et al. (2006) examined the use of postcolonial and participatory research methods (see Appendix B).

Data Analysis and Results

The data analysis procedures (i.e., the statistical tests used in quantitative studies and the results of descriptive and inferential tests applied) are presented in the section labelled "Results" or "Findings," although the data analysis method can be addressed in the "Methods" section and the results under "Results and Discussion," as in the Samuels-Dennis article (2006) (see Appendix C).

Because qualitative studies do not use statistical tests, the procedures for analyzing the themes, concepts, or observational or print data are usually described in the "Methods" or "Data Collection" section and reported in the "Results" or "Findings" section. Smith et al. (2006) reported the data analysis method in the "Methods" section of their qualitative study and reported their findings under "Results" (see Appendix B).

Discussion

The last section of a research study is the "Discussion" section. In this section, researchers tie together all of the pieces of the study and present a picture of the study as a whole. Researchers usually report the results and the discussion in separate sections (see Appendix A); however, some researchers may mix the results and discussion in one section (see Appendices C and D). Note that one method of presentation should not be regarded as better than the other, and journal and space limitations will determine how these sections will be handled. Any new or unexpected findings are usually described in the "Discussion" section.

Recommendations and Implications

In some cases, a researcher reports the implications, based on the findings, for practice and education and recommends future studies in a separate section labelled "Discussion and Implications" (see Appendix C). In other cases, the recommendations appear at the end of the "Discussion" section (see Appendices A, B, and D). Again, one method of presentation should not be regarded as better than the other.

References

All of the references cited in a research or scholarly article are included at the end of the article. The main purpose of the reference list is to support the material presented by identifying the sources in a manner that allows easy retrieval by the reader (APA, 2001). Journals use various referencing styles to organize references. This textbook, for instance, uses the style set out in the *Publication Manual of the American Psychological Association* (APA, 2001).

Communicating Study Results

Communicating the results of a study can take forms other than that of a research article, such as a poster or paper presentation at a conference. Publications and presentations are valid ways of providing the nursing profession with the data and the ability to provide appropriate client care that is based on research findings. Evidence-based nursing care plans and practice protocols, guidelines, or standards are other ways that research results are disseminated to nurses.

Critical Thinking Challenges

- The critical reading of research articles may require a minimum of three or four readings. Is this always the case? What assumptions underlie this claim?
- Why is it necessary to reach an analysis stage of critical reading before critiquing a study?
- To synthesize a research article, what questions must you first be able to answer?
- How would you answer a nursing colleague who stated the following: "Why can't I say in my critique that, based on the findings of this study, the researchers proved their hypotheses?"
- Margaret is a part-time baccalaureate nursing student who works full-time as a registered nurse in an intensive care unit and is a full-time mother of two children under the age of four years. Discuss both the disadvantages and the advantages of Margaret using the critical reading strategies found in Box 3–1.
- If nurses with a baccalaureate degree are not expected to conduct research, how can nursing students be expected to critique each step of the nursing process or an entire study or several studies? Support either a pro or a con position.
- Discuss several strategies that might motivate practising nurses to critically appraise research articles.
- What level of evidence is presented in each of the articles that appear in Appendices A, B, C, and D? Justify your answers.

KEY POINTS

- The best way to develop skills in critiquing research studies is to use critical thinking and critical reading skills.
- Critical thinking when learning the research process, as well as critiquing, requires disciplined, self-directed thinking.
- Critical thinking and critical reading skills enable you to question the appropriateness of the content of a research article, apply standards or critiquing criteria to assess the study's scientific merit for use in practice, and consider alternative ways of handling the same topic.
- Critical reading involves active interpretation and objective assessment of an article and looking for key concepts, ideas, and justifications.
- Critical reading requires four stages of understanding: preliminary (skimming), comprehensive, analysis, and synthesis. Each stage includes strategies to increase your critical reading skills.
- Critically reading for preliminary understanding is gained by skimming or quickly and lightly reading an article to familiarize yourself with its content and to provide you with a general sense of the material.
- Critically reading for a comprehensive understanding is designed to increase your understanding both of the concepts and research terms in relation to the context and of the parts of the study in relation to the whole study, as presented in the article.
- Critically reading for an analysis understanding is designed to break the content into parts so that each part of the study is understood. The critiquing process begins at this stage.
- Critical reading to reach the goal of synthesis understanding combines the parts of a research study into a whole. During this final stage, the reader determines how each step relates to all steps of the research process and how well the study meets the critiquing criteria and the usefulness of the study for practice.
- Critiquing is the process of objectively and critically evaluating the strengths and weaknesses of a research article for scientific merit and application to practice, theory, and education. The need for more research on the topic or clinical problem is also addressed at this stage.
- Each article should be reviewed for level of evidence as a means of judging the application to practice.
- Research articles have different formats and styles depending on journal manuscript requirements and whether they are quantitative or qualitative studies.

- The basic steps of the research process are presented in journal articles in various ways. Detailed examples of such variations can be found in chapters throughout this text.

- Evidence-based practice begins with the careful reading and understanding of research articles.

REFERENCES

Agency for Healthcare Research and Quality (2002). *Systems to rate the strength of scientific evidence* (File inventory, Evidence Report/Technology Assessment No. 47, AHRQ Publication No. 02-E016). Rockville, MD: Author.

American Psychological Association. (2001). *Publication manual of the American Psychological Association* (5th ed.). Washington, DC: Author.

Bottorff, J. L., Johnson, J. L., Moffat, B., Grewal, J., Ratner, P., & Kalaw, C. (2004). Adolescent constructions of nicotine addiction. *Canadian Journal of Nursing Research, 38,* 22–39.

Elder, L., & Paul, R. (2004). *The thinker's guide to the art of strategic thinking.* Dillon Beach, CA: Foundation for Critical Thinking.

Estabrooks, C. A. (1998). Will evidence-based nursing practice make practice perfect? *Canadian Journal of Nursing Research, 30,* 15–36.

Forchuk, C., Martin, M. L., Chan, Y. L., & Jensen, E. (2005). Therapeutic relationships: From psychiatric hospital to community. *Journal of Psychiatric and Mental Health Nursing, 12,* 556–564.

Melnyk, B. M., & Fineout-Overholt, E. (2005). Making the case for evidence-based practice. In B. M. Melnyk & E. Fineout-Overholt (Eds.), *Evidence-based practice in nursing and health care* (pp. 3–25). Philadelphia: Lippincott Williams & Wilkins.

Miles, M. B., & Huberman, A. M. (1994). *Qualitative data analysis* (2nd ed.). Thousand Oaks, CA: Sage.

Paul, R., & Elder, L. (2002). *Critical thinking: Tools for taking charge of your learning and your life.* Englewood, NJ: Prentice-Hall.

Paul, R., & Elder, L. (2003). *The thinker's guide on how to read a paragraph.* Dillon Beach, CA: Foundation for Critical Thinking.

Rogers, M. E. (1990). Nursing: Science of unitary, irreducible, human beings: Update 1990. In E. A. N. Barrett (Ed.), *Visions of Rogers' science-based nursing* (pp. 5–11). New York: National League for Nursing.

Rycroft-Malone, J., Seers, K., Tichen, A., Harvey, G., Kitson, A., & McCormack, B. (2004). What counts as evidence in evidence-based practice? *Journal of Advanced Nursing, 47,* 81–90.

Sackett, D. L., Straus, S. E., Richardson, W. S., Rosenburg, W., & Hayes, R. B. (2000). *Evidence-based medicine: How to practice and teach EBM.* London: Churchill Livingstone.

Samuels-Dennis, J. (2006). Relationship among employment status, stressful life events, and depression in single mother. *Canadian Journal of Nursing Research, 38,* 58–80.

Sandelowski, M. (2004). Using qualitative research. *Qualitative health research, 14*(10), 1366–1386.

Smith, D., Edwards, N., Varcoe, C., Martens, P. J., & Davies, B. (2006). Bringing safety and responsiveness into the forefront of care for pregnant and parenting Aboriginal people. *Advances in Nursing Science, 29*(2), E27–E44.

Tarlier, D. (2005). Mediating the meaning of evidence through epistemological diversity. *Nursing Inquiry, 12,* 126–134.

Judith Haber
Cherylyn Cameron

CHAPTER 4

Developing Research

Questions and Hypotheses

LEARNING OUTCOMES

*After reading this chapter, the student should be able to do
the following:*

- Describe how the research question and hypothesis
  relate to the other components of the research process.
- Describe the process of identifying and refining a
  research question.
- Identify the criteria for determining the significance
  of a research question.
- Discuss the purpose of developing a research question.
- Identify the characteristics of research questions and
  hypotheses.
- Describe the advantages and disadvantages of
  directional and nondirectional hypotheses.
- Compare the use of statistical hypotheses versus
  research hypotheses.
- Discuss the appropriate use of research questions
  versus hypotheses in a research study.
- Identify the criteria used for critiquing a research
  question and a hypothesis.
- Apply the critiquing criteria to the evaluation of a
  research question and a hypothesis in a research report.

KEY TERMS

STUDY RESOURCES

evolve Go to Evolve at

http://evolve.elsevier.com/Canada/LoBiondo/Research/

for Weblinks, content updates, and additional

research articles for practice in reviewing and critiquing.

When nurses ask questions such as "What is happening here?" "What are the client's experiences?" "Why are things done this way?" "I wonder what would happen if . . . ?" "What characteristics are associated with . . . ?" and "What is the effect of . . . on client outcomes?" they are often well on their way to developing a research question or hypothesis.

Formulating the research question and stating the hypothesis are key preliminary steps in the research process. The **research question** (sometimes called the problem statement) presents the idea that is to be examined in the study and is the foundation of the research study. Once the research question is clear, the researcher selects the most appropriate research design. If the research question is primarily explorative, descriptive, or theory generating, then the researcher will opt for qualitative methods. In these studies, a hypothesis is not formulated. However, for those studies in which the researcher is seeking a specific answer to a research question, then a hypothesis is generated and tested.

Hypotheses can be considered intelligent hunches, guesses, or predictions that help researchers seek the solution or answer to the research question. Hypotheses are a vehicle for testing the validity of the theoretical framework assumptions and provide a bridge between **theory** and the real world. In the scientific world, researchers derive hypotheses from theories and subject them to empirical testing. A theory's validity is not directly examined. Instead, through testing hypotheses, researchers can evaluate the merit of a theory.

Consumers of research often find research questions or hypotheses at the beginning of a research article. However, because of space constraints or stylistic considerations in journal publications, the research question or hypothesis may be embedded in the purpose, aims, goals, or even in the results section of the research report. Both the consumer and the producer of research need to understand the importance of research questions and hypotheses as the foundational elements of a research study. This chapter provides methods of developing research questions and hypotheses, the standards for writing them, and a set of criteria for evaluating them.

DEVELOPING AND REFINING A RESEARCH QUESTION: The Researcher's Perspective

A researcher spends a great deal of time refining a research idea into a research question. Unfortunately, the evaluator of a research study is not privy to this creative process because it occurs during the study's conceptualization. The final research question usually does not appear in the research article unless the study is qualitative rather than quantitative. Although this section does not teach you how to formulate a research question, it does provide an important glimpse into the researcher's process of developing a research question.

As illustrated in Table 4–1, research questions or topics are not pulled from thin air. Rather, the researcher's practical experience, critical appraisal of the scientific literature, or interest in an untested theory provides the basis for the generation of a research idea. The research question should reflect a refinement of the researcher's initial thinking. The evaluator of a nursing research study should be able to discern that the researcher has done the following:

1. Defined a specific topic area
2. Reviewed the relevant scientific literature
3. Examined the question's potential significance to nursing
4. Pragmatically examined the feasibility of studying the research question

Defining the Research Question

Brainstorming with teachers, advisors, or colleagues may provide valuable feedback to help the researcher focus on a specific question area. For example, suppose a researcher told a colleague that an area of interest was whether men and women recovered differently after cardiac surgery. The colleague may have said, "What is it about the topic

TABLE 4–1 How Practical Experience, Scientific Literature, and Untested Theory Influence the Development of a Research Idea

Area	Influence	Example
Practical experience	Clinical practice provides a wealth of experience from which research problems can be derived. The nurse may observe the occurrence of a particular event or pattern and become curious about why it occurs, as well as its relationship to other factors in the client's environment.	Coronary heart disease is the leading cause of death among women and is thus a serious health concern. However, women are known to have very low participation rates in cardiac rehabilitation programs. Current rehabilitation programming does not seem to meet the needs of women. Can a rehabilitation program developed by and for women increase the participation of and provide support for women with heart disease? (Arthur, Wright, & Smith, 2001)
Critical appraisal of the scientific literature	The critical appraisal of research studies that appear in journals may indirectly suggest a problem area by stimulating the reader's thinking. Nurses may observe the outcome data from a single study or a group of related studies that provide the basis for developing a pilot study or quality improvement project to determine the effectiveness of this intervention in their own practice.	Several pilot studies found that the successful discharge rate among people with schizophrenia could be improved if supported by discharge models that included peers' support and the overlap of professional care and continuity of care. The researchers recognized a need for larger, better designed studies with more widespread samples to determine whether the models of care were truly effective and to address many unanswered questions (Forchuk, Martin, Chan, & Jensen, 2005) (see Appendix A).
	A research idea may also be suggested by a critical appraisal of the literature that identifies gaps and suggests areas for future study. Research ideas also can be generated by research reports that suggest the value of replicating a particular study to extend or refine the existing body of scientific knowledge.	Abuse of women by significant men in their lives is, unfortunately, a common experience in our society. Research has focused on the process of women leaving their abusive partners and on the actual crisis during the leave taking. However, very little work has been done on the healing and recovery work of these women in the postleaving period (Wuest & Merritt-Gray, 2001).
	Verification of an untested nursing theory provides a relatively uncharted territory from which research questions can be derived. Inasmuch as theories themselves are not tested, a researcher may think about investigating a particular concept or set of concepts related to a particular nursing theory. The deductive process would be used to generate the research question. The researcher would pose questions such as, "If this theory is correct, what kind of behaviour will I expect to observe in particular clients and under which conditions?" or "If this theory is valid, what kind of supporting evidence will I find?"	Single-parent families are known to be at risk for poor health. Most intervention programs focus on health promotion but have failed to address the socioeconomic factors contributing to the risk for poor health. Using the Stress Process Model, Samuels-Dennis (2006) (see Appendix C) wanted to assess the association among income, stressful life events, and employment among single mothers. She found that a significant association exists and that single mothers receiving social assistance reported a greater number of stressful events than participants who were employed.

that specifically interests you?" Such a conversation may have initiated a train of thought that resulted in a decision to explore the recovery processes and gender differences. Figure 4–1 illustrates how a broad area of interest was narrowed to a specific research topic.

Figure 4–1   Development of a research question

Idea Emerges
Socioeconomic determinants of stress among single mothers

Brainstorming
- Why are single-parent families more vulnerable to increased risk of poor health?
- Is the fact that more single-parent families are struggling with poverty related to poor health and to the increased rates of depression among single mothers?

Literature Review
- Income is the most important determinant of health.
- Single mothers face higher rates of poverty.
- Single mothers have almost double the 12-month prevalence rates for depression.
- Single mothers receiving social assistance are at increased risk for psychological distress.

Variables
Independent variable
- Employment status or access to income
Dependent variable
- Stressful life events
- Depression

Research Question
- What is the association among employment status or access to income, stressful life events, and depression among single mothers?

From Samuels-Dennis, J. (2006). Relationship among employment status, stressful life events, and depression in single mothers. *Canadian Journal of Nursing Research, 38*(1), 58–80.

Beginning the Literature Review

Qualitative and quantitative researchers conduct literature reviews differently. For qualitative researchers, the value of the literature review is controversial.

Many researchers believe that a literature review will cause investigators to develop biases or beliefs that will limit their openness to exploring the phenomenon under study. As a general rule, qualitative researchers usually start with a very cursory or general review of the literature to help focus the research question (Speziale & Carpenter, 2007), whereas quantitative researchers begin their study with an extensive review of the literature on their research questions and related topics. The literature review also helps researchers determine whether their study can contribute to the field of nursing.

The databases that researchers use for the literature review (e.g., CINAHL, PsycINFO, MEDLINE, PubMed) should reveal a relevant collection of articles that have been critically examined. Concluding sections in such articles (i.e., the recommendations and implications for practice) often identify remaining gaps in the literature, the need for replication, or the need for extension of the knowledge gleaned on a particular research focus. In the previous example about employment and stressful life events (Samuels-Dennis, 2006), the researcher may have conducted a preliminary review of books and journals for theories and research studies on the impact of employment or access to income on stressful life events and depression in single mothers. These factors, known in research language as variables, should be potentially relevant, of interest, and measurable.

Possible "relevant" factors mentioned in the literature begin with an exploration of the socioeconomic context of single mothers' lives in relation to their psychological well-being. Samuels-Dennis (2006) explored a stress process model as a theoretical framework describing stressors, stress moderators, and stress outcomes. The researcher can then use this information to further define the research question, to address a gap in the literature, and to extend the body of knowledge related to stress in single mothers. At this point, the researcher could write the following tentative research question: "What is the association among employment status or access to income, stressful life events, and depression among single mothers?" After reading this question, you should be able to envision the interrelatedness of the initial definition of the research question, the literature review, and the refined research question. Readers of research reports examine the end product of this process in the form of a research question, hypothesis, or both. Thus, readers need an appreciation of how the researcher fomulates the final research question directing the study (see Appendix C).

Helpful 💡 Hint

Reading the literature review or theoretical framework section of a research article helps to trace the development of the implied research question, the final research question, and the hypothesis.

Significance

In nursing research, before researchers proceed to the final development of the research question, it is crucial that they have examined the question's potential significance to nursing. The research question should have the potential to contribute to and extend the scientific body of nursing knowledge. Guidelines for selecting research questions should meet the following criteria:

- Clients, nurses, the medical community in general, and society will potentially benefit from the knowledge derived from the study.
- The results will be applicable for nursing practice, education, or administration.
- The results will be theoretically relevant.
- The findings will lend support to untested theoretical assumptions, extend or challenge an existing theory, or clarify a conflict in the literature.
- The findings will potentially formulate or alter nursing practices or policies.

If the research question has not met any of these criteria, the researcher needs to extensively revise the question or discard it. For example, in the previously cited research question ("What is the association among employment status or access to income, stressful life events, and depression among single mothers?"), the significance of the question includes the following facts:

- National and provincial health promotion programs have targeted the improvement of the health status of at-risk families with children under 6 years of age.
- Most programs have not focused on the socioeconomic factors that contribute to the risk for poor health in spite of the prevalence of poverty among single mothers.
- Single mothers face depression rates almost double the prevalence of the general population over a 12-month period.

Evidence-Based 🔍 Practice Tip

Without a well-developed research question, the researcher may search for incorrect, irrelevant, or unnecessary information.

Feasibility

The feasibility of a research question must be pragmatically examined. Regardless of how significant or researchable a question may be, owing to pragmatic considerations—such as time; availability of subjects, facilities, equipment, and money; experience of the researcher; and any ethical considerations—the researcher may decide that the question is inappropriate because it lacks feasibility.

THE FULLY DEVELOPED RESEARCH QUESTION

As discussed previously, qualitative researchers ask a research question that outlines a general topic area. Examples include the following:

- What are community-based stakeholders' views on care for pregnant and parenting people? (Smith, Edwards, Varcoe, Martens, & Davies, 2006) (see Appendix B).
- Which aspects of their knowledge about clients do critical care nurses pass along to other health care professionals involved in the care of those clients? (Edwards & Donner, 2007).

- How is knowledge about clients passed along to other health care professionals? (Edwards & Donner, 2007).

When a quantitative researcher finalizes a research question, three characteristics should be evident:

- The *variables* under consideration are clearly identified.
- The *population* being studied is specified.
- The possibility of empirical *testing* is implied.

Because each of these elements is crucial to the formulation of a satisfactory research question, the criteria are discussed in greater detail (see Table 4–2).

Variables

Quantitative researchers refer to the properties they study as **variables**. Such properties take on different values. Thus, as the name suggests, a variable is a property that varies. Properties that differ from each other, such as age, weight, height, religion, and ethnicity, are examples of variables.

Researchers attempt to understand how and why differences in one variable relate to differences in another variable. For example, a researcher may be concerned about the variable of pain in postoperative clients. Pain is a variable because not all postoperative clients have the same amount of pain—or any pain at all. A researcher may also be interested in what other factors can be linked to postoperative pain. For example, anxiety has been discovered to be associated with pain. Thus, anxiety is also a variable because not all postoperative clients have the same amount of anxiety—or any anxiety at all.

When speaking of variables, the researcher is essentially asking, "Is X related to Y? What is the effect of X on Y? How are X_1 and X_2 related to Y?"* The researcher is asking a question about the relationship between one or more independent variables and a dependent variable.

An **independent variable**, usually symbolized by **X**, is the variable that has the presumed effect on the dependent variable. In experimental research studies, the researcher manipulates the independent variable. For example, a nurse may study how different methods of administering pain medication affect the client's perception of pain. The researcher may manipulate the independent variable (i.e., the method of administering pain medication) by using nurse- versus client-controlled administration of analgesia. In nonexperimental research, the independent variable is not manipulated and is assumed to have occurred naturally before or during the study. For example, the researcher may be studying the relationship between the level of anxiety and the perception of pain. The independent variable—the level of anxiety—is not manipulated; it is presumed to occur and is observed and measured as it naturally happens.

The **dependent variable**, represented by **Y**, is often referred to as the consequence or the presumed effect that varies with a change in the independent variable. The dependent variable is not manipulated. It is observed and assumed to vary with changes in the independent variable. Predictions are made based on how changes to the independent variable will affect the dependent variable. The researcher is interested in understanding,

*In some cases, when multiple independent or dependent variables are present, subscripts are used to indicate the number of variables under consideration.

Variables	Population	Testability
Independent variable	Single mothers who are employed	Differential effect of employment on
• Employment status	and on social assistance	stressful life events and depression
Dependent variables		
• Stressful life events		
• Depression		

TABLE 4–2 Components of the Research Question and Related Criteria†

† See Appendix C.

explaining, or predicting the response of the dependent variable. For example, a researcher might assume that the perception of pain (i.e., the dependent variable) will vary with changes in the level of anxiety (i.e., the independent variable). In this case, the researcher is trying to explain the perception of pain in relation to the level of anxiety.

Although variability in the dependent variable is assumed to depend on changes in the independent variable, this assumption does not imply that a causal relationship exists between X and Y or that changes in X cause Y to change. Consider the hypothetical example of nurses' attitudes toward clients with tuberculosis. Assume that the researcher discovered that, compared with younger nurses, older nurses had a more negative attitude about clients with tuberculosis. However, the researcher did not conclude that the nurses' negative attitudes toward clients with tuberculosis were because of their age, although, at the same time, the researcher found a directional relationship between age and negative attitudes about clients with tuberculosis. In other words, as the nurses' ages increased, their attitudes about clients with tuberculosis became more negative. This example highlights the fact that causal relationships are not necessarily implied by the independent and dependent variables; rather, only a relational statement with possible directionality is proposed.

Table 4–3 presents a number of examples to help you learn how to write research questions. Practise substituting other variables for the examples in the table. You will be surprised at the skill you develop in writing and critiquing research questions.

Although one independent variable and one dependent variable are used in the examples in Table 4–3, no restriction exists on the number of variables that can be included in a research question. Remember, however, that questions should not be unnecessarily complex or unwieldy, particularly in beginning research efforts. Research questions that include more than one independent or dependent variable may be divided into subquestions that are more concise.

Finally, note that variables are not inherently independent or dependent. A variable that is

TABLE 4–3 Research Question Format

Type	Format	Example
Quantitative Experimental		
Correlational	Is there a relationship between **X** (independent variable) and **Y** (dependent variable) in the specified population?	Is there a relationship between the effectiveness of pain management strategies and quality of life?
Comparative	Is there a difference in **Y** (dependent variable) between people who have **X** characteristic (independent variable) and those who do not have **X** characteristic?	Is there a difference in prevention of osteoporosis in at-risk breast cancer survivors who receive a combination of long-term progressive strength training exercises, alendronate, calcium, and vitamin D compared with those who do not?
Quantitative	Is there a difference in **Y** (dependent variable) between Group A, which received **X** (independent variable), and Group B, which did not receive **X**?	What is the difference in physical, social, and emotional adjustment in women with breast cancer (and their partners) who have received phase-specific standardized education by video versus phase-specific telephone counselling?
Qualitative		
Phenomenological	What is or was it like to have **X**?	How do older adults learn to live with early stage dementia?

classified as independent in one study may be considered dependent in another study. For example, a nurse may review an article about sexual behaviours that are predictive of the risk for human immunodeficiency virus or acquired immune deficiency syndrome (HIV or AIDS). In this case, HIV/AIDS is the dependent variable. In another article in which the relationship between HIV/AIDS and maternal parenting practices is considered, HIV/AIDS status is the independent variable. Whether a variable is independent or dependent depends on the role it plays in a particular study.

Population

The **population** being studied must be specified in the research question. If the scope of the question has been narrowed to a specific focus and the variables have been clearly identified, the nature of the population will be evident to the reader. For example, a research question may ask, "Is there a relationship between the type of discharge planning for seniors hospitalized with heart failure and their caregivers?" This question suggests that the population under consideration includes seniors hospitalized for heart failure and their caregivers. The question also implies that some of the seniors and their caregivers were involved in a professional–client partnership model of discharge planning, in contrast to other seniors who received the usual discharge planning. The researcher or reader will have an initial idea of the composition of the study population from the outset.

Evidence-Based Practice Tip

Make sure that the population of interest and the setting have been clearly described. If you are going to replicate the study, you will know exactly who the study population needs to be.

Testability

The research question must imply that the problem is testable, that is, measurable by either qualitative or quantitative methods. For example, the research question, "Should postoperative clients control how much pain medication they receive?" is stated incorrectly for a variety of reasons. One reason is that the question is not testable; it represents a value statement rather than a relational problem statement. A scientific or relational question must propose a relationship between an independent variable and a dependent variable in such a way that the variables can be measured. Many interesting and important questions are not valid research questions because they are not amenable to testing.

The question, "Should postoperative clients control how much pain medication they receive?" could be revised from a philosophical question to a research question that implies testability. Examples of the revised research question follow:

- Does a relationship exist between client-controlled analgesia versus nurse-administered analgesia and perception of postoperative pain?
- What is the effect of client-controlled analgesia on pain ratings provided by postoperative clients?

These examples illustrate the relationship between the variables, identify the independent and dependent variables, and imply the testability of the research question.

After the elements of the formal research question have been presented in greater detail, this information can be integrated by formulating a formal research question. Earlier in this chapter, the following unrefined research question was formulated: "What is the association among employment status or access to income, stressful life events, and depression among single mothers?" This research question was originally derived from a general area of interest: understanding of employment as a social determinant of health among single mothers. The topic was more specifically defined by delineating a particular research question. The question crystallized further after a preliminary literature review and emerged in the unrefined form just given. It is now possible to propose a refined research question that specifically states the problem in question form and specifies the relationship of the key variables in the study, the population being studied, and the empirical testability of the question. The following research question can then be formulated: "What is the association among employment status or access to income, stressful life events, and depression among single mothers?" (Samuels-Dennis, 2006). Table 4–2 identifies the components of this research question.

Helpful 💡 Hint

Remember that research questions are often not explicitly stated. The reader must infer the research question from the report's title, the abstract, the introduction, or the purpose.

DEVELOPING AND REFINING A CLINICAL QUESTION: A Consumer's Perspective

Practising nurses and nursing students are challenged to keep their practice up-to-date by searching for, retrieving, and critiquing research articles that apply to practice issues they encounter in their respective clinical settings. Nurses and students strive to use the current best evidence from research in clinical and health care decisions. Although research consumers are not conducting research studies, their search for information from practice is also converted into focused, structured clinical questions. Using criteria similar to those used to frame a research question, focused clinical questions can be used as a basis for searching the literature to identify supporting evidence. The significance of the clinical question becomes apparent as the research evidence from the literature is critiqued. The research evidence is used side by side with clinical expertise and the client's perspective to develop or revise nursing standards, protocols, and policies that are used to plan and implement client care (DiCenso, Guyatt, & Ciliska, 2005). Issues or questions can arise from multiple clinical and managerial situations.

Using the example of pain, albeit from a different perspective, a nurse working in a palliative care setting wondered whether completing pain diaries is a useful thing in the palliative care of clients with advanced cancer. She wondered whether time was being spent developing something that had previously been shown to be useless or even harmful. After all, a client's monitoring of pain in a diary could conceivably heighten the client's awareness and experience of pain. To focus the nurse's search of the literature, she developed the following question: Does the use of pain diaries in the palliative care of clients with cancer lead to improved pain control?

Sometimes, nurses who develop clinical questions from a consumer perspective find it helpful to consider three elements as they frame their focused question: (1) the situation, (2) the intervention, and (3) the outcome, which are defined as follows:

- The situation is the client or question being addressed, such as a single client or a group of clients with a particular health problem (e.g., palliative care of clients with cancer).

- The intervention is the dimension of health care interest, which often asks whether a particular intervention (e.g., pain diaries) is a useful treatment.

- The outcome addresses the effect of the treatment (the intervention) for this client or client population in terms of quality and cost (e.g., decreased pain perception/low cost). The outcome essentially answers whether the intervention makes a difference for the client population.

The individual parts of the question are vital pieces of information to remember when searching for evidence in the literature. One of the easiest ways to keep track of the information is to use a table, as illustrated in Table 4–4. Chapter 5 provides numerous examples of how to effectively search the literature to find answers to questions posed by researchers and research consumers.

| TABLE 4–4 **Consumer Perspective: Elements of a Clinical Question** | | | |
Situation	Intervention	Counterintervention	Outcome
People with advanced cancer	Pain diaries	No pain diaries	Increased pain control

STUDY PURPOSE, AIMS, OR OBJECTIVES

Once the research question is developed and the literature review is critiqued in terms of the level, strength, and quality of evidence available for the particular research question, the purpose, aims, or objectives of the study become focused, and the researcher can decide whether a hypothesis should be tested or a research question answered.

The **purpose** of the study encompasses the aims or goals the investigator hopes to achieve with the research, not the problem to be solved. For example, a nurse working with rehabilitation clients with bladder dysfunction may be disturbed by the high incidence of urinary tract infections. The nurse may propose the following research question: "What is the optimum frequency of changing urinary drainage bags in clients with bladder dysfunction to reduce the incidence of urinary tract infection?" If this nurse were to design a study, its purpose might be to determine the differential effect of a one-week and a four-week urinary drainage bag change schedule on the incidence of urinary tract infections in clients with bladder dysfunction.

The purpose communicates more than just the nature of the question. Through the researcher's selection of verbs, the purpose statement suggests the manner in which the researcher sought to study the question. Verbs such as *discover, explore,* or *describe* suggest an investigation of a little-researched topic that might be more appropriately guided by research questions than by hypotheses. In contrast, verb statements indicating that the purpose is to test the effectiveness of an intervention or to compare two alternative nursing strategies suggest a study with a better-established body of knowledge that is hypothesis testing in nature. Box 4–1 provides other examples of purpose statements.

BOX 4–1	**Examples of Purpose Statements**

- "The purpose of this study was to further our understanding of the effects of nursing-related hospital variables on 30-day mortality rates for hospitalized patients" (Tourangeau, Giovannetti, Tu, & Wood, 2002, p. 71).
- "The objective of this study was to determine the cost and effectiveness of a transitional discharge model (TDM) of care with clients who have a chronic mental illness" (Forchuk et al., 2005, p. 556) (see Appendix A).
- "This investigation sought to describe and compare dependency among dying persons" (Wilson, 2002, p. 81).
- "The purpose of this qualitative study was to extend our understanding of how adolescents view nicotine addiction" (Bottorff et al., 2004, p. 22) (see Appendix D).
- "The purpose of this ethnographic study was to investigate nurses' workplace culture as it relates to tobacco use and control" (Shultz, Bottorff, & Johnson, 2006, p. 317).

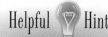

Helpful Hint

The purpose statement often provides the most information about the intent of the research question and hypotheses.

DEVELOPING THE RESEARCH HYPOTHESIS

Like the research question, hypotheses are often not stated explicitly in a research article. The evaluator will often find the hypotheses embedded in the data analysis, results, or discussion section of the research report. The reader then needs to discern the nature of the hypotheses being tested.

Hypotheses flow from the research question, literature review, and theoretical framework. Figure 4–2 illustrates this flow. A **hypothesis** is a statement about the relationship between two or more variables that suggests an answer to the research question. A hypothesis converts the question posed by the research question into a declarative statement that predicts an expected outcome. It explains or predicts the relationship or differences between two or more variables in terms of the expected results or outcomes of a study.

Each hypothesis represents a unit or subset of the research question. For example, a research question might ask: What is the effect of perceived job-related stress on job performance among hospital nurses and the effect of social support from co-workers on job stress, job performance, and the stress–performance relationship? (AbuAlRub, 2004). This question can be divided into the following two subquestions:

1. What is the effect of perceived job stress on job performance among hospital nurses?

2. What is the effect of social support from co-workers on job stress, job performance, and the stress–performance relationship?

A hypothesis can then be generated for each unit of the research question (i.e., the subquestions).

The hypotheses of the research question already mentioned might be stated in the following way:

- *Hypothesis 1:* Hospital nurses with high social support from co-workers have low perceived job stress.
- *Hypothesis 2:* Nurses with high perceived job stress have low job performance.
- *Hypothesis 3:* Nurses with high social support from co-workers have high job performance.
- *Hypothesis 4:* As perceived job stress increases, nurses with high social support from co-workers will perform better than will nurses with less support.

The critiquer of a research report will want to evaluate whether the hypotheses of the study represent subsets of the main research question, as illustrated by these examples.

In quantitative research, hypotheses are formulated before the study is conducted to provide direction for the collection, analysis, and interpretation of data. Hypotheses have the following three purposes:

1. To provide a bridge between theory and reality
2. To be powerful tools for the advancement of knowledge by enabling the researcher to enter new areas of discovery objectively
3. To provide direction for any research endeavour by tentatively identifying the anticipated outcome

Helpful 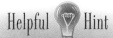 Hint

When hypotheses are not explicitly stated by the author at the end of the "Introduction" section or before the "Methods" section, they will be embedded or implied in the "Results" or "Discussion" section of a research article.

Characteristics

Nurses who are conducting research or critiquing published research studies must have a working knowledge of what constitutes a "good" hypothesis. Such knowledge will provide a standard for evaluating their own work and the work of others.

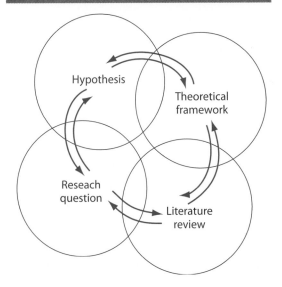

Figure 4–2   Interrelationships of the research question, literature review, theoretical framework, and hypothesis

The following discussion about the characteristics of hypotheses presents criteria to be used when formulating or evaluating a hypothesis.

Relationship Statement   *Hypothesis*

The first characteristic of a hypothesis is that it is a declarative statement identifying the predicted relationship between two or more variables. The hypothesis implies a systematic relationship between an independent variable and a dependent variable. The direction of the predicted relationship is also specified in this statement. Phrases such as *greater than*; *less than*; *positively, negatively*, or *curvilinearly related* (i.e., shaped like ∩ or ∪); and *difference in* describe the directionality proposed in the hypothesis. In the following example of a directional hypothesis, the two variables are explicitly identified, and the relational aspect of the prediction is contained in the phrase "significantly higher . . . than":

> *The rate of continuous smoking abstinence (dependent variable) at six months postpartum, based on self-report and biochemical validation, will be significantly higher in the treatment group (postpartum counselling intervention) than in the control group (independent variable).*

The nature of the relationship, either causal or associative, is also implied by the hypothesis. In a causal relationship, the researcher can predict that the independent variable (X) causes a change in the dependent variable (Y). Rarely is a researcher in a firm enough position to take a definitive stand about a cause-and-effect relationship. For example, a researcher might hypothesize that relaxation training would have a significant effect on the physical and psychological health status of clients who have suffered myocardial infarction. A researcher would have difficulty predicting a strong cause-and-effect relationship, however, because the multiple intervening variables (e.g., age, medication, and lifestyle changes) might also influence the subject's health status.

Variables are more commonly related in non-causal ways. In other words, the variables are related but in an associative way. For example, because strong evidence exists that asbestos exposure is related to lung cancer, a researcher may be tempted to state a causal relationship between asbestos exposure and lung cancer. However, not all individuals exposed to asbestos will have lung cancer and, conversely, not all individuals who have lung cancer have been exposed to asbestos. Thus, a position advocating a causal relationship between these two variables would be scientifically unsound. Instead, only an associative relationship exists between the variables of asbestos exposure and lung cancer, with a strong systematic association between the two phenomena.

Testability

The second characteristic of a hypothesis is its **testability**. The variables of the study must lend themselves to observation, measurement, and analysis. The hypothesis is either supported or not supported after the data have been collected and analyzed. The predicted outcome proposed by the hypothesis will or will not be congruent with the actual outcome when the hypothesis is tested. Hypotheses advance scientific knowledge by confirming or refuting theories.

Hypotheses may fail to meet the criteria of testability because the researcher has not made a prediction about the anticipated outcome, the variables are not observable or measurable, or the hypothesis is couched in terms that are value laden. Table 4–5 illustrates each of these points and provides a remedy for each problem.

Helpful Hint

When a hypothesis is complex (i.e., contains more than one independent or dependent variable), it is difficult for the findings to indicate unequivocally that the hypothesis is supported or not supported. In such cases, the reader must infer which relationships are significant from the "Findings" or "Discussion" section.

TABLE 4–5 Hypotheses That Fail to Meet the Criteria of Testability

Problematic Hypothesis	Problematic Issue	Revised Hypothesis
Coping is related to adaptation.	No predictive statement about the relationship is made, so the relationship is not verifiable.	Coping is positively related to adaptation.
Clients who receive preoperative instruction have less postoperative stress than clients who do not receive such instruction.	The "postoperative stress" variable must be specifically defined so that it is observable or measurable, or the relationship is not testable.	Clients who attend preoperative education classes have less post operative emotional stress than clients who do not attend.
Small-group teaching will be better than individualized teaching for dietary compliance in clients with coronary artery disease (CAD).	"Better than" is a value-laden phrase that is not objective. Moral and ethical questions containing words such as *should, ought, better than,* and *bad for* are not scientifically testable.	Dietary compliance will be greater in clients with CAD receiving diet instruction in small groups than in CAD clients receiving individualized diet instruction.
Nurses' attitudes toward clients with acquired immune deficiency syndrome (AIDS) cause changes in the clients' mood state.	Causal relationships are proposed without sufficient evidence.	Nurses' attitudes toward clients with AIDS will be positively related to the emotional states of the client with AIDS.

Theory Base

A sound hypothesis is consistent with an existing body of theory and research findings. Whether a researcher arrives at a hypothesis inductively or deductively, the hypothesis must be based on a sound scientific rationale. Readers should be able to identify the flow of ideas from the research question to the literature review, to the theoretical framework, and to the hypotheses. Table 4–6 illustrates this process in relation to the research question posed in Samuels-Dennis's (2006, p. 64) study: What is "the association among employment status or access to income, stressful life events, and depression among single mothers?" (see Appendix C). This example makes clear that an explicitly developed, relevant body of scientific data provides the theoretical grounding for the study. The hypotheses, as stated in Table 4–6, are logically derived from the theoretical framework. The research consumer, however, should be cautioned against assuming that the theory–hypothesis link will always be present.

Wording the Hypothesis

As you become more familiar with reading the scientific literature, you will observe that a hypothesis can be worded in a variety of ways. Regardless of the specific format used to state the hypothesis, the statement should be worded in clear, simple, and concise terms. If this criterion is met, the reader will understand the following:

- The variables of the hypothesis
- The population being studied
- The predicted outcome of the hypothesis

Information about hypotheses may be further clarified in the "Instruments," "Sample," or "Methods" section of a research report.

Directional Versus Nondirectional Hypotheses

Hypotheses can be formulated directionally or nondirectionally. A **directional hypothesis** specifies the expected direction of the relationship between the independent and dependent variables. The reader of a directional hypothesis may observe not only that a relationship is proposed but also the nature or direction of that relationship. The following is an example of a directional hypothesis: "Social assistance recipients will report greater depressive symptoms than employed single mothers" (Samuels-Dennis, 2006). Examples of directional hypotheses can also be found in examples 2 to 7 of Table 4–7.

TABLE 4–6	**Flow of Data Among the Research Question, Literature Review, Theoretical Framework, and Hypotheses**		
Research Question	**Literature Review**	**Theoretical Framework**	**Hypotheses**
What is the association among employment status or access to income, stressful life events, and depression among single mothers?	1. Income is defined as the single most important determinant of health. 2. Single mothers have almost double the 12-month prevalence rates of depression of the general population. 3. Single mothers receiving social assistance are at high risk for psychological distress.	The Stress Process Model posits that stress is a dynamic and evolving process that incorporates three core elements: stressors, stress moderators, and stress outcomes	Three hypothesis are included: 1. Social assistance recipients will report greater stressful events than employed single mothers. 2. Social assistance recipients will report greater depressive symptoms than employed single mothers. 3. Employment status and stressful events will predict depression among single mothers.

Based on Samuels-Dennis, J. (2006). Relationship among employment status, stressful life events, and depression in single mothers. *Canadian Journal of Nursing Research, 38*(1), 65.

Although a **nondirectional hypothesis** indicates the existence of a relationship between the variables, it does not specify the anticipated direction of the relationship. The following is an example of a nondirectional hypothesis: ". . . Biophysical and psychosocial factors might influence recovery from cardiac surgery . . ." (King, 2000, p. 492). Other examples of nondirectional hypotheses are illustrated in examples 1 and 8 in Table 4–7.

Nurses who are learning to critique research studies should be aware that both the directional and the nondirectional forms of hypothesis statements are acceptable and definite pros and cons pertain to each form.

Proponents of the nondirectional hypothesis state that this format is more objective and impartial than the directional hypothesis. They argue that the directional hypothesis is potentially biased because the researcher, in stating an anticipated outcome, has demonstrated a commitment to a particular position.

In contrast, proponents of the directional hypothesis argue that researchers naturally have hunches, guesses, or expectations that lead them to speculate about the outcome of their research. The literature review and the conceptual framework provide the theoretical foundation for deriving the hypothesis. Thus, a deductive hypothesis derived from a theory is almost always directional because the theory provides the rationale for proposing the likelihood of a particular outcome. When no theory or related research is available to draw on for a rationale, or when findings from previous research studies are ambivalent, a nondirectional hypothesis may be appropriate.

Directional hypotheses have several advantages, making them appropriate for use in most studies. The advantages are as follows:

- Directional hypotheses indicate to the reader that a theory base has been used to derive the hypotheses and that the phenomena under investigation have been critically thought about and interrelated. Nondirectional hypotheses may also be deduced from a theory base. Because of the exploratory nature of many studies using nondirectional hypotheses, however, the theory base may not be as developed.

- Directional hypotheses provide the reader with a specific theoretical frame of reference, within which the study is being conducted.

- Directional hypotheses suggest to the reader that the researcher is not sitting on a theoretical fence, and, as a result, the analyses of data can be accomplished in a statistically more sensitive way.

For the critiquer, the important consideration is whether a sound rationale exists for the

TABLE 4-7 **Examples of How Hypotheses Are Worded**			
Hypothesis	**Variables**	**Type of Hypothesis**	**Type of Design and Level of Evidence Suggested**
1. A difference in fatigue will exist between two groups of caregivers of preterm infants (i.e., infants on versus not on apnea monitors) during three time periods: prior to discharge, 1 week postdischarge, and 1 month postdischarge). OR There will be a significant difference in menopausal hot flashes between conditions of fasting and experimentally sustained blood glucose concentrations.	IV: Apnea monitor DV: Fatigue OR IV: Blood glucose concentrations DV: Menopausal hot flashes	Nondirectional, research	Nonexperimental; Level IV
2. A positive relationship will exist between phase-specific telephone counselling and emotional adjustment in women with breast cancer and their partners.	IV: Telephone counselling DV: Emotional adjustment	Directional, research	Experimental; Level II
3. A greater decrease in state anxiety scores will result for clients receiving structured informational videos prior to abdominal or chest tube removal than for clients receiving standard information.	IV: Preprocedure structured DVD information IV: Standard information DV: State anxiety	Directional, research	Experimental; Level II
4. The incidence and degree of severity of subject discomfort will be less after administration of medications by the Z-track intramuscular injection technique than after administration of medications by the standard intramuscular injection technique.	IV: Z-track intramuscular injection technique IV: Standard intramuscular injection technique DV: Subject discomfort	Directional, research	Experimental; Level II
5. Therapeutic back massage will reduce the effects of stress experienced by spouses of clients with cancer, as measured by a positive change in mood and a decrease in perceived stress, heart rate, and blood pressure at two postintervention time points, compared with a control group of spouses of clients with cancer.	IV: Therapeutic back massage DV: Change in mood DV: Decrease in perceived stress DV: Decreased heart rate DV: Decreased blood pressure	Directional, research	Experimental; Level II
6. Hospitals with higher registered nurse-to-client ratios will have fewer adverse client events.	IV: Registered nurse-to-client ratio DV: Adverse client events	Directional, research	Nonexperimental; Level IV
7. A positive effect will result from a social support, boosting intervention on levels of stress, coping, and social support among caregivers of children with HIV/AIDS.	IV: Social support boosting intervention DV: Stress DV: Coping DV: Social support	Directional, research	Experimental; Level II
8. A difference in post-test state anxiety scores will emerge in subjects treated with noncontact therapeutic touch rather than in subjects treated with contact therapeutic touch. OR No significant difference will exist in the duration of patency of a 24-gauge intravenous lock in a neonatal client when flushed with 0.5 mL of heparinized saline (2 U/mL), which is standard practice, compared with 0.5 mL of 0.9% normal saline.	IV: Noncontact therapeutic touch IV: Contact therapeutic touch DV: State anxiety OR IV: Heparinized saline IV: Normal saline DV: Duration of patency of intravenous lock	Nondirectional; null OR Nondirectional, research	Experimental; Level II

DV: dependent variable; HIV or AIDS: human immunodeficiency virus or acquired immune deficiency syndrome; IV: independent variable.

researcher's choice of a directional or nondirectional hypothesis.

STATISTICAL HYPOTHESES VERSUS RESEARCH HYPOTHESES

A hypothesis can be further categorized as either a research hypothesis or a statistical hypothesis. A **research hypothesis**, also known as a scientific hypothesis, is a statement about the expected relationship of the variables. A research hypothesis indicates the expected outcome of the study and is either directional or nondirectional. If the researcher obtains statistically significant findings for a research hypothesis, the hypothesis is supported. For example, in a study exploring the relative effectiveness of a transitional discharge model (TDM), Forchuk et al. (2005) (see Appendix A) hypothesized that in the year following discharge from a psychiatric hospital, individuals participating in a TDM would (1) have an improved quality of life and (2) incur fewer health and social services costs compared with individuals receiving standard discharge care. All of the examples in Table 4–7 represent research hypotheses.

A **statistical hypothesis**, also known as a **null hypothesis**, states that no relationship exists between the independent and the dependent variables. The examples in Table 4–8 illustrate statistical hypotheses.

If, in the data analysis, a statistically significant relationship emerges between the variables at a specified level of significance, the null hypothesis is rejected. Rejection of the statistical hypothesis is equivalent to acceptance of the research hypothesis. For example, in the study by King (2000), the relationship between gender and recovery from cardiac surgery was tested using a statistical or null hypothesis. The hypothesis was stated as follows: "The null hypothesis was that gender has no effect on recovery from cardiac surgery" (King, 2000, p. 30). King reported that gender was not a consistent predictor of cardiac surgery recovery; thus, the null hypothesis was accepted.

Some researchers refer to the null hypothesis as a statistical contrivance that obscures a straightforward prediction of the outcome. Others state that the null hypothesis is more exact and conservative statistically and that failure to reject the null hypothesis implies that insufficient evidence exists to support the idea of a real difference. Research hypotheses are generally used more often than statistical hypotheses because research hypotheses are more desirable for stating the researcher's expectation and thus provide readers with a more precise idea of the proposed outcome. In any study that involves statistical analysis, the underlying null hypothesis is usually assumed without being explicitly stated.

TABLE 4–8 **Examples of Statistical Hypotheses**			
Hypothesis	Variables	Type of Hypothesis	Type of Design Suggested
Oxygen inhalation by nasal cannula of up to 6 L/min does not affect oral temperature measurement taken with an electronic thermometer.	IV: Oxygen inhalation by nasal cannula DV: Oral temperature	Statistical	Experimental
There will be no difference in performance accuracy between adult nurse practitioners (ANPs) and family nurse practitioners (FNPs) in formulating accurate diagnoses and acceptable interventions for suspected cases of domestic violence.	IV: Nurse practitioner (ANP or FNP) category DV: Diagnosis and intervention performance accuracy	Statistical	Nonexperimental

DV: dependent variable; IV: independent variable.

RELATIONSHIP AMONG THE HYPOTHESIS, THE RESEARCH QUESTION, AND THE RESEARCH DESIGN

Regardless of whether the researcher uses a statistical or a research hypothesis, a suggested relationship exists among the hypothesis, the research question, and the research design. The type of design, experimental or nonexperimental, will influence the wording of the hypothesis. For example, when an experimental design is used, the research consumer would expect to see hypotheses that reflect relationship statements, such as the following:

- X_1 is more effective than X_2 on Y.
- The effect of X_1 on Y is greater than that of X_2 on Y.
- The incidence of Y will not differ in subjects receiving X_1 and X_2 treatments.
- The incidence of Y will be greater in subjects after X_1 than after X_2.

Such hypotheses indicate that an experimental treatment (i.e., independent variable X) will be used and that two groups of subjects, experimental and control groups, are being used to test whether the difference in the outcome (i.e., dependent variable Y) predicted by the hypothesis exists. Hypotheses reflecting experimental designs also test the effect of the experimental treatment (i.e., independent variable X) on the outcome (i.e., dependent variable Y).

In contrast, hypotheses related to nonexperimental designs reflect associative relationship statements, such as the following:

- X will be negatively related to Y.
- A positive relationship will exist between X and Y.

Thus, the strength of the evidence provided by the results of a study that examined hypotheses with associative relationship statements exists at Level IV (nonexperimental design).

Table 4–8 provides additional examples of this concept. The Critical Thinking Decision Path will help you determine both the type of hypothesis presented in a study and the study's readiness for a hypothesis-testing design.

Evidence-Based Practice Tip

Think about the relationship among the wording of the hypothesis, the type of research design suggested, and the level of evidence provided by the findings of a study using each kind of hypothesis. The research consumer may want to consider which type of hypothesis potentially will yield the strongest results applicable to practice.

Research studies do not always contain hypotheses. As you become more familiar with the scientific literature, you will notice that a significant number of research studies are guided by research questions. Note that exploratory studies usually do not have hypotheses, especially when literature or related research studies are scarce in an area of particular interest to the researcher. The researcher who is interested in finding out more about a particular phenomenon may engage in a fact- or relationship-finding mission, guided only by research questions. The outcome of such an exploratory study may be the amassing of data about the phenomenon, allowing the researcher to formulate hypotheses for a future study, a process sometimes referred to as a hypothesis-generating study.

The article by McDonald, McNulty, Erickson, and Weiskopf (2000) provides an example of an exploratory or hypothesis-generating study. McDonald et al. examined how clients communicate their pain and pain management needs after surgery. The following research questions, which include the variables pain (independent variable X) and postoperative caregiver pain communication (dependent variable Y), illustrate how an investigation designed to generate relationships and fill a gap in the literature was guided:

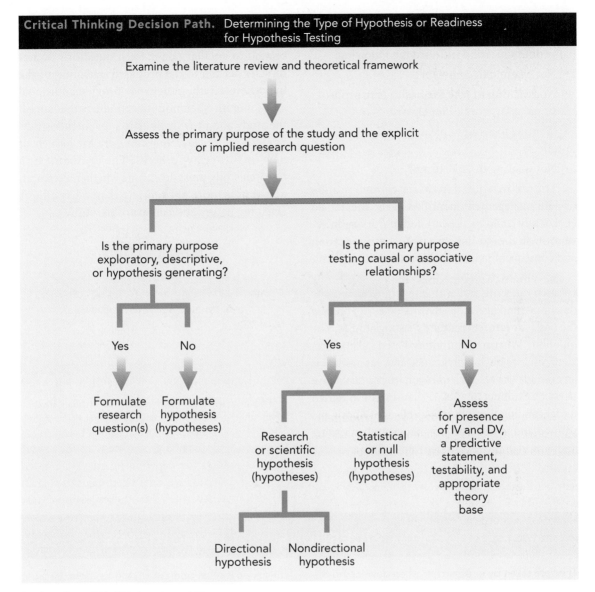

Critical Thinking Decision Path. Determining the Type of Hypothesis or Readiness for Hypothesis Testing

Examine the literature review and theoretical framework

Assess the primary purpose of the study and the explicit or implied research question

Is the primary purpose exploratory, descriptive, or hypothesis generating?

Is the primary purpose testing causal or associative relationships?

Yes — Formulate research question(s)

No — Formulate hypothesis (hypotheses)

Yes — Research or scientific hypothesis (hypotheses) / Statistical or null hypothesis (hypotheses)

No — Assess for presence of IV and DV, a predictive statement, testability, and appropriate theory base

Directional hypothesis   Nondirectional hypothesis

DV: dependent variable; IV: independent variable.

- How do postoperative clients communicate their pain and pain management needs to their health care providers?
- How do demographic variables (e.g., race and gender) relate to pain and the communication of pain management needs to health care professionals?

Because little research has been conducted on the effectiveness of postoperative communication of pain, research questions—rather than hypotheses—are appropriate for this baseline phase of a study. The findings of the McDonald et al. (2000) study highlighted the importance of effective client communication of pain as a variable related to effective pain management by health care professionals. The reasons for clients' decreased pain communication included the following:

- Not wanting to complain
- Not wanting to take the health care professional away from other clients
- Wanting to avoid unpleasant analgesic side effects
- Not wanting to "take drugs"

The research questions in the communication of pain management identified in the McDonald et al. study could be used to design nursing intervention studies to improve pain communication and consequent pain relief in postoperative clients.

Qualitative research studies also are guided by research questions rather than hypotheses, and the descriptive findings of qualitative studies can provide the basis for future hypothesis-testing studies. The question, "What are community-based stakeholders views on care during pregnancy and parenting?" is an example of a research question from a qualitative study by Smith et al. (2006) that sought to enrich understanding about the perspectives of Aboriginal women and families on pregnancy and parenting and how to improve care (see Appendix B).

In other studies, research questions are formulated in addition to hypotheses to answer questions related to ancillary data. Such questions do not directly pertain to the proposed outcomes of the hypotheses. Rather, they may provide additional and sometimes serendipitous findings that enrich the study and provide direction for further study. Sometimes, research questions are the kernels of new or future hypotheses. The evaluator of a research study must determine whether a research question is more appropriate than a hypothesis given the nature and context of the study.

Helpful 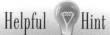 Hint

Remember that research questions are most often used in exploratory, descriptive, qualitative, or hypothesis-generating studies.

Evidence-Based Practice Tip

The answers to questions generated by qualitative data reflect evidence that may provide the first insights about a phenomenon that has not been previously studied.

Critiquing Research Questions and Hypotheses

The care taken by a researcher when developing the research question or hypothesis is often representative of the overall conceptualization and design of the study. A methodically formulated research question provides the basis for hypothesis development. In a quantitative research study, the remainder of the study revolves around testing the hypothesis or, in some cases, the research question. In a qualitative research study, the objective is to answer the research question. This task may be a time-consuming, sometimes frustrating endeavour for the researcher, but, in the final analysis, the product, as evaluated by the consumer, is most often worth the struggle. Because this text focuses on the nurse as a critical consumer of research, the following sections primarily pertain to the evaluation of research questions and hypotheses in published research reports.

Critiquing the Research Question

The Critiquing Criteria box provides several criteria for evaluating this initial phase of the research process—the research question. Because the research question represents the basis for the study, it is usually introduced at the beginning of the research report to indicate the focus and direction of the study. Readers will then be in a position to evaluate whether the rest of the study logically flows from its base. The author will often begin by identifying the background and significance of the issue that led to crystallizing development of the unanswered question. The clinical and scientific background, significance, or both will be summarized, and the purpose, aim, or objective of the study will be identified. Finally, the research question and any related subquestions will be proposed prior to or following the literature review.

The purpose of the introductory summary of the theoretical and scientific background is to provide the reader with a contextual glimpse of how the author critically thought about the research question's development. The introduction to the research question places the study within an appropriate theoretical framework and sets the stage for the unfolding of the study. This introductory section should also include the significance of the study (i.e., why the investigator is conducting the study). For example, the significance may be to answer a question encountered in the clinical area and thereby improve client care, to resolve a conflict in the literature regarding a clinical issue, or to provide data supporting an innovative form of nursing intervention that is more effective and is also cost-effective.

Sometimes readers find that the research question is not clearly stated at the conclusion of the introduction. In some cases, the author only hints at the question, and the reader is challenged to identify the research question. In other cases, the author embeds the research question in the introductory text or purpose statement. To some extent, where or whether the author states the research question depends on the style of the journal. Nevertheless, the evaluator must remember that the main research question should be implied if it is not clearly identified in the introductory section— even if the subquestions are not stated or implied.

When critiquing the research question, the reader looks for the presence of three key elements, which were described and illustrated on page 65. These three key elements are as follows:

- Does the research question express a relationship between two or more variables or, at least, between an independent variable and a dependent variable?
- Does the research question specify the nature of the population being studied?
- Does the research question imply the possibility of empirical testing?

The reader uses these three elements as criteria for judging the soundness of a stated research question. If the question is unclear in terms of the variables, the population, and the implications for testability, then the remainder of the study will likely falter. For example, a research study on anxiety during the perioperative period contained introductory material on anxiety in general, anxiety as it relates to the perioperative period, and the potentially beneficial influence of nursing care in relation to anxiety reduction. The author concluded that the purpose of the study was to determine whether selected measures of client anxiety could be shown to vary when different approaches to nursing care were used during the perioperative period. The author did not state the research questions. A restatement of the problem in question form might be as follows:

$$(Y1) \ (X_1, X_2, X_3)$$

What is the difference in client anxiety level in relation to different approaches to nursing care during the perioperative period?

If this process of developing a research question is clarified at the outset of a research study, the report that follows can develop logically. Readers will have a clear idea of what the report should convey and can knowledgeably evaluate the material that follows. When critically appraising clinical questions, remember that they should be focused and specify the client or problem being addressed, the intervention, and the outcome for a particular client population. The author should provide evidence that the clinical question guided the literature search and that the question suggests the design and level of evidence to be obtained from the study findings.

CRITIQUING CRITERIA

The Research Question

1. Is the research question introduced promptly?

2. Is the question stated clearly and unambiguously in declarative or question form?

3. Does the research question express a relationship between two or more variables or at least between an independent variable and a dependent variable, implying empirical testability?

4. Does the research question specify the nature of the population being studied?

5. Has the research question been substantiated by adequate experiential and scientific background material?

6. Has the research question been placed within the context of an appropriate theoretical framework?

7. Has the significance of the research question been identified?

8. Have pragmatic issues, such as feasibility, been addressed?

9. Have the purpose, aims, or goals of the study been identified?

The Hypotheses

1. Does the hypothesis directly relate to the research question?

2. Is the hypothesis concisely stated in a declarative form?

3. Are the independent and dependent variables identified in the statement of the hypothesis?

4. Are the variables measurable or potentially measurable?

5. Is each of the hypotheses specific to one relationship so that each hypothesis can be either supported or not supported?

6. Is the hypothesis stated in such a way that it is testable?

7. Is the hypothesis stated objectively, without value-laden words?

8. Is the direction of the relationship in each hypothesis clearly stated?

9. Is each hypothesis consistent with the literature review?

10. Is the theoretical rationale for the hypothesis explicit?

11. Are research questions appropriately used (i.e., for an exploratory, descriptive, or qualitative study or in relation to ancillary data analyses)?

Critiquing the Hypotheses

As illustrated in the Critiquing Criteria box, several criteria for critiquing the hypotheses should be used as a standard for evaluating the strengths and weaknesses of the hypotheses in a research report:

1. When reading a research study, research consumers may find the hypotheses clearly delineated in a separate hypothesis section of the research article (i.e., after the literature review or theoretical framework section[s]). In many cases, the hypotheses are not explicitly stated and are only implied in the "Results" or "Discussion" section of the article. In such cases, readers must infer from the purpose statement the hypothesis and the type of analysis used. Readers must also be cognizant of this variation and remember that because hypotheses do not appear at the beginning of the article does not mean they do not exist in the particular study. Even when hypotheses are stated at the beginning of an article, they are re-examined in the "Results" or "Discussion" section when the findings are presented and discussed. Readers should expect hypotheses to be appropriately reflected, depending on the purpose of the study and the format of the article.

2. If a research question is posed at the beginning of the report, the data analysis is designed to answer that question. If a hypothesis or a set of hypotheses is presented, the data analysis should directly answer the hypotheses. The placement of the hypothesis in the research report logically follows the literature review and the theoretical framework because the hypothesis should reflect the culmination and expression

of this conceptual process. The hypothesis should be consistent with both the literature review and the theoretical framework. The flow of this process should be explicit and apparent to the reader. If this criterion is met, the reader feels reasonably assured that the basis for the hypothesis is theoretically sound.

3. As readers examine the actual hypothesis, the following aspects of the statement should be critically appraised:

   • The hypothesis should consist of a declarative statement that objectively and succinctly expresses the relationship between an independent variable and a dependent variable. In wording a complex versus a simple hypothesis, the author may include more than one independent variable and one dependent variable.

   • More than one hypothesis may exist, particularly if more than one independent variable or more than one dependent variable are present. The type of study being conducted determines the number of hypotheses.

   • The reader should be able to understand the variables of the hypothesis. In the interest of formulating a succinct hypothesis statement, the complete meaning of the variables is often not apparent. The researcher may have to choose between having a complete but verbose hypothesis paragraph or a less complete but concise hypothesis. The solution to this dilemma is for the researcher to include a definition section in the research report. The inclusion of **conceptual definitions** and **operational definitions** provides the complete explication of the variables. Other times, the conceptual definitions may be embedded in the theoretical framework or the literature review, whereas the operational definitions will appear in the "Methods" or "Instruments" section of the research report. The reader is then challenged to

evaluate the fit between the conceptual and operational definitions and their relationship to the hypotheses.

   • Although a hypothesis can legitimately be nondirectional, it is preferable for the hypothesis to indicate the direction of the relationship between the variables. When data for the literature review are scarce (i.e., the researcher has chosen to study a relatively undefined area of interest), the nondirectional hypothesis may be appropriate. Because enough information may simply not be available to make a sound judgement about the direction of the proposed relationship, the researcher might only be able to propose that a relationship will exist between two variables. Essentially, readers want to determine the appropriateness of the researcher's choice regarding the directionality of the hypothesis.

4. The notion of testability is central to the soundness of a hypothesis. One criterion related to testability is that the hypothesis should be stated in such a way that it can be clearly supported or not supported. Although the previous statement is important to keep in mind, readers should also understand that, ultimately, theories or hypotheses are never proven beyond doubt through hypothesis testing. Researchers who claim that their data have "proven" the validity of their hypothesis should be regarded with grave reservations. At best, findings that support a hypothesis are considered tentative. If repeated replication of a study yields the same results, more confidence can be placed in the conclusions advanced by the researchers. Although hypotheses are more likely to be accepted with increasing evidence, they are ultimately never proven.

   Another point about testability for research consumers to consider is that the hypothesis should be objectively stated and devoid of any value-laden words. Value-laden hypotheses are not empirically testable.

Quantifiable words, such as *greater than*, *less than*, *decrease*, *increase*, and *positively*, *negatively*, and *curvilinearly related*, convey the idea of objectivity and testability. Readers should immediately be suspicious of hypotheses that are not stated objectively.

5. The evaluator of a research study should be aware that the phrasing of the proposed relationship of the hypothesis suggests the type of research design appropriate for the study. For example, if a hypothesis proposes that treatment X_1 will have a greater effect on Y than treatment X_2, an experimental or quasi-experimental design is suggested. If a hypothesis proposes that a positive relationship will exist between variables X and Y, a nonexperimental design is suggested. Table 4–7 provides additional examples of hypotheses and the type of research design suggested by each hypothesis. The reader of a research report should evaluate whether the selected research design is congruent with the hypothesis. Congruence has important implications for the remainder of the study in terms of the appropriateness of sample selection, data collection, data analysis, interpretation of findings, and, ultimately, the conclusions advanced by the researcher.

6. If the research report contains research questions rather than hypotheses, the reader will want to evaluate whether this choice is appropriate to the study. One criterion for making this decision, as presented earlier in this chapter, is whether the study is of an exploratory, descriptive, or qualitative nature. If it is, then research questions are more appropriate than hypotheses. Ancillary research questions should be evaluated as to whether they answer additional questions secondary to the hypotheses. Sometimes, the substance of an additional research question is more appropriately posed as another hypothesis because it relates in a major way to the original research question.

Critical Thinking Challenges

- Do you agree or disagree with the following statement? "If a research study published in a journal does not clearly state the research question, then it fails to meet the critiquing criteria for research questions as presented in this chapter." Justify your answer.
- Is it possible for "level of anxiety" to be the independent variable in one study and the dependent variable in another study? Support your position.
- Discuss the difference between a classmate predicting that "students who do not study will not do well on a test" and a research study's hypothesis on the topic. Justify your answer.
- How does the wording of the research question or hypothesis suggest the level of evidence that will be provided by the study findings?

KEY POINTS

- Formulation of the research question and stating the hypothesis are key preliminary steps in the research process.

- The research question is refined through a process that proceeds from the identification of a general idea of interest to the definition of a more specific and circumscribed topic.

- A preliminary literature review helps to further define the research question and reveals related factors that appear to be critical to the research topic of interest.

- The significance of the research question must be identified in terms of its potential contribution to clients, nurses, the medical community in general, and society. The applicability of the question for nursing practice and its theoretical relevance must be established. The findings should also have the potential for formulating or altering nursing practices or policies.

- The researcher must examine the feasibility of a research question in light of pragmatic considerations—for example, time; the availability of subjects, money, facilities, and equipment; his or her experience; and ethical issues.

- The final research question consists of a statement about the relationship of two or more variables. The question clearly identifies the relationship between the independent variables and dependent variables, specifies the nature of the population being studied, and implies the possibility of empirical testing.

- Focused clinical questions arise from clinical practice and guide the literature search for the best available evidence to answer the clinical question.

- A hypothesis attempts to answer the question posed by the research question. When testing the validity of the theoretical framework's assumptions, the hypothesis connects the theory and reality.

- A hypothesis is a declarative statement about the relationship between two or more variables that predicts an expected outcome. The characteristics of a hypothesis include a relationship statement, implications regarding testability, and consistency with a defined theory base.

- Hypotheses can be formulated directionally or non-directionally. Hypotheses can be further categorized as either research or statistical hypotheses.

- Research questions may be used instead of hypotheses in exploratory, descriptive, or qualitative research studies. Research questions may also be formulated in addition to hypotheses to answer questions related to ancillary data.

- The critiquing criteria provide a set of guidelines for evaluating the strengths and weaknesses of the research question and hypotheses as they appear in a research report.

- The critiquer assesses the clarity of the research question and the related subquestions, the specificity of the population, and the implications for testability.

- The interrelatedness of the research question, the literature review, the theoretical framework, and the hypotheses should be apparent.

- The reader evaluates the appropriateness of the research design suggested by the research question.

- The purpose of the study (i.e., why the researcher is doing the study) should be differentiated from the research question.

- The reader evaluates the wording of the hypothesis in terms of the clarity of the relational statement, its implications for testability, and its congruence with theory. The appropriateness of the hypothesis in relation to the type of research design is also examined. In addition, the appropriate use of research questions is evaluated in relation to the type of study conducted.

REFERENCES

AbuAlRub, R. F. (2004). Job stress, job performance and social support among hospital nurses. *Journal of Nursing Scholarship, 36*(1), 73–78.

Arthur, H., Wright, D., & Smith, K. (2001). Women and heart disease: The treatment may end but the suffering continues. *Canadian Journal of Nursing Research, 33*, 17–29.

Bottorff, J. L., Johnson, J. L., Moffat, B., Grewal, J., Ratner, P., & Kalaw, C. (2004). Adolescent constructions of nicotine addiction. *Canadian Journal of Nursing Research, 38*, 22–39.

DiCenso, A., Guyatt, G., & Ciliska, D. (2005). *Evidence-based nursing*. Toronto: Elsevier.

Edwards, M., & Donner, G. (2007). The efforts of critical care nurses to pass along knowledge about patients. *Canadian Journal of Nursing Research, 39*, 138–154.

Forchuk, C., Martin, M. L., Chan, Y. L., & Jensen, E. (2005). Therapeutic relationships: From psychiatric hospital to community. *Journal of Psychiatric and Mental Health Nursing, 12*, 556–564.

King, K. (2000). Gender and short-term recovery from cardiac surgery. *Nursing Research, 49*, 29–36.

McDonald, D. D., McNulty, J., Erickson, K., & Weiskopf, C. (2000). Communicating pain and pain management needs after surgery. *Applied Nursing Research, 13*, 70–75.

Samuels-Dennis, J. (2006). Relationship among employment status, stressful life events, and depression in single mothers. *Canadian Journal of Nursing Research, 38*, 58–80.

Schultz, A., Bottorff, J., & Johnson, J. (2006). An ethnographic study of tobacco control in hospital settings. *Tobacco Control, 15*, 317–322.

Smith, D., Edwards, N., Varcoe, C., Martens, P. J., & Davies, B. (2006). Bringing safety and responsiveness into the forefront of care for pregnant and parenting Aboriginal people. *Advances in Nursing Science, 29*(2), E27–E44.

Speziale, H., & Carpenter, D. (2007). *Qualitative research in nursing* (4th ed.). New York: Lippincott.

Tourangeau, A., Giovannetti, P., Tu, J., & Wood, M. (2002). Nursing-related determinants of 30-day mortality for hospitalized patients. *Canadian Journal of Nursing Research, 33*, 71–88.

Wilson, D. (2002). The duration and degree of end-of-life dependency of home care clients and hospital inpatients. *Advanced Nursing Research, 15*, 81–86.

Wuest, J., & Merritt-Gray, M. (2001). Beyond survival: Reclaiming self after leaving an abusive male partner. *Canadian Journal of Nursing Research, 32*, 79–94.

Barbara Krainovich-Miller
Cherylyn Cameron

CHAPTER 5

CINAHL
99, 102, 104, 105
94

Literature Review

Medline
104, 105
102 94

LEARNING OUTCOMES

After reading this chapter, the student should be able to do the following:

- Discuss the relationship of the literature review to nursing theory, research, education, and practice.
- Discuss the purposes of the literature review from the perspective of the research investigator and the research consumer.
- Discuss the use of the literature review for quantitative designs and qualitative approaches.
- Discuss the purpose of reviewing the literature in the development of evidence-based practice protocols.
- Differentiate between conceptual (theoretical) and data-based (research) literature.
- Differentiate between primary and secondary sources.
- Compare the advantages and disadvantages of the most commonly used online databases and traditional print database sources for conducting a relevant literature review.
- Identify the characteristics of a relevant literature review.
- Differentiate between a study's literature review and a systematic review. 97,98 94
- Differentiate between a qualitative systematic review and a quantitative systematic review (meta-analysis).
- Critically read, critique, and synthesize conceptual and data-based resources for the development of a literature review.
- Apply critiquing criteria to the evaluation of literature reviews in selected research studies.

KEY TERMS

computer database 106
conceptual literature 94
Cumulative Index to Nursing and Allied Health Literature (CINAHL)
data-based literature 85
electronic databases 98
empirical literature 98
integrative review 93
literature 85
MEDLINE
meta-analysis 93
primary source 89
print databases 98
print indexes 98
quantitative research 93
refereed (peer-reviewed) journals
research literature
review of the literature 85
scholarly literature 85
scientific literature 94
secondary source 89
systematic review 92
theoretical literature 94
Web browser 99

STUDY RESOURCES

 evolve Go to Evolve at
http://evolve.elsevier.com/Canada/LoBiondo/Research/
for Weblinks, content updates, and additional research articles for practice in reviewing and critiquing.

You may wonder why an entire chapter of a research text is devoted to the review of the **literature**. The main reason is because the literature review is not only a key step in the research process, it is also used in each step of the process. A more personal question you might ask is, "Will knowing more about the literature review help me in my student role or later in my research consumer role as a practising professional nurse?" The answer is that the ability to review the literature is essential both to your current role as a student and to your future role as a research consumer.

The **review of the literature** is an organized critique of the important scholarly literature that supports a study and is a key step in the research process. The term **scholarly literature** refers to published and unpublished data-based (research) reports and conceptual (theoretical) literature. **Data-based literature** refers to reports of original research studies by the researchers who conducted them. For example, all of the studies in Appendices A through D are data-based research reports and, as such, have literature reviews that help to form the basis for each study. Conceptual theoretical literature can include articles that comprise an author's theory or that discuss a particular concept, theory, or topic.

The differences between a data-based report and a conceptual article may seem confusing at first. The key to demystifying the differences is determining whether the author(s) of the article conducted the study or whether the article is the result of an original theory or concept investigated by the author(s). Figure 5–1 shows the relationship of a review of the literature to theory, research, education, and practice. A critical review of the literature accomplishes the following:

- Uncovers conceptual and data-based knowledge related to a particular subject, concept, or clinical problem and is used in all aspects of the research process
- Uncovers new knowledge that can lead to the development, validation, or refinement of theories
- Reveals research questions applicable to the discipline

- Provides the latest knowledge on the topic under review
- Uncovers research findings that support evidence-based practice

The purpose of this chapter is to introduce you to the literature review as it is used in research and other scholarly activities. The primary focus of the discussion is the use of your critical thinking and reading competencies to develop the necessary skills for critically appraising the literature.

REVIEW OF THE LITERATURE

Overall Purpose: Knowledge

Before you can critique the literature review in a research study, it is important to understand the purposes the review of the literature serves (see Box 5–1). The overall purpose of the literature review is to discover what is known about the topic under review. The information uncovered from the critical review of the literature contributes to the development, implementation, and results of the research study.

Purposes of the Literature Review

All 10 objectives listed in Box 5–1 reflect the purposes of a literature review for the conduct of **quantitative research**. Critically reading the literature

Figure 5–1 Relationship of the literature review to theory, research, education, and practice

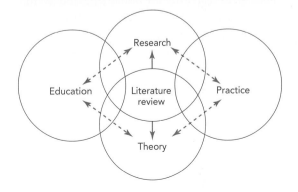

BOX 5–1   Overall Purposes of a Literature Review

MAJOR GOAL

To develop a strong body of knowledge from which to carry out research and other scholarly educational and clinical practice activities.

OBJECTIVES

A review of the literature accomplishes the following:

1. Determines what is known and what is unknown about a subject, concept, or problem.

2. Determines gaps, consistencies, and inconsistencies in the literature about a subject, concept, or problem.

3. Discovers unanswered questions about a subject, concept, or problem.

4. Discovers conceptual traditions used to examine problems.

5. Uncovers a new practice intervention (or interventions) or gains support for current interventions, protocols, and policies.

6. Promotes revision and development of new practice protocols, policies, and projects or activities related to nursing practice.

7. Generates useful research questions and hypotheses for nursing.

8. Determines an appropriate research design, methodology, and analysis for answering the research question(s) or hypothesis (hypotheses) based on an assessment of the strengths and weaknesses of earlier works.

9. Determines the need for replication or refinement of a study.

10. Synthesizes the strengths and weaknesses and findings of available studies on a topic or problem.

is essential to meeting these objectives. The main goal of a literature review is to develop the foundation of a sound study, but it is also used for other scholarly, educational, and clinical practice activities. Table 5–1 summarizes the main focus of the literature review in the steps of the research process for quantitative and qualitative designs. Box 5–2 lists the characteristics of a literature review that meet critiquing criteria; these characteristics are discussed throughout the chapter.

Purposes of the Literature Review

Sometimes, the goal of the literature review is specifically related to writing a paper for a student assignment or to searching for potential evidence that supports a nursing practice. As a practising nurse, you will be called on to develop evidence-based practice protocols, and conducting a literature review is essential to this practice outcome. Table 5–2 illustrates a few examples of research consumer activities. For example, a student assignment related to the development of an evidence-based practice protocol, a practice standard, or a policy change would involve retrieving and critically reviewing a

number of data-based (research) articles, systematic reviews, and conceptual (theoretical) articles to determine the degree of support found in the literature. A critical review of the literature essentially uncovers data that contribute evidence to support current practice and clinical decision making or to support making changes in practice.

Evidence-Based Practice Tip

The clinical question provides a focus that can guide the literature review.

Research Conduct and Consumer of Research Purposes: Differences and Similarities

How does the literature review differ when it is used for research purposes versus consumer of research purposes? In a research study, the literature review is used to develop a sound research proposal. The literature review includes a critical evaluation of both data-based and conceptual literature related to the proposed study and concludes with a statement relating the proposed study's purpose to the reviewed

TABLE 5–1   Examples of the Uses of Literature Review for the Research Process: Quantitative and Qualitative

Quantitative Process	Qualitative Process
The review of the literature is used for all quantitative research designs.	The use of the literature review depends on the selected qualitative approach or method, designs or types, and phases of the research study. An extensive database is not usually available, and conceptual data can be limited, so a qualitative design is used.
The review of the literature is defined as a step in the research process. When a research study is written as a proposal or published, the literature review is often written as a separate aspect of the study—even if it is not labelled as such. The actual review of the literature (i.e., the results of the review), however, is used in developing all steps of the research process.	The following examples highlight the predominant use of the literature review for the particular qualitative approach:
The review of the literature is essential to developing the following parts of the research process:	<ul><li>Phenomenological—compares findings with information from the literature review for the purpose of enhancing knowledge</li><li>Grounded theory—constantly compares literature with the data being generated</li><li>Ethnographic—more conceptual than data based; provides a framework for study</li><li>Case study—conceptual and data-based literature are embedded in the report</li><li>Historical—the literature review is the source of data</li></ul>
<ul><li>Clinical question</li><li>Need or significance</li><li>Research question or hypothesis (hypotheses)</li><li>Theoretical or conceptual framework</li><li>Design or methodology</li><li>Specific instruments (validity and reliability)</li><li>Data collection method</li><li>Type of analysis</li><li>Findings (interpretation)</li><li>Implications of the findings</li><li>Recommendations based on the findings</li></ul>	

research. From a broader perspective, the major focus of reviewing the literature as a consumer is to uncover multiple sources on a given topic. From a student perspective, a critical review of the literature is essential to acquiring knowledge for the development of scholarly papers, presentations, debates, and evidence-based practice. Students use data-based and conceptual literature resources to support rationales for nursing interventions written for a nursing diagnosis. The literature reviews for conducting and consuming research are similar: both reviews should be critical, framed in the context of previous

BOX 5–2   Characteristics of a Relevant Literature Review

Each reviewed source of information reflects critical thinking and scholarly writing; is relevant to the study, topic, or project; and, in its content, satisfies the following criteria:

- The purposes of a literature review are met.
- The summary of each data-based or conceptual article is succinct and adequately represents the review source.
- Established criteria for related study designs are used to analyze the study for strengths, weaknesses, or limitations, as well as for conflicts or gaps in information that relate directly or indirectly to the area of interest.

- Evidence of synthesis of the critiques of each source of information is presented; in other words, the parts (i.e., each critique) are put together to form a new whole for or connection to what is to be studied, replicated, developed, or implemented.
- The review consists of mainly primary sources and contains a sufficient number of data-based sources.
- Summaries or critiques of studies are presented logically, ending with a conclusion or synthesis of the reviewed material that indicates why the study or project should be implemented.

TABLE 5–2   Examples of Uses of the Literature for Research Consumer Purposes: Educational and Practice Settings

Educational Setting	Clinical or Professional Setting
Undergraduate Students • To develop academic scholarly papers (i.e., to research a topic, problem, or issue) • To prepare oral presentations or debates on a topic, problem, or issue; to prepare clinical projects **Graduate Students (Master's and Doctoral)** • To develop research proposals • To develop research- or evidence-based practice protocols and other scholarly projects **Faculty** • To develop and revise curricula • To develop theoretical papers for presentations or publication • To develop research proposals • To conduct research • To participate in the development of systematic reviews • To collaborate with practice colleagues in the development of evidence-based practice protocols	**Nurses in the Clinical Setting** • To implement research-based nursing interventions and evidence-based practice protocols • To develop hospital-specific nursing protocols or policies related to client care • To develop, implement, and evaluate hospital-specific quality assurance projects or protocols related to client outcome data **Professional Nursing Organizations and Governmental Agencies** • To develop Canadian Nurses Association's major documents (e.g., Code of Ethics for Registered Nurses [Canadian Nurses Association, 2002]) • To develop practice guidelines (e.g., Registered Nurses' Association of Ontario's Best Practice Guidelines) • To develop health care policies (e.g., Health Canada's Office of Nursing Policy report on health care in Canada [Health Canada, 2003b]).

data-based and conceptual literature, and pertinent to the objectives presented in Box 5–1. The amount of literature required to be reviewed, however, may differ between a research proposal and an academic paper or clinical project. Table 5–2 lists a number of research consumer projects conducted in educational and clinical settings. For research consumers, a critical literature review is central to developing and implementing activities. A practice protocol or nursing intervention implemented in a health care setting should be based on a critical review of data-based (research) literature. For example, the Registered Nurses' Association of Ontario has developed and published Best Practice Guidelines for frequently occurring health problems. One such guideline is the *Assessment & Management of Stage I to IV Pressure Ulcers*, which was developed to identify best practices related to assessment and care of pressure ulcers (Registered Nurses' Association of Ontario, 2007). For the development of these Best Practice Guidelines, a large team of researchers and clinicians conducted an extensive review and critique of all of the available data-based and conceptual literature on each topic.

LITERATURE REVIEW: Understanding the Perspective of the Research Investigator

The literature review is essential to all steps of the quantitative research process and to some qualitative designs. From the researcher's perspective, the review is broad, systematic, and in-depth, but it is not usually exhaustive. Rather, the literature review is a critical collection and evaluation of the important published literature in journals, monographs, books, and book chapters, as well as unpublished data-based print and computer-accessed materials (e.g., doctoral dissertations and master's theses), audiovisual materials (e.g., audiotapes and DVDs), and sometimes personal communications (e.g., conference presentations and one-on-one interviews). From the researcher's perspective, the objectives in Box 5–1 direct the questions the researcher asks while reading the literature to determine the useful research question(s) and the implementation of a particular study. As a consumer of research, the following brief overview of the use of the literature review in relation to the steps of the quantitative research process will help you understand the researcher's focus. A critical review of the relevant literature has the following impact on the quantitative research process:

- *Theoretical or conceptual framework:* A critical literature review reveals conceptual traditions, concepts, and theories or conceptual models from nursing and other related fields that can be used to examine problems. This framework presents the context for studying the problem and can be viewed as a map for understanding the relationships between or among the variables in quantitative studies. The literature review provides a rationale for the variables and explains linkages or relationships between the individual variables for the theoretical framework of the study. In addition, the literature review should demonstrate use of mainly primary sources; there are, of course, exceptions when a **secondary source** appears. (A secondary source is scholarly material that is written by someone other than the originator of the theory or research.) Note that the studies selected for the literature review should offer the strongest and most consistent level of evidence available on the topic.

- *Research questions and hypotheses:* The literature review helps to determine what is known and what is not known; to uncover gaps, consistencies, or inconsistencies; and to reveal unanswered questions in the literature about a subject, concept, theory, or problem. The review allows for refinement of research questions and hypotheses.

- *Design and method:* The literature review reveals the strengths and weaknesses of the designs and methods of previous research studies. The review is crucial to choosing an appropriate design, data collection method, sample size, valid and reliable instruments, and effective data analysis method(s), as well as to helping to develop an appropriate consent form that addresses ethical concerns. A critical literature review reveals the appropriateness

of a study's design and can help the researcher determine whether a previous study should be replicated or refined. The review also can reveal instruments that lack validity and reliability, thus identifying the need for instrument refinement or development through research testing. Often, because of space limitations, researchers do not include this information in their journal articles.

- *Outcome of the analysis (i.e., findings, discussion, implications, and recommendations):* The literature review is used to accurately interpret and discuss the results or findings of a study. To accomplish this goal, the researcher returns to the literature and uses conceptual and data-based literature. The researcher then indicates in this section of the journal article that a particular finding was supported by one or several prior research studies (i.e., data-based articles), and by several theories on the topic (i.e., conceptual articles or books), which are documented in the literature review. The literature review also helps to develop the implications of the findings for practice, education, and further research. Figure 5–2 relates the literature review to all aspects of the quantitative research process.

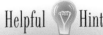 Helpful Hint

The critical reading strategy (see Chapter 3) referred to as "scanning an article's abstract" is very useful in helping to determine whether the article is data based or conceptual.

PRIMARY AND SECONDARY SOURCES

As previously mentioned, a credible literature review reflects the use of mainly **primary source** materials. Table 5–3 provides general definitions and examples of primary and secondary sources, and highlights the differences between primary and secondary sources. Most primary sources are found

Figure 5–2　Relationship of the literature review to the steps of the quantitative research process

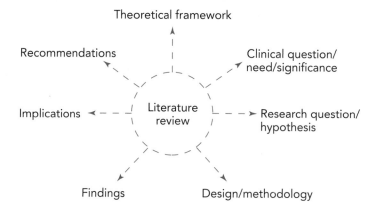

in published literature. A **secondary source** often represents a response to or a summary and critique of a theorist's or researcher's work; an in-depth analysis of a topic, issue, problem, or concept; or an educational article on a specific practice. Box 5–3 lists peer-reviewed journals that contain both primary and secondary research, and Table 5–4 gives examples of primary and secondary print sources in addition to the data-based articles found in Appendices A through D.

Generally speaking, secondary sources are consulted for two reasons. The first reason is that a primary source is unavailable. Note, however, that unavailability of primary sources is rarely the case because computer searches, interlibrary loans, and access to electronic databases (which now

TABLE 5–3　Primary and Secondary Sources	
Primary Source: Essential	**Secondary Source: Useful**
The author is the person who conducted the study, developed the theory (model), or prepared the scholarly discussion on a concept, topic, or issue of interest (i.e., the original author).	The author is someone *other than* the original author (i.e., the person who conducted the original work—whether it is data based or conceptual) who writes or presents the author's original work. These sources are usually published in the form of a summary and critique (i.e., analysis and synthesis) of someone else's scholarly work.
Primary sources can be published or unpublished.	Secondary sources can be published or unpublished.
A data-based example is an investigator's report of his or her research study (i.e., purpose or aims, questions/hypothesis[es], design or method, sample or setting, findings, results [e.g., articles in Appendices A, B, C, and D]), which is a primary source of data-based reports.	Examples include response, commentary, or critique articles of a research study, a theory or model, or a professional view of an issue; a review of an article published in a refereed scholarly journal; abstracts of a published work written by someone other than the original author; a doctoral dissertation's review of the literature
A conceptual or theoretical example is a theorist's work reported in the literature by the author in an article, a chapter of a book, or a book (Watson, 1988, 1999).	Alligood and Tomey (2006) described the work of nursing theorists and discussed the significance of the theory in their textbook, *Nursing Theory: Utilization and Application*.
HINT: Critical evaluation of mainly primary sources is essential to a thorough and relevant review of the literature.	HINT: Use secondary sources sparingly; noting that secondary sources—especially of studies that include a research critique—are particularly valuable learning tools for beginning consumers of research.

BOX 5–3 Examples of Nursing Journals for Literature Reviews*

Advances in Nursing Science
Applied Nursing Research
Canadian Journal of Neuroscience Nursing
 (formerly AXON)
Canadian Journal of Nursing Leadership
Canadian Journal of Nursing Research
Canadian Journal of Public Health
Canadian Journal on Aging
Canadian Nurse
Canadian Oncology Nursing Journal
Canadian Operating Room Journal
Clinical Nurse Specialist
Clinical Nursing Research
Evidence-Based Nursing
Geriatric Nursing
International Journal of Nursing Studies
Issues in Comprehensive Pediatric Nursing
Issues in Mental Health Nursing
Journal of Advanced Nursing
Journal of Clinical Nursing

Journal of Neonatal Nursing
Journal of Nursing Administration (JONA)
Journal of Nursing Care Quality
Journal of Nursing Education
Journal of Nursing Scholarship (formerly Image:
 Journal of Nursing Scholarship)
Journal of Obstetric, Gynecologic and Neonatal
 Nursing
Journal of Professional Nursing
Journal of Qualitative Research
Journal of Transcultural Nursing
Nurse Educator
Nursing Management
Nursing Outlook
Nursing Research
Nursing Science Quarterly
Qualitative Health Research
Research in Nursing & Health
Scholarly Inquiry for Nursing Practice
Western Journal of Nursing Research

*Main focus of these journals: Provide peer-reviewed articles, primary sources of research studies and conceptual articles, and resources for some secondary sources (e.g., extensive reviews of literature on a particular concept) and issues, as well as responses or critiques of data-based and conceptual articles. Most of the journals in this list are refereed; all can be searched through the Cumulative Index to Nursing and Allied Health Literature (CINAHL), PubMed, and MEDLINE, as well as other health-related computer and print databases. Note also that many of the articles found in these journals are available online.

TABLE 5–4 Conceptual and Data-Based Examples of Primary and Secondary Journal Articles, Books, Chapters in Books, and Documents

Primary	Secondary
Journal Article	**Journal Commentary**
Forchuk, C., Martin, M. L., Chan, Y. L., & Jensen, E. (2005). Therapeutic relationships: From psychiatric hospital to community. *Journal of Psychiatric and Mental Health Nursing, 12,* 556–564. (see Appendix A)	Edwards, N., & Aminzadeh, F. (2003). [Commentary on the article "Prediction of fracture in nursing home residents" by C. J. Girman, J. M. Chandler, S. I. Zimmerman, et al.]. *Evidence-Based Nursing, 6*(2): 58.
Book	**Book**
Watson, J. (1999). *Postmodern nursing and beyond.* Toronto: Churchill Livingstone. (conceptual)	Alligood, M., & Tomey, A. (2006). *Nursing theory: Utilization and application.* Toronto: Elsevier.
Chapter in a Book	**Chapter in a Book**
Thorne, S. (2006). Theoretical foundations of nursing practice. In J. Ross-Kerr & M. Wood (Eds.), *Canadian fundamentals of nursing* (3rd ed., pp. 66–79). Toronto: Elsevier.	Jesse, R. (2006). Watson's philosophy in nursing practice. In M. Alligood & A. Tomey (Eds.). *Nursing theory: Utilization and application* (pp. 103–130). Toronto: Elsevier.
Doctoral Dissertation	**Documents**
Cameron, C. (2003). *The lived experience of transfer students in a collaborative baccalaureate nursing program.* Unpublished doctoral dissertation, University of Toronto, Toronto, Canada.	Registered Nurses' Association of Ontario. (2006). *Nursing Best Practice Guideline: Establishing therapeutic relationships.* Toronto: Author. Retrieved September 17, 2007, from http://www.rnao.org/Page.asp?PageID=924&ContentID=801
Document	Health Canada. (2003a). *The report of the National Advisory Committee on SARS and Public Health.* Ottawa: Health Canada.
Canadian Nurses Association. (2002). *Code of ethics.* Ottawa: Canadian Nurses Association.	

often feature full-text articles) are now standard practice. Moreover, most libraries have the ability to copy an article and mail or fax it to the person requesting the information. The other reason secondary sources are consulted is that they offer different ways of looking at an issue or problem. Secondary sources can help you develop the ability to see topics, problems, and issues from another person's point of view, which is an essential aspect of critical reading (Paul & Elder, 2001). As previously mentioned, however, secondary sources should not be overused, especially for literature reviews.

Secondary sources published in refereed journals usually provide a critical evaluation of, or a response to, a theory or research study. These sources typically include implications for practice and the work's contributions to the development of nursing science. For example, some issues of the *Western Journal of Nursing Research* contain a critique, entitled "Commentary," that follows a published study; the author of the study is given an opportunity to respond to the critique. The *Annual Review of Nursing Research* (see Fitzpatrick, Shandor, & Holditch-Davis, 2003) is another source of critiqued research. Another secondary source for research evidence information presented in a distilled format is the journal *Evidence-Based Nursing*. In this journal, strict criteria for the quality and validity of research are applied to reviewed studies, and practising clinicians assess the strength of evidence and clinical relevance of the best studies. The key details of these essential studies are presented in a succinct, informative abstract with an expert commentary on the clinical application of the research study's findings.

Secondary sources, especially those mentioned above, are credible and time-saving tools that can help nurses keep up with the latest evidence for practice. As stressed earlier, however, although asking faculty, advisors, or librarians about secondary sources is an effective way to secure an appropriate primary resource, those conducting literature reviews must read *primary* sources and use standardized critiquing criteria to develop research critiquing competencies.

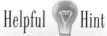

Helpful Hint

Remember that a secondary source of a theory- or data-based study usually does not include all of the theory's concepts or aspects of a study, and definitions may not be fully presented. If concepts or variables are included in a secondary source, the definitions may have been collapsed or paraphrased. If the purpose, findings, and recommendations are presented in a secondary source, even if it is a literature review, these may have been collapsed or paraphrased to such a degree that they no longer represent the researcher's original study. If the critique (whether positive or negative) is based on the condensed summary or abstract, it is less useful to the consumer. Remember, one study on a topic does not prove anything. Be cautious when a nurse colleague tells you to change your practice based on the results of one study. Read a primary data-based study and a secondary source critique on the same study and compare your critique with the critique of the secondary source.

SYSTEMATIC REVIEWS

In addition to the literature review that appears within a study and published reviews of the literature that summarize, critique, and synthesize prior research, another type of literature review exists: a **systematic review**. A systematic review is a methodology that adheres to explicit and rigorous methods to identify, critically appraise, and synthesize relevant primary or original studies (Mulrow, Cook, & Davidoff, 1997). In general, "systematic reviews differ from other types of (literature) reviews in that they [systematic reviews] adhere to a strict scientific design in order to make them more comprehensive, to minimize the chance of bias, and so ensure their reliability" (*Systematic Reviews*, pp. 3–7). Systematic reviews or evidence summaries produce the best available objective evidence on a topic (Albanese & Norcini, 2002). Generally, since 1995, systematic reviews have used rigorous scientific methods.

However, this type of evidence still must be examined through your evidence-based practice "lens." Thus, evidence that you have derived through your critical analysis and synthesis or through another researcher's systematic review must be integrated with an individual clinician's expertise and clients' wishes (DiCenso, 2003; Sackett, Straus, Richardson, Rosenberg, & Haynes, 2000).

The main purpose of systematic reviews is to offer clinicians the best available evidence to make sound clinical judgements for their clients. Systematic reviews are key to developing evidence-based practice protocols. Two types of systematic reviews exist: quantitative and qualitative. A **qualitative systematic review** does not use statistical methods to combine the findings. An example of a qualitative systematic review is found in the studies by Scott et al. (2003), which examined interventions for improving communication with children and adolescents about a family member's cancer. A systematic review that employs statistical methods to combine the findings of at least two or more studies is usually referred to as a **meta-analysis** or **quantitative systematic review**.

An analysis of the Cochrane Reviews, using the *Cumulative Index to Nursing and Allied Health Literature* (CINAHL), revealed 10 systematic reviews related to nursing. Of the 10 reviews, 3 had used quantitative meta-analyses: "Cot-Nursing versus Incubator Care for Preterm Infants" (Gray & Flenady, 2001), "Nursing Interventions for Smoking Cessation" (Rice & Stead, 2004), and "Home Care by Outreach Nursing for Chronic Obstructive Pulmonary Disease (COPD)" (Smith, Appleton, Adams, Southcott, & Ruffin, 2001). The other seven systematic reviews, classified as Cochrane Reviews, used qualitative criteria to judge the studies because of a lack of sufficient data for quantitative analysis, such as a small number of studies or too many methodological problems (e.g., Forster, Smith, Young, Knapp, House, & Wright, 2000). Both qualitative and quantitative systematic reviews share the following characteristics:

- *Explicity:* Systematic reviews indicate the question the review will address, the method of retrieving primary sources, the selection process, the critiquing criteria, and the techniques to be used to synthesize the findings.

- *Reproducibility:* The use of explicit criteria enables another researcher to use the criteria and draw the same conclusion.
- *Efficiency:* Systematic reviews are an essential information management tool; they condense large amounts of primary or original studies into a manageable objective format.

Evidence-Based Practice Tip

Reading systematic reviews, if available on your clinical question or topic, will enhance your ability to implement evidence-based nursing practice because they generally offer the strongest and most consistent level of evidence.

Although you will encounter the term *systematic review* most frequently when retrieving literature, you will likely also encounter two other terms that could be confused with a traditional literature review: **evidence synthesis** and **integrative review**. Evidence synthesis, which is used by the Agency for Healthcare Research and Quality (2000), employs essentially the same rigorous process as the systematic review; whereas an integrative review, although similar to a systematic review, is a broader, sometimes less rigorous, nonquantitative method to systematically combine the results from a body of studies. The review by Li, Mazurek, and McCann (2004) of nine intervention studies of families with hospitalized elderly relatives is an example of an integrative review.

Although a traditional review is not the same as a systematic review, when conducting a literature search, systematic reviews should be included as often as possible because they represent the best available evidence on that topic (see the section on Level I evidence in Table 3–3 of Chapter 3). Because nursing research is a growing field, you may find that your particular clinical or research question is not addressed by systematic reviews, which typically have a medical focus. If you are having difficulty locating a systematic review, access

The Cochrane Database of Systematic Reviews (http://www.cochrane.org/reviews/clibintro.htm)."

The *British Medical Journal* (*BMJ*), another international source for the best available clinical evidence for effective health care, will be useful for nurses at basic and advanced practice levels when conducting a review of the literature on a clinical topic. *BMJ* provides print updates twice a year, including a CD, and updates are extended monthly at http://www.clinicalevidence.com. Remember that although you may believe that the literature review you wrote for a class assignment was systematically researched and written, you should not confuse it with a systematic review.

REVIEW OF THE LITERATURE:
Research Consumer Perspective

As a consumer of research, you are not expected to write a complete review of the literature on your own. However, you are expected to know how to conduct a literature review and critically evaluate it. Understanding the purpose(s) of a literature review for research and research consumer purposes will enable you to meet beginner's goals. In your basic research course, you develop novice competencies in understanding and evaluating research findings that have implications for your practice. Embedded in the purposes of a literature review is the ability to do the following:

- Efficiently retrieve an adequate amount of scholarly literature using electronic databases. Some electronic databases that can be accessed via the Internet are *Cumulative Index to Nursing and Allied Health Literature* (CINAHL), MEDLINE, and the Cochrane Database of Systematic Reviews; a multitude of health information is also available on the World Wide Web. You should also explore traditional print resources for material not entered into common electronic databases.

- Critically evaluate data-based and conceptual material based on accepted critiquing criteria for reviewing the respective literature.

- Synthesize the critically evaluated literature according to your level of educational competence.

When reading a literature review, use the objectives listed in Box 5–1 (on p. 86) to help you focus the activity. Table 5–5 presents an overview of the steps required when conducting a literature search. In the right-hand column, you will find some useful tips and strategies or rationales for successfully completing these steps. This process is the same whether the purpose is critiquing or writing a literature review; the process reflects the cognitive processes and manual techniques of retrieving and critically reviewing literature sources. The remainder of this chapter presents the essential material for accomplishing these goals.

SCHOLARLY LITERATURE

Conceptual and Data-Based Literature: Synonyms and Sources

Synonyms for conceptual and data-based scholarly literature are presented in Table 5–6. The term **theoretical literature** is most often interchanged with **conceptual literature**, whereas the terms **empirical literature**, **scientific literature**, and **research literature** are interchanged with **data-based literature**. Table 5–7 presents definitions and examples of conceptual and data-based literature.

The usual sources of theoretical or conceptual literature are books, chapters of books, and journal articles. The most common sources of data-based literature are journal articles, critique reviews, abstracts published in conference proceedings, professional and governmental reports, and unpublished doctoral dissertations. Many data-based and conceptual articles are available online in full-text format. Full-text articles are usually available when you conduct an electronic search of databases; if your college or university subscribes

TABLE 5–5 Steps and Strategies for Searching the Literature

Steps of the Literature Review	Strategy
Step I: Determine the concept, issue, topic, or problem.	Keep focused on the types of clients you deal with in your practice setting. You know what works and what does not work in the delivery of nursing care. In your student role, keep focused on the assignment's objective; use the literature to support opinions or develop a concept under discussion.
Step II: Identify variables and terms.	Ask your reference librarian for help and read the data-based guidebooks usually found near the computers used for student searches; include "research" as one of your variables.
Step III: Conduct a computer search using fee-based recognized databases (electronic [online or CD-ROM], print, or both).	Do the search yourself or with the help of your librarian; use at least two health-related databases, such as CINAHL, MEDLINE, or PubMed.
Step IV: Weed out irrelevant sources before printing.	Scan through your search, read the abstracts provided, and mark only those that fit your topic; select "references," "search history," and "full-text articles" if available, prior to printing your search, downloading it, or e-mailing it to yourself.
Step V: Organize sources from printout for retrieval.	Organize your sources by journal type and year and reread the abstracts to determine whether the articles chosen are relevant and worth retrieving.
Step VI: Retrieve relevant sources.	If an article is available online or in journals or microfiche, scan its abstract before printing or copying it to determine whether it is worth your time and money to retrieve.
Step VII: Copy or print articles.	Save yourself time and money; purchase a library copy card ahead of time or bring adequate change to complete the task. Copy the entire article (including the references), making sure that you can clearly read the name of the journal, year, volume number, and pages. Having a copy of the article will save an immense amount of time when preparing your paper.
Step VIII: Conduct preliminary reading and weed out irrelevant sources.	Review the critical reading strategies (see Chapter 3). For example, read the abstract at the beginning of the Samuels-Dennis (2006) article.
Step IX: Critically read each source (summarize and critique each source).	Use the critical reading strategies from Chapter 3 (e.g., use a standardized critiquing tool); take the time to summarize each source (no more than one page long); include the reference in APA style at the top or bottom of each abstract; and attach the copied article to the back of the summary.
Step X: Synthesize critical summaries of each article.	Decide how you will present your synthesis of the reviewed articles (e.g., chronologically, according to type [data based or conceptual]) and compile the synthesized material and a reference list.

TABLE 5–6 Literature Review Synonyms

Conceptual Literature	Data-Based Literature
Theoretical literature	Empirical literature
Scholarly nonresearch literature	Scientific literature
Scholarly literature	Research literature
Soft versus hard science	Scholarly research literature
Literature review article	Research study
Analysis article	Concept analysis (as methodology)
Integrative review	Study

TABLE 5–7 Types of Information Sources for a Literature Review*	
Conceptual Literature	**Data-Based Literature**
Published articles; documents; chapters in books; or books discussing theories, conceptual frameworks or conceptual models, concept(s), constructs, or theorems	Published quantitative and qualitative studies, including concept analysis or methodology studies on a concept; such material is found in journals, monographs, or books that are directly or indirectly related to the problem of interest
Literature reviews of a concept that include both conceptual and data-based critiques	Unpublished studies, such as master's theses and doctoral dissertations
Proceedings, audiotapes, and DVDs from scholarly conferences containing abstracts of a conceptual paper or the entire conceptual presentation	Unpublished research abstracts or entire studies from print, audio, and online sources: proceedings of conferences, compendiums, home pages of professional organizations, or listservs
Web-based online articles and information from professional organizations and provincial and federal agencies	

*Many of the examples given are or will be available online.

to a journal, you can obtain the article online; if not, request it through an interlibrary loan. An example of a free, peer-reviewed, international, online publication that addresses pertinent topics affecting nursing practice, research, and education and the wider health care sector is *The Online Journal of Issues in Nursing* (*OJIN*) (see http://www.ana.org/ojin/). Both MEDLINE and CINAHL index this journal. The Sigma Theta Tau International Honor Society of Nursing also has a new online knowledge magazine, *Excellence in Nursing Knowledge* (*ENK*). The inaugural issue is posted at http://www.nursingknowledge.org/enk. Although quarterly summaries are free, a small fee is charged for each issue.

Examples of Theoretical Material

Some conceptual or theoretical articles do not use the term *conceptual* in the title, yet, on close review, these articles do, in fact, provide extensive literature reviews of both conceptual and data-based articles on a specific concept or variable; they are usually not exhaustive reviews. You may see the terms *literature review* and *review of the literature* used interchangeably; the term *integrative review* is also used, but many literature review articles do not employ the broad criteria of an integrative review previously discussed.

Evidence-Based Practice Tip

The differences between data-based and conceptual articles will become clear as you learn about the various types of quantitative and qualitative designs and discover that some research journals include theoretical articles and research articles. As a rule of thumb, even if a research study does not obtain significant findings, it is still considered a data-based article. Also, conceptual articles do not use terminology such as design, sample, experimental and control group, or methodology as headings. When in doubt, ask your reference librarian or a faculty member to help you. Asking for clarification is a true sign of a critical thinker (Paul & Elder, 2001).

For example, Moorhead, Johnson, and Maas (2004) conducted a literature review of both data-based and conceptual articles related to the effect of nursing research on diagnostic-specific outcomes. Greenway's (2004) conceptual article on using the ventrogluteal site for intramuscular (IM) injection reviewed 21 data-based and conceptual articles from the United Kingdom, the United States, and Canada. This review included Beyea and Nicoll's (1996) classic literature review related to the administration of IM injections, which reviewed more than 90 studies related to IM injections from the 1920s to 1995. Greenway stated that the purpose of this literature review was to change nursing's common practice from using the dorsogluteal site for IM injections to the evidence-based ventrogluteal site.

Another example of a literature review is the review by Fisher (2004) on health disparities and mental retardation. Although search strategies to retrieve both conceptual and data-based articles between 1992 and 2002 were specified, specific critiquing criteria of 33 of the 54 data-based studies retrieved were not identified.

Do not assume that because an article's abstract uses terms such as *purpose*, *organizing framework*, *findings*, and *conclusions* that it is a research study. For example, these terms were used in the abstract of the conceptual article by Ferguson (2004) that examined the concepts of external validity and generalizability related to research findings.

Data-Based Material

The discipline of nursing has an ever-growing body of data-based or research literature that focuses on testing various concepts, theories, or models, as well as a variety of variables related to the practice of nursing. Data-based articles are primary sources. For example, studies have tested components of Peplau's theory of "interpersonal relations in nursing" (1952, 1991), such as the work of Forchuk (1994), Forchuk and Voorberg (1991), Forchuk et al. (2000), Forchuk, Martin, Chan & Jensen (2005), and Peden (1993, 1996, 1998). The following are data-based articles that appear in the appendices of this book and focus on various aspects of client problems and nursing interventions:

- Forchuk et al. (2005) determined the cost and effectiveness of a transitional discharge model of care for clients who have a chronic mental illness (see Appendix A).
- Smith, Edwards, Varcoe, Martens, and Davies (2006) investigated the experiences of two Aboriginal organizations in improving care for pregnant and parenting Aboriginal people (see Appendix B).
- Samuels-Dennis (2006) assessed the association of employment, stressful life events, and depression among single mothers (see Appendix C).

- Bottorff, Johnson, Moffat, Grewal, Ratner, and Kalaw (2004) explored how adolescents view nicotine addition (see Appendix D).

Data-based articles may specifically indicate in their titles that a study was conducted, but more often they do not. You can determine whether an article is data based in several ways. First, read the title and look for keywords that suggest testing (e.g., effect, relationship, evaluation, exploration, cross-sectional, or longitudinal) or, in quantitative studies, look for the description and interpretation of human phenomena. Next, check which journal published the article. A number of journals predominantly publish research articles (e.g., *Canadian Journal of Nursing Research*, *Applied Nursing Research*, and *Research in Nursing and Health*).

Although these tips can be helpful in determining whether the article is data based, the only 100% reliable method of determining whether an article is data based is to read the abstract and the article. The abstracts of the studies that appear in Appendices A, B, C, and D indicate that each of these studies represents reports of completed studies. Another helpful tip to enable you to implement an evidence-based practice is to include "research" as one of your electronic search strategies (see the section of this chapter on conducting electronic searches). If you are still not clear whether the article is data based from reading the abstract or scanning the article, review the criteria for evaluating a qualitative study and a quantitative study (see p. 28).

Refereed Journals

A major portion of most literature reviews consists of journal articles. Journals are a ready source of the latest information on almost any conceivable subject. Unfortunately, books and texts—despite the inclusion of multiple data-based sources—take much longer to publish than journals. Therefore, journals are the preferred mode of communicating the latest theory or the results of a research study.

As a beginning consumer of research, you should use **refereed (peer-reviewed) journals** as your first source of primary scholarly literature.

A refereed journal is one in which a panel of external and internal reviewers (i.e., peer reviewers) or editors review submitted manuscripts for possible publication. The external reviewers for nursing journals are drawn from a pool of nurse scholars who are experts in various fields. In most cases, peer reviews are "blind," meaning that the manuscript (i.e., a research study or conceptual article) to be reviewed does not include the name of the author(s). The review panels use a set of scholarly criteria to judge whether a manuscript is worthy of publication; these criteria are similar to those used to judge the strengths and weaknesses of a study (see Chapters 18 and 19). Consequently, the credibility of the reported research or conceptual article is enhanced through the peer-review process.

For example, *Cochrane Systematic Reviews* published Nixon, O'Brien, Glazier, and Tynan's (2004) systematic review on aerobic exercise interventions for adults living with human immunodeficiency virus (HIV) or acquired immune deficiency syndrome (AIDS). The authors reviewed studies conducted between 1991 and 2002 and rejected some based on exclusion criteria. If you were conducting a literature review on this same topic, you would include Nixon et al.'s (2004) systematic review as well as studies not retrieved for their review; in other words, your search would cover studies published after 2002.

CONDUCTING A SEARCH AS A CONSUMER OF RESEARCH

In your student role, when you are preparing an academic paper, you read the required course materials and the additional literature retrieved from the library. Students often think that they know how to do research. Perhaps you have thought the same thing because you "researched" a topic for a paper in the library. In this situation, however, it would be more accurate to say that you have been "searching" the literature to uncover data-based and conceptual information to prepare an academic term paper on a certain topic.

Although reviewing the literature for research purposes requires the same critical thinking and reading skills as research consumer activities, a literature review for a research proposal is usually much more extensive and comprehensive, and the critiquing process is more in-depth. From an academic standpoint, the requirements of a literature review for a particular assignment differ depending on the level and type of course and the specific objective of the assignment. These factors determine whether a student's literature search requires a minor (or limited), selected, major, cursory, or extensive review. Regardless, discovering knowledge is the goal of any "search"; therefore, a consumer of research must know how to search the literature. Reference librarians are excellent people to ask about various sources of scholarly literature. If you are unfamiliar with the process of conducting a scholarly computer search, your reference librarian can certainly help.

Before the 1980s, literature searches were usually conducted by hand (a tedious and time-consuming process) using **print indexes** or **print databases**. Print indexes actually represent only a small portion of the available electronic literature because the electronic format has virtually unlimited space. Print indexes, however, are useful for finding sources that have not been entered into electronic databases. **Electronic databases** are used to find journal sources (periodicals) of data-based and conceptual articles on a variety of topics (e.g., doctoral dissertations), as well as the publications of professional organizations and various governmental agencies. Box 5–4 lists examples of the more commonly used electronic databases.

Most college and university libraries have an electronic card catalogue, such as BobCat, to find books, journals (titles only), DVDs and other media items, scripts, monographs, conference proceedings, masters' theses, dissertations, and archival materials. Card catalogues are rarely used except for dates not entered into electronic sources, which are most often accessed via the Web for direct online use. Your school library most likely enables

BOX 5–4	**Common Databases**

INDEXES

Cumulative Index to Nursing and Allied Health Literature (CINAHL)

- Initially called Cumulative Index to Nursing Literature
- First published in 1956
- Print version known as the "Red Books"
- The electronic version is available as part of the OVID online service

Index Medicus (IM)

- Published by the National Library of Medicine in the United States
- Oldest health-related index, first published in 1879
- Includes literature from medicine, allied health, biophysical sciences, humanities, veterinary medicine, and nursing from 1960 to the present
- The electronic version, MEDLINE, covers 1966 to the present and is available on the Web via OVID or PubMed

International Nursing Index (INI)

- Quarterly publication of the American Journal of Nursing Company in cooperation with the National Library of Medicine
- Started in 1966
- Includes over 200 journals of all languages and nursing publications in non-nursing journals

NURSING STUDIES INDEX

- Developed by Virginia Henderson
- Publishes nursing literature and literature from other disciplines, from 1900 to 1959

Hospital and Health Administration Index (HHAI)

- Formerly known as the Hospital Literature Index (HLI)
- First published in 1945 by the American Hospital Association in cooperation with the National Library of Medicine
- Includes over 700 journals and related journals from the IM
- Main focus is hospital administration and delivery of care

Current Index to Journals in Education (CIJE)

- First published in 1969 in cooperation with the Educational Resources Information Center (ERIC)
- The electronic version, ERIC, is available on the Web

Psychological Abstracts

- Covers 1927 to the present
- The electronic version, PsychINFO, is available on the Web

Abstract Reviews

- *Dissertation Abstracts International, Master's Abstracts, Nursing Abstracts, Psychological Abstracts,* and *Sociological Abstracts*

you to access electronic databases from your residence whether it is on or off campus.

CINAHL remains the most relevant and frequently used electronic database for nursing literature from 1982 to the present. CINAHL includes sources from the date each particular database added an electronic version; each electronic database usually indicates the starting date of entries. Print versions of CINAHL, known as the "Red Books," cover all nursing and related literature from 1956 to the present. Note that print resources are still necessary if a

search requires materials not entered into an electronic database before a certain year.

You are probably familiar with accessing a **Web browser** (e.g., Internet Explorer) to access search engines such as Google to find information or articles. However, "surfing" the Web is not a good use of your time for scholarly literature searches. Table 5–8 indicates reliable sources of online information. Review it carefully to determine whether a particular Web source is a reliable source of primary data-based studies. Note, however, that most

Web sites are not a primary source of data-based reports. Through utilization of the Web browser, you may also access scholarly material such as audiotapes, DVDs, personal communications (e.g., letters, telephone interviews, or in-person interviews), unpublished doctoral dissertations, and

TABLE 5–8 **Selected Examples of Web Sites and Outcomes for Literature Searches**		
Site	**Sources**	**Outcomes for Literature Review**
Online Journal of Issues in Nursing: site can be accessed from **http://www.ana.org** and vice versa; online journal owned by Kent University College of Nursing and published in partnership with the American Nurses Association's (ANA) *Nursing World*	Service offered without charge; join by simply entering your e-mail address; the site will keep you posted of new articles; this peer-reviewed electronic journal provides a free discussion forum of issues in nursing	Limited for scholarly review of data-based literature when used as the only source; access only to literature that is published on the *Online Journal Issues in Nursing*; a source of complete articles from this site's journal; articles can be printed; an interesting site for students in beginning courses in nursing (especially in courses in issues and trends) or practising nurses; offers access to nursing's professional nursing association (ANA); journal can be accessed via CINAHL
Sigma Theta Tau International (STTI), Honor Society of Nursing: **http://www.nursingsociety.org**	Visit to update yourself on the news and activities of the society; three online research sources are available through links to Virginia Henderson International Library: *Registry of Nursing Research* (*RNR*), *Online Journal of Knowledge Synthesis for Nursing* (*OJKSN*), and *Nursing Knowledge Indexes*	For a fee, an online literature search via MEDLINE can be requested (see Box 5–5 for the advantages of using CINAHL with MEDLINE); limited for scholarly review of data-based literature if used as the only search tool; *OJKSN* literature is limited to studies published in the STTI online journal; the *RNR* contains over 11,000 English-language international nursing studies, which are not peer-reviewed
National Institute of Nursing Research: **http://www.nih.gov/ninr**	Promotes science for nursing practice, funding for nursing and interdisciplinary research, and nurse scientist training programs; provides links to many nursing organizations and search sites; an excellent site for graduate students	Able to link to CRISP (Computer Retrieval of Information on Scientific Projects) and PubMed (the National Library of Medicine's search service), which accesses literature via MEDLINE and PreMEDLINE and other related material from online journals; a *limited* site for the beginning consumer of research for conducting scholarly review of nursing data-based literature because MEDLINE alone does not include all nursing literature; searching CINAHL and MEDLINE on your own would be your first choice; a useful site for graduate students in addition to CINAHL and MEDLINE and a third database related to your topic
Clinical Evidence: **http://www.clinicalevidence.org**	Fee-based subscription from the British Medical Journal Publishing Group; an online full-text compendium of summaries of current knowledge on clinical conditions based on literature sources and reviews; updated and expanded every six months; each issue is peer-reviewed by a renowned group of international experts	Costly for individuals to subscribe; determine whether your institution's (work or school) library is a subscriber; a limited site for the beginning consumer of research because the site is a "secondary" source of information; instead, choose CINAHL, MEDLINE, and another electronic database (see Box 5–6)

TABLE 5-8 **Selected Examples of Web Sites and Outcomes for Literature Searches (cont'd)**		
Site	**Sources**	**Outcomes for Literature Review**
Cochrane Library: **http://www.cochrane.org**	An electronic publication designed to supply high-quality evidence to inform people providing and receiving care and those responsible for research, teaching, funding, and administration at all levels; includes the Cochrane Database of Systematic Reviews (COCH), Database of Abstracts of Reviews of Effectiveness, the Cochrane Controlled Trials Register, the Cochrane Methodology Register, Health Technology Assessment database (HTA), and the NHS Economic Evaluation Database (NHS EED); considered a database rather than a Web site	Abstracts of Cochrane Reviews are available without charge and can be browsed or searched; Cochrane Library uses many databases in its reviews, including CINAHL and MEDLINE; some are primary sources (e.g., systematic reviews or meta-analyses); others (if commentaries of single studies) are secondary sources; an important source for clinical evidence but limited as a provider of primary documents for literature reviews
Canadian Association for Nursing Research (CANR): **http://www.canr.ca/**	As an interest group of the Canadian Nurses Association, the purpose is to support nursing research through the sharing of studies, methods, funding sources, and other resources	Members may join for a fee, which is reduced for students; membership includes a reduced subscription price for the *Canadian Journal of Nursing Research*; the site provides many links to sources of funding
Statistics Canada: **http://www.statcan.ca/**	Collects data on the Canadian population related to demographic trends, labour, health, trade, and education; data on health trends identify populations at risk and suggest associations among health determinants, health status, and population characteristics; research papers on a variety of topics are also published.	Free source of primary data essential for comprehensive demographic data and socioeconomic trends; updated daily

masters' theses. These materials are not as commonly used as data-based studies but may provide useful information.

Most searches using electronic databases include under the citation itself the option of including a hyperlink to the abstract, the complete reference, OVID full text, or a remote link. When possible, print the full text, which will include the abstract and the complete references. If the text is not available, choose the option *complete reference*, which will include the abstract. Reading the abstract is critical to determining whether you need to retrieve the article through another mechanism. Examples of fee-based databases are listed in Table 5–9.

Helpful Hint

Make an appointment with your educational institution's reference librarian to take advantage of his or her expertise in accessing electronic databases.

When you are doing your electronic search, have an empty or formatted disk at hand so you can download your search and not take up unnecessary room on your computer's hard drive, or e-mail your search to yourself.

Take time to set up your home or residence computer for electronic library access.

If the full text of an article is unavailable through your electronic search, choose the complete reference option so you can read the abstract to determine whether the article is data based.

TABLE 5–9 Examples of Fee-Based Online Databases

Electronic Databases	Sources: Data-Based and Conceptual Literature
CINAHL (*Cumulative Index to Nursing and Allied Health Literature*) • 1982 to present • Available as part of the OVID online service	Citations of articles in journals in the nursing and allied health care fields (e.g., medical technology, health care administration) and publications of the ANA and NLN
MEDLINE (medical literature analysis and retrieval system online) • 1966 to present • Available as part of the OVID online service • On the Web via the PubMed search service	Produced by the National Library of Medicine; citations and some abstracts to articles on health-related topics for over 3600 biomedical and nursing journals; the search service provides access to over 11 million citations in MEDLINE and PreMEDLINE and other related databases, with links to participating online journals
PsychINFO	Covers professional and academic literature in psychology and related disciplines; worldwide coverage of over 1300 journals in 20 languages, and books and chapters in books in English

AACN: American Association of Critical Care Nurses; ANA: American Nurses Association; NLN: National League for Nursing

---

BOX 5–5   Advantages of Using Multiple Online Fee-Based Databases, CINAHL and MEDLINE, for Nurse Consumers of Research*

QUICK

Online information can be instantly accessed, especially if you have a LAN or cable connection (as opposed to a modem or telephone connection). Internet access depends on a number of factors (e.g., the server may be "down," or the number of users can affect your ability to access the information [i.e., the number of users slows down access]). For students in a university or college, access is free via your library.

Overall, using multiple online databases saves time and increases the credibility of the search.

INCREASED ACCESS TO MULTIPLE SOURCES

Using multiple databases allows you to cover a broad scope of sources. CINAHL accesses more than 900,000 records from 1982 to the present (e.g., journals, books, chapters in books, abstracts, software, audiovisuals, index articles from 1777 journals); you can download full text from 33 journals online. MEDLINE is the National Library of Medicine's database of indexed journal citations and abstracts and now covers nearly 4500 journals published in the United States and more than 70 other countries. Available for online searching since 1971, MEDLINE includes references to articles indexed from 1966 to the present. New citations are added weekly.

ALLOWS KEYWORD SEARCHING

Synonyms and related terms are considered; you can use the thesaurus for each database. For data-based literature, include the terms *systematic reviews* and *meta-analysis*. Keep refining your search by combining terms with Boolean connectors (e.g., *and*, *or*, and *not*). CINAHL uses American Nurses Association–approved taxonomy terms.

SOURCE OF ABSTRACTS AND SOME FULL-TEXT ARTICLES AVAILABLE: IMPORTANT SOURCES OF DATA-BASED LITERATURE

CINAHL and MEDLINE provide access to clinical trials, meta-analyses, systematic reviews, methodologies, conceptual frameworks, and variables. All research instruments are identified.

FREQUENT UPDATES

These updates are conducted monthly or weekly.

DOCUMENT RETRIEVAL

Documents can be retrieved via e-mail, downloaded to disk, or delivered via fax or mail for CINAHL direct and PubMed.

*Access time and all features are not available with the print index. From CINAHL Information Systems. (2006). *Recent statistics for the CINAHL database*. Glendale, CA: CINAHL Information Systems. Retrieved September 15, 2007, from http://www.cinahl.com/ and the National Library of Medicine. PubMed information retrieved from http://www.ncbi.nlm.nih.gov/PubMed/

PERFORMING A COMPUTER SEARCH

Why a Computer Search?

Perhaps you are still not convinced that computer searches are the best way to acquire information for a review of the literature. Maybe you have gone to the library, taken out a few of the latest journals, and tried to find some related articles. This temptation is understandable, especially if your assignment requires you to use only five articles. Think about it from another perspective and ask yourself: "Is this approach the most appropriate and efficient way to find the latest and strongest research on a topic that affects client care?" If you take the time to learn how to conduct a sound electronic search, you will have the essential competency needed for your career in nursing. The Critical Thinking Decision Path will help you avoid the pitfall of missing important studies because you chose the hands-on strategy of looking at the index of the most recent journals. Box 5–5 presents the advantages of using at least two electronic databases (CINAHL and MEDLINE).

Helpful 💡 Hint

The use of at least two electronic health-related databases, such as CINAHL and MEDLINE (see Box 5–5), is recommended.

How Far Back Must the Search Go?

Students often ask "How many articles do I need?" "How much is enough?" and "How far back in the literature do I need to go?" When conducting a search, you must specify the range of years for the search (e.g., 1991 to 2003) and the variables (i.e., keywords) and other factors (e.g., "research," "abstract," or "full text"), or you may end up with hundreds or thousands of citations. Retrieving too many citations is usually a sign that your search technique needs improvement. Each electronic database offers an explanation of every feature; it is worth your time to click on each icon and

explore the explanations to increase your confidence and skills.

For most academic or evidence-based practice papers or projects, go back in the literature at least three years but preferably five years—although a research project may warrant going back 10 or more years if the topic has not been extensively researched or the historical perspective is important. Extensive literature reviews on particular topics or a concept clarification methodology study helps you to limit the length of your search.

As you scroll through and mark the citations you wish to include in your downloaded or printed search, make sure you review all fields of the citation manager. In addition to indicating which citations you want and choosing which fields to search (e.g., citation plus abstract or ASCII full text, if available), an opportunity exists to indicate whether you want the "search history" included. It is always a good idea to include this information in your paper. If your instructor suggests that some citations were missed, you can then produce your search and together determine what variable(s) you overlooked so that you do not make the same error the next time. Scrolling through and marking the citations is also your opportunity to indicate whether you want to e-mail the literature search to yourself.

What Do I Need to Know?

Helpful 💡 Hint

First, think of conducting a CINAHL computer search. It can facilitate all steps of critically reviewing the literature, especially Steps III, IV, and V (see Table 5–5).

Each database typically includes a specific search guide that provides information on the organization of the entries and the terminology used. The following suggestions and strategies incorporate general search strategies, as well as those related to CINAHL and MEDLINE. Finding the right variables, concepts, and terms to "plug in" as keywords for a computer search is an important aspect of conducting a search. Both CINAHL and MEDLINE

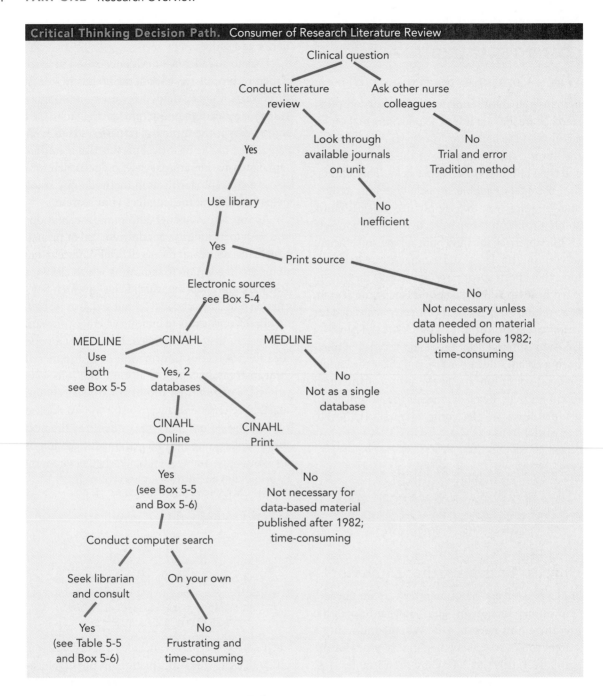

Critical Thinking Decision Path. Consumer of Research Literature Review

are user friendly: they have "explode" features, which means that you can search multiple headings with a single command. Another feature of CINAHL programming is its mapping capability. If the term you use is not exactly the same as the term used in the database, the program maps or connects you to a term nearest to what you typed in (CINAHL Information Systems, 2004). Both databases have assigned index terms, known in CINAHL as *medical headings* and in MEDLINE as *MeSH*. It is important to combine index terms and to expect to do a number of search histories. This description may sound as if the literature search will take a great deal of time, but it does not. Once you type in your keywords and choose "perform search," the results come up almost instantly. If you are still having difficulty, do not hesitate to ask your reference librarian.

Box 5–6 offers a quick overview of how user friendly these two databases are. The box provides helpful hints that take you through the steps of a search. Implementing an evidence-based nursing practice requires developing efficient electronic search skills. This particular protocol is based on using CINAHL and MEDLINE. Of course, the specifics may differ in your institution, but more similarities than differences exist. The example

given in Table 5–10 indicates the number of citations retrieved using two databases at once, CINAHL and MEDLINE. After choosing the tab on the menu entitled "Choose more than one database," the keywords "anxiety disorders" and "treatment" were entered and limited to the years 1996 to 2004; then the search was performed. As indicated in Table 5–10, the first search (#1) revealed 18,255 citations, which is a good indication that the keywords did not narrow the search sufficiently. This is far too many citations to scroll through. In addition to the number of citations retrieved, the first few citations usually appear. In this example, the first few were found in the CINAHL database. In

---

BOX 5–6   Helpful Hints: Using CINAHL and MEDLINE Online via OVID

- Connect to your library's electronic databases via your Internet server. Choose "Health Sciences Related Database" or determine which general category houses CINAHL on the menu. Then hit "Enter."

- An alphabetical list of databases usually appears. Scroll down to "CINAHL." In the next column, the source of the database is indicated (e.g., on the Web); place your cursor on this term and hit "Enter."

- The "Choose a Database" menu will appear. You can either choose one database or select the tab that indicates that you can choose more than one database. It is recommended that you use at least two databases. Choose "Select more than one database to search."

- Once the next menu pops up, mark each of the databases you wish to search (e.g., CINAHL [1982 to current] and MEDLINE [1996 to current]).

- The top of the next screen will indicate that you are using the CINAHL and MEDLINE databases. The screen will ask you to type in the keyword or phrase for your search history. Do not hesitate to explore the various icons that appear at the top of the menu. You can search by author, title, or particular journal. Another useful icon is the "?" or "Help" icon.

- Type in your keyword or phrase (e.g., "nursing intervention and depression"). Do not use complete sentences. (Ask your librarian for the manual guide for each database.)

- Each word is searched separately, and "hits" (i.e., a set of corresponding items) are created for each word.

- Before choosing "Perform search," make sure you mark "Save search history," limit the years of publication according to the objectives of your assignment, and indicate whether you are limiting the search to "Research," "Abstracts," or both, or "Full text available."

- See the results in Table 5–10 that used the terms "depression" and "treatment": 18,255 citations were retrieved. This first history did not "limit," as is suggested here. Before performing the search, the program may ask you to limit your search by providing keywords or phrases to mark either "focus" or "explode" (i.e., narrowing or broadening your search).

- Add additional variables to narrow your search (e.g., "nursing intervention"). Mark any additional limitations by typing in the "Keyword" box "#1" and "nursing intervention" and marking the appropriate "limit to" categories.

- Using the Boolean connector *and* between each of the above words you wish to use plus additional variables narrows your search. Using the Boolean connector *or* broadens your search.

- Boolean connectors save time because you do not have to retype each search word.

- Once the search results appear and you determine that they are manageable, you can decide whether to review them on screen, print them, save them to disk, or e-mail them to yourself.

the second search (#2), the keywords were combined (e.g., "depression and treatment" and "nursing intervention and adults"). The third search was limited to the years 1999 to 2004 and yielded 12,216 citations. Table 5–10 indicates that the fourth search history (#4) revealed a more useful number of retrievals (nine). Using the Boolean connector "and" with "nursing" along with checking "research" resulted in 14 research citations for search number two (see the explanation of the Boolean connector "and" in Box 5–6). Although none of the citations was full text, at this point, you can easily read through the abstracts to determine whether the articles should be retrieved through library retrieval, that is, very quickly if your library subscribes to the journal or through interlibrary loan. Having copies of the articles will allow you to organize them for priority critical reading.

The final number of nine (see Table 5–10) is a manageable number of results to review on screen by quickly reading the abstracts and marking some for print retrieval. Remember to mark off the appropriate circles in the "citation," "fields," "citation format," and "action" columns and to check off the box "include search history" before printing your search. The "complete reference" option should be checked in the "fields" column; although this option makes for a long printing job, you will often come across a classic document or one that was not entered in the **computer database** because it was published before 1982. If you intend to download your search or to e-mail the results, make sure you include this option. When you upload the search onto your computer, you will be able to retrieve all of your references and the references of each entry, into your word-processing program. Think how much time you will save! Your reference list will be typed, and you will only have to edit the material according to the style, such as APA, required by your instructor.

TABLE 5–10 Example of a CINAHL, MEDLINE, and OVID Search

STEP 1: INITIAL TRY

#	Search History	Results	Display
1	(depression and treatment). mp. [mp = ti, sh, ab, it, ot, rw]	18,255	Display

0 Saved Searches   0 Save Search History   0 Delete Searches   0 Remove Duplicates

Enter Keyword or Phrase

	Perform Search

Limit to:
 Abstracts   Consumer Health Journals   English Language
 Full Text Available   Review Articles Human   Latest Update   Research
Publication Year

	⇓		⇑	

Ask A Librarian

STEP 2: SECOND TRY

#	Search History	Results	Display
2	Limit 14 to research (limit not valid in OVID, MEDLINE; records were retained)	16,874	Display
3	Limit 15 to years 1999–2004	12,216	Display
4	Limit 16 to nursing research.mp. [mp = ti, sh, ab, it, ot, rw]	9	Display

Modified from CINAHL, MEDLINE, OVID search.

You can also use the thesaurus to "focus" (narrow) or "explode" (broaden) your search. "Focus" limits the search to articles that contain the subject heading you identified, whereas "explode" permits you to search related subject headings with a single command.

How Do I Complete the Search?

Now the truly important aspect of the search begins: your critical reading of the retrieved materials. Critically reading scholarly material, especially data-based articles, requires several readings and the use of critiquing criteria (see Chapters 3, 9, and 19). Do not be discouraged if all of the retrieved articles are not as useful as you first thought; even the most experienced researcher discovers this. If most of the articles are not useful, be prepared to do another search but discuss the variables you will use with your instructor, the reference librarian, or both; you may also want to add a third database. In the previous example of interventions with adults diagnosed with depression (see Table 5–10), the third database of choice could be PsychINFO (see Table 5–9). Remind yourself how quickly you will be able to do the search, now that you are experienced.

Helpful Hint

Read the abstract carefully; review the discussion on critical reading strategies in Chapter 3 to determine whether the article is a data-based article. It is also a good idea to review the references of your articles; if any of the references seem relevant, you can retrieve them.

LITERATURE REVIEW FORMAT: What to Expect

Becoming familiar with the format of the literature review helps research consumers use critiquing criteria to evaluate the review. To decide which style you will use so that your review is presented in a logical and organized manner, you must consider the following:

- The research question or topic
- The number of retrieved sources reviewed
- The number and type of data-based versus conceptual materials

Some reviews are written according to the variables being studied and are presented chronologically under each variable. Other reviews present the material chronologically with subcategories or variables discussed within each period. Still other reviews present the variables and include subcategories related to the study's type or design or related variables.

An example of a literature review that is logically presented according to the variables under study was completed by Tourangeau, Giovannetti, Tu, and Wood (2002). The researchers stated that they were briefly describing hospital variables that were associated with client mortality. Beginning with research on hospitals that formed the basis of their understanding, they focused on later studies that considered nursing-related factors. The authors labelled the section "Literature Review."

In contrast to the styles of previous quantitative studies, the literature reviews of qualitative studies are usually handled in a different manner (see Chapters 7 and 8). Often, little is known about the topic under study, or the very nature of the qualitative design dictates that a review of the literature be conducted after the study is completed; the researchers then compare the literature review with their findings. In some cases, the reviewed literature is used during the analysis process. For example, Bournes and Mitchell's (2002) phenomenological study presented the experiences of family members in a critical care waiting room. These researchers used the reviewed literature related to the study in their "Discussion" section.

Evidence-Based Practice Tip

Sort the research articles you retrieve according to the levels of evidence defined in Chapter 3. Remember that articles that are systematic reviews, especially meta-analyses, generally provide the strongest and most consistent evidence to include in a literature review.

Critiquing **Criteria** for a **Review** of the **Literature**

As you analyze (critique) a scholarly report, you must use appropriate criteria. If you are reading a research study, it must be evaluated in terms of each step of the research process. The characteristics of a relevant review of the literature (see Box 5–2) and the purposes of the review of the literature (see Box 5–1) provide the framework for developing the evaluation criteria for a literature review. Difficulties that research consumers might have regarding this task and related strategies are presented after a discussion of the critiquing criteria. For a more in-depth discussion of critiquing criteria, see Chapters 18 and 19.

Critiquing the literature review of data-based or conceptual reports is a challenging task even for experienced consumers of research, so do not be surprised if you feel a little intimidated by the prospect of critiquing the published research of doctorally educated researchers. Critiquing criteria have been developed for all aspects of the quantitative research process, for various quantitative designs

and qualitative approaches, and for research consumer projects for educational and clinical settings. Critiquing criteria for the review of the literature are usually presented from the perspective of the quantitative research process. Because the focus of this book is on the baccalaureate nurse in the research consumer role, the critiquing criteria for the literature review incorporate this frame of reference. The processes used in qualitative studies are presented in Chapter 8, and Chapter 19 presents an overview of evaluating quantitative research studies.

When critiquing the literature, the reader needs to determine the overall value of the data-based or conceptual report. Does the review of the literature permeate the report? Does the review of the literature contribute to the significance of the report in relation to nursing theory, research, education, or practice (see Figure 5–1)? The overall question to be answered is, "Does the review of the literature uncover knowledge?" This question is based on the

CRITIQUING CRITERIA

1. What gaps or inconsistencies in knowledge does the literature review uncover?

2. How does the review reflect critical thinking?

3. Are all of the relevant concepts and variables included in the review?

4. Does the summary of each reviewed study reflect the essential components of the study design (e.g., in a quantitative design, the type and size of the sample, instruments, validity and reliability; in a qualitative design, does the summary indicate the type [e.g., phenomenological])?

5. Does the critique of each reviewed study include the strengths, weaknesses, or limitations of the design; conflicts; and gaps or inconsistencies in information related to the area of interest?

6. Are both conceptual literature and data-based literature included?

7. Are primary sources mainly used?

8. Is a written summary of the reviewed scholarly literature provided?

9. Does the synthesis summary follow a logical sequence that leads the reader to the rea-

son(s) why the particular research or nonresearch project is needed?

10. Does the organization of the reviewed studies (e.g., chronologically, according to concepts or variables, or by type, design, or level of study) flow logically, enhancing the reader's ability to evaluate the need for the particular research or nonresearch project?

11. Does the literature review follow the purpose(s) of the study or nonresearch project?

overall purpose of a review of the literature, which is to uncover knowledge (see Box 5–1). The major goal turns into the question, "Did the review of the literature provide a strong body of knowledge to carry out the reported research or scholarly educational or clinical practice setting project?" The Critiquing Criteria box provides questions for the consumer of research to ask about the literature review. Whenever possible, read both qualitative and quantitative (meta-analysis) systematic reviews of a clinical question. Remember that although these reviews are a form of research, they also represent a body of research that has been critiqued (analyzed) and summarized through synthesis to represent the best available evidence on a particular clinical problem.

Questions related to the logical presentation of the reviewed articles can be more challenging for beginning consumers of research. The more you read scholarly articles, the easier it is to answer these questions. At times, the type of question being asked lends itself to presenting the reviewed studies chronologically (i.e., perhaps beginning with early or landmark data-based or conceptual literature).

Questions must be asked about whether each explanation of a step of the research process met or did not meet these guidelines (criteria). For instance, Box 5–1 illustrates the overall purposes of a literature review. The second objective states that the review of the literature is to determine gaps, consistencies, and inconsistencies in the literature about a subject, concept, or problem. The Critiquing Criteria box summarizes general critiquing criteria for a review of the literature. Other sets of critiquing criteria may phrase these questions differently, perhaps more broadly. For example, questions may be the following: "Does the literature search seem adequate?" and "Does the report demonstrate scholarly writing?" These questions may seem difficult to answer; one place to begin, however, is by determining whether the source is a refereed journal. It is reasonable to assume that a scholarly refereed journal publishes manuscripts that are adequately searched, use mainly primary sources, and are written

in a scholarly manner. However, not every study reported in a refereed journal will meet all of the critiquing criteria for a literature review and other components of the study in an equal manner. Because of style differences and space constraints, each citation summarized is often very brief, or related citations may be summarized as a group and lack a critique. You still must answer the critiquing questions. Consultation with a faculty advisor may be necessary to develop skill in answering this question.

A literature review in a research article should reflect a synthesis, or pulling together of, the main points or value of all of the sources reviewed in relation to the study's research question (see Box 5–1). The relationships between and among these studies must be explained. The synthesis of a written review of the literature usually appears at the end of the review section, before the research question or hypothesis-reporting section. If not labelled as a literature review, it is usually evident in the last paragraph. Therefore, demonstrating synthesis becomes an essential critiquing criterion for the review of the literature.

Critiquing a review of the literature is an acquired skill. Continued reading and rereading and seeking advice from faculty are essential to developing critiquing skills. Synthesizing the body of literature you have critiqued is even more challenging; in fact, in this era of evidence-based practice, teams of researchers usually conduct systematic reviews. These specialized teams can critique reviews and synthesize literature that meets the proper criteria to be included in the review. If you are not familiar with systematic reviews, take this opportunity to read both a meta-analysis (quantitative systematic review) and a qualitative metasynthesis (a qualitative type of systematic review) (Jensen & Allen, 1996; Melnyk & Fineout-Overholt, 2005). Critiquing the literature will help you transfer new knowledge from your synthesis of research findings into practice. This process is vital to the "survival and growth of the nursing profession and is essential to evidence-based practice" (Pravikoff & Donaldson, 2001).

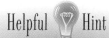

Critical Thinking Challenges

- How can the review of the literature be both an individual step of the research process and a research component used in each step of the process? Support your answer with examples.

- How does a researcher justify using both conceptual and data-based literature in a literature review, and would you—for research consumer purposes (e.g., developing an academic scholarly paper)—use the same types of literature?

- A classmate in your research class tells you that she has access to the Internet and can do all of her searches from home. What essential questions do you need to ask her to determine whether database sources can be accessed?

- An acute care agency's nursing research committee is developing a research-based practice protocol for client-controlled analgesia. One suggestion is to use a Best Practice Guideline on pain, and another is to conduct a review of the literature from the past six years on pain control. How would you settle the question? Which of these suggestions will most effectively contribute to the goal of a research-based protocol?

KEY POINTS

- The review of the literature is defined as a broad, comprehensive, in-depth, systematic critique of scholarly publications, unpublished scholarly print and online materials, audiovisual materials, and personal communications.

- The review of the literature is used for development of research studies and for other research consumer activities, such as development of evidence-based practice protocols and scholarly conceptual papers for publications.

- In relation to conducting and writing a literature review, the main objectives for the consumer of research are to acquire the ability to do the following: (1) conduct an appropriate electronic or print data-based search on a topic; (2) efficiently retrieve a sufficient amount of scholarly materials for a literature review in relation to the topic and scope of the project; (3) critically evaluate (i.e., critique) data-

based and conceptual material based on accepted critiquing criteria; (4) critically evaluate published reviews of the literature based on accepted standardized critiquing criteria; and (5) synthesize the findings of the critique materials for relevance to the purpose of the selected scholarly project.

- Primary data-based and conceptual resources are essential for literature reviews.

- Secondary sources from peer-reviewed journals are part of a learning strategy for developing critical critiquing skills.

- Strategies for efficiently retrieving scholarly literature for nursing include consulting the reference librarian and using at least two computer databases (e.g., CINAHL and MEDLINE).

- Literature reviews are usually organized both according to variables and chronologically.

- Critiquing criteria for scholarly literature reflect the purposes and characteristics of a relevant literature review and are presented in the form of questions.

- Whenever possible, read systematic reviews (meta-analyses and meta-syntheses) which represent the best available evidence on a clinical topic.

- Critiquing and synthesizing a number of data-based articles, including systematic reviews, are essential to implementing evidence-based nursing practice.

REFERENCES

Agency for Healthcare Research and Quality. (2000). *Garlic: Effects on cardiovascular risks and disease, protective effects against cancer, and clinical adverse effects* (Evidence Report/Technology Assessment No. 20 [AHRQ 01-E023]). Rockville, MD: Author.

Albanese, M., & Norcini, J. (2002): Systematic reviews: What are they and why should we care? *Advanced Health Science Education, 7*, 147–151.

Alligood, M., & Tomey, A. (2006). *Nursing theory: Utilization and application.* St. Louis, MO: Elsevier.

Beyea, S. C., & Nicoll, L. H. (1996). Administering IM injections the right way. *American Journal of Nursing, 96,* 34–35.

Bottorff, J. L., Johnson, J. L., Moffat, B., Grewal, J., Ratner, P., & Kalaw, C. (2004). Adolescent constructions of nicotine addiction. *Canadian Journal of Nursing Research, 38,* 22–39.

Bournes, D., & Mitchell, G. (2002). Waiting: The experience of persons in a critical care waiting room. *Research in Nursing and Health, 25,* 58–67.

Cameron, C. (2003). *The lived experience of transfer students in a collaborative baccalaureate nursing program.* Unpublished doctoral dissertation, University of Toronto.

Canadian Nurses Association. (2002). *Code of ethics.* Ottawa: Canadian Nurses Association.

CINAHL Information Systems. (2004). Table 5–2 retrieved April 24, 2008, from http://www.cinahl.com

DiCenso, A. (2003). Leadership perspectives. Evidence-based nursing practice: How to get there from here. *Canadian Journal of Nursing Leadership, 16*(4), 20–26.

Edwards, N., & Aminzadeh, F. (2003). [Commentary on the article "Prediction of fracture in nursing home residents" by C. J. Girman, J. M. Chandler, S. I. Zimmerman, et al.] *Evidence Based Nursing, 6*(2): 58.

Ferguson, L. (2004). External validity, generalizability, and knowledge utilization. *Journal of Nursing Scholarship, 36*(1), 16–22.

Fisher, K. (2004). Health disparities and mental retardation. *Journal of Nursing Scholarship, 26*(1), 48–53.

Fitzpatrick, J. J., Shandor, M. M., & Holditch-Davis, D. (Eds.). (2003). *Annual review of nursing research: Vol. 21. Research on child health and pediatric issues.* New York, Springer.

Forbes, D., & Clark, K. (2003). The Cochrane Library can answer your nursing care effectiveness questions. *Canadian Journal of Nursing Research, 35*(3), 19–25.

Forchuk, C. (1994). The orientation phase of the nurse-client relationship: Testing Peplau's theory. *Journal of Advanced Nursing Practice, 20,* 532–537.

Forchuk, C., Martin, M. L., Chan, Y. L., & Jensen, E. (2005). Therapeutic relationships: From psychiatric hospital to community. *Journal of Psychiatric and Mental Health Nursing, 12,* 556–564.

Forchuk, C., & Voorberg, N. (1991). Evaluating a community mental health program. *Canadian Journal of Nursing Administration, 4*(6), 16–20.

Forchuk, C., Westwell, J., Martin, M., Bamber-Azzapardi, W., Kosterewa-Tolman, D., & Hu, M. (2000). The developing nurse–client relationship: Nurses' perspectives. *Journal of the American Psychiatric Nurses Association, 6*(1), 3–10.

Forster, A., Smith, J., Young, J., Knapp, P., House, A., & Wright, J. (2000). Information provision for stroke patients and their caregivers. *Cochrane Library (Oxford)(ID #CD001919), 6*(1), 3–10.

Gray, P. H., & Flenady, V. (2001). Cot-nursing versus incubator care for preterm infants. *The Cochrane Database of Systematic Reviews, (1).* DOI: 10.1002/14651858.CD003062.

Greenway, K. (2004). Using the ventrogluteal site for intramuscular injection. *Nursing Standards, 18*(25), 39–42.

Health Canada. (2003a). *The report of the National Advisory Committee on SARS and Public Health.* Ottawa: Health Canada. Retrieved on September 16, 2007, from http://www.hc-sc.gc.ca/english/protection/warnings/sars/learning/

Health Canada. (2003b). *Health care in Canada.* Ottawa: Health Canada, Office of Nursing Policy.

Jensen, L. A., & Allen, M. N. (1996). Meta-synthesis of qualitative findings. *Qualitative Health Research, 6,* 553–560.

Jesse, R. (2006). Watson's philosophy in nursing practice. In M. Alligood & A. Tomey (Eds.). *Nursing theory: Utilization and application* (pp. 103–130). St. Louis, MO: Elsevier.

Li, H., Mazurek, M. B., & McCann, R. (2004). Review of intervention studies of families with hospitalized elderly relatives. *Journal of Nursing Scholarship, 36*(1), 54–59.

Melnyk, B. M., & Fineout-Overholt, E. (2005). *Evidence-based practice in nursing and healthcare: A guide to best practice.* Philadelphia: Lippincott Williams & Wilkins.

Moorhead, S., Johnson, M., & Maas, M. (Eds.). (2004). *Iowa outcomes project: Nursing outcomes classification (NOC)* (3rd ed). St. Louis, MO: Mosby/Elsevier Science.

Mulrow, C. D., Cook, D .J., & Davidoff, F. (1997). Systematic reviews: Critical links in the great chain of evidence. *Annals Internal Medicine, 126,* 389–391.

Nixon, S., O'Brien, K., Glazier, R. H., & Tynan, A. M. (2004). Aerobic exercise interventions for adults living with HIV/AIDS. *The Cochrane Database of Systematic Reviews, (1).* DOI: 10.1002/14651858.CD001796.pub2.

Paul, R., & Elder, L. (2001). *Critical thinking: Tools for taking charge of your learning and your life.* Englewood Cliffs, NJ: Prentice-Hall.

Peden, A. R. (1993). Recovering in depressed women: Research with Peplau's theory. *Nursing Science Quarterly, 6,* 140–146.

Peden, A. R. (1996). Recovering from depression: A one-year follow-up. *Journal of Psychiatric & Mental Health Nursing, 3,* 289–295.

Peden, A. R. (1998). Evolution of an intervention—The use of Peplau's process of practice-based theory development. *Journal of Psychiatric & Mental Health Nursing, 5,* 173–178.

Peplau, H. E. (1952). *Interpersonal relations in nursing: A conceptual frame of reference for psychodynamic nursing.* New York: Putnam and Sons.

Peplau, H. E. (1991). *Interpersonal relations in nursing: A conceptual frame of reference for psychodynamic nursing.* New York: Springer.

Pravikoff, D., & Donaldson, N. (2001, March). The online journal of clinical innovations. *Online Journal of Issues in Nursing, 5*(1). Retrieved September 13, 2008, from http://www.nursingworld.org/MainMenuCategories/ANAMarketplace/ANAPeriodicals/OJIN/TableofContents/volume62001/Number2May31/ArticlePreviousTopic/ClinicalInnovations.aspx

Registered Nurses' Association of Ontario. (2006). *Nursing Best Practice Guideline: Establishing therapeutic relationships*. Toronto: Author. Retrieved September 17, 2007, from http://www.rnao.org/Page.asp?PageID=924&ContentID=801

Registered Nurses Association of Ontario. (2007, March). *Nursing Best Practice Guideline: Assessment and management of stage I to IV pressure ulcers*. Retrieved September 2, 2008, from http://www.rnao.org/Storage/29/2371_BPG_Pressure_Ulcers_I_to_IV.pdf

Rice, V. H. & Stead, L. F. (2004). Nursing interventions for smoking cessation. Cochrane tobacco addiction group, *The Cochrane Database of Systematic Reviews* (3). DOI: 10.1002/14651858.CD002294.pub2.

Sackett, D. L, Straus, S. E., Richardson, W. S., Rosenberg, W., & Haynes, R. B. (2003). *Evidenced-based medicine: How to practice and teach EBM* (2nd ed.). Edinburgh: Churchill Livingston.

Samuels-Dennis, J. (2006). Relationship among employment status, stressful life events, and depression in single mothers. *Canadian Journal of Nursing Research, 38*(1), 58–80.

Scott, J. T, Prictor, M. J., Harmsen, M., Broom, A., Entwistle, V., Sowden, A., et al. (2003). Interventions for improving communication with children and adolescents about a family member's cancer. *The Cochrane Database of Systematic Reviews* (4). DOI: 10.1002/14652858.CD004511.

Smith, B., Appleton, S., Adams, R., Southcott, A., & Ruffin, R. (2001). Home care by outreach nursing for chronic obstructive pulmonary disease. *The Cochrane Database of Systematic Reviews* (3). DOI: 10.1002/14651858.

Smith, D., Edwards, N., Varcoe, C., Martens, P. J., & Davies, B. (2006). Bringing safety and responsiveness into the forefront of care for pregnant and parenting aboriginal people. *Advances in Nursing Science, 29*(2), E27–E44.

Thorne, S. (2006). Theoretical foundations of nursing practice. In J. Ross-Kerr & M. Wood (Eds.), *Canadian fundamentals of nursing* (3rd ed., pp. 66–79). Toronto: Elsevier.

Tourangeau, A., Giovannetti, P., Tu, J., & Wood, M. (2002). Nursing-related determinants of 30-day mortality for hospitalized patients. *Canadian Journal of Nursing Research, 33*, 71–88.

Watson, J. (1988). *Nursing: Human science and human care*. New York: National League for Nursing.

Watson, J. (1999). *Postmodern nursing and beyond*. Toronto: Churchill Livingston.

Judith Haber

Mina D. Singh

CHAPTER 6

Legal and Ethical Issues

LEARNING OUTCOMES

After reading this chapter, the student should be able to do the following:

- Describe the historical background that led to the development of ethical guidelines for the use of human subjects in research.
- Identify the essential elements of an informed consent form.
- Evaluate the adequacy of an informed consent form.
- Describe the research ethics board's role in the research review process.
- Identify populations of subjects who require special legal and ethical research considerations.
- Appreciate the nurse researcher's obligations to conduct and report research in an ethical manner.
- Describe the nurse's role as client advocate in research situations.
- Discuss the nurse's role in ensuring that Health Canada guidelines for testing of medical devices are followed.
- Discuss animal rights in research situations.
- Critique the ethical aspects of a research study.

KEY TERMS

animal rights
anonymity
assent
beneficence
benefits
confidentiality
consent
ethics
informed consent
justice
process consent
product testing
research ethics board (REB)
respect for persons
risk–benefit ratio
risks

STUDY RESOURCES

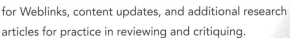 Go to Evolve at
http://evolve.elsevier.com/Canada/LoBiondo/Research/
for Weblinks, content updates, and additional research
articles for practice in reviewing and critiquing.

Nurses are in an ideal position to promote clients' awareness of the role played by research in the advancement of science and improvement in client care. In Canada, our professional code of ethics (Canadian Nurses Association [CNA], 2008) outlines the ethical standards for practice, which can include research and informing clients of their rights with regard to research. Not only do the codes represent rules and regulations regarding practice, but when research becomes the domain of a nurse, these codes can be applied to the participation of human research subjects to ensure that nursing research is conducted legally and ethically. The CNA states that nurses must strive to uphold human rights and call attention to any violations of these rights. The *Code of Ethics for Registered Nurses* is currently being revised and is scheduled to be released in June 2008 (Storch, 2007). According to Kikuchi (2004, cited in Storch, 2007) the revised CNA code should include "clarification of the meaning of social justice, health and well-being with a stronger focus on human rights" (p. 37). These rights can also be translated to clients' or subjects' rights in research, and nurses can be advocates to ensure that ethical concepts in nursing research are upheld.

Researchers and caregivers of clients who are research subjects must be fully committed to the tenets of informed consent and clients' rights. The principle "the ends justify the means" must never be tolerated. Researchers and caregivers of research subjects must take every precaution to protect people being studied from physical or mental harm or discomfort (although it is not always clear what constitutes harm or discomfort).

The focus of this chapter is the legal and ethical considerations that must be addressed before, during, and after the conduct of research to ensure that the research does not harm the client. Informed consent, research ethics boards (REBs), and research involving vulnerable populations—older adults, pregnant women, children, prisoners, Aboriginal people, and persons with acquired immune deficiency syndrome (AIDS), as well as animals—are discussed. The nurse's role as client advocate, whether functioning as researcher, caregiver, or research consumer, is addressed.

ETHICAL AND LEGAL CONSIDERATIONS IN RESEARCH: A Historical Perspective

Past Ethical Dilemmas in Research

Ethical and legal considerations regarding medical research first arose in the United States and received focused attention after the Second World War. When it was learned that the defence of war criminals intended to justify the atrocities committed by Nazi physicians by claiming their actions were in the name of "medical research," the US secretary of state and the secretary of war stepped in. They asked the American Medical Association to appoint a group to develop a code of ethics for research to serve as a standard for judging the medical atrocities committed by physicians on concentration camp prisoners. These experiments included the sterilization of people considered enemies of the state (Benedict & Georges, 2006).

The code of ethics developed as 10 rules that became known as the *Nuremberg Code* (see Box 6–1). The Code's definitions of the terms *voluntary*, *legal capacity*, *sufficient understanding*, and *enlightened decision* have been the subject of numerous court cases and US presidential commissions involved in setting ethical standards in research (Creighton, 1977). The code that was developed requires informed consent in all cases but makes no provisions for any special treatment of children, older adults, or people who are mentally incompetent. Several other international standards have followed; the most notable is the Declaration of Helsinki, which was adopted in 1964 by the World Medical Assembly and revised in 1975 (Levine, 1979).

The research heritage in the United States and Canada is well documented and is used here to illustrate the human consequences of not adhering to ethical standards when conducting research.

BOX 6–1 Articles of the Nuremberg Code

1. The voluntary consent of the human subject is absolutely essential.

2. The study should be conducted so as to yield fruitful results for the good of society, unprocurable by other means of study, and not random and unnecessary in nature.

3. The experiment should be so designed and based on the results of animal experimentation and knowledge of the natural history of the disease or other problems under study that the anticipated results will justify the performance of the experiment.

4. The experiment should be conducted to avoid all unnecessary physical and mental suffering and injury.

5. No experiment should be conducted where there is a prior reason to believe that death or disabling injury will occur.

6. The degree of risk to be taken should never exceed that determined by the humanitarian importance of the problem to be solved by the experiment.

7. Proper preparations should be made and adequate facilities provided to protect the subject against . . . injury, disability, or death.

8. The experiment should be conducted only by scientifically qualified persons.

9. The human subject should be at liberty to bring the experiment to an end.

10. During the experiment, the scientist . . . if he or she has probable cause to believe that a continuation of the experiment is likely to result in injury, disability, or death to the experimental subject . . . will bring [the experiment] to a close.

From United States Government. (2008). *"Trials of war criminals before the Nuremberg Military Tribunals under Control Council Law No. 10"*, Vol. 2, pp. 181–182. Washington, DC: US Government Printing Office, 1949. Retrieved April 10, 2008, from http://www.hhs.gov/ohrp/references/nurcode.htm

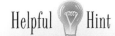

Helpful Hint

The qualitative researcher must be especially diligent with respect to protecting the privacy and confidentiality of participants because when the subjects' verbatim quotations are used in the results or findings section of the research report to highlight the findings, the small sample size may make it easy to identify an individual participant. Moreover, when researchers and REBs are engaging in naturalistic observation, the Tri-Council policy statement indicates that "[they] should pay close attention to the ethical implications of such factors as: the nature of the activities to be observed; the environment in which the activities are to be observed (in particular, whether it is to be staged for the purposes of the research); and the means of recording the observations. Naturalistic observation that does not allow for the identification of the subjects, and what is not staged, should normally be regarded as of minimal risk" (Government of Canada, 2003).

major charge of the commission was to identify the basic principles that should underlie the conduct of biomedical and behavioural research involving human subjects and to develop guidelines to ensure that research is conducted in accordance with those principles (Levine, 1986). Three ethical principles were identified as relevant to the conduct of research involving human subjects: **respect for persons**, **beneficence**, and **justice** (see the definitions in Box 6–2). These three principles have formed the basis of many ethical guidelines in Canada.

In Canada, for the protection of human participants in all types of research, Health Canada has adopted the *Good Clinical Practice: Consolidated Guidelines* (Health Canada, 1997). The collaboration of the three major funding agencies, the Canadian Institutes of Health Research (CIHR), the Natural Sciences and Engineering Research Council of Canada (NSERC), and the Social Sciences and Humanities Research Council (SSHRC), has led to a joint statement for the protection of human subjects. This document, the *Tri-Council Policy Statement: Ethical Conduct for Research Involving Humans* (Government of Canada, 2003), has also

Some examples are highlighted in Table 6–1 and incorporated into Table 6–2 to demonstrate violation of human rights that occurred in these studies.

In the United States, the *National Research Act*, passed in 1974 (Public Law 93-348), created the National Commission for the Protection of Human Subjects of Biomedical and Behavioral Research. A

TABLE 6–1 Highlights of Unethical Research Studies Conducted in the United States and Canada

Research Study	Year(s)	Focus of Study	Ethical Principle Violated
Tuskegee Syphilis Study, Tuskegee, Alabama	1932–1973	For 40 years, the US Public Health Service conducted a study using two groups of poor Black male sharecroppers. One group consisted of those who had untreated syphilis; the other group was judged to be free of the disease. Treatment was withheld from the group with syphilis even after penicillin became generally available and accepted as effective treatment for syphilis in the 1950s. Steps were even taken to prevent the subjects from obtaining penicillin. The researcher wanted to study the untreated disease.	Many of the subjects who consented to participate in the study were not informed about the purpose and procedures of the research. Others were unaware that they were subjects. The degree of risk outweighed the potential benefit. Withholding of known effective treatment violates the subjects' right to fair treatment and protection from harm (Levine, 1986).
Sterilization experiments in Auschwitz concentration camp	1940–1944	Sterilization experiments	Basic human rights and rights to fair and ethical treatment were violated, and the subjects did not give informed consent. Nurses who were prisoners were forced to participate in the experiments, which was against their *prima facie* duty to protect (Benedict & Georges, 2006).
Dr. Ewen Cameron's psychiatric experiments, Allan Memorial Psychiatric Institute, Montreal, Quebec	1950s–1960s	The US Central Intelligence Agency (CIA) funded psychic driving or brainwashing experiments on clients with psychiatric illnesses (Collins, 1988, cited in Charron, 2000). Psychic driving is a psychiatric procedure pioneered by Dr. Cameron in which electroconvulsive therapy and psychedelic drugs, such as LSD, are used in an attempt at mind control. To develop the psychic driving, increasingly higher levels of electroconvulsive therapy (ECT) were applied to clients as often as three times a day. This treatment would continue for 30 days. Considerable damage was done to clients after such severe treatment. Clients were unable to walk or feed themselves and were incontinent (Gillmor, 1987, cited by Charron, 2000).	The ethical principles of respect for persons and beneficence were severely violated. Dr. Cameron used clients with diminished autonomy (clients with psychiatric illnesses), even though, as a physician, he was obliged to protect them. The ECT treatments did more harm than good.
Hyman v. Jewish Chronic Disease Hospital, Jewish Chronic Disease Study, New York City	1965	Doctors injected aged senile clients with cancer cells to study the clients' response to rejection of the cells.	Informed consent was not obtained, and no indication was given that the study had been reviewed and approved by an ethics committee. The two physicians involved claimed that they did not wish to evoke emotional reactions or refusals to participate by informing the subjects of the nature of the study (Hershey & Miller, 1976).

TABLE 6–1 Highlights of Unethical Research Studies Conducted in the United States and Canada—cont'd

Research Study	Year(s)	Focus of Study	Ethical Principle Violated
Midgeville, Georgia case	1969	Investigational drugs were used on mentally disabled children without first obtaining the opinion of a psychiatrist.	The study protocol or institutional approval of the program was not reviewed before implementation (Levine, 1986).
San Antonio Contraceptive Study, San Antonio, Texas	1969	In a study examining the side effects of oral contraceptives, 76 impoverished Mexican American women were randomly assigned to an experimental group receiving birth control pills or a control group receiving placebos. Subjects were not informed about the placebo and the attendant risk of pregnancy. Eleven subjects became pregnant, ten of whom were in the placebo control group.	Principles of informed consent were violated; full disclosure of the potential risk, harm, results, and side effects was not evident in the informed consent document. The potential risk outweighed the benefits of the study. The subjects' right to fair treatment and protection from harm was violated (Levine, 1986).
Willowbrook Hospital, New York State	1972	Children with mental incompetence (N = 350) were not admitted to Willowbrook Hospital, a residential treatment facility, unless parents consented to their children being subjects in a study examining the natural history of infectious hepatitis and the effect of gamma globulin. The children were deliberately infected with the hepatitis virus under various conditions; some received gamma globulin, whereas others did not.	The principle of voluntary consent was violated. Parents were coerced into consenting to their children's participation as research subjects. Subjects or their guardians have a right to self-determination; in other words, they should be free of constraint, coercion, and undue influence of any kind. Many subjects feel pressured to participate in studies if they are in powerless, dependent positions (Rothman, 1982).
Schizophrenia Medication Study, University of California-Los Angeles	1983	In a study examining the effects of withdrawing psychotropic medications in 50 clients under treatment for schizophrenia, 23 subjects suffered severe relapses after their medication was stopped. The goal of the study was to determine whether some clients with schizophrenia might do better without medications that had deleterious side effects.	Although all subjects signed informed consent documents, they were not informed about how severe their relapses might be or that they could suffer worsening symptoms with each recurrence. Principles of informed consent were violated; full disclosure of the potential risk, harm, results, and side effects was not evident in the informed consent document. The potential risk outweighed the benefits of the study. The subjects' right to fair treatment and protection from harm was violated (Hilts, 1995).
Ivory Coast, Africa, AIDS/AZT case	1994	In research supported by the US government and conducted in the Ivory Coast, Dominican Republic, and Thailand, some pregnant women infected with HIV were given placebo pills rather than AZT, a drug known to prevent mothers from passing the virus to their babies. Babies born to these mothers were in danger of contracting a fatal disease.	Subjects who consented to participate and who were randomized to the control group were denied access to a medication regimen with a known benefit. This denial violates the subjects' right to fair treatment and protection (French, 1997; Wheeler, 1997).

AIDS: acquired immune deficiency syndrome; AZT: azidothymidine; HIV: human immunodeficiency virus.

TABLE 6–2　Protection of Human Rights

Basic Human Right	Definition
Right to self-determination	This right is based on the ethical principle of respect for persons; people should be treated as autonomous agents who have the freedom to choose without external controls. An autonomous agent is one who is informed about a proposed study and is allowed to choose to participate or not to participate (Brink, 1992). Moreover, subjects have the right to withdraw from a study without penalty. Subjects with diminished autonomy are entitled to protection. They are more vulnerable because of age, legal or mental incompetence, terminal illness, or confinement to an institution. A justification for the use of vulnerable subjects must be provided.
Right to privacy and dignity	Based on the principle of respect, privacy is the freedom of a person to determine the time, extent, and circumstances under which private information is shared or withheld from others.
Right to anonymity and confidentiality	Based on the principle of respect, anonymity exists when the subject's identity cannot be linked, even by the researcher, to his or her individual responses (American Nurses Association, 1985). Confidentiality means that the individual identities of subjects will not be linked to the information they provide and will not be publicly divulged.

Violation of Basic Human Right	Example
A subject's right to self-determination is violated through the use of coercion, deception, and covert data collection. • Coercion occurs when an overt threat of harm or excessive reward is presented to ensure subjects' compliance. • Deception occurs when subjects are misinformed about the purpose of the research. • Covert data collection occurs when people become research subjects and are exposed to research treatments without knowing it. • The potential for violation of the right to self-determination is greater for subjects with diminished autonomy, who have decreased ability to give informed consent and are vulnerable.	Subjects may feel that their care will be adversely affected if they refuse to participate in research. The Willowbrook Hospital Study (see Table 6–1) is an example of how coercion was used to obtain the consent of parents of vulnerable children with mental retardation, who would not be admitted to the institution unless they participated in a study in which they were deliberately injected with the hepatitis virus. The Jewish Chronic Disease Hospital Study (see Table 6–1) is an example of a study in which clients and their doctors did not know that cancer cells were being injected. In the Milgram (1963) study, subjects were deceived when asked to administer electric shocks to another person, who was an actor pretending to feel the shocks. Subjects administering the shocks were very stressed by participating in this study, although they were not administering shocks at all. This study is an example of deception.
The US *Privacy Act* of 1974 was instituted to protect subjects from privacy violations. These violations occur most frequently during data collection, when invasive questions are asked that might result in the loss of a job, friendships, or dignity, or might create embarrassment and mental distress. These violations also may occur when subjects are unaware that information is being shared with others.	Subjects may be asked personal questions, such as "Were you sexually abused as a child?" "Do you use drugs?" "What are your sexual preferences?" When questions are asked using hidden microphones or hidden tape recorders, the subjects' privacy is invaded because they have no knowledge that the data are being shared with others. Subjects' right to control access of others to their records is also violated.

TABLE 6-2 Protection of Human Rights—cont'd

Violation of Basic Human Right	Example
Anonymity is violated when the subjects' responses can be linked to their identity.	Researchers who choose to identify data by using the subject's name are breaching the basic human right of anonymity. Instead, researchers should assign subjects a code number that is used for identification purposes. Subjects' names are never used when reporting findings.
Confidentiality is breached when a researcher, by accident or direct action, allows an unauthorized person to gain access to study data that contain information about the subject's identity or responses, which creates a potentially harmful situation for the subject.	Breaches of confidentiality occur when a researcher, by accident or direct action, allows an unauthorized person personality variables can be harmful to subjects. Data should be analyzed as group data so that individuals cannot be identified by their responses. Breaches of confidentiality with regard to sexual preference, income, drug use, prejudice, or

Basic Human Right	Definition
Right to fair treatment	Based on the ethical principle of justice, people should be treated fairly and should receive what they are due or owed.
	Fair treatment refers to the equitable selection of subjects and their treatment during the research study. This treatment includes selection of subjects for reasons directly related to the problem studied versus selection of subjects owing to convenience, the compromised position of the subjects, or their vulnerability. Fair treatment also extends to the treatment of subjects during the study, including fair distribution of risks and benefits of the research regardless of age, race, or socioeconomic status.
Right to protection from discomfort and harm	Based on the ethical principle of beneficence, people must take an active role in promoting good and preventing harm both in the world around them and in research studies.
	Discomfort and harm can be physical, psychological, social, or economic in nature.
	The five categories of studies based on levels of harm and discomfort are as follows:
	1. No anticipated effects
	2. Temporary discomfort
	3. Unusual level of temporary discomfort
	4. Risk of permanent damage
	5. Certainty of permanent damage

Violation of Basic Human Right	Example
Injustices with regard to subject selection have occurred as a result of social, cultural, racial, and gender biases in society.	The Tuskegee Syphilis Study (1973), the Jewish Chronic Disease Study (1965), the San Antonio Contraceptive Study (1969), and the Willowbrook Hospital Study (1972) (see Table 6–1) all provide examples of unfair subject selection and the use of vulnerable populations
Historically, research subjects often have been obtained from groups of people who were regarded as having less "social value," such as people living in poverty, prisoners, slaves, people who are mentally incompetent, and people who are dying. Often subjects were treated carelessly, without consideration of physical or psychological harm.	Investigators should not be late for data collection appointments, should terminate data collection on time, should not change agreed-upon procedures or activities without consent, and should provide agreed-upon benefits, such as a copy of the study findings or a participation fee.

TABLE 6–2   Protection of Human Rights—cont'd

Violation of Basic Human Right—cont'd	Example
Subjects' right to be protected is violated when researchers know in advance that harm, death, or disabling injury will occur, and, thus, the benefits do not outweigh the risks.	Temporary physical discomfort involving minimal risk includes fatigue or headache; emotional discomfort includes the expense involved in travelling to and from the data collection site. Studies examining sensitive issues, such as rape, incest, or spouse abuse, might cause unusual levels of temporary discomfort by opening up current or past traumatic experiences. In these situations, researchers assess distress levels and provide debriefing sessions, during which the subject may express feelings and ask questions. The researcher has the opportunity to make referrals for professional intervention.
	Studies with the potential to cause permanent damage are more likely to be medical in nature rather than nursing in nature, as physiological damage may occur. A recent clinical trial of a new drug, a recombinant activated protein C (Zovan) for treatment of sepsis, was halted when interim findings from the phase 3 clinical trials revealed a reduced mortality rate for the treatment group versus the placebo group. Evaluation of the data led to termination of the trial to make available a known beneficial treatment to all clients.
	In some research, such as the Tuskegee Syphilis Study or Nazi medical experiments, subjects experienced permanent damage or death. The participants in Dr. Cameron's study (see Table 6–1) were not protected from harm as the continued electroconvulsive therapy increasingly did more damage.

been accepted by Health Canada. The guiding principles, set out in Article *i*, *Contexts of an Ethical Framework*, are as follows:

- Respect for Human Dignity
- Respect for Free and Informed Consent
- Respect for Vulnerable Persons
- Respect for Privacy and Confidentiality
- Respect for Justice and Inclusiveness
- Balancing Harms and Benefits
- Minimizing Harm
- Maximizing Benefit

Current and Future Ethical Dilemmas in Research

The ethical dilemmas in research for the twenty-first century concern biotechnology, the use of animals for research, and the creation of an organizational culture that values and nurtures research **ethics** and the rights of people who engage in research either as investigators or subjects (Pranulis, 1996). For example, in only 12 years,

---

BOX 6–2   Basic Ethical Principles Relevant to the Conduct of Research

RESPECT FOR PERSONS

People have the right to self-determination and to treatment as autonomous agents. Thus they have the freedom to participate or not participate in research. Persons with diminished autonomy are entitled to protection.

BENEFICENCE

Beneficence is an obligation to do no harm and maximize possible benefits. Persons are treated in an ethical manner when their decisions are respected, they are protected from harm, and efforts are made to secure their well-being.

JUSTICE

Human subjects should be treated fairly. An injustice occurs when benefit to which a person is entitled is denied without good reason or when a burden is imposed unduly.

From Elder, G. (1981). Social history & life experience. In D. H. Eichorn, J. A. Clausen, N. Haan, & P. H. Mussen (Eds.), *Present and past in middle life* (pp. 3–31). New York: Academic Press. Copyright © 1981 Academic Press. Reprinted by permission.

the Human Genome Project, an international research project launched by the United States in 1988, has provided a vast amount of data on deoxyribonucleic acid (DNA), including the molecular details about the DNA of more than 26 organisms. In a postgenomic world, the focus is on studying (1) groups of genes rather than single genes; (2) functions of genes rather than structures of genes; and (3) proteomes, the proteins based on genes (Wheeler, 1999). Nanoscience, a new scientific frontier, and its related nanotechnology, makes substances by manipulating materials at the atomic level. To engage in genome research, genetic engineering and genetic information must exist (Carrol & Ciaffa, 2008), which can raise ethical concerns relating to the purpose of the engineering. If the purpose is to treat a disease, then the research is ethically acceptable, but if germline intervention exists, there are "more significant ethical concerns, because risks will extend across generations, magnifying the impact of unforeseen consequences" (Carroll & Ciaffa, 2008). Ethical concerns also arise vis-à-vis the privacy of genetic information, mandatory testing of newborns, and mandatory genetic screening.

Other areas of research that engender much discussion and controversy are fetal tissue research and use of women who are of child-bearing potential as subjects in drug or therapeutic studies. The Tri-Council (i.e., the CIHR, the NSERC, and the SSHRC) worked over a period of two years to make stem cell research a reality in Canada, with the appropriate ethical guidelines (CIHR, 2007). In the past, women of child-bearing potential were denied access to participation as subjects in studies of a drug or potential therapy because of the unknown, potentially harmful effects on fetuses of drugs and other therapies that were in various stages of testing. Guidelines related to the inclusion of pregnant women as research subjects have been even more stringent than previous guidelines, leading to the exclusion of women from many important drug and research studies over the years. Similarly, inclusion of ethnic minorities in federally funded research studies also is a priority area of research (Campbell, 1999b; Julion, Gross, & Barclay-

McLaughlin, 2000). The Tri-Council policy statement also has a well-articulated policy on the ethical guidelines for research with the Aboriginal population to ensure protection of the rights of the community (CIHR, 2007).

EVOLUTION OF ETHICS IN NURSING RESEARCH

The evolution of ethics in nursing research can be traced back to 1897 and the constitution of the Nurses' Associated Alumnae Organization in the United States. One of the first purposes of this organization was to establish a code of ethics for the nursing profession. In 1901, Isabel Hampton Robb wrote *Nursing Ethics: For Hospital and Private Use*. In describing the moral laws by which people must abide, she stated the following:

> *Etiquette, speaking broadly, means a form of behavior or manners expressly or tacitly required on particular occasions. It makes up the code of polite life and includes forms of ceremony to be observed, so that we invariably find in societies that certain etiquette is required and observed either tacitly or by expressed agreement.*

Although Robb's comments reflect the norms of Victorian society, they also highlight a historical concern for ethical actions by nurses as health care providers (Robb, 1900).

In Canada, most disciplines have developed their own code of ethics with guidelines for research. The CNA's first document on ethical principles related to nursing research, *Ethical Guidelines for Nurses in Research Involving Human Participants*, was released in 1983 (CNA, 1983). It was revised in 1994 and 2002 and is now called *Ethical Research Guidelines for Registered Nurses* (CNA, 2002).

Clearly, ignorance and naïveté vis-à-vis ethical and legal guidelines for the conduct of research must never be an excuse for a nurse's failure to be familiar with and act on behalf of clients, whose human rights must be safeguarded at all times.

Nurse researchers are often among the most responsible and conscientious investigators when it comes to respecting the rights of human subjects. All nurses should be aware that in addition to the ethical research guidelines of the CNA, nurse researchers associated with universities or hospitals may also have a supplemental set of ethical guidelines to follow.

PROTECTION OF HUMAN RIGHTS

Human rights are the claims and demands that have been justified in the eyes of an individual or by a group of individuals. The term *human rights* refers to the following five rights outlined in the CNA's (2002) guidelines and linked to the Tri-Council's principles of respect for research participants:

1. Right to self-determination
2. Right to privacy and dignity
3. Right to anonymity and confidentiality
4. Right to fair treatment
5. Right to protection from discomfort and harm

These rights apply to everyone involved in a research project, including research team members involved in data collection, practising nurses involved in the research setting, and subjects participating in the study. As consumers of research read a research article, they must realize that any issues highlighted in Table 6–2 should have been addressed and resolved before a research study is approved for implementation.

Procedures for Protecting Basic Human Rights

INFORMED CONSENT

Informed consent, illustrated by the ethical principles of respect and the related right to self-determination, is outlined in Box 6–3. Nurses need to understand the elements of informed consent to be knowledgeable participants when either obtaining informed consent from clients or critiquing this process as it is presented in research articles.

Informed consent is the legal principle that, in theory, governs the client's ability to accept or reject individual medical interventions designed to diagnose or treat an illness. The Tri-Council (Government of Canada, 2003) states that free and informed consent is at the heart of ethical research and is a process of dialogue and information sharing to allow participants the choice

BOX 6–3	Elements of Informed Consent

The elements of informed consent include the following:

1. A statement that the study involves research
2. An explanation of the purposes of the research, delineating the expected duration of the subject's participation
3. A description of the procedures to be followed and identification of any procedures that are experimental
4. A description of any reasonably foreseeable risks or discomforts to the subject
5. A description of any benefits to the subject or to others that may reasonably be expected from the research
6. A disclosure of appropriate alternative procedures or course of treatment, if any, that might be advantageous to the subject
7. A statement describing the extent to which the anonymity and confidentiality of the records identifying the subject will be maintained
8. For research involving more than minimal risk, an explanation as to whether any medical treatments are available if injury occurs and, if so, what they consist of or where further information may be obtained
9. An explanation about who to contact for answers to questions about the research and researcher subjects' rights and who to contact in the event of a research-related injury to the subject
10. A statement that participation is voluntary, that refusal to participate will not involve any penalty or less benefit to which the subject is otherwise entitled, and that the subject may discontinue participation at any time without penalty or loss of otherwise entitled benefits

From Code of Federal Regulations: Protection of human subjects, 45 CFR 46, *OPRR Reports*, revised March 8, 1983.

to participate in research. Free and informed consent must be given without manipulation, undue influence, or coercion.

For example, Jack, DiCenso, and Lohfeld (2005) adhered to the principles of informed consent in their study to develop a theory to describe the process by which mothers of children at risk engage with public health nurses and family visitors. They stated that all participants received a written and verbal description of the study and gave informed consent to participate. Included in this informed consent was the provision that the mothers' participation was voluntary and that they could withdraw from the study at any time without negative consequences to their home visting services.

No investigator may involve a human as a research subject until the legally effective informed consent has been obtained from either the subject or a legally authorized representative of the subject, and prospective subjects must have time to decide whether to participate in a study. The researcher must not coerce the subject into participating, nor may researchers collect data on subjects who have explicitly refused to participate in a study.

An ethical violation of this principle is illustrated by the case of *Halushka v. University of Saskatchewan et al.* (1965) 52 WWR 608 (Sask CA). In this landmark case, a university student volunteered for a study testing a new anaesthetic, for which he would be paid $50.00. He consented to be in the study based on the following information disclosed to him: the test would last a few hours, the test was safe and had been conducted many times before, and the student had nothing to worry about. He was informed that the procedure would include placement of electrodes on his arms, legs, and head and insertion of a catheter into a vein in his arm. He signed a consent form releasing the physicians and the university from liability for any untoward effects or accidents, which were explained to him as "falling down at home after the test" (McLean, 1996, p. 49). The test proceeded with administration of an untested anaesthetic, and the student suffered a cardiac arrest. He was unconscious for four days in hospital and left

with a residual inability to concentrate. The physicians and the university were found negligent for failing to "disclose that there was risk involved with the use of an anaesthetic and that this particular drug had not been previously tested by them" (McLean, 1996, p. 49).

When composing an informed consent form, researchers must ensure that the language is understandable. For example, the reading level should be no higher than Grade 8 for adults and the use of technical research language should be avoided (Rempusheski, 1991). The elements that need to be contained in an informed consent are listed in Box 6–3 (page 122). Note that many institutions require additional elements. An example of an informed consent form is presented in Figure 6–1.

In a qualitative research study investigating the process of caregiving by daughters of cardiac clients, Gage-Rancoeur and Purden (2003) informed the clients and the clients' daughters of the purpose of the study and that their participation was voluntary. In addition, the participants were told they could withdraw at any time, all documentation would be stored in a safe place, and their anonymity would be maintained by their names not being published or appearing anywhere in the documentation. Moreover, the researcher reassured the participants that only a limited number of people would have access to the data, and the transcripts, audiotapes, and any other data collected would be destroyed six months to one year after the completion of the study.

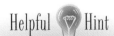

Helpful Hint

Remember that research reports rarely provide readers with detailed information regarding the degree to which the researcher adhered to ethical principles, such as informed consent, because of space limitations in journals, which make it impossible to describe all aspects of a study. Failure to mention procedures to safeguard subjects' rights does not necessarily mean that such precautions were not taken.

Most investigators obtain **consent** through personal discussion with potential subjects. This

Informed Consent

The University of British Columbia School of Nursing
T201-2211 Westbrook Mall
Vancouver, BC Canada V6T 2B5

Tel: (604) 822-7417
Fax: (604) 822-7466

Consent Form

Title of Research Project: The Nature of Self-Care Decision Making in Type 1 Diabetes

Principal Investigator:

Dr. Barbara Paterson
Associate Professor
School of Nursing
University of British Columbia
Telephone (604) XXX-XXXX

Co-investigator:

Dr. Sally Thorne
Professor
School of Nursing
University of British Columbia
Telephone (604) XXX-XXXX

Co-investigator:

Dr. Sandra LeFort
Professor
Memorial University
St. John's, Newfoundland
Telephone (709) XXX-XXXX

Associate:

Dr. Cynthia Russell
College of Nursing
University of Tennessee, Memphis
Memphis, TN 38163
Telephone (901) XXX-XXX

You are being invited to participate in a research study designed to explore self-care decision making in individuals who have type 1 diabetes. The study consists of three individual interviews and tape recording your daily decisions regarding the management of your disease for a period of one week in a year. Upon your written consent, the researchers will review your clinic chart to obtain information about your treatment and past medical history prior to the first interview. Although the researchers have received permission from the clinic staff to access the charts at the clinic, you must give written approval before they can read your chart. If you agree to participate in this study, you will be given a permission form to indicate that you give the researchers permission to read your chart. The study will also entail measuring your glycosylated hemoglobin

Figure 6–1 Example of an informed consent form

(HbA1c) level at the beginning of the study and two months following your last interview. This will require that you go to a laboratory in your area to have 1 to 3 mL (about half a teaspoon) of blood taken from a vein, usually in the inside of the elbow or the back of the hand. You will be given the results of these tests by a member of the research team immediately upon receipt of the results from the laboratory. The results of these tests and a description of the study will be sent to your physician in the outpatient clinic as soon as possible after the research team receives them. The project manager of the research project, a nurse experienced in diabetes care, will discuss the implications of the results with you and recommend follow-up by a physician when indicated. You will also be given written guidelines for follow-up regarding the results (e.g., if you have an above-normal HbA1c level, you should discuss this with the doctor because it indicates that at times during the last three months, you have had more sugar in your body than it could use).

The first interview will be a maximum of two hours in length. At that interview, you will be asked to complete a short survey about what you think and feel about diabetes. The other interviews will occur in one hour. A maximum of five hours of your time over the course of one year will be required if you decide to participate in this project.

Participation in the study is voluntary. You may withdraw from the study at any time or refuse permission for the use of your tapes, written records, or interview transcripts. You are being invited to participate in this research project because you have type 1 diabetes, you live in British Columbia, you are at least 18 years of age, and you are able to speak and write in English. As well, you do not have a condition that makes thinking or remembering difficult for you, you have no history of depression requiring treatment or of major mental illness within the past year, and you do not need home nursing or hospital or nursing home care. You understand that if you do not wish to participate in this project, it will not affect the health care you receive.

If you agree to take part in the study, you will be interviewed by a researcher and will be asked to tell about your experience with the disease to date, as well as some specific information about yourself. The interviewer will begin by asking you some short-answer questions about yourself and your family (e.g., "When were you born?"). The interviewer will record in writing your answers to these questions on a record designed for this purpose. During this interview, the interviewer will give you a tape recorder and discuss the process for recording your decisions in the research study. Following the interview, you will be assigned one week during the year to record your daily decisions about your disease management (e.g., February 5–12). In the scheduled week, you will be asked to carry a voice-activated, pocket-sized tape recorder to record your thinking during decisions you make regarding diet, medication, physical activity, rest, stress management, skin care, and/or other disease-related situations. A member of the research team will pick up your tape in the early evening of day three and day seven of the week.

If you have to make alternate arrangements for the pick-up of the tape because of work or other circumstances, you can arrange this with any member of the research team. You will be interviewed within two hours of the tape pick-up by a researcher regarding the decisions you recorded during the previous days. At the completion of the research, you will be asked to attend a group in which other participants will join you to hear and discuss the results of the research. All interviews will be taped and transcribed.

Figure 6–1 Example of an informed consent form—cont'd

Informed Consent—cont'd

Your name will not be used in the transcriptions of the tapes or interviews. Your tapes and interviews will be identified only by a code number assigned to you. Only the research team will have access to the tapes and transcriptions; the tapes and transcriptions will be stored in a locked filing cabinet to which only the principal investigator has a key. The tapes and transcriptions will be destroyed in ten years, following the completion of the study. The tapes will be erased, and the transcriptions will be incinerated. The findings of the research may be published, but your name will not be associated with the study.

There are no known risks to the research. If you agree to participate, you will contribute information that may be beneficial to other individuals with chronic illness. You will receive a written summary of the results of the research upon its completion. Before you sign this form, please ask any questions regarding aspects of the study that remain unclear. You may contact the principal investigator, Dr. Barbara Paterson, if you have any questions regarding the study. She will attempt to answer any questions you may have prior to, during, or following the study.

If you agree to participate in the study and you complete the requirements of the study, you will receive the tape recorder with which you recorded your decisions. You may also contact the Research Subject Information Line in the UBC Office of Research Services at 604-XXX-XXXX if you have any questions or concerns about your rights or treatment in the research study at any time. For additional information, you may also contact Joan Johnson or Patti Phillip at the North Shore Health Region at 604-XXX-XXXX. For additional information regarding your rights as a research subject, please contact Dr. Richard Lupton, vice president of medicine, North Shore Health Region, at 604-XXX-XXXX.

Authorization

I, _____, have read and decided to participate in the research study described above. My signature indicates that I give permission for the information I provide in tapes or interviews to be used for publication in research articles, journals, books, and/or teaching materials. Additionally, my signature indicates that I have received a copy of the consent form.

Name of the person consenting (please print): _____

Signature: _____ Date: _____

Name of person witnessing (please print): _____

Witness: _____ Date: _____

Figure 6–1 Example of an informed consent form—cont'd

process allows the person who is the potential subject to obtain immediate answers to questions. However, consent forms, written in narrative or outline form, highlight elements that both inform and remind subjects of the nature of the study and their participation (Dubler & Post, 1998; Haggerty & Hawkins, 2000). When one individual is scheduled to participate in many interviews, the participant for each data collection point must give **process consent**, which can be verbal.

Assurance of **anonymity** and **confidentiality** (defined in Table 6–2), which is conveyed in writing, is sometimes difficult in unique research situations that capture the public's attention. For example, when physicians at Loma Linda University Hospital in California transplanted a baboon's heart into a 2-week-old infant, her identity was protected as she was known only as Baby Fae. Maintaining anonymity and confidentiality is particularly important for qualitative researchers because the researcher often functions as the data collection instrument and meets the participant. The consent form must be signed and dated by the subject. The presence of witnesses is not always necessary but does constitute evidence that the subject concerned actually signed the form. In cases in which the subject is a minor or is physically or mentally incapable of signing the consent, the legal guardian or representative must sign. The investigator also signs the form to indicate commitment to the agreement of the concepts above.

In the Jack et al. (2005) study described previously, the participants' anonymity and confidentiality were guaranteed, but in cases in which the researcher suspected child abuse or neglect, the participants were clearly informed that the researcher has a legal responsibility to report any suspicions to the child welfare agency. Another strategy that can be used to ensure confidentiality is to ask the transcribers in a qualitative study to sign a confidentiality agreement as Heaman, Chalmers, Woodgate, and Brown (2007) did in their study examining relationship work in an early childhood home visiting program.

Generally, the signed informed consent form is given to the subject. The researcher should also keep a copy. Some research, such as a retrospective chart audit, may not require informed consent, only institutional approval. Or, in some cases, when minimal risk is involved, the investigator may have to provide the subject only with an information sheet and a verbal explanation. In other cases, such as a volunteer convenience sample, completion and return of research instruments provide evidence of consent. The REB will advise on exceptions to these guidelines, such as cases in which the REB might grant waivers or amend its guidelines in other ways. The REB makes the final determination regarding the most appropriate documentation format. Research consumers should note whether and what kind of evidence of informed consent has been provided in a research article.

Helpful Hint

Note that researchers often do not obtain written, informed consent when the major means of data collection is through self-administered questionnaires. The researcher usually assumes implied consent in such cases; in other words, the return of the completed questionnaire reflects the respondent's voluntary consent to participate.

RESEARCH ETHICS BOARDS

Research ethics boards (REBs) are boards that review research projects to assess whether ethical standards are met in relation to the protection of the rights of human subjects. The Tri-Council and most funding agencies require that universities, hospitals, and other health agencies applying for a grant or contract for any project or program that involves the conduct of biomedical or behavioural research involving human subjects must submit with their application assurances that they have established an REB that reviews the research projects and protects the rights of the human subjects (Government of Canada, 2003). The Tri-Council also requires that the REB have at least five members, including both men and women. Membership must include at least two members who have broad expertise in research, at least one member who is aware of ethics for biomedical research, at least one member who knows the law, and at least one member who is a community member and has no affiliation with the institution but is recruited from the community served by the institution (Government of Canada, 2003).

The REB is responsible for protecting subjects from undue risk and loss of personal rights and dignity. For a research proposal to be eligible for consideration by an REB, it must already have been approved by a departmental review group, such as a nursing research committee, that attests to the proposal's scientific merit and congruence with institutional policies, procedures, and mission. The REB reviews the study's protocol to ensure that it meets the requirements of ethical research that appear in Box 6–4. Most boards provide guidelines or instructions for researchers that include steps to be taken to receive REB approval. For example, guidelines for writing a standard consent form or criteria for qualifying for an expedited rather than a full REB review may be available. The REB has the authority to approve research, require modifications, or disapprove a research study, based on the guidelines outlined in Box 6–5. A researcher must receive REB approval before beginning to conduct research. REBs have the authority to suspend or terminate approval of research that is not conducted in accordance with REB requirements or that has been associated with unexpected serious harm to subjects (Pallikkathayll, Crighton, & Aaronson, 1998). An example of an REB approval is provided by Baker (2007) in a study exploring globalization and the cultural safety of an immigrant Muslim community in Canada following the terrorist attacks on September 11, 2001. These researchers sought ethical approval from the Ethical Review Committee of the Université de Moncton.

REBs in Canada also provide for reviewing research in an expedited manner when the risk to research subjects is minimal. An expedited review usually shortens the length of the review process. Keep in mind, however, that although a researcher may determine that a project involves minimal risk, the research cannot be conducted until the REB makes the final determination. Many qualitative research projects are eligible for an expedited review because the research is noninvasive and focuses on methods such as observation, interviews, and questionnaires. Note that an expedited review does not automatically exempt the researcher from obtaining informed consent.

Not all research requires an ethical review, however. Although, to follow protocol, researchers can submit a proposal to their own REB, the Tri-Council (Government of Canada, 2003) states that this step is not necessary for the following types of research:

- Research about a person living in the public area or an artist, based on public information, documents, records, performances, archival materials, or third-party interviews
- Annual renewals of approved projects in which little or no change has occurred in the ongoing research
- Research involving review of client records by hospital personnel

Adapted from: Government of Canada. (2003). Article 1.6 of *Tri-Council policy statement: Ethical conduct for research involving humans, 2003* (with 2000, 2002 updates). Retrieved September 29, 2007, from http://www.pre.ethics.gc.ca/english/pdf/TCPS%20June2003_E.pdf

The CIHR Web site has a complete listing of updated information concerning ethical guidelines involving human subjects. In addition, all researchers should consult their agency's research offices to ensure that the application being prepared for REB approval adheres to the most current requirements. Nurses who are critiquing published research should be familiar with current regulations to determine whether ethical standards have been met. The Critical Thinking Decision Path illustrates the ethical decision-making process an REB might use in evaluating the risk–benefit ratio of a research study.

PROTECTING THE BASIC HUMAN RIGHTS OF VULNERABLE GROUPS

Researchers are advised to consult their agency's REB for the most recent guidelines when considering research involving vulnerable groups, such as

BOX 6–4   **Canadian Nurses Association Ethical Research Guidelines for Registered Nurses**

These guidelines are the primary values in the Canadian Nurses Association's *Code of Ethics for Registered Nurses* (2008), and they form the structural framework for the *Ethical Research Guidelines for Registered Nurses* (Canadian Nurses Association [CNA], 2002). Below each guideline are examples of principles for implementation.

GUIDELINE 1: PROMOTING SAFE, COMPASSIONATE, COMPETENT, AND ETHICAL CARE
Implementation
Nurses engaged in research must comply with the *Code of Ethics for Registered Nurses* (2008) and conduct themselves with honesty and integrity in all their interactions with research subjects and research colleagues (CNA, 2002, p. 6).

Nurses involved as principal investigators, clinical research coordinators or research assistants must base their research on relevant knowledge of research methods and continue to acquire new skills and knowledge to develop and maintain their level of competence in research (CNA, 2002, p. 6).

GUIDELINE 2: PROMOTING HEALTH AND WELL-BEING
Implementation
Nurses engaged in nursing practice must hold people's optimum health and well-being as first and foremost in their interactions with all those they serve (CNA, 2002, p. 7).

Nurses should recognize the importance of bringing a nursing perspective to health research and engage with other health professionals in interdisciplinary health research promoting health and well-being (CNA, 2002, p. 8).

GUIDELINE 3: PROMOTING AND RESPECTING INFORMED DECISION-MAKING
Nurses caring for people involved in research should do their part in ensuring that consent is free and informed. The investigator, or the individual designated by the investigator, should fully inform the subject of all pertinent aspects of the study including the type and level of commitment required and potential benefits and risks (CNA, 2002, p. 9).

Nurses caring for persons must be alert to any signs that these individuals feel pressured or coerced into participating in a research study. If they suspect that these individuals feel pressured or coerced, nurses must advise the investigator and/or the agency's REB (CNA, 2002, p. 9).

GUIDELINE 4: PRESERVING DIGNITY
Implementation
Nurses demonstrate equal respect for persons who choose to become research subjects and for those who choose not to participate (CNA, 2002, p. 12).

Nurse should respect the process by which communities determine whether and under what conditions research can be conducted (e.g. First Nations communities) (CNA, 2002, p. 13).

GUIDELINE 5: MAINTAINING PRIVACY AND CONFIDENTIALITY
Implementation
Nurses caring for persons involved in research must be attentive to the subject's privacy and exercise caution in use, access, collection, and disclosure of information. They should be aware of relevant provincial legislation about the confidentiality of health and research information (CNA, 2002, p. 14).

In all cases where research data must be released, nurses should release only the minimum amount of data required and restrict the number of people to whom data is released (CNA, 2002, p. 14).

GUIDELINE 6: PROMOTING JUSTICE
Implementation
Nurses must seek to ensure that all persons have access to opportunities, subject to availability, to be involved as research subjects (CNA, 2002, p. 15).

Nurses should promote participatory research where research subjects can work in partnerships with researchers in design, implementation and dissemination of research (CNA, 2002, p. 15).

GUIDELINE 7: BEING ACCOUNTABLE
Implementation
Nurses engaged in research must conduct the research within their own level of competence. Even if others assume that nurses know and should be able to perform certain research interventions required in the study, nurses must advise researchers and clinical staff if they do not feel they have the level of competence needed to perform these tasks. If placed in such a position, they should seek information and help from investigators and other knowledgeable researchers (CNA, 2002, p. 17).

Nurses engaged in research and nurse educators should seek to ensure their students learn about research design, research ethics and the need for ethics approval. They should also help students be aware of their level of competence in conducting research (CNA, 2002, p. 17).

From Canadian Nurses Association. (2002b). *Ethical research guidelines for registered nurses.* Ottawa: Author. Reprinted with permission; Canadian Nurses Association. (2008). *Code of Ethics for Registered Nurses.* Ottawa: Author. Retrieved September 9, 2008, from http://www.cna-aiic.ca/CNA/documents/pdf/publications/Code_of_Ethics_2008_e.pdf

BOX 6–5 **Partial Guidelines for Research Ethics Board Approval of Research Studies**	**Critical Thinking Decision Path.** Evaluating the Risk–Benefit Ratio of a Research Study

To approve research, the REB must determine that the following guidelines have been satisfied:

1. There is an analysis of balance and distribution of harms and benefits.

2. The design of any research project that poses more than minimal risk is capable of addressing questions being asked in the research.

3. There is a proportionate approach based on the general principle that the more invasive the research, the greater the care should be in assessing the research.

4. There is a formal informed consent process.

From Government of Canada (Medical Research Council of Canada, Natural Sciences and Engineering Research Council of Canada, and Social Sciences and Humanities Research Council of Canada). (2003). Sections C and D of *Tri-council policy statement: Ethical conduct for research involving humans, 2003 (with 2000, 2002 updates)*. Retrieved September 29, 2007, from http://www.pre.ethics.gc.ca/english/pdf/TCPS%20June2003_E.pdf

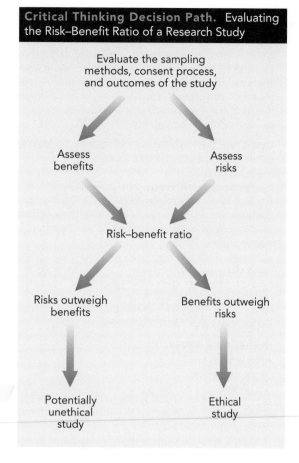

older adults, children, pregnant women, the unborn, those who are emotionally or physically disabled, prisoners, the deceased, students, and persons with AIDS (Baskin, Morris, Ahronheim, Meier, & Morrison, 1998; Campbell, 1999a, 1999b; Haggerty & Hawkins, 2000; Lutz, 1999; National Bioethics Advisory Commission, 1998). In addition, researchers should consult the REB before planning research that potentially involves an oversubscribed research population, such as clients who have undergone organ transplantation, clients with AIDS, or "captive" and convenient research populations, such as prisoners. Note that the use of special populations does not preclude undertaking research; safeguards must be undertaken, however, to protect the rights of these subjects (Government of Canada, 2003; Levine, 1995). Davis (1981) reminded us that a society can be judged by the way it treats its most vulnerable people—a point worth remembering in research that involves children, older adults, and other vulnerable groups.

Pediatric research can be particularly problematic. Mitchell (1984) discussed the US National Commission's concept of assent versus consent in regard to pediatric research. **Assent** contains the following three fundamental elements:

1. A basic understanding of what the child will be expected to do and what will be done to the child

2. A comprehension of the basic purpose of the research

3. An ability to express a preference regarding participation

An example of research using assent in a pediatric group is illustrated by the study of Rennick, Morin, Kim, Johnston, Dougherty, and Platt (2004). These researchers were interested in identifying children at high risk for psychological problems following hospitalization in a pediatric intensive care unit. The children were categorized as being either at high or low risk for developing persistent psychological sequelae based on illness severity and the number of invasive procedures to which they were exposed. The children gave assent verbally or in writing, and their parents provided written consent for their children to participate.

In contrast to assent, consent requires a relatively advanced level of cognitive ability. Informed consent reflects competency standards requiring abstract appreciation of and reasoning regarding the information provided. The issue of assent versus consent is an interesting one. For example, at what age can children be expected to make meaningful decisions about participating in research. In terms of the work by Piaget regarding cognitive ability, children age 6 years and older can participate in giving assent. Children age 14 years and older, although not legally authorized to give sole consent unless they are emancipated minors, can make such decisions as capably as adults (Mitchell, 1984).

If the research involves more than minimal risk and does not offer a direct benefit to the individual child, then both parents must grant permission. When individuals reach maturity, usually at 18 years of age in the case of research, they may render their own consent. They may do so at a younger age if they have been legally declared emancipated minors. Questions regarding assent, consent, and the age of the individual should be addressed by the REB or research administration office and not left to the discretion of the researcher to answer.

Special ethical considerations also exist when conducting research with older adults. As an advocate for vulnerable older adults who are of increasing dependence and declining cognitive ability, the American Geriatrics Society Ethics Committee (1998) states that older adults are precisely the class of persons who were historically and are potentially vulnerable to abuse and for whom the law must struggle to fashion specific protections. The issue of the legal competence of older adults is often raised (Flaskerud & Winslow, 1998), but no issue exists if the potential subject can supply legally effective informed consent. Competence is not a clear "black or white" situation. The complexity of the study may affect an individual's ability to consent to participate. The capacity to give informed consent should be assessed in each individual for each research protocol being considered (American Geriatrics Society Ethics Committee, 1998). For example, an elderly person may be able to consent to participate in a simple observation study but not in a clinical drug trial.

The issue of the necessity of requiring the older adult to provide consent often arises. Dubler (personal communication, 1993) referred to research regulations that indicate some or all of the elements of informed consent may be waived for the following reasons:

1. The research involves no more than minimal risk to the subjects
2. The waiver or alteration will not adversely affect the rights and welfare of the subjects
3. The research could not feasibly be carried out without the waiver or alteration

No vulnerable population may be singled out for study merely for convenience. For example, neither people with mental illness nor prisoners may be studied simply because they are available and convenient groups. Prisoners may be studied if the study pertains to them—for example, studies concerning the effects and processes of incarceration. Similarly, people with mental illness may participate in studies that focus on expanding knowledge about psychiatric disorders and treatments. Students also are often a convenient group. They must not, however, be singled out as research subjects because of convenience; the research questions must have some bearing on their status as students.

Researchers and client caregivers involved in research with vulnerable people are well advised to seek advice from appropriate REBs, clinicians, lawyers, ethicists, and others. In all cases, the burden should be on the investigator to show the REB that it is appropriate to involve vulnerable subjects in research.

Keep in mind that researchers rarely mention explicitly that the study participants were vulnerable subjects or that special precautions were taken to appropriately safeguard the human rights of this vulnerable group. Research consumers need to be attentive to the special needs of individuals who may be unable to act as their own advocates or are unable to adequately assess the risk–benefit ratio of a research study.

RESEARCH INVOLVING ABORIGINAL PEOPLE

When developing ethical guidelines, attention is paid to the culture and traditions of Aboriginal people in Canada. To this end, the Tri-Council (Government of Canada, 2003) has developed the following "good practices" for researchers and REBs to consider when engaged in research:

- *To respect the culture, traditions and knowledge of the Aboriginal group;*
- *To conceptualize and conduct research with the Aboriginal group as a partnership;*
- *To consult members of the group who have relevant expertise;*
- *To involve the group in the design of the project;*
- *To examine how the research may be shaped to address the needs and concerns of the group;*
- *To make best efforts to ensure that the emphasis of the research, and the ways chosen to conduct it, respect the many viewpoints of different segments of the group in question;*
- *To provide the group with information respecting the following:*
  - *Protection of the Aboriginal group's cultural estate and other property;*
  - *The availability of a preliminary report for comment;*

- *The potential employment by researchers of members of the community appropriate and without prejudice;*
- *Researchers' willingness to cooperate with community institutions;*
- *Researchers' willingness to deposit data, working papers and related materials in an agreed-upon repository.*
- *To acknowledge in the publication of the research results the various viewpoints of the community on the topics researched; and*
- *To afford the community an opportunity to react and respond to the research findings before the completion of the final report, in the final report or even in all relevant publications.*

Adapted from: Canadian Institutes of Health Research. (2007). *CIHR guidelines for health research involving Aboriginal people (Section 6.2).* Retrieved September 29, 2007, from http://www.cihr-irsc.gc.ca/e/29134.html

In the study by Smith, Edwards, Varcoe, Martens, and Davies (2006) (see Appendix B), using a participatory action research approach assisted the researchers in acknowledging many of the considerations above by involving leaders of the community and other key informants in the research design. In some cases, however, these "good practices" are not fully implemented. For example, Smylie et al. (2005) raised concerns about ethical issues in certain studies in which community members were not consulted in the formulation of the study and cautioned researchers that using "Aboriginality" as a social construct is not paying attention to the heterogeneity in the various groups.

To understand the evidence being collected, and to make informed choices about what First Nations leaders need to improve the social and economic conditions of their people, an ethical framework, called OCAP (Ownership, Control, Access, and Possession), was developed by the First Nations Statistics Initiative. This initiative is important because a perceived mistrust exists between First Nations people and researchers, and researchers choose participants and studies based on their own interests rather than on the needs of the people (Anonymous, 2003).

SCIENTIFIC FRAUD AND MISCONDUCT

Fraud

Periodically, articles reporting the unethical actions of researchers appear in the professional and lay literature. Data may have been falsified or fabricated, or subjects may have been coerced into participating in a research study (Kevles, 1996; Tilden, 2000; US Department of Health and Human Services, 2000). In a climate of "publish or perish" in academic and scientific settings and declining research dollars, increasing pressure is put on academics and scientists to produce significant research findings. Job security and professional recognition are coveted, essential, and often predicated on being a productive scientist and a prolific writer. These pressures have been known to overpower some people, who then take shortcuts, fabricate data, and falsify findings to advance their positions (Rankin & Esteves, 1997; Tilden, 2000).

The risks of engaging in fraudulent research are many, including harming research subjects or basing clinical practice on false data. As advocates of client welfare and professional practice, nurses should be aware that sometimes they might observe or suspect a researcher's misconduct. In such cases, nurses must be advised to contact the appropriate group, such as the REB, to ensure that this matter receives appropriate attention and review.

Misconduct

Of equal importance is the issue of basing nursing practice on reports that appear in journals when subsequent research and reports on those subjects change the scientific basis for practice. Journals may print corrections or further research in follow-up reports that are buried, obscure, or under-reported. Physician Lawrence K. Altman (1988) stated that "such shortcomings are critically important because the thousands of journals that cover a range of specialties are the central reservoir of scientific knowledge. They are the standard references for crediting discoveries and determining treatments" (p. C3). It is incumbent on nurses as client advocates and research consumers to keep up-to-date on scientific reports related to nursing practice and to adjust their practice as directed by ever-evolving, evidence-based research findings. In addition, researchers have a responsibility to keep current to with federal compliance regulations on prevention, detection, and inquiry into and adjudication of scientific misconduct.

Unauthorized Research

At times, ad hoc or informal and unauthorized research is conducted, including **product testing**. Although the testing may seem harmless, again, it is not the purview of the investigator to make that determination. Nurses must carefully avoid being involved in unauthorized research for a number of reasons, including the following (Raybuck, 1997):

- These treatments or methods of care are usually not monitored as closely for untoward effects, hence exposing the client to unwarranted risk.
- Clients' rights to informed consent in clinical trials are not protected.
- The success or failure of these unrecorded trials contributes nothing to the organized scientific knowledge of the efficacy or complications of the treatment.
- The lack of independent quality supervision allows deviations from the adopted experimental program that may eliminate the program's effectiveness.

PRODUCT TESTING

Nurses are often approached by manufacturers to test products on clients. Often, nurses assume the role of research coordinator in clinical drug or product trials (Raybuck, 1997). Consequently, nurses should be aware of the Health Products branch guidelines and regulations for testing of medical devices before they initiate any form of clinical testing. Medical devices are classified according to the extent of control necessary to ensure the safety and effectiveness of each device (see Health Canada, n.d.).

LEGAL AND ETHICAL ASPECTS OF ANIMAL EXPERIMENTATION

The laws that have been written to protect **animal rights** in research emanate from an interesting history of attitudes toward animals and the value people place on them. In 1963, the Medical Research Council of Canada (now CIHR) requested that a committee be established to investigate the care and use of experimental animals. The Canadian Council on Animal Care (CCAC) was formed and became a nonprofit, autonomous, and independent body in 1982 (CCAC, 2005). It is now funded by the CIHR and the NSERC and conducts assessment visits to each institution every three years—often unannounced. The CCAC requires that institutions conducting animal-based research, teaching, or testing establish an animal care committee and that this committee be functionally active. The CCAC has a detailed guide regarding developing terms of reference for animal care committees (CCAC, 2006).

Recently, the CIHR scrutinized the proposed amendments to the Cruelty to Animal Provisions of the *Criminal Code of Canada*, Bill-C15. The objective of these changes is to strengthen but simplify the existing penal code and "to enhance the effectiveness of the offence provisions for clearly abusive, brutal and cruel treatment of animals." The CIHR supported this objective in principle and, with the NSERC, prepared a joint submission to the House of Commons Standing Committee on Justice and Human Rights in the fall of 2001, recommending amendments to clarify certain provisions of the bill with respect to their application to health research. This section serves only as an introduction to the concept of legal and ethical issues related to animal experimentation. Principles of protection of animal rights in research have evolved over time. Animals, unlike humans, cannot give informed consent, but other conditions related to their welfare must not be ignored. Nurses who encounter the use of animals in research should be alert to their rights.

RESEARCH INVOLVING HUMAN GAMETES, EMBRYOS, OR FETUSES

Human genome and other reproductive research have caused much ethical debate and concern; thus, the Tri-Council (Government of Canada, 2003) developed the following guidelines:

- Research Involving Human Gametes
  - Researchers shall obtain free and informed consent from the individual whose gametes are to be used in research (Article 9.1).
  - In research, it is not ethical to use ova or sperm that have been obtained through commercial transactions, including exchange for service (Article 9.2).
  - It is not ethically acceptable to create, or intend to create, hybrid individuals by such means as mixing human and animal gametes or transferring somatic or germ cell nuclei between cells of humans and other species (Article 9.3).
- Research Involving Human Embryos
  - It is not ethically acceptable to create human embryos specifically for research purposes (Article 9.4; see under conditions).
  - It is not ethically acceptable to undertake research that involves ectogenesis, cloning human beings by any means, including somatic cell transfer, formation of animal or human hybrids, or the transfer of embryos between humans and other species (Article 9.5).

- Research Involving Fetuses
  - Research may be undertaken on methods to treat, in utero, a fetus that is suffering from genetic or congenital disorders.

- Research Involving Fetal Tissue
  - Research involving the use of fetal tissue should be guided by respect for the woman's dignity and integrity.

Critiquing the Legal and Ethical Aspects of a Research Study

Research articles and reports often do not contain detailed information regarding either the degree to which or all of the ways in which the investigator adhered to the legal and ethical principles presented in this chapter. Space considerations in articles preclude extensive documentation of all legal and ethical aspects of a research study. Lack of written evidence regarding the protection of human rights does not imply that appropriate steps were not taken.

The Critiquing Criteria box provides guidelines for evaluating the legal and ethical aspects of a research report. Although research consumers reading a research report will not see all areas explicitly addressed in the research article, they should be aware of them and should determine that the researcher has addressed them before gaining REB approval to conduct the study. A nurse who is asked to serve as a member of an REB will find the critiquing criteria useful in evaluating the legal and ethical aspects of the research proposal.

Information about the legal and ethical considerations of a study is usually presented in the "Methods" section of a research report. The subsection on the sample or data collection methods is the most likely place for this information. The author most often indicates in a few sentences that informed consent was obtained and that approval from an REB or similar committee was granted. It is likely that a manuscript will not be accepted for publication without such a discussion, which also makes it almost impossible for unauthorized research to be published. Therefore, when a research article provides evidence of having been approved by an external review committee, the reader can feel confident that the ethical issues raised by the study have been thoroughly reviewed and resolved.

CRITIQUING CRITERIA

1. Was the study approved by an REB or other agency committee members?

2. Is there evidence that informed consent was obtained from all subjects or their representatives? How was it obtained?

3. Were the subjects protected from physical or emotional harm?

4. Were the subjects or their representatives informed about the purpose and nature of the study?

5. Were the subjects or their representatives informed about any potential risks that might result from participation in the study?

6. Was the research study designed to maximize the benefit(s) and to minimize the risks to human subjects?

7. Were subjects coerced or unduly influenced to participate in this study? Did they have the right to refuse to participate or withdraw without penalty? Were vulnerable subjects used?

8. Were appropriate steps taken to safeguard the privacy of subjects? How have data been kept anonymous or confidential?

To protect subject and institutional privacy, the locale of the study frequently is described in general terms in the sample subsection of the report. For example, the article might state that data were collected at a 500-bed tertiary care centre in Ontario, without mentioning the centre's name. Protection of subject privacy may be explicitly addressed by statements indicating that the anonymity or confidentiality of the data was maintained or that grouped data were used in the data analysis.

Determining whether participants were subjected to physical or emotional risk is often accomplished indirectly by evaluating the study's methods section. The reader evaluates the **risk–benefit ratio**, that is, the extent to which the **benefits** of the study are maximized and the **risks** are minimized such that subjects are protected from harm during the study (Dubler & Post, 1998; Pruchino & Hayden, 2000).

For example, a study by Chalmers, Sequire, and Brown (2002) reported the attitudes, beliefs, and personal behaviours of baccalaureate students in regard to tobacco use. The researchers adhered to the principles of informed consent and confidentiality and ensured that the team remained sensitive to the issues of power differences between the students and the faculty engaged in the study. In addition, the students were reassured that their participation or nonparticipation in the study would not affect their education.

In another example, the study by Morse, Penrod, Kassab, and Dellasega (2000) investigated the efficiency and effectiveness of approaches to nasogastric tube insertion during trauma care. To conduct this study, the procedure was videotaped. Approval was granted by the local REB, and all staff, clients, and visiting support individuals were approached for consent to participate. Extra care was undertaken for the preservation of anonymity as all identifying information was removed and any sound bites mentioning names, addresses, or other identification were erased from the videotapes. The obligation to balance the risks and benefits of a study is the responsibility of the researcher. However, the research consumer reading a research report also should be confident that subjects have been protected from harm.

When considering the special needs of vulnerable subjects, research consumers should be sensitive to whether the special needs of individuals who are unable to act on their own behalf have been addressed. For instance, has the right of self-determination been addressed by the informed consent protocol identified in the research report? For example, a study by Dahinten (2003) investigated the relationship of gender and peer sexual harassment in adolescence. The study was approved by the Ethics Board at the University of British Columbia, and written consent was obtained from the school administration. Owing to the sensitive nature of the topic and the young ages (approximately 14 to 16 years) of the participants, written consent was obtained from the parents. The students were informed that their consent to participate was implied if they filled out the questionnaire on the day of the study. The findings of this study have implications for school health programming and for decreasing the deleterious effects of peer harassment.

When qualitative studies are reported, verbatim quotations from informants often are incorporated into the findings section of the article. In such cases, the reader will evaluate how effectively the author protected the informant's identity, either by using a fictitious name or withholding information such as age, gender, occupation, or other potentially identifying data. (See Chapter 8 for special ethical issues related to qualitative research.)

Although the need for guidelines for the use of human and animal subjects in research is evident and the principles themselves are clear, many instances arise in which nurses must use their best judgement, as both client advocates and researchers, when evaluating the ethical nature of a research project. In any research situation, the basic guiding principle of protecting the client's human rights must always apply. When conflicts arise, nurses must feel free to raise suitable questions with appropriate resources and personnel. In an institution, raising questions may include contacting the researcher first; then, if there is no resolution, raising the matter with the director of nursing research and the chairperson of the REB. In cases in which ethical considerations in a research article are in question, clarification from a colleague, agency, or the researcher's REB is indicated. Nurses should pursue their concerns until satisfied that the client's rights and their rights as professionals are protected.

Critical Thinking Challenges

Barbara Krainovich-Miller

- As part of a needs assessment for future health care delivery planning, the Ministry of Health is interested in determining the number of babies infected with the human immunodeficiency virus (HIV). A provincewide study is funded that will include the testing of all newborns for HIV, but the mothers will not be told that the test is being done, nor will they be told the results. Using the basic ethical principles found in Box 6–2, defend or refute this practice.

- The REB of your health care agency does not include a nurse, and you think it should. You discuss this matter with your supervisor, who states that including a nurse is not necessary because the REB uses strict guidelines. What essential arguments and explanations should your proposal address for including a nurse on your institution's REB?

- A qualitative researcher intends to conduct a phenomenological study on caring and to use informants who are severely and persistently mentally ill and attend an outpatient clinic. The REB denies the study, indicating that informed consent cannot be obtained and that these clients will not be able to tolerate an interview. What assumptions have the members of this REB made? If you were the researcher and you were given the opportunity to address their concerns, what would you say? Include information from Table 6–2.

- How do you see computer electronic databases and Web sites assisting researchers in conducting ethical studies? Do you think that REBs can use this technology to assist them in their goals?

Research. The findings, contained in the Belmont Report, discuss the three basic ethical principles of respect for persons, beneficence, and justice that underlie the conduct of research involving human subjects (National Commission for the Protection of Human Subjects of Biomedical and Behavioral Research, 1978). US federal regulations developed in response to the Commission's report provide guidelines for informed consent and REB protocols.

- Protection of human rights includes the rights to (1) self-determination, (2) privacy and dignity, (3) anonymity and confidentiality, (4) fair treatment, and (5) protection from discomfort and harm.

- Procedures for protecting basic human rights include gaining informed consent, which illustrates the ethical principle of respect, and obtaining REB approval, which illustrates the ethical principles of respect, beneficence, and justice.

- Special consideration should be given to studies involving vulnerable populations, such as children, older adults, prisoners, and those who are mentally or physically disabled.

- Scientific fraud or misconduct represents unethical conduct and must be monitored as part of professional responsibility. Informal, ad hoc, or unauthorized research may expose clients to unwarranted risk and may not protect subject rights adequately.

- Nurses who are asked to be involved in product testing should be aware of Health Canada guidelines and regulations for testing medical devices before becoming involved in product testing and, perhaps, violating guidelines for ethical research.

- Animal rights need to be protected, and regulations for animal research have evolved over time. Nurses who encounter the use of animals in research should be alert to their rights.

- As consumers of research, nurses must be knowledgeable about the legal and ethical components of a research study so that they can evaluate whether a researcher has ensured appropriate protection of human or animal rights.

KEY POINTS

- Ethical and legal considerations in research first received attention after the Second World War, during the Nuremberg trials, which resulted in the Nuremberg Code. This Code became the standard for research guidelines protecting the human rights of research subjects.

- The US *National Research Act*, passed in 1974, created the National Commission for the Protection of Human Subjects of Biomedical and Behavioral

REFERENCES

Altman, L. K. (1988, May 31). A flaw in the research process: Uncorrected errors in journals. *New York Times*, p. C3.

American Geriatrics Society Ethics Committee. (1998). Informed consent for research on human subjects with dementia. *Journal of the American Geriatric Society, 46*, 1308–1310.

American Nurses Association. (1985). *Code for nurses with interpretive statements.* Kansas City, MO: Author.

Anonymous. (2003). "OCAP: Ownership, control, access and possession" and research ethics. *The Aboriginal Nurse, 18,* 10–11.

Baker, C. (2007). Globalization and the cultural safety of an immigrant Muslim community. *Journal of Advanced Nursing, 57,* 296–305.

Baskin, S. A., Morris, J., Ahronheim, J. C., Meier, D. E., & Morrison, R. S. (1998). Barriers to obtaining consent in dementia research: Implications for surrogate decision-making. *Journal of the American Geriatric Society, 46,* 287–290.

Benedict, S., & Georges, J. M. (2006). Nurses and the sterilization experiments of Auschwitz: A postmodernist perspective. *Nursing Inquiry, 13,* 277–288.

Brink, P. J. (1992). Autonomy versus do no harm. *Western Journal of Nursing Research, 14,* 264–266.

Campbell, P. W. (1999a, June 25). Federal officials fault two New York institutions for research risks to children. *Chronicle of Higher Education,* p. A43.

Campbell, P. W. (1999b, March 5). Lawmakers push NIH to focus research on minority populations and cancer. *Chronicle of Higher Education,* pp. A32–A33.

Canadian Council on Animal Care. (2005). *About the CCAC.* Retrieved September 29, 2007, from http://www.ccac.ca/en/CCAC_Main.htm

Canadian Council on Animal Care. (2006). *Terms of reference for animal care committees.* Retrieved September 29, 2007, from http://www.ccac.ca/en/CCAC_Programs/Guidelines_Policies/POLICIES/TERMS00E.HTM

Canadian Institutes of Health Research. (2007). *CIHR guidelines for health research involving Aboriginal people.* Retrieved September 29, 2007, from http://www.cihr-irsc.gc.ca/e/29134.html

Canadian Nurses Association. (1983). *Ethical research guidelines for nurses in research involving human participants.* Ottawa: Author.

Canadian Nurses Association. (2002). *Ethical research guidelines for registered nurses.* Ottawa: Author.

Canadian Nurses Association. (2008). *Code of ethics for registered nurses.* Ottawa: Author. Retrieved September 9, 2008, from http://www.cna-aiic.ca/CNA/documents/pdf/publications/Code_of_Ethics_2008_e.pdf

Carroll, M. L. & Ciaffa, J. (2008). *The human genome project: A scientific and ethical overview.* Retrieved on April 11, 2008, from http://www.actionbioscience.org/genomic/carroll_ciaffa.html

Chalmers, K., Sequire, M., & Brown, J. (2002). Tobacco use and baccalaureate nursing students: A study of their attitudes, beliefs and personal behaviours. *Journal of Advanced Nursing, 40*(1), 17–24.

Charron, M. (2000). *Ewen Cameron and the Allan Memorial Psychiatric Institute: A study in research and treatment ethics.* Retrieved September 19, 2004, from http://www.sfu.ca/˜wwwpsyb/issues/2000/summer/charron.htm

Code of Federal Regulations: Protection of human subjects, 45 CFR 46, *OPRR Reports,* revised March 8, 1983.

Collins, A. (1988). *In the sleep room: The story of the CIA brainwashing experiments in Canada.* Toronto: Lester & Orpen Dennys.

Creighton, H. (1977). Legal concerns of nursing research. *Nursing Research, 26,* 337–340.

Dahinten, S. (2003). Peer sexual harassment in adolescence: The function of gender. *Canadian Journal of Nursing Research, 35,* 56–73.

Davis, A. (1981). Ethical issues in gerontological nursing research. *Geriatric Nursing, 2,* 267–272.

Dubler, N. N., & Post, L. F. (1998). Truth telling and informed consent. In J. C. Holland (Ed.), *Textbook of psycho-oncology* (pp. 1085–1095). New York: Oxford Press.

Elder, G. (1981). Social history & life experience. In D. H. Eichorn, J. A. Clausen, N. Haan, & P. H. Mussen (Eds.), *Present and past in middle life* (pp. 3–31). New York: Academic Press.

Flaskerud, J. H., & Winslow, B. J. (1998). Conceptualizing vulnerable populations' health-related research. *Nursing Research, 47,* 69–78.

French, H. W. (1997, October 9). AIDS research in Africa: Juggling risks and hopes. *New York Times,* pp. A1, A12.

Gage-Rancoeur, D., & Purden, M. A. (2003). Daughters of cardiac patients: The process of caregiving. *Canadian Journal of Nursing Research, 35,* 90–105.

Gillmor, D. (1987). *I swear by Apollo: Dr. Ewen Cameron and the CIA-brainwashing experiments.* Montreal: Eden Press.

Government of Canada (Medical Research Council of Canada, Natural Sciences and Engineering Research Council of Canada, and Social Sciences and Humanities Research Council of Canada). (2003). *Tri-Council policy statement: Ethical conduct for research involving humans, 2003 (with 2000, 2002 updates).* Retrieved September 29, 2007, from http://www.pre.ethics.gc.ca/english/pdf/TCPS%20June2003_E.pdf

Haggerty, L. A., & Hawkins, J. (2000). Informed consent and the limits of confidentiality. *Western Journal of Nursing Research, 22,* 508–514.

Health Canada. (n.d.). *Health Products and Food Branch: Background.* Retrieved November 30, 2003, from http://www.hc-sc.gc.ca/hpfb-dgpsa/sched_a_background_e.html

Health Canada. (1997). *Good clinical practice: Consolidated guideline. Therapeutic products directorate guidelines: ICH harmonized tripartite guidelines. International conference on harmonization of technical requirements for the registration of pharmaceuticals for human use.* Ottawa: Ministry of Public Works and Government Services Canada.

Heaman, M., Chalmers, K., Woodgate, R., & Brown, J. (2007). Relationship work in an early childhood home visiting program. *Journal of Pediatric Nursing, 22,* 319–330.

Hershey, N., & Miller, R. D. (1976). *Human experimentation and the law.* Germantown, MD: Aspen.

Hilts, P. J. (1995, March 9). Agency faults a UCLA study for suffering of mental patients. *New York Times,* pp. A1, A11.

Jack, S.M., DiCenso, A., & Lohfeld, L. (2005). A theory of maternal engagement with public health nurses and family visitors. *Journal of Advanced Nursing, 49,* 182–190.

Julion, W., Gross, D., & Barclay-McLaughlin, G. (2000). Recruiting families of color from the inner city: Insights from the recruiters. *Nursing Outlook, 48,* 230–237.

Kevles, D. J. (1996, July 5). An injustice to a scientist is reversed, and we learn some lessons. *Chronicle of Higher Education,* pp. B1–B2.

Levine, R. J. (1979). Clarifying the concepts of research ethics. *Hastings Center Report, 93*(3), 21–26.

Levine, R. J. (1986). *Ethics and regulation of clinical research* (2nd ed.). Baltimore–Munich: Urban and Schwartzenberg.

Levine, R. J. (1995, November 10). Consent for research on children. *Chronicle of Higher Education,* pp. B1–B2.

Lutz, K. F. (1999). Maintaining client safety and scientific integrity in research with battered women. *Image, 31*(1), 89–93.

McLean, P. (1996, November). Biomedical research and the law of informed consent. *The Canadian Nurse, 92,* 49–50.

Milgram, S. (1963). Behavioral study of obedience. *Journal of Abnormal and Social Psychology, 67,* 371–378.

Mitchell, K. (1984). Protecting children's rights during research. *Pediatric Nursing, 10,* 9–10.

Morse, J. M., Penrod, J., Kassab, C., & Dellasega, C. (2000). Evaluating the efficiency and effectiveness of approaches to nasogastric tube insertion during trauma care. *American Journal of Critical Care, 9,* 325–333.

National Bioethics Advisory Commission. (1998). *Report and recommendations on research involving persons with mental disorders that may affect decisional capacity.* Rockville, MD: Author.

National Commission for the Protection of Human Subjects of Biomedical and Behavioral Research. (1978). *Belmont report: Ethical principles and guidelines for research involving human subjects* (DHEW Pub. No. 05). Washington, DC: US Government Printing Office, 78-0012.

Pallikkathayll, L., Crighton, F., & Aaronson, L. S. (1998) Balancing ethical quandaries with scientific rigor: Part I. *Western Journal of Nursing Research, 20,* 388–393.

Pranulis, M. F. (1996). Protecting rights of human subjects. *Western Journal of Nursing Research, 18,* 474–478.

Pruchino, R. A., & Hayden, J. M. (2000). Interview modality: Effects on costs and data quality in a sample of older women. *Journal of Aging and Health, 12*(1), 3–24.

Rankin, M., & Esteves, M. D. (1997). Perceptions of scientific misconduct in nursing. *Nursing Research, 46,* 270–276.

Raybuck, J. A. (1997). The clinical nurse specialist as research coordinator in clinical drug trials. *Clinical Nurse Specialist, 11*(1), 15–19.

Rempusheski, V. F. (1991). Elements, perceptions, and issues of informed consent. *Applied Nursing Research, 4,* 201–204.

Rennick, J. E., Morin, I., Kim, D., Johnston, C., Dougherty, G., & Platt, R. (2004). Identifying children at risk for psychological sequelae after pediatric intensive care unit hospitalisation. *Pediatric Critical Care Medicine, 5,* 358–363.

Robb, I. H. (1901). *Nursing ethics: For hospital and private use.* Milwaukee, WI: GN Gaspar.

Rothman, D. J. (1982). Were Tuskegee and Willowbrook studies in nature? *Hastings Centre Report, 12*(2), 5–7.

Smith, D., Edwards, N., Varcoe, C., Martens, P. J., & Davies, B. (2006). Bringing safety and responsiveness into the forefront of care for pregnant and parenting Aboriginal people. *Advances in Nursing Science, 29*(2), E27–E44.

Smylie, J., Tonelli, M., Hemmelgarn, B., Yeates, W. M., Joffres, M. R., Tataryn, I. V., et al. (2005). The ethics of research involving Canada's Aboriginal populations. *Canadian Medical Association Journal, 172,* 977–979.

Storch, J. (2007). Enduring values in changing times: The CNA codes of ethics. *The Canadian Nurse, 103*(4), 29–37.

Tilden, V. P. (2000). Preventing scientific misconduct— Times have changed. *Nursing Research, 49,* 243.

US Department of Health and Human Services (Office of Research Integrity). (2000). Retrieved April 21, 2008, from http://www.ori.dhhs.gov

United States Government. (2008). *"Trials of war criminals before the Nuremberg Military Tribunals under Control Council Law No. 10,"* Vol. 2, pp. 181–182. Washington, DC: US Government Printing Office, 1949. Retrieved April 10, 2008, from http://www.hhs.gov/ohrp/references/nurcode.htm

Wheeler, D. L. (1997, August 13). Three medical organizations embroiled in controversy over use of placebos in AIDS studies abroad. *Chronicle of Higher Education*, pp. A15–A16.

Wheeler, D. L. (1999, August 13). For biologists, the post-genomic world promises vast and thrilling new knowledge. *Chronicle of Higher Education*, pp. A17–A18.

PART TWO

Qualitative Research

Creating Qualitatively Derived Theory

Qualitative inquiry begins with a question that asks about meaning, or "What is going on here?" Data are collected and analyzed by seeking patterns; then concepts are developed, and the association between these concepts is identified to create theory. The type of theory may be classified as descriptive, explanatory, or even predictive. The most significant characteristic of qualitatively derived theory (QDT) is, however, that it is built from a qualitative method that primarily uses observational or interview data and has been systematically and rigorously verified throughout the process of construction. Thus, QDT is a reasonable representation of reality rather than a conjecture that must be tested or a hypothetical extension of what is already known, as is theory used in quantitative inquiry. QDT remains theory (rather than fact) because of the level of abstraction created; in other words, the concepts developed from the data are not exact replicas of the data but are concepts representing clusters of behaviours. This analytical process of synthesization and abstraction classifies the theory as a *theory*.

For example, my present research focuses on exploring suffering. Suffering is important to nursing because it is a universal and normal response to the losses associated with illness and

dying—loss of health, loss of a pain-free existence, loss of independence and autonomy, loss of normal relationships with others, and even the loss of self. Although the causes of suffering are numerous, suffering produces similar behavioural patterns. I have described the behavioural patterns of suffering as switching between two states: enduring (in which emotions are suppressed) and emotional suffering (in which emotions are released).

Enduring behaviours enable a person to contain suffering, maintain control, and get through the immediate crisis. Because of differences in what is being suffered, behavioural strategies to ensure enduring differ. These strategies may be classified as *enduring to die, enduring to live*, and *enduring to survive*.

Once the threat to the self is past, the person may then move to a state of emotional suffering, in which the emotions are released. The person may "fall apart"—cry, sob, and talk incessantly about what has been lost. These behaviours trigger feelings of compassion and a desire in others to provide comfort. Over time, hope "seeps in," and emotional suffering is replaced with a new perspective on life—the transcended or reformulated self in which the person lives life more fully and has a desire to "give back" and to help others who are suffering.

Comforting interventions ease and relieve the suffering and facilitate the person's progression through the suffering experience. These comforting interventions—or modes of symptom management—may be as complex as facilitating hope or as simple and immediate as the appropriate use of empathy. The interventions may be targeted to clients, the family or caregiver, the community, or the nurse. The model is not linear but one in which the person vacillates between enduring and emotional suffering. Appropriate comforting interactions are *client led*, in a complex *comforting interaction model* of the nurse reading and responding to the client's behavioural cues. The nurse then selects an appropriate response, observes the client's response to the intervention, and repeats or continues the intervention, or tries a new intervention, until the suffering or distress is minimized.

This theory of suffering developed from interviews with bereaved relatives, clients who experienced trauma from motor vehicle accidents or burns, and persons experiencing a variety of chronic and acute illnesses.

An example of the comforting interaction model may be seen in the trauma room. Major trauma often dictates that analgesics are inadequate to deal with agonizing pain or are withheld from the victims of major trauma until medical assessment is completed. Clients frequently arrive in the trauma room distressed, terrified, or even "out of control." Real-time observation and videotaped microanalytical data reveal that nursing interventions are aimed at keeping the client in control. This is done primarily using modes of touch (usually firm palm touch), body posturing, and patterns of speech labelled *talking the client through*. Enabling the client to maintain control allows urgent emergency care to be administered as quickly and as safely as possible, and, in this situation, may be considered life-saving.

Client interviews conducted several weeks after the resuscitation revealed that clients could hear the nurse's voice and "just held on." Our videotapes showed that this intonation of speech is sing-song, high-pitched, loud, and used with short sentences that encourage, reassure, inform, and instruct the client. With Adele Proctor (a speech-language pathologist and researcher), I used linguistic analysis to document nurses' intonation and labelled the type of speech used as the *comfort talk register (CTR)*. We believe that the CTR occurs cross-culturally, as do baby talk and birthing talk registers.

Studies such as the one described above demonstrate that comforting strategies are also essential during the conduct of painful clinical procedures such as nasogastric tube insertion. Without such comforting, clients exhibit more distress and may even perceive the care as assault. Comforting strategies are particular to the client's state of suffering and vary according to the client's responsiveness. If an inappropriate comforting strategy is used, the client withdraws, and his or her behaviour escalates. However, most often, if nurses use an inappropriate comforting strategy, the client's immediate response signals the nurse to change the comforting strategy, so the *comforting interaction model* is self-correcting.

Have these studies had an effect on nursing practice? As a researcher, I do not know. Ask yourself, whose responsibility is it to move such findings from a journal article to the bedside? Is it the responsibility of the researcher? The author of nursing textbooks? The clinical instructor? The practising nurse? Or should such changes simply be legislated by those who prepare standards for nursing practice, license professionals and health care institutions, and write nursing policy and procedures?

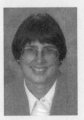

Janice M. Morse
RN, PhD
Professor, Faculty of
    Nursing
Director, International
    Institute for Qualitative
    Methodology, Faculty
    of Nursing
University of Alberta
Edmonton, Alberta

ADDITIONAL READINGS

Morse, J. M. (2001). Toward a praxis theory of suffering. *Advances in Nursing Science, 24*(1), 47–59.

Morse, J. M., Havens, G., DeLuca, A., & Wilson, S. (1997). The comforting interaction: Developing a model of nurse–patient relationship. *Scholarly Inquiry for Nursing Practice, 11*, 321–343.

Morse, J. M., & Proctor, A. (1998). Maintaining patient endurance: The comfort work of trauma nurses. *Clinical Nursing Research, 7*, 250–274.

Penrod, J., Morse, J. M., & Wilson, S. (1999). Comforting strategies used during nasogastric tube insertion. *Journal of Clinical Nursing, 8*, 31–38.

Proctor, A., Morse, J. M., & Khonsari, E. S. (1996). Sounds of comfort in the trauma center: How nurses talk to patients in pain. *Social Sciences & Medicine, 42*, 1669–1680.

Marlene Zichi Cohen
Cherylyn Cameron

CHAPTER 7

Introduction to Qualitative Research

LEARNING OUTCOMES

After reading this chapter, the student should be able to do the following:

- Identify assumptions underlying the qualitative methods of grounded theory; case study; historical, ethnographic, and participatory action research; and phenomenological approaches to research.
- Identify the links between qualitative research and evidence-based practice.
- Discuss significant issues that arise in conducting qualitative research in relation to topics such as ethics, criteria for judging scientific rigour, combination of research methods, and use of computers to assist data management.

STUDY RESOURCES

evolve Go to Evolve at
http://evolve.elsevier.com/Canada/LoBiondo/Research/
for Weblinks, content updates, and additional
research articles for practice in reviewing
and critiquing.

KEY TERMS

behavioural/materialistic 145
  perspective
case study 147
cognitive perspective 149
context 149
ethnographic research 149
ethnography 149
grounded theory 146
hermeneutics 150
historical research 148
intersubjectivity 151
metasynthesis 159
narrative analysis 152
naturalistic research 145
orientational qualitative inquiry 152
participatory action research 153
phenomenological research 150
phenomenology 150
propositions 147
qualitative research 145
reflexivity 157
symbolic interactionism 146
text 145
triangulation 156

Qualitative research is an important term to understand because it is a broad label that includes many approaches. The term implies a focus on the qualities of a process or entity and meanings that are not empirically examined or measured in terms of quantity, amount, frequency, or intensity. Qualitative research can mean the analysis of respondents' answers to open-ended questions. The term also can refer to what is thought of as **naturalistic research**, a general label for qualitative research methods that involve the researcher going to a natural setting, that is, to where the phenomenon being studied is taking place. Qualitative research includes many methods: grounded theory, case study, historical research, ethnography, phenomenology, participatory action research, and many others. These methods have both similarities and differences. Because all methods involve data that are text rather than numbers, all include some content analysis of the text. The term **text** means that data are in a textual form, that is, narrative or words written from interviews that were recorded and then transcribed or notes written from the researcher's observations. However, the methods differ in the philosophical bases on which they are built and in purpose and outcome. This chapter addresses the philosophies underlying the qualitative research methods most commonly used by nurses.

Nurse researchers determine the approach they will take based on their worldview and the nature of the research question. Beginning is never easy and requires many forms of preparation. Beginning research is like beginning a marriage. With luck, both are worth the time and trouble, and what you learn about yourself along the way is often the most important part of the process. In research, as in marriage, having a wonderful partner with whom to share the process is both useful and helpful. This partner will make the journey more fun and a better and richer experience. Nursing research, like nursing itself, concerns many different and complex phenomena. Good research is seldom simple; therefore, conducting research alone is seldom feasible. As a nurse, you will be in an ideal position to identify practice problems. When these problems require research solutions, if you find a team to help solve them, both your clients and your nursing practice will benefit.

So, as you begin your research "marriage," how might you choose among the many different qualitative research methods? Of course, the first lesson learned in research classes is that the research design should match the question being asked. Another important consideration is the philosophy that underlies a research method and how it matches the objectives of the study. Understanding the philosophy on which research is based also is important in evaluating research as a consumer and user of research in your nursing practice.

Figure 7–1 illustrates one of the reasons your research "marriage" might lead you to select a qualitative method. As this cartoon shows, Garfield is

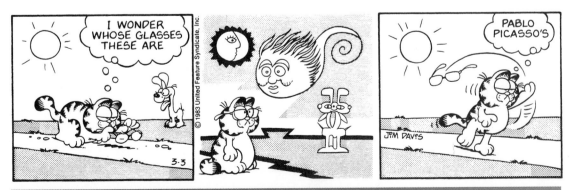

Figure 7–1 Shifting perspectives: Seeing the world as others see it

putting on glasses, and the scene changes as he realizes the glasses belong to Picasso. This is the goal of qualitative methods: to be able to see the world as others perceive and attach meaning to it.

This chapter provides an overview of the major research traditions commonly used in qualitative nursing research, including grounded theory, case study, historical research, ethnographic research, and phenomenological research. Each of these research traditions is discussed as shown in Figure 7–2, based on views that move along a continuum from the positivist view to the constructivist view. Remember that the constructivist paradigm (multiple realities) is the basis of most qualitative research, and the positivist or contemporary empiricist paradigm (single reality) is the basis of most empirical analytical or quantitative research. The philosophical foundation and assumptions of qualitative research are discussed in Chapter 2. You may wish to quickly review pages 28 to 29 to refresh your memory. Make sure that you can differentiate between positivism and constructivism. In addition, several other qualitative research methods are briefly described here.

GROUNDED THEORY

Grounded theory is a research method designed to explore the social processes that guide human interaction and to inductively develop a theory based on observations of the world of selected people. The theory has been described as the "most influential paradigm for qualitative research in the social sciences today" (Denzin, 1997, p. 16). Grounded theory moves along the philosophical continuum from the positivist view toward the constructivist view (see Figure 7–2). This method is based on the sociological tradition of the Chicago School of **Symbolic Interactionism**, a tradition that reflects on issues related to human behaviour. Glaser and Strauss (1967) developed the method of grounded theory and published the classic first text describing the methodology: *The Discovery of Grounded Theory*. Strauss and Corbin (1990) explained that grounded theory

> *is one that is inductively derived from the study of the phenomenon it represents. That is, it is discovered, developed, and provisionally verified through systematic data collection and analysis of data pertaining to that phenomenon. Therefore, data collection, analysis, and theory stand in reciprocal relationship with each other. One does not begin with a theory, then prove it. Rather one begins with an area of study and what is relevant to that area is allowed to emerge.* (p. 23)

Many qualitative research traditions describe and develop explanatory models and theories related to a human phenomenon under study; grounded theory is distinctive from the other traditional qualitative research methods because its primary focus is on generating theory about dominant social processes. The three major premises that

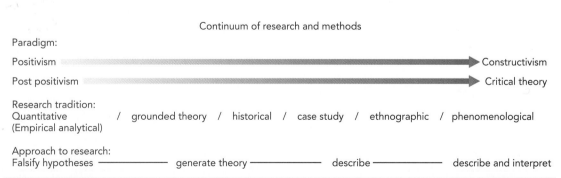

Figure 7–2 Continuum of philosophical foundations and qualitative research methods

continue to underlie grounded theory research are outlined in Box 7–1.

The purpose of grounded theory, as the name implies, is to generate a theory from data. Researchers can then develop middle theories from social phenomena. Grounded theory has contributed substantively to nursing's body of knowledge. Often, the theories generated from grounded research are then tested empirically. In an example of a grounded theory study, researchers interviewed and observed for over a year families with children with neurodegenerative, life-threatening illnesses for the purpose of describing and developing a theory of illness trajectory that explains the experiences families face with a child's death at an unknown time (Steele, 2000). The basic social process examined in this study was "navigating uncharted territory," with four dimensions described as "entering unfamiliar territory, shifting priorities, creating meaning, and holding the fort" (Steele, 2000, p. 55). During the trajectory of certain death, Steele found that families lived on plateaus of relative stability until, eventually, they fell off the plateau and descended into decline and toward the child's inevitable death (2000).

Qualitative data are gathered through interviews and observation. Analysis of the data generates substantive codes that are clustered into categories. **Propositions** about the relationships among and between the categories create a conceptual framework that guides further data collection. Additional data thought likely to answer generated hypotheses are collected until all categories are "saturated," meaning that no new information is generated (see Chapter 8). The goal of generating a theory implies that laws drive at least some portion of reality. The truth is sought from relevant groups, for example, those who are dying.

The context is very important, as was shown in a classic work by Glaser and Strauss (1965). They noted that, at the time of their work, clients were unwilling to talk openly about the process of their own dying, physicians were unwilling to disclose impending death to clients, and nurses were expected not to make these disclosures. This lack of communication led Glaser and Strauss to their study of the problem of awareness of dying. They described various types of awareness contexts, problems of awareness, and practical uses of awareness theory. Their early fieldwork led to hypotheses and the gathering of additional data, and the framework was refined with further analysis until they formed a systematic substantive theory.

CASE STUDY

Case study as a research method involves an in-depth description of the essential dimensions and processes of the phenomenon being studied. Case study research has been given several definitions and can be thought of as the collection of detailed, relatively unstructured information from several sources, usually including the reports of those being studied. Stake (2003) stated that "as a form of research, case study is defined by interest in individual cases, not by the methods of inquiry used" (p. 134).

Case studies can be used for a variety of purposes, including to present data gathered with another method, as a teaching device, or as a research method (Yin, 1994). Hammersley (1989) linked case studies to the Chicago School of Sociology, where grounded theory was developed.

BOX 7–1 | **Major Premises of Grounded Theory**

1. Humans act toward objects on the basis of the meaning those objects have for them. Meaning is embedded in context and, therefore, it cannot be separated from the context or from the consequences of the meanings in a particular setting.

2. Social meanings arise from social interactions with others over time and are embedded socially, historically, culturally, and contextually. Therefore, the focus of grounded theory is on social interactions.

3. People use interpretive processes to handle and change meanings in dealing with their situations.

Case studies have been used in various disciplines, including nursing, political science, sociology, business, social work, economics, and psychology. Nurses have a long and continuing tradition of using case studies for teaching and learning about clients (e.g., Parsons, 1911). Nightingale (1858/1969) stressed the importance of coming to know clients and of basing practice on experience. She noted that knowing how to provide care requires the nurse to learn about the client's life. In case studies, these details are described, and the lessons that can be learned from the particular client are made clear. Persons who have had a particular experience can provide insights that are both valuable and unavailable to those who have not had the experience. Obtaining these descriptions through the use of case studies can serve a variety of functions: sensitization to make practitioners and researchers aware of clients' experiences; conceptualization to make clear the concepts included in an experience or general label; policy decision making; and theory building by identifying hypotheses for testing with further research (Cohen & Saunders, 1996).

The *American Journal of Nursing* features case studies on a regular basis. When this feature was added to the journal, the editor noted that case studies are a way of providing in-depth, evidence-based discussion of clinical topics along with practical information and guidelines for improving practice (Mason, 2000). The journal features case studies written by staff nurses and includes a commentary on some aspect of the case. A case study on advocacy by Miller, Cohen, and Kagan (2000) was the first example of this new feature. Case studies help us understand complex phenomena about which little is known. They can be exploratory and descriptive, as in Whyte's famous example (1943/1955) describing one neighbourhood. A case study can involve one case or multiple cases.

Yin (2003) described three types of case study design: explanatory, exploratory, and descriptive. The explanatory case study considers cause-and-effect relationships, whereas an exploratory case study is a precursor to further studies by defining questions for future studies. The descriptive case

provides a complete, thick (detailed) description of a phenomenon.

An example of a case study is the work by Chircop and Keddy (2003), who explored the experiences of four women with environmental illness. Their illness had a severe impact on their health, families, and significant others. Additionally, these women carried the dual burden of providing proof of their illness and taking refuge from the hostile environment causing their symptoms. Nurses who understand the challenges faced by people with environmental illness may be able to provide more comprehensive and holistic care.

HISTORICAL RESEARCH

Historical research methods allow the researcher to get inside an event and to understand the thoughts of participants in the event within the context of time, place, and other influencing situations. Essentially, historical researchers are narrators and interpreters of past events. Using a variety of sources, such as journals, books, magazines, films, newspapers, and eyewitness accounts, historical researchers seek to understand the past. Reflecting on past events can open new ideas and understanding to guide the future. The three theoretical frameworks that guide historical research are as follows (Speziale & Carpenter, 2007):

1. Biographical history explores the life of an individual to understand the impacts of the time and culture on the person's life.

2. Social history explores the prevailing values and beliefs in a particular period by examining everyday events.

3. Intellectual history explores the ideas of a particular individual or a group of people.

An example of biographical history is the book about Gertrude Richard Ladner (i.e., her family and nursing life), in which the authors presented new ideas about nursing and family life in the late nineteenth and early twentieth centuries in Western Canada (Zerr, Zilm, & Grant, 2006). Although the authors believed that Ladner represented the ordinary life of women and nurses in that time, they discovered that she was more than a handmaiden for the physicians with whom she worked. Many of the details included in the book were gathered from her personal journal, providing a record of the work of nurses, their day-to-day experiences, and nursing knowledge that informed their practice.

ETHNOGRAPHIC RESEARCH

Ethnographic research has a long history in the qualitative research tradition. Anthropologists developed **ethnographic research**, a tradition viewed as beginning with the British anthropologist Bronislaw Malinowski, who was influenced by William Rivers, a physician, anthropologist, and psychologist (Stocking, 1983). Ethnographic research is defined as a method that scientifically describes cultural groups. Scotch (1963) first described medical anthropology as the field of research that focuses on health and illness within a cultural system. Nurses also conduct medical ethnographies that focus on health and illness within a cultural system (Roper & Shapira, 2000). Although early work addressed the cultural patterns of village life, often in distant locations, nurses now often conduct focused ethnographies, the study of distinct problems within a specific context among a small group of people or the study of a group's social construction and understanding of a health or illness experience (Roper & Shapira, 2000). Leininger (1985) developed an ethnographic research method called ethnonursing, which she defined as "an open discovery process using diverse strategies and enablers to document, describe, and understand people's experiences, care meanings, and symbols of care related to their beliefs, values, health and cultural lifeways" (Leininger, 2005).

Ethnography (ethnographic research) describes cognitive models or patterns of behaviour of people within a culture. It seeks to understand another way of life from the "native's" perspective. The following values underlie ethnography:

- Culture is fundamental to ethnographic studies. Culture includes behavioural/materialist and cognitive perspectives. The **behavioural/ materialist perspective** sees culture as observed through a group's patterns of behaviour and customs, its way of life, and what it produces. In the **cognitive perspective**, culture consists of the beliefs, knowledge, and ideas people use as they live. Culture refers to the structures of meaning through which we shape experiences.

- Understanding culture requires a holistic perspective that captures the breadth of the beliefs, knowledge, and activities of the group being studied.

- **Context is** important for an understanding of a culture. Understanding this context requires intensive face-to-face contact over an extended period of time. People are studied where they live, in their natural settings, or where an experience occurs, such as in a hospital or community setting.

- The aim of ethnographic research is to combine the emic perspective—the insider's view of the world—with the etic perspective—the view the researcher (outsider) brings—to develop a scientific generalization about different societies. In other words, generalizations are drawn from special examples or details from participant observation.

An example of ethnographic work that has been useful to nurses is the notion of explanatory models. This idea was developed most by cognitive anthropologists, especially Kleinman (1980). Explanatory models use an interactive approach, emphasizing variations between clients' and practitioners' models of illness. They offer explanations of sickness and treatment, guide choices among available therapies and therapists, and give social meaning to the experience of sickness. These cognitive models vary over time and in response to a particular illness episode.

Varcoe (2001) used an ethnographic design to describe nursing practice in relation to violence against women in two hospital emergency units in large Canadian cities. She discovered that practice is shaped by stereotypical thinking with a focus on physical problems. Her study provides information for the development of educational programs for nurses and for organizational changes to support more effective nursing practice. A more recent study, also conducted in a hospital setting, explored workplace culture relevant to tobacco use and control. The authors discovered that although the policies related to the restriction of smoking were well integrated into the organizational culture, cessation strategies were not supported. The authors concluded that tobacco control in hospitals should also include addressing clients' use, nicotine dependence, and resources to assist with addiction issues (Schultz, Bottorff, & Johnson, 2006).

Several ethnographic schools of thought exist, three of which are of particular interest to nurse researchers: critical, feminist, and ethnogeriatric. Critical ethnography does not use different methods but focuses on beliefs and practices that limit human freedom, justice, and democracy (Usher, 1996). Critical ethnographic researchers make their values explicit. In other words, they document tacit rules that govern human interaction and behaviour. They also explore how dominant social groups oppress those in the minority or those without power. Finally, many critical ethnographers consider the study participants to be co-investigators and explore problems and possible solutions with them.

Feminists, like critical ethnographers, focus on oppression and power but apply their work to women. They also consider and analyze the impact of race, class, culture, ethnicity, sexual preference, and other identities as forces that cause and sustain oppression (Macquire, 1996). For example, Elliott, Berman, and Kim (2002), in their critical ethnographic study, examined how menopause is experienced by Korean Canadian women. McDonald (2006) interviewed 15 lesbian women recruited from a university in Western Canada to understand the experience of lesbians disclosing their sexuality.

Ethnogeriatrics, as the name implies, focuses on examining the "health and aging issues in the context of cultural beliefs, values, and practices among racial and ethnic minority elders"

(Fitzpatrick & Wallace, 2006, p. 179). Ethnogeriatric researchers are interested in the disparities facing racial and ethnic minority older adults and hope to develop nursing knowledge and culturally appropriate interventions to guide health care systems to be more inclusive of this client population.

PHENOMENOLOGICAL RESEARCH

Phenomenological research is used to answer questions of personal meaning. This method is most useful when the task is to understand an experience in the way those having the experience understand it and is well suited to the study of phenomena important to nursing. For example, what is the experience of men facing prostate surgery? What is the meaning of pain for people with chronic arthritis? Phenomenological research is an important method with which to begin when studying a new topic or a topic that has been studied but needs a fresh perspective.

Phenomenological research is based on phenomenological philosophy, which has changed over time and with philosophers. Various phenomenological methods exist, including the following:

1. Descriptive phenomenology, which focuses on the description of the lived world and is based on Edmund Husserl's philosophy;

2. Heideggerian phenomenology, which expands description to understanding achieved through interpretation; and

3. Hermeneutic philosophy, which focuses on interpretation of phenomena.

Derived from the Greek word *hermeneuein*, the term **hermeneutics** refers to a theoretical framework to understand or interpret human phenomena. Hermeneutic researchers believe that interpretation cannot be absolutely correct or true but must be viewed from the perspective of the historical or cultural context and the original purpose of the text. Researchers "use qualitative methods to establish context and meaning for what people do." Hermeneutists are much clearer about the fact that they are "constructing the reality on the basis of their interpretations of data with the help of the participants who provided data in the study" (Patton, 2002, p. 115). Hermeneutic researchers clearly outline their own perspectives and how they may influence the interpretation and analysis of the data. Many nursing studies use the hermeneutic approach to understand a particular phenomenon and scientific interpretation of phenomena from text or the written word (Speziale & Carpenter, 2007).

Patton described many of the different phenomenological approaches in his text, *Qualitative Research and Evaluation Methods* (2002). Although he acknowledged the complexity and differing traditions of these approaches, he also stated the following:

> *What these various phenomenological and phenomenographic approaches share in common is a focus on exploring how human beings make sense of experience and transform experience into consciousness, both as individuals and as shared meaning. This requires methodologically, carefully, and thoroughly capturing and describing how people experience some phenomenon—how they perceive it, describe it, feel about it, judge it, remember it, make sense of it, and talk about it with others. To gather such data, one must take undertake in-depth interviews with people who have directly experienced the phenomenon of interest; that is, they have "lived experience" as opposed to secondhand experience. (p. 104)*

The five important concepts or values in phenomenological research (Cohen, 1987) are as follows:

1. Phenomenological research was developed to understand meanings. The goal was to develop a rigorous science in the service of humanity. This science seeks to go to the roots or foundations of a topic to be clear about what the basic concepts are and what they mean.

2. **Phenomenology** was based on a critique of positivism, or the positivist view, which was

seen as inappropriate to the study of some human concerns. Carefully considering representative examples was the test of knowledge.

3. The object of study is the life-world (*Lebenswelt*), or lived experience, not contrived situations. In other words, as the philosopher Husserl said, we go to the things themselves. We are concerned with the appearance of things (*phenomena*) rather than the things themselves (*noumena*). For example, think about a desk in a classroom. The desk is a real physical object, the noumena, which we all see. If that were not the case, we would bump into the desk every time we passed it. In addition, your view of that desk, the phenomenon, changes as you move in the room. If you sit at the desk, you see only the top of it. However, as you move away, you can see the desk's legs, and so on. Nurses are often interested in various aspects of people's experiences or views of health, illness, and treatment.

4. **Intersubjectivity**, the belief that others share a common world with us, is an important tenet in phenomenology. Although phenomena differ, they also share similarities based on the similarities in people. The most fundamental of those similarities is that we all have a body in space and time. In other words, our physical bodies and historical sense lead to similarities in how we experience phenomena. An essence to the shared experience or basic elements of the experience are common among people or members of a specific society.

5. The phenomenological reduction, also called bracketing, is controversial and more important in some phenomenological approaches than in others (i.e., descriptive methods). Phenomenological reduction means that researchers must be aware of and examine their prejudices or values. The term *bracketing* comes from the mathematical metaphor of putting "brackets" around our beliefs so

that they can be put aside and we can "see" the experience as the person having it sees it, rather than as it changes as filtered through our prejudices.

An example of a phenomenological study is research conducted with persons with advanced cancer who had been referred to a palliative care service because, although they did not report experiencing pain, they had a variety of other symptoms. These symptoms were found to improve when the clients took pain medications. When they were asked to describe their experience, it became clear that similarities and differences existed among these persons that helped to explain why they did not report pain (Cohen et al., 2004). Understanding these experiences provides evidence that can assist nurses in providing comprehensive care in a holistic manner, rather than focusing only on fragmented tasks that need to be accomplished in providing nursing care. Although assessing pain by asking clients to rate their pain on a 0 to 10 scale is a useful beginning, it is clearly only a beginning to pain assessment. Our goal is to come to understand the world as the person who has had the experience sees it. We shift our perspective to see the world as clients see it—an approach that is central to providing competent nursing care to meet client needs.

NARRATIVE ANALYSIS

Narrative analysis extends the hermeneutic tradition to include in-depth interview transcripts, memoirs, stories, and creative nonfiction. This discipline also draws from the phenomenological tradition in its interest in the lived experience and perceptions of experience. Based on the "stories" of people, at times including those of the researcher, narrative analysis attempts to interpret and understand experiences in terms of cultural and social meanings (Patton, 2002). As Lindsay (2006) noted, "Thinking narratively about experience by including the personal and social over time in particular places is personal, reflective and relational work

that is autobiographically meaningful and socially significant" (p. 62). Lindsay and Smith (2003) conducted a narrative analysis when they reflected on and wrote narratively about their relationship as nursing instructor and nursing student. They retold and shared their recollections and interactions and reconstructed their experiences; through this process, they shed light on how students become nurses, construct knowledge, and enact caring–healing practices.

ORIENTATIONAL QUALITATIVE INQUIRY

In **orientational qualitative inquiry** approaches, researchers begin with an ideology or orientation to direct the inquiry, including the research question, methodology, fieldwork, and analysis of the findings. Ideologies include feminist, queer, and critical theories (Patton, 2002). For example, a feminist researcher presumes that gender influences all relationships and societal processes. The researcher will attend to "women's ways of knowing" and include the participants throughout the research. Emerging from feminist theory, queer theory focuses on sexual orientation and activities. For example, Holmes, O'Byrne, and Gastaldo explored why homosexual men continue to have unprotected sex in the face of the associated health risks (2006, 2007). Critical theorists focus on issues of power and justice and how injustice and subjugation shape people's experiences and their view of the world. Rather than studying to understand, the critical theorist attempts to critique society, name injustices, and change society. Nurses are particularly interested in addressing and changing oppressive practices that influence health and health care (Browne, 2000). Smith, Edwards, Varcoe, Martens, and Davies (2006) took a critical postcolonial stance in their study on Aboriginal pregnancy and parenting experiences. The postcolonial stance views issues of power through the lens of the legacy of the colonialization of Aboriginal peoples and the neocolonial present (see Appendix B).

PARTICIPATORY ACTION RESEARCH

Based on orientational research, **participatory action research** also seeks to change society. This methods holds that all forms of knowledge, including indigenous knowledge, are of value and can be applied to practical problems. The researcher studies a particular setting to identify problem areas to improve practice (Glesne, 2006) After identifying possible solutions, action is taken to implement changes in partnership with the stakeholders. Careful attention is given to evaluating the process to ensure that the changes have the desired effect. Participatory action research requires careful collaboration with the research participants and focuses on practical problems particular to a practice setting (Speziale & Carpenter, 2007). Stringer and Genat (2004) defined action research as

> a systematic, participatory approach to inquiry that enables people to extend their understanding of problems or issues and to formulate actions directed towards the resolution of those problems or issues . . . action research seeks local understandings that are specifically relevant to the particular context of a study. (p. 4)

For example, Smith et al. (2006) (see Appendix B) worked with a broad group of stakeholders to identify the themes of pregnancy and parenting experiences among Aboriginal people. Each of the themes and subthemes was discussed and analyzed, resulting in a series of mutually developed innovations to improve health care. The key strategies identified were reaching out and being visible, empowerment and education, including fathers and family, and feeding the body, mind, and soul. All of these strategies were viewed as practical mechanisms to establish safe and responsive care to embrace the local communities' cultural values, norms, and practices.

In this section of the chapter, we have explored several different traditions and methods of qualitative research; however, many emerging researchers are combining a number of related or different methods to frame their naturalistic study. Remember that qualitative inquiry is evolving and changing. As Glesne (2006) noted, "The open, emergent nature of qualitative inquiry means a lack of standardization; there are no clear criteria to package into neat research steps" (p. 19). As you read more qualitative research studies, you will note many interesting designs, all open to the complexity of the human experience. The Smith et al. (2006) study in Appendix B, for example, combines a postcolonial standpoint, participatory research principles, and a case study design. But in their study, Ford-Gilboe, Wuest, and Merritt-Gray (2005) applied a feminist perspective to their grounded theory on the basic social processes of health promotion among single-parent families recovering from intimate family violence.

EVIDENCE-BASED PRACTICE

Traditionally, randomized clinical trials and other types of intervention studies have been the major focus of evidence-based practice, as exemplified by the systematic reviews conducted by the Cochrane Collaboration. Typically, the selection of studies to be included in systematic reviews is guided by levels of evidence models that focus on the effectiveness of interventions according to their strength and the consistency of their predictive power. Because the levels of evidence models are hierarchical in nature, which perpetuates intervention studies as the "gold standard" of research design, the value of qualitative studies and the evidence offered by their results have been understated. Historically, qualitative studies have been ranked lower in a hierarchy of evidence, along with descriptive, evaluative, and case studies, as weaker forms of research designs. This linear application does not seem to fit with the multiple purposes, designs, and methods of qualitative research.

Because nursing is a practice discipline, the most important purpose of nursing research is to put research findings to use. Levels of evidence include qualitative or case studies and systematically obtained evaluation data as sources of evidence to use in practice. Yet, qualitative methods are the best way to start to answer questions that have not been addressed or to look for options when a new perspective is needed in practice. The answers to questions provided by qualitative data reflect important evidence that may offer the first systematic insights into a phenomenon and the setting in which it occurs. Broadening evidence models beyond a narrow hierarchical perspective has already begun as groups of experts consider how qualitative evidence can be evaluated and included more in systematic reviews (Pearson, 2002; Powers, 2005). Such work promises to be an important contribution to expanding the evidence base nurses use for clinical decision making.

Attention to metasynthesis or metastudy of qualitative research is becoming more important in the literature on qualitative research (Paterson, Thorne, Canam, & Jillings, 2001). Metasynthesis involves examining reports of qualitative research, interpreting the results to reveal similarities and differences, and creating new knowledge. An example of a metasynthesis was a review of studies that sought to understand nonvocal, mechanically ventilated clients' experiences with communication (Carroll, 2004). Reviews of this kind are useful and important to show clinicians how they can use findings from qualitative research in their practice.

Remember, the definition of evidence-based practice has three components: clinically relevant evidence, clinical expertise, and client preferences. Qualitative research does not test interventions but does require researchers both to apply their clinical expertise to the choice of the research question and study design and to gain a solid understanding of the client's experience. Although qualitative research uses different methodologies and has different goals from quantitative research, it is important to explore how and when to use the evidence provided by findings of qualitative studies in practice.

Evidence-Based Practice Tip

Qualitative research findings can be used in many applications, including improving the ways in which clinicians communicate with clients and with each other.

ISSUES IN QUALITATIVE RESEARCH

Ethics

Inherent in all research is the demand for the protection of human subjects. This requirement exists for both quantitative and qualitative research approaches and is discussed in Chapter 6. The basic tenets of ethical practice hold true for the qualitative approach. However, several characteristics of qualitative methodologies, outlined in Table 7–1, generate unique concerns and necessitate an expanded view of protecting human subjects.

NATURALISTIC SETTING

The central concern that arises when research is conducted in naturalistic settings focuses on the need to gain consent. The need to acquire informed consent is a basic responsibility of the researcher, but it is not always easy in naturalistic settings. For example, when research methods include observing groups of people interacting over time, the complexity of

TABLE 7–1 **Characteristics of Qualitative Research Generating Ethical Concerns**	
Characteristics	**Ethical Concerns**
Naturalistic setting	Some researchers using methods that rely on participant observation may believe that consent is not always possible or necessary.
Emergent nature of the design	Planning for questioning and observation emerges over the duration of the study. Thus, it is difficult to inform participants precisely of all potential threats before they agree to participate.
Researcher–participant interaction	Relationships developed between the researcher and the participant may blur the focus of the interaction.
Researcher as instrument	The researcher is the study instrument, collecting data and interpreting the participant's reality.

gaining consent is apparent. These complexities generate controversy and debate among qualitative researchers. The balance between respect for human participants and efforts to collect meaningful data must be continuously negotiated. The reader should look for evidence that the researcher has addressed this issue of balance by recording attention to human participant protection.

EMERGENT NATURE OF THE DESIGN

The emergent nature of the research design emphasizes the need for ongoing negotiation of consent with the participant. In the course of a study, situations change, and what was agreeable at the beginning may become intrusive. Sometimes, as data collection proceeds and new information emerges, the study shifts direction in a way that is not acceptable to the participant.

For example, if the researcher is present in a family's home during a time in which marital discord arises, the family may choose to renegotiate the consent. From another perspective, Morse (1998) discussed the increasing involvement of participants in the research process, which sometimes resulted in participants' request to have their names published in the findings or be included as co-authors. If the participant originally signed a consent form and then chose an active identified role, Morse suggested that the participant then sign a "release for publication" form.

The underlying point of this discussion is that the emergent qualitative research process demands ongoing negotiating of researcher–participant relationships, including the consent relationship. The opportunity to renegotiate consent establishes a relationship of trust and respect, characteristic of the ethical conduct of research.

RESEARCHER–PARTICIPANT INTERACTION

The nature of the researcher–participant interaction over time introduces the possibility that the research experience may become therapeutic—a case of research becoming practice. Basic differences exist between the intention of the nurse when conducting research and when engaging in practice (Smith & Liehr, 1999). In practice, the nurse has caring–healing intentions. In research, the nurse intends to "get the picture" from the perspective of the participant. "Getting the picture" may be a therapeutic experience for the participant. Sometimes talking to a caring listener about things that matter energizes healing, even though this result was not intended. From an ethical perspective, the qualitative researcher is promising only to listen and to encourage the other's story. If this experience is therapeutic for the participant, it becomes an unplanned benefit of the research.

Several ethical dilemmas may emerge from the qualitative researcher's interaction with participants. Glesne (2006) described several roles that the qualitative researcher may assume, such as exploiter, intervenor or reformer, advocate, and friend. All researchers use participants to some extent to meet their own needs, such as status and recognition from ensuing publications, with no recognition of the participants. Further, the researcher is in a position of power (researchers who conduct studies in collaboration with others share the power). Often, the rationale for the "exploitation" lies in the good that may come of sharing the knowledge gained from the research. Issues of reciprocity are particularly troublesome for ethnographic researchers, who are immersed in fieldwork for long periods of time (Lipson, 1994).

Other dilemmas are faced when the researcher attempts to intervene in a situation. For example, if the researcher becomes aware of potentially dangerous drug abuse among a group of young adults, should the researcher intervene, with the possible consequence of breaching the confidentiality and, ultimately, the trust of the participants? Finally, as trust and respect are established, researchers may find themselves in the role of confidant, which may, in some cases, lead to friendship. Although some qualitative researchers find the role of friend acceptable if based on trust, caring, and collaboration, an inherent danger exists that the data are given in the context of friendship and not for the purposes of research (Glesne, 2006). Investigators may also find it difficult to leave and say goodbye to participants. Fournier, Mill, Kipp, and Walusimbi (2006) indicated that more attention needs to be given to psychological preparation, focused on exiting the relationship. In participatory action research, the researcher also needs to consider whether there are any long-term obligations to sustain the project (Fournier et al., 2006)

Helpful Hint
Researchers are privileged to enter the lives of others and must treat the ensuing relationship with the utmost respect.

RESEARCHER AS INSTRUMENT

Qualitative research demands that the researcher become immersed in the field. Understanding comes from trying to comprehend how others think, act, and feel (Patton, 2002). Because researchers are interpreting what they observe and experience, personal history, experiences, knowledge, and bias may distort the data. The responsibility to remain true to the data requires that the researchers acknowledge any personal bias and interpret findings in a way that accurately reflects the participant's reality. Researchers need to become aware of and monitor their own subjectivity to decrease any distortion of the data. This responsibility is a serious ethical obligation. To accomplish this, researchers should prepare for differences in other cultures and groups by reading, interacting, and seeking out experiences outside of their own norms (Roper & Shapira, 2000). Qualitative researchers frequently write journals during their research activity to monitor and become aware of their personal biases and feelings (Glesne, 2006). Through this process of **reflexivity** in qualitative research, researchers constantly challenge themselves to understand how their perspective may be shaping the method, interviews, analysis, and interpretations. Additionally, many researchers may return to the participants at critical interpretive points and ask for clarification or validation. Patton (2002) advocated the stance of neutrality; in other words, the researcher does not enter the field with

predisposed notions but is open to understanding "the world as it unfolds" (p. 51).

Speziale and Carpenter (2007) recommended that researchers identify their own thoughts, feelings, and perceptions by compartmentalizing them in the process referred to as bracketing, defined earlier (see pages 151–152). Bracketing is important in both the descriptive phenomenological and the ethnographic traditions and is necessary for the researcher to be "open" and receptive to the phenomenon under study. Bracketing is based on the assumption that people can separate their personal knowledge about a specific phenomenon from their experiences and background. For this reason, bracketing may not always be possible, but, at a minimum, researchers should be aware as much as possible of their own assumptions and how they may colour their observations and interpretations and thus influence the results of the study.

Triangulation

Triangulation has become a buzzword in qualitative research over the past several years. The buzz has progressed from viewing triangulation as merely a strategy for ensuring data accuracy (more than one data source presents the same picture) to viewing it as an opportunity to more fully address the complex nature of the human experience. From this perspective, **triangulation** can be defined as the expansion of research strategies in a single study or multiple studies to enhance diversity, enrich understanding, and accomplish specific goals. Richardson (2000) suggested that the triangle be replaced by the crystal as a more appropriate metaphor for the multimethod approach.

Five basic types of triangulation were described (Denzin, 1978; Janesick, 1994):

1. Data: the use of a variety of data sources in a study. For example, the researcher collects data at different times, in different settings, and from different groups of people.

2. Investigator: the use of several different researchers or evaluators from divergent backgrounds

3. Theory: the use of multiple perspectives to interpret a single set of data

4. Methodological: the use of multimethods to study a single problem

5. Interdisciplinary triangulation: the use of other disciplines to increase understanding of the phenomenon (i.e., nursing and sociology)

Although support exists for the use of multiple research methods, controversies surround the appropriateness of combining qualitative and quantitative research approaches and of combining multiple qualitative methods in one study (Barbour, 1998; Giddings & Grant, 2007). Mixed methods research can take two approaches: the mixing of different research methodologies (defined as the theoretical assumptions underlying the research approach) or the mixing of different research methods (defined as the tools for collecting and analyzing data) (Giddings & Grant, 2007). Mixing methodologies can be more difficult if the assumptions and values underlying the research approaches (i.e., the methodologies being mixed) are from different paradigm boundaries. Giddings and Grant (2007) also argued that because most mixed methods studies favour the forms of analysis associated with positivism, this form of research is a Trojan horse for positivism. In other words, results from mixed methods research are more likely to be associated with positivism.

In spite of the dangers of mixing methodologies and methods, serious readers of nursing research will not take long to determine that approaches and methods are being combined to contribute to theory building, to guide practice, and to facilitate instrument development. Several mixed methodology research designs have been developed—many from the seminal work of nurse researchers such as Morgan (1998) and Morse (1991). Note that researchers need to determine the primary method (qualitative or quantitative). For example, if the purpose of the study is to describe, discover, or explore, then the theoretical drive will be inductive, with principal methods that are qualitative. However, if the purpose of the research is to confirm a theory or hypothesis, the underpinning of the research is deductive and, subsequently, a quantitative drive will be used. This recognition is imperative because it drives the design of the study from the size of the sample to the analysis of the data.

Several models were identified by Morgan (1998) and include (a) small, preliminary, qualitative data providing information useful in the development of a larger quantitative study; (b) limited use of quantitative methods to guide the researcher in decisions

TABLE 7–2 **Types of Multimethod Designs**			
Paradigm	**Design**	**Order**	
Inductive	Qualitative + qualitative	Simultaneous	One is dominant and forms the basis for the study; used when more than one perspective is required
	Qualitative → qualitative	Sequential	One is dominant and forms the basis for the study; the second supplements the first
	Qualitative + quantitative	Simultaneous	Inductive drive; used when some portion of the phenomenon can be measured
	Qualitative → quantitative	Sequential	Inductive drive; can confirm earlier qualitative findings
Deductive	Quantitative + quantitative	Simultaneous	One is dominant and forms the basis for the study; validates the finding of each instrument used
	Quantitative → quantitative	Sequential	One is dominant and forms the basis for the study; used to elicit further details
	Quantitative + qualitative	Simultaneous	Deductive theoretical drive; used when some aspect of the phenomenon is not measurable
	Quantitative → qualitative	Sequential	Deductive theoretical drive; often used when the findings are unexpected, the qualitative portion tries to find explanations

pertaining to the larger qualitative project; (c) qualitative methods used to interpret results from a quantitative study; and (d) quantitative methods used to confirm results from the qualitative study. Morse (2003) identified eight different types of multimethod designs with simultaneous or sequential use of qualitative and quantitative methods (see Table 7–2).

Mixed methods research provides researchers with a wider range of tools and options to study phenomena. The variety of methods provide different views and different levels of data.

Table 7–3 synthesizes three studies reporting multimethod analyses. The table notes the conceptual focus of the work, the study purposes, and whether the study suggests implications for theory, practice, and instrument development.

From the perspective of crystallization, Swanson's (1999) work is the most complete (see Table 7–3) because she addressed implications for practice, instrument development, and theory building focused on the issue of caring for women who have had a miscarriage. Her research program included an initial theory-building phase (studies 1 and 2), an instrument development phase (studies 3, 4, and 5), and a phase of testing a practice intervention (study 6). Swanson used the phenomenological method for studies 1 and 2 and quantitative methods for each of her other studies. She does not use more than one method in any of her studies, but her use of multimethods during the course of her 15-year research program can be likened to examining different facets of one crystal—in this case, the experience of miscarrying. The crystallization process has contributed to theory building, nursing practice, and instrument development. Her practice contribution is highlighted by a case exemplar (Swanson, 1999), which synthesized her years of work with women living through the experience of miscarrying their baby.

Both Cameron (2003) and Valkenier, Hayes, and McElheran (2002) used mixed methodology, with the quantitative portion providing a sample and interview questions providing the qualitative portion. Cameron (2003) combined qualitative (interviews) and quantitative (questionnaire) methods to explore the lived experience of transfer students in a collaborative baccalaureate nursing program in Ontario (see Table 7–3). Data from the quantitative survey supported the findings emerging from the qualitative methods. The qualitative methods provided depth and substance to the findings from the questionnaire—like differing facets of a crystal. The study reported by Valkenier et al. (2002) (see Table 7–3) evaluated the impact of a Canadian nursing respite program. The quantitative analysis measured variables (overall cost of child care, nature of nursing care, changes in activities of daily living, and changes in caregiving demands for parents) related to outcome measures. Taking a subset of 10 mothers who were caring for technology-dependent children in their home, the researchers explored how the respite services affected the mothers' lives through the use of unstructured interviews and observations.

The studies of Swanson (1999), Cameron (2003), and Valkenier et al. (2002) (see Table 7.3) presented a range of approaches for combining methods in research studies. The mixed-methods field continues to evolve, as nurse researchers strive to determine which research combinations promise an enhanced understanding of human complexity and a substantial contribution to nursing science. Consumers of nursing research are encouraged to follow this ongoing debate.

SYNTHESIZING QUALITATIVE EVIDENCE: METASYNTHESIS

Qualitative researchers often need to synthesize critical masses of qualitative findings. Qualitative **metasynthesis** is a type of systematic review applied to qualitative research. Unlike quantitative research, which uses statistical approaches to aggregate or average data using meta-analysis (see Chapter 11), metasynthesis integrates qualitative research findings on a common topic and is based on comparative analysis and interpretative synthesis of qualitative research findings that seek to retain the essence and unique contribution of each study (Sandelowski & Barroso, 2003). Essentially, metasynthesis allows researchers to build up a critical mass of qualitative research evidence that

TABLE 7-3 Research Using Multimethod Approaches

Author, Year	Conceptual Focus	Multimethod Approach	Study Purpose	Theory-Building Implications	Practice Implications	Instrument Development Implications
Swanson, 1999	Miscarriage and caring	Six studies, each using one method	**Study 1:** To define common themes for women who had recently miscarried	Yes	Yes	
			Study 2: To describe the human experience of miscarriage and the meaning of caring	Yes	Yes	
			Study 3: To use descriptive data to create a survey instrument based on women's experience of miscarriage			Yes
			Study 4: To evaluate the relevance of the survey items to create a miscarriage scale			Yes
			Study 5: To assess the reliability and validity of the miscarriage scale			Yes
			Study 6: To test the effects of caring, measurement, and time on women's well-being in the first year after miscarriage	Yes	Yes	Yes
Cameron, 2003	Transition resilience	One study using multimethods	To explore the lived experience of students transferring from college to university in a collaborative nursing program	Yes	Yes	Yes
Valkenier, Hayes, & McElheran, 2002	Stress coping	One study using multimethods	To explore the experience of mothers receiving nursing respite services with complex conditions	Yes	Yes	

is relevant to clinical practice (Melnyk & Fineout-Overholt, 2005). Sandelowski (2004) cautioned that the use of qualitative metasynthesis is laudable and necessary but requires researchers who use metasynthesis methods to clearly understand qualitative methodologies and the nuances of the various qualitative methods. Research consumers will follow with interest the progress of researchers who seek to develop criteria for appraising a set of qualitative studies and to then apply those criteria to guide the incorporation of these studies into systematic literature reviews.

Critiquing the Foundation of Qualitative Research

A final example illustrates the differences in the methods discussed in this chapter and provides you with the beginning skills of how to critique qualitative research. The information in this chapter, coupled with the information presented in Chapter 8, provides the underpinnings of critical analysis of qualitative research. Consider the question of nursing students learning how to conduct research. The empirical analytical approach (quantitative research) might be used in an experiment to determine whether one teaching method led to better learning outcomes than another. The students' knowledge might be tested, the teaching conducted, and then a post-test of knowledge given. Scores on these tests would be analyzed statistically to determine whether the different methods produced a difference in the results.

The grounded theorist would be interested in the process and for this example would consider the process of learning research. The researcher might attend the class to observe what occurs and then ask students to describe how their learning changed over time. They might be asked to describe becoming researchers or becoming more knowledgeable about research. The goal would be to describe the stages or process of this learning.

A case study could be written about a particular research class to provide a detailed description of the class or perhaps a particular individual in the class. The case would then be used to explicate what is important in this setting.

Ethnographers would consider the class as a culture and could join to observe and interview students. Questions would be aimed at discovering the students' values, behaviours, and beliefs in learning research. The goal would be to understand and describe the group members' shared meanings.

Phenomenologists would be interested in the meaning of the students' experiences. The phenomenologists would attempt to unearth the meaning of students' experiences by asking students to describe the experience of learning research, that is, to give concrete specific examples. The goal would be to understand and describe the meaning of this experience for the students.

Many other research methods exist. Although you need to be aware of the basis of the research methods used, it is most important that the method chosen will provide the best approach to answering the question being asked. Some research methods, such as focus groups developed from marketing research, are not explicitly based on philosophy, but they have been useful as a method of collecting data to answer nursing research questions. For example, Bottorff, et al. (2004) recruited six adolescents for a focus group to explore issues of tobacco use (see Appendix D).

A helpful metaphor about the need to use a variety of research methods was employed by Seymour Kety, a key figure in the development of biological research in psychiatry who was the scientific director of the US National Institute of Mental Health (NIMH) for many years. He invited readers to think about a civilization whose inhabitants, although very intelligent, had never seen a book (Kety, 1960). On discovering a library, the inhabitants set up a scientific institute for studying books that included anatomists, physical chemists, molecular biologists, behavioural scientists, and psychoanalysts. Each discipline discovered important facts, such as the structure of cellulose, the frequency of collections of letters of varying length, and so on. But the meaning of a "book" continued to escape them. Kety argued that a truer picture of a topic under study would emerge only from research conducted by a variety of disciplines and techniques, each with its own virtues and particular limitations. Qualitative research methods could be added to understand how books are used by different groups—the meaning of books for individuals, for example.

This idea can serve as summary of an important point of this chapter. It is not that one research method is better than others but rather that a variety of methods exist, based on different worldviews. Considering what we need to know to do the important and complex work of nursing, we must guide our practice with knowledge from both nonscientific and scientific realms and, within science, from a wide variety of methods.

CRITIQUING CRITERIA

1. Is the philosophical basis of the research method consistent with the study's purpose?

2. Are the researchers' values apparent? Do they influence the research or the results of the study?

3. Is the phenomenon focused on human experience within a natural setting?

Critical Thinking Challenges

- Why is it important for researchers to consider their own values before conducting research? Include an example in your answer.
- If a grounded theory research study developed a theory—for example, on why certain cultural groups do not use pain medication—why would it be necessary to test the theory with other methods?
- Can the metaphor "We do not always get closer to the truth as we slice and homogenize and isolate [it]" be applied to both qualitative and quantitative methods? Justify your answer.
- What is the value of qualitative research in evidence-based practice? Give an example.

KEY POINTS

- All research is based on philosophical beliefs or paradigms.
- Paradigms are useful or not useful in reaching research goals but are not correct or incorrect.
- Values should be kept as separate as possible from the conduct of research.
- Grounded theory is based on symbolic interactionism and is focused on processes or social interactions.
- Case studies are based on the Chicago School of Sociology and are ways to study complex, real-life situations.

- Ethnographical research, developed by anthropologists, is used to understand cultures.
- Phenomenological research is based on phenomenological philosophy and is designed to understand the meaning of a lived experience.
- Hermeneutic philosophy focuses on interpretation of phenomena from texts.
- Narrative analysis extends the hermeneutic tradition to include in-depth interview transcripts, memoirs, stories, and creative nonfiction.
- In orientational qualitative inquiry approaches, the researcher begins with an ideology or orientation (e.g., a feminist, Marxist, or critical theory) to direct the inquiry.
- Rather than just studying to understand a phenomenon, participatory action research seeks to change society by identifying problem areas and implementing changes.
- Ethical issues in qualitative research involve issues related to the naturalistic setting, the emergent nature of the design, researcher–participant interaction, and the researcher as instrument.

REFERENCES

Barbour, R. S. (1998). Mixing qualitative methods: Quality assurance or qualitative quagmire? *Qualitative Health Research, 8*, 352–361.

Bottorff, J. L., Johnson, J. L., Moffat, B., Grewal, J., Ratner, P., & Kalaw, C. (2004). Adolescent constructions of nicotine addiction. *Canadian Journal of Nursing Research, 38*, 22–39.

Browne, A. J. (2000). The potential contribution of critical social theory to nursing science. *Canadian Journal of Nursing Research, 32*(2), 35–55.

Cameron, C. (2003). *The lived experience of transfer students in a collaborative baccalaureate nursing program.* Unpublished doctoral dissertation, University of Toronto.

Carroll, S. (2004). Nonvocal ventilated patients' perceptions of being understood. *Western Journal of Nursing Research, 24,* 454–471.

Chircop, A. & Keddy, B. (2003). Women living with environmental illness. *Health Care for Women International, 24*(5), 371-383

Cohen, M. Z. (1987). A historical overview of the phenomenological movement. *Image, 19*(1), 31–34.

Cohen, M. Z., & Saunders, J. (1996). Using qualitative research in advanced practice. *Advanced Practice Nursing Quarterly, 2*(3), 8–13.

Cohen, M. Z., Williams, L., Knight, P., Snider, J., Hanzik, K., & Fisch, M. (2004). Symptom masquerade: Understanding the meaning of symptoms. *Support Care Cancer, 12,* 184–190.

Denzin, N. K. (1997). Coffee with Anselm. *Qualitative Family Research, 11*(1), 16–18.

Denzin, N. K. (1978) *The research act: A theoretical introduction to sociological methods* (2nd ed). New York: McGraw-Hill.

Elliott, J., Berman, H., Kim, S. (2002). A critical ethnography of Korean-Canadian women's experience with menopause. *Health for Women International, 23,* 377–388.

Fitzpatrick, J. J., & Wallace, M. (Eds.). (2006). *Encyclopedia of nursing research* (2nd ed.). New York: Springer.

Ford-Gilboe, M., Wuest, J., & Merritt-Gray, M. (2005). Strengthening capacity to limit intrusion: Theorizing family health promotion in the aftermath of woman abuse. *Qualitative Health Research, 15,* 477–501.

Fournier, B., Mill, J., Kipp, W., & Walusimbi, M. (2006). Discovering voice: A participatory action research study with nurses in Uganda. *International Journal of Qualitative Methdods, 6*(2). Retrieved August 3, 2007, from http://www.ualberta.ca/~iigm/

Giddings, L. S., & Grant, B. M. (2007). A Trojan horse of positivism? A critique of mixed methods research. *Advances in Nursing Science, 30,* 52–60.

Glaser, B., & Strauss, A. (1965). *Awareness of dying.* Chicago: Aldine de Gruyter.

Glaser, B., & Strauss, A. (1967). *The discovery of grounded theory: Strategies for qualitative research.* New York: Aldine de Gruyter.

Glesne, C. (2006). *Becoming qualitative researchers: An introduction* (3rd ed.). Don Mills, ON: Longman.

Hammersley, M. (1989). *The dilemma of qualitative research: Herbert Blumer and the Chicago Tradition.* London: Routledge.

Holmes, D., O'Byrne, P., & Gastaldo, D. (2006). Raw pleasure as limit experience: A Foucauldian analysis of unsafe anal sex between men. *Social Theory and Health, 4,* 319–333.

Holmes, D., O'Byrne, P., & Gastaldo, D. (2007). Setting the space for sex: Architecture, desire and health issues in gay bathhouses. *International Journal of Nursing Studies, 44*(2), 273–284.

Janesick, V. J. (1994) The dance of qualitative research design. In N. K. Denzin & Y. S. Lincoln (Eds.), *Handbook of qualitiative research* (pp. 209–219). Thousand Oaks, CA: Sage.

Kety, S. (1960). A biologist examines mind and behavior. *Science, 132,* 1861–1870.

Kleinman, A. (1980). *Patients and healers in the context of culture.* Berkeley, CA: University of California Press.

Leininger, M. (1985). Life-health-care history: Purposes, methods and techniques. In M. M. Leininger (Ed.), *Qualitative research methods in nursing* (pp. 119–132). New York: Strune & Stratton.

Leininger, M. (2005). Overview of Leininger's ethnonursing research method and process. Retrieved December 16, 2007, from http://www.madeleine-leininger.com/eng/documents/ethnonursingresearch.pdf

Lindsay, G. (2006). Constructing a nursing identity: Reflecting on and reconstructing experience. *Reflective Practice, 7,* 59–72.

Lindsay, G., & Smith, F. (2003). Narrative inquiry in a nursing practicum. *Nursing Inquiry, 10,* 121–129.

Lipson, G. L. (1994). Ethical issues in ethnography. In J. Morse (Ed.), *Critical issues in qualitative research methods* (pp. 333–355). Thousand Oaks, CA: Sage.

Macquire, P. (1996). Considering more feminist participatory participatory research: What's congruency got to do with it? *Qualitative Inquiry, 2,* 106–118.

Mason, D. (2000). On centennials and millennia [Editorial]. *American Journal of Nursing, 100,* 7.

McDonald, C. (2006). Lesbian disclosure: Disrupting the taken for granted. *Canadian Journal of Nursing Research, 38,* 42–57.

Melnyk, B. M., & Fineout-Overholt, E. (2005). *Evidence-based practice in nursing and healthcare.* Philadelphia: Lippincott Williams & Wilkins.

Miller, S. H., Cohen, M. Z., & Kagan, S. H. (2000). The measure of advocacy. *American Journal of Nursing, 100,* 61–64.

Morgan, D. (1998). Practical strategies for combining qualitative and quantitative methods: Applications to health research. *Qualitative Health Research, 8,* 362–377.

Morse, J. M. (1991). Approaches to qualitative-quantitative research methodological triangulation. *Nursing Research, 40,* 120–123.

Morse, J. M. (1998). The contracted relationship: Ensuring protection of anonymity and confidentiality. *Qualitative Health Research, 8,* 301–303.

Morse, J. M. (2003). Principles of mixed methods and multimethod research design. In A. Tashakkori & C. Teddlie (Eds.), *Handbook of mixed methods in social & behavioural research* (pp. 189–208). Thousand Oaks, CA: Sage.

Nightingale, F. (1969). *Notes on nursing: What it is and what it is not.* New York: Dover. (Original work published 1858)

Parsons, S. (1911). The case method of teaching nursing. *American Journal of Nursing, 11,* 1009–1011.

Paterson, B., Thorne, S., Canam, C., & Jillings, C. (2001). *Meta-study of qualitative research: A practical guide to meta-analysis and meta-synthesis.* Thousand Oaks, CA: Sage.

Patton, M. (2002). *Qualitative research & evaluation methods* (3rd ed.). Thousand Oaks, CA: Sage.

Pearson, A. (2002). Nursing takes the lead: Redefining what counts as evidence in Australian health care. *Reflective Nurse Leader, 28*(4), 18–21.

Powers, B. A. (2005). Critically appraising qualitative evidence. In B. M. Melnyk & E. Fineout-Overholt (Eds.), *Evidence-based practice in nursing and healthcare* (pp. 127–162). Philadelphia: Lippincott.

Richardson, L. (2000). Writing: A method of inquiry. In N. K. Denzin & Y. S. Lincoln (Eds.), *Handbook of qualitative research* (2nd ed., pp. 923–948). Thousand Oaks, CA: Sage.

Roper, J., & Shapira, J. (2000). *Ethnography in nursing research.* Thousand Oaks, CA: Sage.

Sandelowski, M. (2004). Using qualitative research. *Qualitative Health Research, 14,* 1366–1386.

Sandelowski, M., & Barroso, J. (2003). Creating meta-summaries of qualitative findings. *Nursing Research, 52,* 226–233.

Schultz, A., Bottorff, J., & Johnson, J. (2006). An ethnographic study of tobacco control in hospital settings. *Tobacco Control, 15,* 317–322.

Scotch, N. (1963). Medical anthropology. *Biennial Review of Anthropology, 3,* 30–68.

Smith, D., Edwards, N., Varcoe, C., Martens, P. J., & Davies, B. (2006). Bringing safety and responsiveness into the forefront of care for pregnant and parenting Aboriginal people. *Advances in Nursing Science, 29*(2), E27–E44.

Smith, M. J., & Liehr, P. (1999). Attentively embracing story: A middle range theory with practice and research implications. *Scholarly Inquiry for Nursing Practice: An International Journal, 13,* 187–204.

Speziale, H., & Carpenter, D. (2007). *Qualitative research in nursing: Advancing the humanistic imperative* (4th ed.). New York: Lippincott

Stake, R. E. (2003). Case studies. In N. Denzin & Y. Lincoln (Eds.), *Strategies of qualitative inquiry* (2nd ed., pp. 134–164).Thousand Oaks, CA: Sage.

Steele, R. (2000). Trajectory of certain death at an unknown time: Children with neurodegenerative life-threatening illness. *Canadian Journal of Nursing Research, 32,* 49–67.

Stocking, G. (1983). *Observers observed: Essays on ethnographic fieldwork.* Madison, WI: University of Wisconsin Press.

Strauss, A., & Corbin, J. (1990). *Basics of qualitative research: Grounded theory procedures and techniques.* Newbury Park, CA: Sage.

Stringer, E., & Genat, W. (2004). *Action research in health.* New Jersey: Pearson.

Swanson. K. M. (1999). Research-based practice with women who have had miscarriages. *Image, 31,* 339–345.

Usher, P. (1996). Feminist approaches to research. In D. Scott & R. Usher (Eds.), *Understanding educational research* (pp. 120–143). New York: Routledge.

Valkenier, B., Hayes, V., & McElheran, P. (2002). Mothers' perspectives of an in-home nursing respite service: Coping and control. *Canadian Journal of Nursing Research, 34,* 87–109.

Varcoe, C. (2001). Abuse obscured: An ethnographic account of emergency nursing in relation to violence against women. *Canadian Journal of Nursing Research, 32,* 95–115.

Whyte, W. (1955). *Street corner society: The social structure of an Italian slum.* Chicago: University of Chicago Press. (Original work published 1943)

Yin, R. (1994). *Case study research: Design and methods* (2nd ed.). Thousand Oaks, CA: Sage.

Yin, R. (2003). Applications of case study research (2nd ed). Thousand Oaks, CA: Sage.

Zerr, S. J., Zilm, G., & Grant, V. (2006). *Labor of love. A memoir of Gertrude Richards Ladner 1879 to 1976.* Delta, BC: ZGZ Publication.

Patricia R. Liehr

Geri LoBiondo-Wood

Cherylyn Cameron

CHAPTER 8

Qualitative Approaches to Research

LEARNING OUTCOMES

After reading this chapter, the student should be able to do the following:

- Identify connections between and among the researcher's worldview, research question, and research method.
- Recognize the uses of qualitative research for nursing.
- Identify the processes of phenomenological, grounded theory, ethnographic, and case study methods.
- Recognize appropriate use of historical methods.
- Recognize appropriate use of participatory research methods.
- Apply the critiquing criteria to evaluate a report of qualitative research.

STUDY RESOURCES

evolve Go to Evolve at
http://evolve.elsevier.com/Canada/LoBiondo/Research/
for Weblinks, content updates, and additional
research articles for practice in reviewing
and critiquing.

KEY TERMS

The discipline of nursing has a body of knowledge that provides the foundation for practice and research. Nursing is both a science and an art. **Qualitative research** combines the scientific and artistic aspects of nursing to enhance understanding of the human health experience. Qualitative research is a general term encompassing a variety of philosophic underpinnings and research methods. According to Denzin and Lincoln (2000), "qualitative researchers study things in their natural settings, attempting to make sense of, or interpret, phenomena in terms of the meanings people bring to them" (p. 3). Natural settings are the environments where people live every day. So, the researcher doing qualitative research goes wherever the participants are—in their homes, schools, communities, and sometimes the hospital or an outpatient setting.

This chapter focuses on the most commonly used qualitative research methods: phenomenology, grounded theory, ethnography, and case study. Historical research and newer methodologies, such as participatory and narrative methods, are also discussed. Each method, although distinct from the others, shares characteristics that identify it as a method within the qualitative research approach.

In the previous chapter, the authors located these qualitative methods along a continuum ranging from the "positivist" to the "constructivist" view (see Figure 7–2). The authors emphasized the importance of one's paradigmatic perspective, sometimes called a worldview. Embedded in one's worldview are beliefs that guide the choice of an issue for research study and the creation of a research study question. For example, if your view fits best with the positivist paradigm, you likely believe in the composite nature of humans, allowing isolation of body systems for accurate measurement purposes. If you hold this perspective, you will pose a research question to be addressed by an empirical analytical or quantitative method. If, on the other hand, your view fits best with the constructivist paradigm, you likely believe in the unitary nature of human life—that humans are intricately connected to each other and their environment. If you hold this perspective, you will most often pose a research question that can be best addressed with a qualitative method.

One research method is not better than another; one is not good, whereas another is excellent and yet another poor. The only judgement of excellence relates to the fit between one's worldview, the research question, and the research method. If congruence exists between the worldview, the question, and the method, then the researcher has made an excellent choice of method. For example, if a researcher's worldview comes from the constructivism paradigm and a question about the effect of slow-stroke back massage on blood pressure is posed, the fit between the worldview and the research question is good. Massage is an intervention that can be manipulated by the researcher, and blood pressure is an outcome variable that can be measured. When researchers study the effects of an intervention on an outcome variable, they generally use empirical analytical quantitative methods, grounded in the positivist worldview.

In this chapter, you are invited to look through the lens of the constructivist view to learn about phenomenological, grounded theory, ethnographic, case study, historical, and participatory action research. You are encouraged to "change glasses" as each method is introduced—to imagine studying an issue of interest from the perspective of each of these methods. No matter which methods a researcher uses, it is important to embrace the wholeness of humans, focusing on human experience in natural settings. The researcher using these methods believes that humans uniquely attribute meaning to their experience, and experience evolves from life context. **Life context** is the matrix of human–health–environment relationships emerging over the course of day-to-day living.

For example, one person's experience of pain is distinct from another's and can be known by the individual's subjective description of it. The researcher interested in studying the lived experience of pain for the adolescent with rheumatoid arthritis will spend time in the adolescent's natural settings, such as the home and school. Effort will be directed toward uncovering the meaning of pain as it extends beyond the facts of the number of medications taken or a rating on a reliable and valid scale. These methods are grounded in the belief that factual objective data do not capture the human experience. Rather, the meaning of the adolescent's pain will emerge within the context of personal history, current relationships, and future plans as the adolescent lives daily life in dynamic interaction with his or her environment.

The researcher using qualitative methods begins collecting bits of information and piecing them together, building a mosaic or picture of the human experience being studied. As with a mosaic, when one steps away from the work, the whole picture emerges, transcending the bits and pieces. When presenting the study findings, the researcher strives to capture the human experience and present it so that others can understand it. Often, findings are shared as a narrative or story.

QUALITATIVE APPROACH AND NURSING SCIENCE

Qualitative research is particularly well suited to study the human experience of health, a central concern of nursing science. Because qualitative methods focus on the whole of human experience and the meaning ascribed by individuals living the experience, these methods extend understanding of health beyond traditionally measured units to include the complexity of the human health experience as it occurs in everyday life. This closeness to what is "real" and "everyday" promises guidance for nursing practice; it is also important for instrument and theory development. In Figure 8–1, three examples are cited to emphasize the capacity of qualitative methods to (1) guide nursing practice, (2) contribute to instrument development, and (3) develop nursing theory.

Qualitative Research Guiding Practice

In a study of caring for critical care clients, Hurlock-Chorostecki (2002) stated that "despite extensive knowledge of pain and pain management, critical-care nurses commonly withhold analgesia from patients for extended periods prior to and during weaning from mechanical ventilation" (p. 33). Because of the ethical and practical problems of studying clients enduring weaning from mechanical ventilation, Hurlock-Chorostecki interviewed nurses to understand how they made decisions related to pain management during weaning. Ten nurses working in critical care participated.

A constant comparative analysis method was used to analyze the data. Hurlock-Chorostecki (2002) used the research method of grounded theory to develop a theory of nurse decision making. The researcher described the theory as a circular model to represent the continuous nature of the decision-making process. In this theory, six circles represent the skill level of the decision maker, with the inner circles representing the highest skill level. Each skill level is subdivided into two styles of nursing, identified as diagnostic and humanistic. The diagnostic nurse believes that pain is a function of the client's medical diagnosis, whereas the humanistic nurse believes that pain exists when the client indicates so. The researcher suggested that nurse decision making, in this context, is a continuous, dynamic process.

Nurses with greater experience used the broadest scope of knowledge gathering and intervention, with two major influences affecting their decision making: a priori beliefs about the nature of pain (diagnostic or humanistic view) and beliefs about the nurse's role during weaning from mechanical ventilation. In this study, the author provided a theory explaining the role that experience plays and the forces influencing decision making among critical care nurses. This emerging theory can provide a method for critical care nurses to reflect on their practice, particularly in relation to pain management during weaning from mechanical ventilation. Additionally, the theory can guide the professional

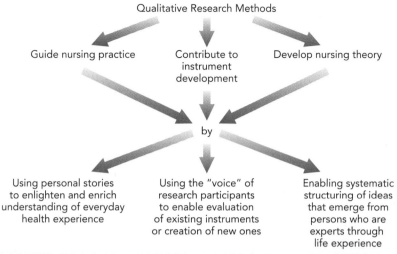

Figure 8–1 Qualitative approach and nursing science

development activities and orientation programs for novice nurses.

Qualitative Research Contributing to Instrument Development

As part of a larger study determining the quality of life of terminally ill cancer clients, Cohen and Leis (2002) evaluated the content validity of quality of life (QOL) questionnaires. The McGill Quality of Life Questionnaire (MQOL) developed by Cohen and Leis measured the QOL, defined as subjective well-being, of people with life-threatening illness. Although the instrument seemed to be an improvement over other instruments, the content validity had not been demonstrated.

Sixty clients with cancer receiving palliative care were studied across six sites in three Canadian cities. Half of the participants lived at home, whereas the rest resided in inpatient palliative care units. Demographic data included an average age of 68 years, and two-thirds of the participant population were females with many types of cancer, the three most common types of which were gastrointestinal, lung, and gynecological. Semi-structured interviews were used to solicit the determinants of the clients' QOL. Primary interview questions included "What is

important to your quality of life?" and "What makes a good day?" Content analysis was used to pull out first the themes and then the broad domains.

Fifty emergent themes were placed into broad categories and then reduced to five broad domains. The five domains were labelled "own state" (physical condition, physical functioning, psychological state, cognitive functioning), "quality of palliative care," "physical environment," "relationships," and "outlook." These five domains were used to evaluate the comprehensiveness of the MQOL. The researchers were interested in whether the QOL instrument addressed all of the domains emerging from the interviews. The researchers concluded that many existing instruments cover many of the domains; however, the MQOL included all of the content. The MQOL was revised to reflect the new data. In this study, qualitative research was used to strengthen an existing instrument, making it more relevant to the clients for whom it was intended.

Qualitative Research Contributing to Theory Building

As a consumer of nursing research, you will notice that the qualitative method most readily linked with theory building is the grounded theory method. An example of this method is Schreiber, Stern, and Wilson's (2000) study of depression in 12 Black West Indian Canadian women. The researchers asked participants, "What is it like to go through depression as a Black West Indian Canadian?" In addition to interviews, participant observation occurred, in keeping with the grounded theory method. Schreiber et al. emphasized that this experience was heavily influenced by major contexts: visible minority status in a Eurocentric society, the social stigma of depression imposed by the participants' own cultural group, gender expectations within their cultural group, and Christian upbringing.

According to the authors, "the goal of the women was to be able to manage their depression with grace and to live up to the cultural imperative to be strong." *Being strong* was the overarching social process used by these women in managing their depression. Being strong included the subprocesses of "dwelling on it," "diverting [themselves]," and "regaining [their] composure." *Dwelling on it* referred to the women's recognition that suffering and struggle were integral to being a woman, and they could do little about it. As ways of dwelling on it, the authors described patterns of separating from others, gaining a sense of competence by showing compassion when confronted with insensitive behaviour, and recognizing the depression for what it was, which enabled the women to divert themselves. *Diverting self*, the second subprocess, was the beginning of efforts to manage depression. These efforts included seeking God's comfort, seeking professional help, socializing, exercising, and thinking positively. The authors suggested that diverting self led to the third subprocess, regaining composure. *Regaining composure* was characterized by "recognizing God's strength within" and moving on with everyday living.

These central subprocesses of being strong were enhanced by the willingness of some women to consider other ways to manage their depression. The authors labelled this effort "trying new approaches" and emphasized the challenging nature of new approaches for women embedded in the Black West Indian Canadian cultural context. The authors provided a model of "being strong," depicting the relationships between subprocesses and contexts. This qualitative study enabled creation of the structure of "being strong," which contributes to nursing's body of knowledge and offers guidance for further research and practice.

QUALITATIVE RESEARCH METHODS

Thus far, an overview of the qualitative research approach has been presented, focusing on its importance for nursing science. An effort has been made to highlight how the choice of a qualitative approach reflects one's worldview and research question and how qualitative methods contribute to guiding practice, testing instruments, and building theory. These topics provide a foundation for examining the six qualitative methods discussed in this chapter. The Critical Thinking Decision Path introduces the consumer of nursing research to a process for recognizing differing qualitative methods by distinguishing areas of interest for each method and noting how the research question might be introduced for each method. The phenomenological, grounded theory, ethnographic, case study, historical, and participatory action methods are described in detail for the consumer of nursing research.

Parse, Coyne, and Smith (1985) suggested that research methods, whether quantitative or qualitative, include the following five basic elements:

1. Identifying the phenomenon
2. Structuring the study
3. Gathering the data
4. Analyzing the data
5. Describing the findings

Each qualitative method is defined here, followed by a discussion of these five basic elements. The factors that distinguish the methods are highlighted, and research examples are presented, providing the beginning consumer of research with directions for critiquing.

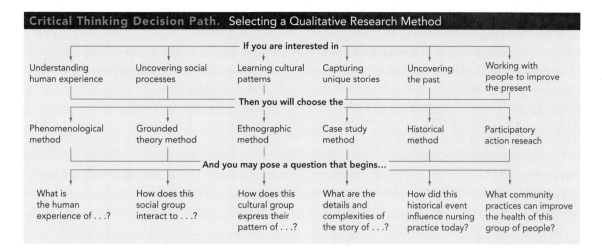

Critical Thinking Decision Path. Selecting a Qualitative Research Method

If you are interested in

| Understanding human experience | Uncovering social processes | Learning cultural patterns | Capturing unique stories | Uncovering the past | Working with people to improve the present |

Then you will choose the

| Phenomenological method | Grounded theory method | Ethnographic method | Case study method | Historical method | Participatory action reseach |

And you may pose a question that begins...

| What is the human experience of . . .? | How does this social group interact to . . .? | How does this cultural group express their pattern of . . .? | What are the details and complexities of the story of . . .? | How did this historical event influence nursing practice today? | What community practices can improve the health of this group of people? |

Phenomenological Method

The **phenomenological method** is a process of learning and constructing the meaning of human experience through intensive dialogue with persons who are living the experience. The researcher's goal is to understand the meaning of the experience as it is lived by the participant. Meaning is pursued through dialogue, which extends beyond a simple interview and requires thoughtful responses on the part of the researcher.

In the previous chapter, the authors introduced the nursing research consumer to the traditional philosophical bases that provide a foundation for phenomenological research. Each philosophical base (Husserl's eidetic phenomenology, Heidegger's interpretive phenomenology, Dutch hermeneutical phenomenology) calls for slight differences in research methods. Furthermore, American forms of phenomenological research have been distinguished from the traditional Husserl's, Heidegger's, and Dutch forms (Caelli, 2000). Caelli suggested that nursing tends to use American forms, which focus on understanding the reality of experience for the person as he or she engages with the phenomenon, rather than focusing on the more objective phenomenon itself, as is the case in traditional forms of phenomenological research (2000). Whatever the form of phenomenological research, the consumer of nursing research will find the researcher asking a question about lived experience.

IDENTIFYING THE PHENOMENON

Because the focus of the phenomenological method is the **lived experience**, the researcher is likely to choose this method when studying a dimension of day-to-day existence for a particular group of individuals. For instance, the nurse may be interested in the experience of anger for persons who have heart disease or the experience of success for baccalaureate nursing students. Kelly (2006), for example, studied the experiences of battered Latina women, and Charlebois and Bouchard (2007) studied the experience of grandparents having a grandchild diagnosed with cancer.

STRUCTURING THE STUDY

To describe structuring, the following topics are addressed: the research question, the researcher's perspective, and sample selection. The issue of human subjects' protection has been suggested as a dimension of structuring (Parse et al., 1985). Specific ethics concerns are addressed in Chapters 6 and 7.

Research Question. The question that guides phenomenological research always asks about an experience of everyday living. Phenomenological research guides the researcher to ask the participant about a past or present experience. The research question is not exactly the same as the question used to initiate dialogue with the participant, but often both questions are very similar. For example, Bournes and Mitchell (2002) wanted to explore the experiences of persons waiting for friends or relatives in a critical care unit. The statement that introduced their research dialogue with participants was, "Please tell me about your experiences of waiting" (p. 60). In the study by Charlebois and Bouchard (2007), the research purpose was to "describe and better understand the meaning given by Quebec grandparents to the experience of having a grandchild with cancer" (p. 26). Participants were grandparents of children who were between the ages of 4 and 12 years and had been diagnosed with cancer within the last two months. The statement the researchers posed to the participants to initiate dialogue was, "Please describe the circumstances surrounding the disclosure of your grandchild's diagnosis (p. 27). As demonstrated in the two examples, the question used to begin dialogue with the participant(s) needs to be clear and understandable for the participant.

Helpful 💡 Hint

Although the research question may not always be explicitly reported, it may be identified by evaluating the study purpose or the question or statement posed to the participants.

Researcher's Perspective.   When using the phenomenological method, the researcher's perspective is bracketed. **Bracketing** means that the researcher identifies personal biases about the phenomenon of interest to clarify how personal experience and beliefs may colour what is heard and reported. The researcher is expected to set aside personal biases—to bracket them—when engaged with the participants. By becoming aware of personal biases, the researcher is more likely to be able to pursue issues of importance as introduced by the participant, rather than leading the participant to issues the researcher deems important.

In Chapter 7, the authors suggested that bracketing was more important for some phenomenological methods than others. Many researchers are now embracing the researcher's subjectivity because once it is recognized and monitored, it can contribute to the research (Glesne, 2006). However, the researcher using phenomenological methods usually uses a strategy to identify personal biases and hold them in abeyance while querying the participant.

The reader may find it difficult to identify bracketing strategies because they are seldom explicitly identified in a research article. Sometimes, the researcher's view of the world provides insight into biases that have been considered and bracketed. In Gates's (2000) article, the author indicated that she was interested in understanding the experience of caring for a loved one based on her own experience of caring for her mother with advanced dementia. Gates acknowledged that her experiences of caring profoundly affected her perspective.

By tuning into the subjectivity of one's own perspectives, researchers can examine their personal assumptions and create new personal understandings. Many qualitative researchers monitor their subjectivity by writing a series of journals to scrutinize their perspectives, just as one would analyze the research data (Glesne, 2006). This process allows researchers not only to monitor their own subjectivity but also to learn more about their own beliefs, values, and interests.

Sample Selection.   The reader of a phenomenological study will find that the selected sample either is living the experience the researcher is querying or has lived the experience in the past. Because phenomenologists believe that an individual's history is a dimension of the present, a past experience exists in the present. Even when a participant is describing an experience occurring in the present, remembered information is being gathered.

In the study describing the experiences of grandparents whose grandchildren have cancer, participants were recruited from an organization with the mandate to promote wellness for families with cancer. The eight grandparents who agreed to participate had grandchildren who had been diagnosed within the last two months (Charlebois & Bouchard, 2007). This sample size is typical of phenomenological studies, which usually have fewer than 20 participants.

DATA GATHERING

Written or oral data may be collected when using the phenomenological method. The researcher may pose the query in writing and ask for a written response or may schedule a time to interview the participant and record the interaction. In either case, the researcher may return to ask for clarification of written or recorded transcripts.

To some extent, the particular data collection procedure is guided by the choice of a specific analysis technique. Different analysis techniques require a different number of interviews. Data saturation usually guides decisions regarding how many interviews are enough. **Data saturation** is the situation of "having heard the themes before." The researcher knows that saturation has been reached when the ideas surfacing in the dialogue have been previously heard from other participants. For example, Cameron (2003) interviewed nursing students in a collaborative baccalaureate nursing program to understand their lived experience when moving from college to university. Initially, the research proposal planned for interviewing 9 to 10 students; however, 13 students were interviewed because new ideas and experiences continued to emerge.

DATA ANALYSIS

All qualitative data analysis "seeks to organize and reduce data gathered into themes or essences, which, in turn, can be fed into descriptions, models, or theories" (Walker & Myrick, 2006, p. 547). Several specific techniques are available for data analysis when the phenomenological method is used. For detailed information about specific techniques, the reader is referred to original sources (Colaizzi, 1978; Giorgi, Fischer, & Murray, 1975; Spiegelberg, 1976; van Kaam, 1969). Although the techniques for each are slightly different, a general pattern is the movement from the participant's description to the researcher's synthesis of all participants' descriptions. The steps typically include the following:

1. Thorough reading and sensitive presence with the entire transcription of the participant's description

2. Identification of shifts in participant thought, resulting in division of the transcription into thought segments

3. Specification of the significant phrases in each thought segment, using the words of the participant

4. Distillation of each significant phrase to express the central meaning of the segment in the words of the researcher

5. Grouping together of segments that contain similar central meanings for each participant

6. Preliminary synthesis of grouped segments for each participant with a focus on the essence of the phenomenon being studied

7. Final synthesis of the essences that have surfaced in all participants' descriptions, resulting in an exhaustive description of the lived experience

Charlebois and Bouchard (2007) analyzed the results of their interviews using thematic analysis following the basic steps described above. Paton, Backlund, Thirsk and Barnes (2007) used Heideggerian hermeneutics for their interpretation of the data gathered from interviews with women exploring their day-to-day experiences of living with heart failure. Through the process of moving back and forth with the text or "playing" with the story, understandings of the phenomenon are created. The researchers met frequently to discuss the understandings, commonalities, and diversities as they reviewed the text. Through discussion, questioning, and probing, an understanding of the participants' experience emerged, including recalibrating time and space, balancing wishing and hoping and the acknowledging of loss, and "preserving" through uncertainty.

DESCRIBING THE FINDINGS

When using the phenomenological method, the nurse researcher provides the research consumer with a path of information leading from the research question through samples of participants' words to the researcher's interpretation, culminating in the final synthesis that elaborates the lived experience as a narrative. When reading the report of a phenomenological study, the reader will find that detailed descriptive language is used to convey the complex meaning of the lived experience. For example, Paton et al. (2007) quoted from participants experiencing heart failure to support the identified themes. Direct participant quotations enable the reader to evaluate the connection between what the participant said and how the researcher labelled what was said. For example, one of the themes included "acknowledging loss as persevering through uncertainty" (p. 12). To support this theme, the following quotation was included:

> I was really angry because I couldn't do what I wanted to do, go places I wanted to go and I always walked and then I couldn't walk and I couldn't walk and it just drove me nuts. So I had to learn to live with it [heart failure] . . . . But I am stubborn and I said "if I can't do that then I will do the best I can with what I have", so that is what I am doing. I have developed a new philosophy of one day at a time. I still have freedom. I still have freedom! (p. 12)

Evidence-Based Practice Tip

Phenomenological research is an appropriate approach for accumulating evidence when studying a new topic about which little is known.

Grounded Theory Method

The **grounded theory method** is an inductive approach involving a systematic set of procedures to arrive at a theory about basic social processes. The emergent theory is based on observations and perceptions of the social scene and evolves during data collection and analysis in the actual research process (Strauss & Corbin, 1994). The aim of the grounded theory approach is to discover underlying social forces that shape human behaviour. This method is used to construct theory where no theory exists or when the existing theory fails to explain a set of circumstances.

According to Denzin (1998), grounded theory is the qualitative perspective most widely used by social scientists today, largely because the theory sets forth clearly defined steps for the researcher.

Although developed originally as a sociologist's tool to investigate interactions in social settings (Glaser & Strauss, 1967), the grounded theory method is not bound to that discipline. Investigators from different disciplines may study the same phenomenon from varying perspectives (Denzin & Lincoln, 1998; Strauss & Corbin, 1994, 1997). For example, in a study of chronic illness, a nurse might be interested in coping patterns within families, a psychologist in personal adjustment, and a sociologist in group behaviour in health care settings. The theory generated by each discipline will reflect the discipline and serve to explain the phenomenon of interest to the discipline (Liehr & Marcus, 2002). In grounded theory, usefulness stems from the transferability of theories from one study to another situation, making the key objective the development of more formal theories that are faithful to the cases from which they were derived (Sandelowski, 2004).

IDENTIFYING THE PHENOMENON

Researchers typically use the grounded theory method when they are interested in social processes from the perspective of human interactions, or "patterns of action and interaction between and among various types of social units" (Denzin & Lincoln, 1998). The basic social process is often expressed as a "gerund," indicating change across time as social reality is negotiated. (A gerund is "a noun formed from a verb, in English ending in -ing, and designating an action or state" [Barber, 2004, p. 629].) For example, Wuest and Merritt-Gray (2001) studied the survival process of women leaving abusive relationships (their subtitle begins "Reclaiming Self after Leaving . . ."). Worthington and Myers (2003) examined the situation and social processes that underlie the anxiety associated with human immunodeficiency virus (HIV) testing (their title begins "Factors Underlying Anxiety . . .").

STRUCTURING THE STUDY

Research Question.   Research questions appropriate for the grounded theory method are those that address basic social processes. These questions tend to be action or change oriented, such as "What factors underlie HIV testing anxiety, and what implications do such factors have for HIV testing provision, and diagnostic testing service provision generally?" (Worthington & Myers, 2003, p. 637). In a grounded theory study, the research question can be a statement or a broad question that permits in-depth explanation of the phenomenon. Ford-Gilboe, Wuest, and Merritt-Gray (2005) stated that their purpose "was to develop a substantive theory that explains the variation in health promotion processes of mother-headed [single-parent families] with a history of woman abuse" (p. 479).

Researcher's Perspective.   In a grounded theory study, the researcher brings some knowledge of the literature to the study, but the consumer will notice that an exhaustive literature review has not been done. Theory is allowed to emerge directly from the data and to reflect the contextual values that are integral to the social processes being studied. In this way, the theory product that emerges is "grounded in" the data.

For example, Ford-Gilboe et al. (2005) used broad questions to encourage participants to discuss their health promotion after leaving the abusive relationship. Thus, grounded theory is likely to be sensitive to contextual values and not merely to the researcher's values (Strauss & Corbin, 1997).

Sample Selection.   Sample selection involves choosing participants who are experiencing the circumstance and selecting events and incidents related to the social process under investigation. For example, using theoretical sampling, Ford-Gilboe et al. (2005) recruited 40 single-parent families from New Brunswick and Ontario who had left abusive relationships. The participants were women from a variety of cultural or ethnic and socioeconomic backgrounds, as well as families from both rural and urban areas. Children who were over 12 years of age were also included in the interviews if parental permission was obtained.

In the grounded theory method, the sample size is not predetermined. People are interviewed and data are collected until the data are saturated, meaning that no new conceptual information emerges (Speziale & Carpenter, 2007).

DATA GATHERING

In the grounded theory method, the consumer will find that data are collected through interviews with and skilled observations of individuals interacting in a social setting. The interviews are recorded and then transcribed, and the observations are recorded as field notes. Open-ended questions are used initially to identify concepts for further focus. Ford-Gilboe et al. (2005) used broad questions to encourage dialogue about their health promotion practices over a period of two interviews. In contrast, Worthington and Myers (2003) used a semi-structured interview schedule to guide the participants in their descriptions of their HIV testing experience from the circumstances leading to the testing through to the post-test experience.

DATA ANALYSIS

A major feature of the grounded theory method is that data collection and analysis occur simultaneously. The process requires systematic, detailed record keeping using field notes and transcribed interviews. Hunches about emerging patterns in the data are noted in memos, and the researcher directs activities in the field by pursuing these hunches. This technique, called **theoretical sampling**, is used to select experiences that will help the researcher test ideas and gather complete information about developing concepts. The researcher begins by noting indicators or actual events, actions, or words in the data. Concepts, or abstractions, are developed from the indicators (Charmaz, 2000; Strauss, 1987).

The initial analytical process is called open coding (Strauss, 1987). Data are examined carefully line by line, divided into discrete parts, and compared for similarities and differences (Strauss &

Corbin, 1990). Through a process known as the **constant comparative method**, data are compared with other data continuously as they are acquired during research. Codes in the data are clustered to form categories. The categories are expanded and developed or collapsed into one another. Theory is constructed through this systematic process. As a result, data collection, analysis, and theory generation have a direct reciprocal relationship (Charmaz, 2000; Strauss & Corbin, 1990).

Ford-Gilboe et al. (2005), for example, carefully described the analysis process used in their study. Because the research team was separated geographically, the initial interviews were coded line by line using the constant comparative method at team meetings. As the codes and categories began to emerge, the team members worked individually, sharing their work through monthly teleconferences and memos. Finally, the relationship among the categories was articulated, tested, and then refined among the team. Using a feminist participatory methodology, the researchers brought the emergent theory back to the participants for confirmation and further refinement.

Related literature, both technical and nontechnical, is reviewed continuously throughout data collection and analysis. All literature is treated as data and is compared with the researcher's developing theory as it progresses. When critiquing a study using grounded theory, the reader should expect to find, at the end of the report, the researcher's grounded theory formally related to and incorporated with existing knowledge. For example, Ford-Gilboe et al. (2005) used the literature to illuminate the concepts and the relationships between them as an emerging theory. Many of their findings were supported by previous researchers. Worthington and Myers (2003) also reviewed the research literature to integrate their findings with the literature.

DESCRIBING THE FINDINGS

Grounded theory studies are reported in sufficient detail to provide the reader with the steps in the process and the logic of the method and the theory that has emerged. Ford-Gilboe et al. (2005) guided the reader through the steps of data collection, theoretical sampling, constant comparisons, and theoretical coding.

Grounded theory studies use descriptive language and diagrams of the process to ensure that the theory reported in the findings remains connected to the data. For example, Ford-Gilboe et al. (2005) included several figures in their research report and used the following quotation to support the theme of "family ideals" as one of the conditions that influence strengthening capacity to limit intrusion:

> *I grew up in an abusive family . . . . My Mom was away from my Dad,* so I wanted to make sure that my kids at least knew their father . . . . *I wanted to get something on paper saying that I have joint custody or I have interim custody so that he couldn't take off with them. That's all I wanted. I* told him, *"Those are your kids too just as much as mine, but I need some papers."* . . . *Once we get this done, you can have your visitation. (Emphasis ours, p. 485)*

Evidence-Based 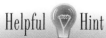 Practice Tip

When thinking about the evidence generated by the grounded theory method, consider whether the theory is useful in explaining, interpreting, or predicting the study phenomenon of interest.

Ethnographic Method

Derived from the Greek term *ethnos*, meaning people, race, or cultural group, the **ethnographic method** focuses on scientific description and interpretation of cultural or social groups and systems (Creswell, 1998). The reader should know that the goal of the ethnographer is to understand the natives' view of their world, or the **emic view**. The emic

Helpful 💡 Hint

In a report of research using the grounded theory method, the reader can expect to find a diagrammed model of a theory that synthesizes the researchers' findings in a systematic way.

(insider's) view is contrasted to the **etic view** (or outsider's view) obtained when the researcher uses quantitative analyses of behaviour. The ethnographic approach requires that the researcher enter the world of the study participants to observe what happens, listen to what is said, ask questions, and collect whatever data are available. The term *ethnography* refers to both the research technique and the product of that technique, the study itself (Creswell, 1998; Tedlock, 2000). Vidick and Lyman (1998) traced the history of ethnography, with roots in the disciplines of sociology and anthropology, as a method born out of the need to understand "other" and "self." Nurses use the method to study cultural variations in health and client groups as subcultures within larger social contexts (Liehr & Marcus, 2002).

IDENTIFYING THE PHENOMENON

The phenomenon under investigation in an ethnographic study can vary in scope from a long-term study of a very complex culture, such as that of the Aborigines (Mead, 1949), to a shorter-term study of a phenomenon within subunits of cultures. For example, a researcher may study the health and healing philosophies of nurses and alternative healers (Engebretson, 1996), the ways in which First Nations women encounter mainstream health care services (Browne & Fiske, 2001), or a cross-cultural comparison of health-promoting practices among immigrant women from India (Choudhry, 1998). Kleinman (1992) noted the clinical utility of ethnography in describing the "local world" of groups of clients who are experiencing a particular phenomenon, such as suffering. The local worlds of clients have cultural, political, economical, institutional, and social–relational dimensions similar to larger, complex societies. A study of cross-cultural relationships between nurses and Filipino Canadian clients is used here as an example to introduce the reader to ethnography (Pasco, Morse, & Olson, 2004).

STRUCTURING THE STUDY

Research Question.   When reviewing a report of ethnographic research, notice that questions are asked about lifeways or particular patterns of behaviour within the social context of a culture or subculture. **Culture** is the system of knowledge and linguistic expressions used by social groups that allows the researcher to interpret or make sense of the world (Aamodt, 1991).

Ethnographic nursing studies address questions that concern how cultural knowledge, norms, values, and other contextual variables influence one's health experience. For example, Pasco et al.'s (2004) research question was implied in their purpose statement and can be stated as follows: "What are the culturally embedded values that implicitly guide Filipino Canadian clients' interactions in developing nurse–client relationships?" Choudhry (1998) asked, "What cultural norms and values influence women's health and their health promotion activities?" Other ethnographic questions Choudhry asked included the following: "What is the meaning of health and well-being to immigrant women from India?" "What value do these women place on their health?" and "What factors influence the use of culture to maintain and promote health in the Canadian context?" (p. 270).

In Schultz, Bottorff, and Johnson's study on tobacco control in hospital settings (2006), the researchers asked, "Think of everything you would do for a patient during a shift (pause) and now when I say tobacco what do you think of?" (p. 318). This last question does not imply "culture" in the same way as a question about Filipino clients or migrant workers. However, the question fits a broader definition of culture, in which a particular social context is conceptualized as a culture. In this case, hospitals are seen as a culture appropriate for ethnographic study.

Researcher's Perspective.   When using the ethnographic method, the researcher's perspective is that of an interpreter entering an alien world and attempting to make sense of that world from the insider's point of view (Agar, 1986). Like phenomenologists and grounded theorists, ethnographers make their own beliefs explicit and *bracket*, or set aside, their personal biases as they seek to understand the worldview of others. In her study of immigrant women from India, Choudhry (1998) described herself as researcher as instrument (see Chapter 7). She had also been an immigrant from India 30 years prior to the study, and her experiences assisted in explaining the "world of these women" (p. 271).

To fully understand the emic view, researchers must do more than just observe: they must become participants in the setting (Speziale & Carpenter, 2007). For example, Varcoe (2001) spent more than two years in an emergency department, working alongside nurses and tallying more than 200 hours of observation. Although Varcoe was an experienced critical care nurse, she did not participate in nursing interventions but provided comfort and emotional support to clients.

Sample Selection.   The ethnographer selects a cultural group that is living the phenomenon under investigation. The researcher gathers information from general informants and from key informants. **Key informants** are individuals who have special knowledge, status, or communication skills and who are willing to teach the ethnographer about the phenomenon (Creswell, 1998). For example, Pasco et al. (2004), who selected participants through purposive sampling, spent time with 23 Filipino Canadian clients who were hospitalized for a range of health problems and had been living in Canada for a minimum of five years. These informants were recruited because they were uniquely capable of sharing cultural perspectives of interest to the researchers.

Purposeful sampling simply means that participants are selected "purposefully" because they are "information-rich cases for study" (Patton, 2002, p. 46). Snowballing, as an extension of purposeful sampling, is an approach to collect more information-rich informants by asking established participants, "Who else may have something to contribute or have knowledge of . . . ?" (Patton, 2002).

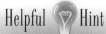 Helpful Hint

Managing personal bias is expected of researchers using all of the methods discussed in this chapter.

DATA GATHERING

Ethnographic data gathering involves participant observation or immersion in the setting, informant interviews, and the researcher's interpretation of cultural patterns (Crabtree & Miller, 1992). According to Boyle (1991), ethnographic research in nursing, as in other disciplines, always involves "face-to-face interviewing, with data collection and analysis taking place in the natural setting." Thus, fieldwork is a major focus of the method.

Other techniques may include obtaining life histories and collecting material items reflective of the culture. Photographs and films of the informants in their world can be used as data sources. Spradley (1979) identified three categories of questions for ethnographic inquiry: (1) descriptive or broad open-ended questions; (2) structural or in-depth questions that expand and verify the unit of analysis; and (3) contrast questions, or questions that further clarify and provide criteria for exclusion.

Data gathering for the study of Filipino Canadian clients began with a request for participants to tell the researcher about their hospital experience; however, "follow-up interviews were more structured with questions validating and extending analytic notes" (Pasco et al., 2004, p. 241). Many participants spoke both English and Filipino during their interviews.

Choudhry (1998) collected data from face-to-face interviews conducted in the women's homes. Each interview was informal and semi-structured, with open-ended questions such as "What is the meaning of health?" (p. 271). Socialization during the interview was important. Tea and snacks were offered as a gesture of hospitality, an important cultural custom among East Indians. Choudhry also attended many cultural and social events to observe the women's health promotion activities. Interviews were audiotaped, transcribed, and translated into English. Observations were documented in field notes within 24 hours of the visit.

Field notes are critical to the qualitative researcher; they are the primary recording tool and contain descriptions of the settings, interviews, ideas, hunches, and reflections. Notes about emerging patterns are documented as they occur to the researcher. Many qualitative researchers also use their field notes to explore their own subjectivity and bias (Glesne, 2006).

DATA ANALYSIS

As with the grounded theory method, data are collected and analyzed simultaneously. Data analysis proceeds through several levels as the researcher looks for the meaning of cultural symbols in the informants' language. Analysis begins with a search for **domains**, or symbolic categories that include smaller categories. Language is analyzed for semantic relationships, and structural questions are formulated to expand and verify data. Analysis proceeds through increasing levels of complexity until the data, grounded in the informant's reality and synthesized by the researcher, lead to hypothetical propositions about the cultural phenomenon under investigation. The reader is encouraged to consult Creswell (1998) for a detailed description of ethnographic analysis.

Pasco et al. (2004) provided few details about their analysis, except to state that initial categories of data were used to direct follow-up interviews, moving toward a model depicting types of nurse–client relationships and levels of interaction. In contrast, Schultz et al. (2006) described their ethnographic analysis. First, the data set, composed of field notes from observation, documents, records of conversations, and photographs, was analyzed through a process of repetitive review to identify key concepts that profiled the use of tobacco across two hospital settings in British Columbia. In the second stage, the data were coded using the key concepts. This process allowed the researchers to compare the findings between the two sites. Further review allowed the researchers to finalize the concepts.

DESCRIBING THE FINDINGS

Ethnographic studies yield large quantities of data amassed as field notes of observations, interview transcriptions, and other artifacts, such as photographs. Charmaz (2000) provided guidelines for ethnographic writing that provide an excellent framework for the consumer of nursing research

wishing to critique descriptions of ethnographic studies. The five techniques recommended in Charmaz's guidelines are pulling the reader in, recreating experiential mood, adding surprise, reconstructing ethnographic experience, and creating closure for the study.

When critiquing, be aware that the report of findings usually provides examples from data, thorough descriptions of the analytical process, and statements of the hypothetical propositions and their relationship to the ethnographer's frame of reference. Evidence provided by complete ethnographies may be published as monographs.

Pasco et al. (2004) developed a taxonomy diagrammed as a matrix of levels of progressive nurse–client interaction (formality, adjustment, acceptance, mutual comfort, oneness) and characteristics of interaction (nature of interaction, clients' needs, clients' feelings, clients' trust, clients' response to nursing care). The final product also included a glossary of Filipino terms that identified words pertinent to nurse–client interaction. For instance, *hindi ibang tao* means "one of us," and *ibang tao* means "not one of us"—critical ideas for nurse–client interaction with this group of Filipino Canadian participants. The evidence provided by the ethnographic information in this study can guide the provision of culturally competent care with this client population.

Evidence-Based Practice Tip

Evidence generated by ethnographic studies will answer questions about how cultural knowledge, norms, values, and other contextual variables influence the health experience of a particular client population in a specific setting.

Case Study Method

Case study research, which is rooted in sociology, is currently described slightly differently by Yin (1994), Stake (1995, 2003), Merriam, and Creswell (1998), major thinkers who wrote about this method (Aita & McIlvain, 1999). For the purposes of introducing the nursing research consumer to this method, Stake's view is emphasized here. The **case study method** reviews the peculiarities and the commonalities of a specific case—familiar ground for practising nurses. Stake (2003) noted that case study is not a methodological choice but rather a choice of what to study. Case study can include quantitative data, qualitative data, or both, but it is defined by its focus on uncovering an individual case.

Stake distinguished intrinsic from instrumental case study. **Intrinsic case study** is undertaken to have a better understanding of the case—nothing more and nothing less. As Stake noted, "The researcher at least temporarily subordinates other curiosities so that the stories of those 'living the case' will be teased out" (2003, p. 136). **Instrumental case study** is defined as research undertaken when the researcher is pursuing insight into an issue or wants to challenge a particular generalization.

Smith, Edwards, Varcoe, Martens, and Davies (2006) used case study research methods to describe two Aboriginal community-based stakeholders' perspectives on the care of families who were pregnant and parenting. Working with 16 key informants from policy, leadership, and provider positions, perspectives were gathered though telephone or face-to-face interviews. Several communities were identified by the stakeholders as potential participants in the second phase of the study. Once two sites were selected, fieldwork commenced to gather the community stakeholders' perspectives during interviews and small focus groups.

IDENTIFYING THE PHENOMENON

Although some definitions of case study demand that the focus of research be contemporary, Stake's (1995, 2003) defining criterion of attention to the single case broadens the scope of phenomenon for study. By *single case*, Stake is designating a focus on an individual, a family, a community, or an organization as a complex phenomenon that demands close scrutiny for understanding. Although the strength of case studies lies in the detailed and thick description of the phenomenon under study, an obvious limitation exists in generalization (which is always

difficult in qualitative research). Some researchers will use a case method approach but will explore the experiences of more than one person. For our purposes, we are interested in examining a case study that uses a multiple case design (Yin, 1994). This case study, by Smith et al. (2006), explored the experiences of two Aboriginal communities in British Columbia, one urban and one rural, and the participants' experiences with pregnancy and parenting (see Appendix B). The researchers noted that poor access to prenatal care for Aboriginal people is well known and used case study to explore this issue.

STRUCTURING THE STUDY

Research Question.   The research question for case study is one that provokes the curiosity of the researcher. Stake (2003) suggested that research questions be developed around issues that serve as a foundation to uncover complexity and pursue understanding. In our case study example, Smith et al. (2006) stated their research question as follows: "What are community based stakeholders' views on care during pregnancy and parenting?" (p. E28). By understanding the systematic disenfranchisement of Aboriginal people owing to colonization, the authors worked with the community to extend the notion of safety in health care and to improve responsiveness.

Although researchers pose questions to begin, the beginning questions are never all-inclusive. Rather, the researcher uses an iterative process of "growing questions" in the field. In other words, as data are collected to address these questions, other questions will emerge to guide the researcher down another path in the process of untangling the complexities. Thus, research questions evolve over time and recreate themselves in case study research.

Researcher's Perspective.   When the researcher begins with questions developed around suspected issues of importance, the perspective of the researcher is reflected in the questions. This approach is sometimes referred to as an etic perspective. As the researcher begins engaging the phenomenon of interest, the story unfolds and leads the way, shifting from an etic (researcher) to an emic (story) perspective (Stake, 2003). The reader may recognize a shift from an etic to an emic perspective when stories spin off from the original questions posed by the researcher.

Sample Selection. Sample selection is one of the areas in which scholars in the field present differing views, ranging from choosing only the most common cases to choosing only the most unusual cases (Aita & McIlvain, 1999). Stake (2003) advocated selecting cases that may offer the best opportunities for learning. For example, if several clients who have received heart transplant are available for study, practical factors will influence who offers the best opportunity for learning. A person who lived in the area and could be easily visited at home or in the medical centre would be a better choice than someone living in another country. The researcher may want to choose someone with a family because most clients with transplants live in a family setting. No choice is perfect when selecting a case. The researcher has much to learn about any individual, situation, or organization when doing case study research, regardless of the contextual factors influencing the unit of analysis.

Smith et al. (2006) designed a two-phase study to collect the community views on care during pregnancy and parenting. In the first phase, 16 key informants from a variety of policy, leadership, and provider positions were purposefully selected using network sampling techniques. This technique, also known as snowballing, uses social networks to find people who have knowledge of the phenomenon under study. In the second phase, two Aboriginal health care delivery organizations, one urban and one rural, were selected as settings. Again, using the network sampling technique, a variety of community members, providers, and leaders were chosen. Seventy-three key informants were interviewed, 16 from phase 1 and the remainder from phase 2. The authors included a table showing the sample composition based on study phase, Aboriginal identity, and gender (see Smith et al., 2006, p. E33).

DATA GATHERING

Data are gathered using interview, observation, document review, and any other methods that enable understanding of the complexity of the case. The researcher will do what is needed to get a sense of the environment and the relationships that provide the context for the case. Stake (1995) advocated development of a data-gathering plan to guide the progress of the study from definition of the case through decisions regarding reporting. The consumer of research may find little or no explicit information about data gathering in the report.

Smith et al. (2006) gathered primary data using one-to-one exploratory interviews and small-group discussions. The interviews lasted from 45 to 120 minutes each and were taped and transcribed. Because of the sensitive nature of case studies, particularly in settings with postcolonial histories of oppression, racism, and inequitable health and social conditions, researchers such as Smith et al. (2006) took time "to create a safe, trusting, respectful environment and dynamic in the researcher-participant relationship and to emphasize the importance of many ways of knowing, particularly feelings or embodied knowledge" (p. E32). The researchers also used supplementary documents, such as government reports, proceedings from community meetings and annual reports, and field notes, in their data set.

DATA ANALYSIS AND DESCRIBING FINDINGS

Data analysis is closely tied to data gathering and description of findings as the case study story is generated. As Stake noted, "Qualitative case study is characterized by researchers spending extended time, on site, personally in contact with activities and operations of the case, reflecting, revising meanings of what is going on" (2003, p. 150). Reflecting and revising meanings are the work of the case study researcher, who has recorded data, searched for patterns, linked data from multiple sources, and arrived at preliminary thoughts regarding the meaning of collected data. This reflective dynamic evolution is the iterative process of creating the case study story. The reader of a qualitative case study will have difficulty determining how data analysis was conducted because the research report generally does not list research activities. Findings are embedded in (1) a chronological development of the case, (2) the researcher's story of coming to know the case, (3) a one-by-one description of case dimensions, and (4) vignettes that highlight case qualities (Stake, 1995).

Smith et al. (2006) used a postcolonial standpoint and the principles of participatory research as they analyzed the data. The researchers used an interpretive descriptive method, and NVivo software was used to manage the data. Important themes were identified after cycles of coding, collapsing, and reorganizing. Four main themes and 14 subthemes emerged and were shared with the participants for validation through distribution of hard copies and a series of luncheons and workshops. The themes identified and validated by the participants were pregnancy as an opportunity for change, safe health care places and relationships, responsive care, and making interventions safe and responsive (see Appendix B). Quotations were used to illustrate each theme. For example, the theme of pregnancy as an opportunity for change, which refers to the Aboriginal peoples' efforts to follow a healing path and thus create a better future for their children, was illustrated with the following quotation:

> *I was abused. I was neglected. I was physically abused by my parents, my friends. This is something that I don't want to happen to the next generation of children. I want things to be different for my kids. I want them to succeed—I can see that they are going to succeed. They are doing well and they are going to have a chance. (Smith et al., 2006, p. E35).*

Evidence-Based Practice Tip

Case studies provide an in-depth evidence-based discussion of clinical topics that can be used to guide practice.

Historical Research Method

The **historical research method** is a systematic approach to understanding the past through collection, organization, and critical appraisal of facts. One of the goals of the researcher using historical methodology is to shed light on the past so that it can guide the present and the future. Nursing's attention to historical methodology was initiated by Teresa E. Christy, who elaborated the method (1975) and the need (1981) for historical research long before most nurse scholars accepted it as a legitimate research method. More recently, Lusk (1997) summarized important information for the nurse interested in understanding historical research. She provided guidance for choosing a topic, acquiring data, addressing ethical issues, analyzing data, and reporting findings.

When critiquing a study that used the historical method, expect to find the research question embedded in the phenomenon to be studied. The question is stated implicitly rather than explicitly. Data sources provide the sample for historical research. The more clearly a researcher delineates the historical event being studied, the more specifically data sources can be identified. Data may include written or video documents, interviews with persons who witnessed the event, photographs, and any other artifacts that shed light. Sometimes, pivotal information cannot be retrieved and must be eliminated from the list of possible sources. To determine which data sources were used in a published study, the reader will look at the reference list. Sources of data may be primary or secondary. **Primary sources** are eyewitness accounts provided by various sorts of communication appropriate to the time. **Secondary sources** provide a view of the phenomenon from another's perspective rather than a first-hand account.

The reliability of data is established by internal criticism, whereas the validity of data is established by external criticism. **External criticism** judges the authenticity of the data source. The researcher seeks to ensure that the data source is what it seems to be. For example, if the researcher is reviewing a letter purportedly written by Florence Nightingale, some of the validity issues are the following:

- Are the ink, paper, and wax seal on the envelope representative of Nightingale's time?
- Is the wax seal one that Nightingale used in other authentic data sources?
- Is the writing truly Nightingale's?

Only if the data source passes the test of external criticism does the researcher begin internal criticism. **Internal criticism** concerns the reliability of information within the document (Christy, 1975). To judge reliability, the researcher must become familiar with the time in which the data emerged. A sense of the context and language of the time is essential to understanding a document. The meaning of a word in one era may not be equivalent to the meaning in another era. Knowing the language, customs, and habits of the historical period is critical for judging reliability.

The researcher assumes that a primary source provides a more reliable account than a secondary source (Christy, 1975). The further a source moves from providing an eyewitness account, the more questionable is its reliability. The researcher using historical methods attempts to establish fact, probability, and possibility (see Box 8–1).

Helpful 💡 Hint

When critiquing the historical method, do not expect to find a report of data analysis but simply a description of findings synthesized into a continuous narrative.

Evidence-Based 🔍 Practice Tip

The presentation of a historical study should be logical, consistent, and easy to follow.

Participatory Action Research

Participatory action research (PAR) as described in Chapter 7, is a research method that combines exploration of, reflection on, and action on social and health problems. **Community-based participatory**

| BOX 8–1 | Establishing Fact, Probability, and Possibility with the Historical Method |

FACT

Two independent primary sources that agree with each other

or

One independent primary source that receives critical evaluation and one independent secondary source that is in agreement and relieves critical evaluation and no substantive conflicting data

PROBABILITY

One primary source that receives critical evaluation and no substantive conflicting data

or

Two primary sources that disagree about particular points

POSSIBILITY

One primary source that provides information but is not adequate to receive critical evaluation

or

Only secondary or tertiary sources

Adapted from Christy, T. E. (1975). The methodology of historical research: A brief introduction. *Image, 24*(3), 189–192.

research (CBPR) is a method that systematically accesses the voice of a community to plan context-appropriate action. CBPR "provides an alternative to traditional research approaches that assume a phenomenon may be separated from its context for purposes of study . . . . CBPR recognizes the importance of involving members of a study population as active and equal participants, in all phases of the research project, if the research process is to be a means of facilitating change" (Holkup, Tripp-Reimer, Salois, & Weinert, 2004, p. 162). Change or action is the intended "end product" of CBPR, and PAR is related to CBPR. Some scholars would consider CBPR a sort of action research and would group both action research and CBPR within the tradition of critical science (Fontana, 2004). From this point forward, PAR is used to describe both action research and CBPR.

In *Action Research in Health*, Stringer and Genat (2004) distilled the research process into three phases: *look*, *think*, and *act*. The *look* phase is about "building the picture" by getting to know stakeholders so that the problem is defined on their terms and the problem definition reflects the community context. The *think* phase addresses interpretation and analysis of what was learned in the *look* phase, where the researcher is charged with connecting the ideas of the stakeholders so that they provide evidence that is understandable to the community group. The *act* phase involves planning, implementing, and evaluating, based on information collected and interpreted in the other phases of research.

Marcus, a nurse researcher, and her community and university colleagues reported a study to prevent substance use and human immunodeficiency virus/acquired immune deficiency syndrome (HIV/AIDS) in African American adolescents (Marcus et al., 2004). The research team used Stringer and Genat's (2004) phases of look, think, and act to frame their study within an African American church community in the Southwest United States.

In the *look* phase, university research team members and church leaders formed a coalition, which met to consider the existing community situation and to evaluate the effectiveness of services already provided by the church to address substance use and HIV/AIDS in the adolescent congregation. Weekly meetings were convened to discuss evidence provided by relevant literature and application of the literature to the community situation. The coalition's *look* phase indicated that community youth could benefit from attention to substance use and HIV and AIDS prevention and that the best course of action may be to begin with one community church, realizing that follow-up work could expand to the larger metropolitan community.

In the *think* phase, the coalition continued its work by analyzing and interpreting what was learned in the first phase of the research process. Analysis and interpretation were simultaneously connected with discussion of actions that could be taken. The collaborators initiated plans for Project BRIDGE to take African American adolescents to a new level of understanding about everyday decisions that could seriously affect their health. Project BRIDGE integrated a faith component into structured programs supporting wise choices to reduce substance use and HIV/AIDS exposure.

As plans for Project BRIDGE were formulated, the coalition was already moving into the *act* phase of research, based on the strength of evidence generated in the previous phases. In the action phase, Project BRIDGE was delivered to sixth, seventh, and eighth graders within the structure of the community church environment. The church–university coalition members participated in all components of delivery and continued to meet to evaluate ongoing development, effectiveness, need for adjustment, and outcomes. Project BRIDGE is one example of PAR that involved community members as equal participants in all phases of research to engage in context-appropriate action for affecting substance use and HIV/AIDS prevention in African American youth.

IDENTIFYING THE PHENOMENON

PAR evolved from the work of Kurt Lewin (1948), who viewed action research as a means to solve practical social problems and to enact change for the improvement of communities. PAR is heavily used as a research methodology in education, and health professions are using PAR methods to improve health care services in communities. PAR has been applied to health and wellness programs, program evaluation, care plans, community nursing, and health care delivery and policy. Studies have ranged from issues and conditions stemming from chronic illness, pregnancy and childbirth, pain management, and incontinence to rehabilitation (Stringer & Genat, 2004). Fournier, Mill, Kipp, and Walusimbi (2007) were interested in the experiences of Ugandan nurses and their role in caring for people with AIDS. Their study is used in the following section to illustrate PAR.

STRUCTURING THE STUDY

Research Question.   The first step in structuring the PAR study, as in other qualitative methods, is to frame the research question and to identify who is affected by or has an effect on the problem. Owing to the emergent nature of PAR, researchers can begin with a tentative problem and questions and then refine or reframe them as they enter the field. Recall the look–think–act cycle of Stringer and Genat (2004) described earlier. In the look phase, the researcher explores the problem by "asking who is involved, what is happening, and how, where and when events and activities occur" (p. 36). Reflecting on their observations, researchers, in collaboration with the stakeholders, can fine-tune the final research question, which serves as a guide to the study. For example, Fournier et al. (2007) explored the experiences of nurses from Uganda who cared for people with HIV and AIDS. As part of the research project, they worked with the participants to define their issues, suggest solutions, and act on them and then to reflect on the process and outcomes.

Researcher's Perspective.   When using PAR methods, the researcher is no longer the expert but acts more as a consultant. As Smith et al. (2006) stated in their case study that used participatory methodology on pregnant and parenting Aboriginal families, "participatory research views all forms of knowledge as valuable" (p. E21). The participants are co-researchers and are engaged in the research process as it emerges. This involvement requires processes that are democratic, participatory, empowering, and life-enhancing (Stringer & Genat, 2004). Participatory action researchers, like ethnographers, immerse themselves in the field for deep understanding and to build trust and credibility. For example, Fournier (Fournier et al., 2007), a faculty lecturer from the University of Alberta, spent five months over two trips onsite in Uganda.

SAMPLE SELECTION

Because it is not possible to include everyone who may have a "stake" or interest in the research question, researchers purposively select a sample of participants who represent varied perspectives, experiences, and backgrounds. Participants may be people who have the widest range of differences in their experiences, particularly interesting backgrounds or experiences, those who are typical, and those with particular knowledge of the phenomenon under study. For example, Fournier et al. (2007) selected nurses who worked on a variety of health care units and regularly cared for people with AIDS.

DATA GATHERING

In the look phase, data are gathered from a variety of sources, with interviews as the principal means to understanding the experiences of the participants. PAR also includes observation in the field, gathering and reviewing of relevant documents, and the examination of relevant materials and equipment. A literature review may add information to enhance the understanding of the data emerging from the interviews and other sources. Fournier et al. (2007) used the photovoice method in their work with nurses in Uganda. Photovoice, developed by Caroline Wang (2005), is

> *a process by which people can identify, represent, and enhance their community through a specific photographic technique. . . . It uses the immediacy of the visual image and accompanying stories to furnish evidence and to promote an effective, participatory means of sharing expertise to create healthful public policy.*

The participants took pictures of what they considered to be nurse's work. During photovoice meetings, the nurses shared stories about their pictures. Viewing their work from behind the camera and sharing stories allowed the nurses to critically assess their work. They discovered that they were not working at their fullest potential because the hospital administration did not value their input or opinions.

DATA ANALYSIS

The next phase is the (think) phase, in which the researchers think about and reflect on all of the data gathered. The purpose of data analysis is to distill and reduce the volumes of information into a manageable and organized set of concepts or ideas. The process in PAR must directly capture the experiences of the participants and be distilled in such a way "that it makes sense to them all" (Stringer & Genat, 2004).

Stringer and Genat (2004) identified two approaches to analysis. The first, based on "epiphanic moments" (Denzin, 1998), focuses on the significant experiences as the primary units of analysis, giving voice to the participants' experiences. A second process categorizes and codes data to reveal patterns and themes. Regardless of the process used, PAR allows the participants to make sense of their experience and then to use the new understanding to make a positive change.

In Fournier et al.'s (2007) project, the nurses fully participated in the analysis. They each reviewed the stories and developed themes independently. A group leader was selected to facilitate a group meeting to develop broader themes from the input of each nurse. Fournier, the principal investigator, spent an additional two months further analyzing the data with the next two authors of the study.

DESCRIBING THE FINDINGS

Following Stringer and Genat's look–think–act framework, the next step is to present the outcomes to the participants and other nonparticipant stakeholders so that they understand what is happening. Several dissemination mechanisms may be used because formal academic writing is not available for most lay participants. The results may be shared in written reports, presentations, or performances. Written narrative accounts and storytelling are often used to describe the findings. The next and most important step is to apply the findings to solve the research problem or issue that instigated the study. This action portion of PAR

parallels the nursing process of identification of goals and objectives, intervention, and, finally, evaluation. The action plans should include the following (Stringer & Genat, 2004):

Why: a statement of the overall purpose

What: a set of objectives to be obtained

How: a sequence of tasks and steps for each objective

Who: the people responsible for each task and activity

Where: the place where the tasks will be done

When: the time for initiation and completion

The researcher should also arrange for ongoing evaluation of the process. As with the exploratory phase, stakeholders are intimately involved in each step of the action plan, from identifying the plan to implementing it. The participants in Fournier et al.'s (2007) study indicated that one of their issues was inadequate knowledge about antiviral medications. This finding resulted in an unexpected outcome: the researchers determined that they would develop a research proposal. These nurses, who formed supportive and strong bonds, began to take leadership roles in the hospital, particularly in addressing ethical issues.

Evidence-Based Practice Tip

Although qualitative in its approach, PAR leads to an action component in which a nursing intervention is implemented and evaluated for its effectiveness in a specific client population.

QUALITATIVE APPROACH: Nursing Methodology

The qualitative methodologies elaborated throughout this chapter are derived from other disciplines, such as sociology, anthropology, and philosophy. The discipline of nursing borrows these methodologies to conduct research. However, as the discipline matures, methodology based on nursing ontology (belief system) emerges. Madeleine Leininger (1996), Rosemarie Rizzo Parse (1997), and Margaret Newman (1997) are nurse theorists who have created research methods specific to their theories. Table 8–1 compares the methodologies of these theorists. Each method was developed over years and tested by other researchers. Each researcher attempts to advance nursing knowledge through inquiry that is congruent with the specific nursing theory.

TABLE 8–1 **Nursing Research Methodology**			
	Leininger	**Parse**	**Newman**
Theory	Culture care	Human becoming	Health as expanding consciousness
Research methodology	Ethnonursing is centred on learning from people about their beliefs, experiences, and culture care information (Leininger, 1996).	Parse's research methodology is the study of universal health experiences through true presence both with participants sharing life stories and with transcribed data to uncover meaning (Parse, 1997).	Newman's method focuses on pattern recognition and uses multiple interviews, involving collaboration, to arrive at recognized life patterns (Newman, 1997).
Research example	Use of culture care theory with Anglo- and African American elders in a long-term care setting (McFarland, 1997)	The lived experience of serenity: Using Parse's research method (Kruse, 1999)	Pattern of expanding consciousness in women in midlife: Creative movement and narrative as modes of expression (Picard, 2000)

Critiquing Qualitative Research

Although general criteria for critiquing qualitative research are proposed in the Critiquing Criteria box, each qualitative method has unique characteristics that influence what the research consumer may expect in the published research report. The criteria for critiquing are formatted to evaluate the selection of the phenomenon, the structure of the study, data gathering, data analysis, and description of the findings. Each question of the criteria focuses on factors discussed throughout this chapter. Critiquing qualitative research is a useful activity for learning the nuances of this research approach. As a research consumer, you are encouraged to identify a qualitative study of interest and apply the criteria for critiquing. Keep in mind that qualitative methods are the best way to start to answer clinical or research questions that previously have not been addressed in research studies or that do not lend themselves to a quantitative approach. The answers provided by qualitative data reflect important evidence that may provide the first insights into a client population or clinical phenomenon.

The term *qualitative research approach* is an overriding description of multiple methods with distinct origins and procedures. In spite of distinctions, each method shares a common nature that guides data collection from the perspective of the participants to create a story that synthesizes disparate data pieces into a comprehensible whole and promises direction for building nursing knowledge.

CRITIQUING CRITERIA

IDENTIFYING THE PHENOMENON

1. Is the phenomenon focused on human experience within a natural setting?

2. Is the phenomenon relevant to nursing, health, or both?

STRUCTURING THE STUDY

Research Question

3. Does the question specify a distinct process to be studied?

4. Does the question identify the context (participant group/place) of the process that will be studied?

5. Does the choice of a specific qualitative method fit with the research question?

Researcher's Perspective

6. Are the biases of the researcher reported?

7. Do the researchers provide a structure of ideas that reflect their beliefs?

Sample Selection

8. Is it clear that the selected sample is living the phenomenon of interest?

Data Gathering

9. Are data sources and methods for gathering data specified?

10. Is evidence presented that participant consent is an integral part of the data gathering process?

Data Analysis

11. Can the dimensions of data analysis be identified and logically followed?

12. Does the researcher paint a clear picture of the participant's reality?

13. Is evidence presented that the researcher's interpretation captured the participant's meaning?

14. Have other professionals confirmed the researcher's interpretation?

Describing the Findings

15. Are examples provided to guide the reader from the raw data to the researcher's synthesis?

16. Does the researcher link the findings to existing theory or literature, or is a new theory generated?

Critical Thinking Challenges

- Discuss how the qualitative researcher knows when data saturation has occurred. Offer explanations from your life experiences that are similar to the experience of data saturation.

- How would you answer your classmate in research class who insists that it is impossible for researchers to "bracket" their personal biases about the phenomenon they are going to study? Use examples from your own clinical experience in your response.

- Defend why qualitative studies do not include hypotheses. Include in your argument whether you think qualitative studies warrant the same recognition as true experimental studies.

- Would it be legitimate qualitative research to conduct an interview using an Internet chat room? Justify your position and address ethical considerations.

- Of what value is the level of evidence provided by the findings of qualitative research studies?

KEY POINTS

- Qualitative research is the investigation of human experiences in natural settings, pursuing meanings that inform theory, practice, instrument development, and further research.

- Qualitative research studies are guided by research questions.

- Data saturation occurs when the information being shared with the researcher becomes repetitive.

- Qualitative research methods include five basic elements: identifying the phenomenon, structuring the study, gathering the data, analyzing the data, and describing the findings.

- The phenomenological method is a process of learning and constructing the meaning of human experience through intensive dialogue with persons who are living the experience.

- The grounded theory method is an inductive approach that implements a systematic set of procedures to arrive at theory about basic social processes.

- The ethnographic method focuses on scientific descriptions of cultural groups.

- The case study method focuses on a selected phenomenon over a short or long period of time to provide an in-depth description of the phenomenon's essential dimensions and processes.

- The historical research method is the systematic compilation of data and the critical presentation, evaluation, and interpretation of facts regarding people, events, and occurrences of the past.

- PAR is a method that systematically accesses the voice of a community to plan context-appropriate action.

REFERENCES

Aamodt, A. A. (1991). Ethnography and epistemology: Generating nursing knowledge. In J. M. Morse (Ed.), *Qualitative nursing research: A contemporary dialogue* (pp. 29–40). Newbury Park, CA: Sage.

Agar, M. H. (1986). *Speaking of ethnography.* Beverly Hills, CA: Sage.

Aita, V. A., & McIlvain, H. E. (1999). An armchair adventure in case study research. In B. Crabtree & W. L. Miller (Eds.), *Doing qualitative research* (2nd ed., pp. 253–268). Thousand Oaks, CA: Sage.

Barber, K. (Ed.). (2004). *The Canadian Oxford dictionary* (2nd ed.). Toronto: Oxford University Press.

Bournes, D., & Mitchell, G. (2002). Waiting: The experience of persons in a critical care waiting room. *Research in Nursing and Health, 25,* 58–67.

Boyle, J. S. (1991). Field research: A collaborative model for practice and research. In J. M. Morse (Ed.), *Qualitative nursing research: A contemporary dialogue.* Newbury Park, CA: Sage.

Browne, A., & Fiske, J. (2001). First Nations women's encounters with mainstream health care services. *Western Journal of Nursing Research, 23,* 126–147.

Caelli, K. (2000). The changing face of phenomenological research: Traditional and American phenomenology in nursing. *Qualitative Health Research, 10,* 366–377.

Cameron, C. (2003). *The lived experience of transfer students in a collaborative baccalaureate nursing program.* Unpublished doctoral dissertation, University of Toronto.

Charlebois, S., & Bouchard, L. (2007). "The worst experience": The experience of grandparents who have a grandchild with cancer. *Canadian Oncology Nursing Journal, 1,* 26–30.

Charmaz, K. (2000). Grounded theory: Objectivist and constructivist methods. In N. K. Denzin & Y. S. Lincoln (Eds.), *Handbook of qualitative research* (2nd ed., pp. 509–535). Thousand Oaks, CA: Sage.

Choudhry, U. K. (1998). Health promotion among immigrant women from India living in Canada. *Journal of Nursing Scholarship, 30,* 269–274.

Christy, T. E. (1975). The methodology of historical research: A brief introduction. *Image, 24,* 189–192.

Christy, T. E. (1981). The need for historical research in nursing. *Image, 4,* 227–228.

Cohen, S., & Leis, A. (2002). What determines the quality of life of terminally ill cancer patients from their own perspective? *Journal of Palliative Care, 18,* 48–59.

Colaizzi, P. (1978). Psychological research as a phenomenologist views it. In R. S. Valle & M. King (Eds.), *Existential phenomenological alternatives for psychology* (pp. 48–71). New York: Oxford University Press.

Crabtree, B. F., & Miller, W. L. (1992). *Doing qualitative research.* Newbury Park, CA: Sage.

Creswell, J. W. (1998). *Qualitative inquiry and research design: Choosing among five traditions.* Thousand Oaks, CA: 1998.

Denzin, N. K. (1998). The practices and politics of interpretation. In N. K. Denzin & Y. S. Lincoln (Eds.), *Collecting and interpreting qualitative materials* (pp. 458–498). Thousand Oaks, CA: Sage.

Denzin, N. K., & Lincoln, Y. S. (1998). *The landscape of qualitative research.* Thousand Oaks, CA: Sage.

Denzin, N. K., & Lincoln, Y.S. (2000). Introduction: The discipline and practice of qualitative research. In N. K. Denzin & Y. S. Lincoln (Eds.), *Handbook of qualitative research* (2nd ed., pp. 1–29). Thousand Oaks, CA: Sage.

Engebretson, J. (1996). Comparison of nurses and alternative healers. *Image, 28,* 95–99.

Fontana, J. S. (2004). A methodology for critical science in nursing. *Advances in Nursing Science, 27,* 93–101.

Ford-Gilboe, M., Wuest, J., & Merrit-Gray, M. (2005). Strengthening capacity to limit intrusion: Theorizing family health promotion in the aftermath of woman abuse. *Qualitative Health Research, 15,* 477–601.

Fournier, B., Mill, J., Kipp, W., & Walusimbi, M. (2007). Discovering voice: A participatory action research study with nurses in Uganda. *International Journal of Qualitative Methdods, 6*(2). Retrieved August 3, 2008, from http://www.ualberta.ca/~iigm/

Gates, K. (2000). The experience of caring for a loved one: A phenomenological study. *Nursing Science Quarterly, 13,* 54–59.

Giorgi, A., Fischer, C. L., & Murray, E. L. (Eds.). (1975). *Duquesne studies in phenomenological psychology.* Pittsburgh, PA: Duquesne University Press.

Glaser, B. G., & Strauss, A. L. (1967). *The discovery of grounded theory: Strategies for qualitative research.* Chicago: Aldine.

Glesne, C. (2006). *Becoming qualitative researchers: An introduction* (3rd ed.). Don Mills, ON: Longman.

Holkup, P. A., Tripp-Reimer, T., Salois, E. M., & Weinert, C. (2004). Community-based participatory research: An approach to intervention research with a Native American community. *Advances in Nursing Science, 27*, 162–175.

Hurlock-Chorostecki, C. (2002). Management of pain during weaning from mechanical ventilation: The nature of nurse decision-making. *Canadian Journal of Nursing Research, 34*, 33–47.

Kelly, U. (2006). "What will happen if I tell you?" Battered Latina women's experiences of health care. *Canadian Journal of Nursing Research, 38*, 78–95.

Kleinman, A. (1992). Local worlds of suffering: An interpersonal focus for ethnographies of illness experience. *Qualitative Health Research, 2*, 127–134.

Kruse, B. G. (1999). The lived experience of serenity: Using Parse's research method. *Nursing Science Quarterly, 12*, 143–150.

Leininger, M. M. (1996). Culture care theory. *Nursing Science Quarterly, 9*, 71–78.

Lewin, K. (1948). *Resolving social conflicts.* New York: Harper.

Liehr, P., & Marcus, M. T. (2002). Qualitative approaches to research. In G. LoBiondo-Wood & J. Haber (Eds.), *Nursing research: Methods, critical appraisal, and utilization* (5th ed., pp. 139–164). St Louis: Mosby.

Lusk, B. (1997). Historical methodology for nursing research. *Image, 29*, 355–359.

Marcus, M. T., Walker, T., Swint, J. M., Smith, B. P., Brown, C., Busen, N., et al. (2004). Community-based participatory research to prevent substance abuse and HIV/AIDS in African American adolescents. *Journal of Interprofessional Practice, 18*, 186–192.

McFarland, M. R. (1997). Use of culture care theory with Anglo- and African American elders in a long-term care setting. *Nursing Science Quarterly, 10*, 186–192.

Mead, M. (1949). *Coming of age in Samoa.* New York: New American Library/Mentor Books. (Original work published 1928)

Merriam, S. B. (1998). *Qualitative research and case study applications in education.* San Francisco, CA: Jossey-Bass Publishers.

Newman, M. A. (1997). Evolution of the theory of health as expanding consciousness. *Nursing Science Quarterly, 10*, 22–25.

Parse, R. R. (1997). Transforming research and practice with the human becoming theory. *Nursing Science Quarterly, 10*, 171–174.

Parse, R. R., Coyne, A. B., & Smith, M. J. (1985). *Nursing research: Qualitative and quantitative methods.* Bowie, MD: Brady.

Pasco, A. C. Y., Morse, J. M., & Olson, J. K. (2004). Cross-cultural relationships between nurses and Filipino Canadian patients. *Journal of Nursing Scholarship, 36*, 239–246.

Paton, B. I., Backlund, J., Thirsk, L. M., & Barnes, M. (2007). Recalibrating time and space: Women's challenges of living with heart failure. *Canadian Journal of Cardiovascular Nursing, 17*, 7–14.

Patton, M. (2002). *Qualitative research and evaluation methods* (3rd ed.). Thousand Oaks, CA: Sage.

Picard, C. (2000). Pattern of expanding consciousness in midlife women: Creative movement and narrative as modes of expression. *Nursing Science Quarterly, 13*, 150–157.

Sandelowski, M. (2004). Using qualitative research. *Qualitative Health Research, 14*, 1366–1386.

Schreiber, R., Stern, P. N., & Wilson, C. (2000). Being strong: How Black West-Indian Canadian women manage depression and its stigma. *Journal of Nursing Scholarship, 32*, 39–45.

Schultz, A., Bottorff, J., & Johnson, J. (2006). An ethnographic study of tobacco control in hospital settings. *Tobacco Control, 15*, 317–322.

Smith, D., Edwards, N., Varcoe, C., Martens, P. J., & Davies, B. (2006). Bringing safety and responsiveness into the forefront of care for pregnant and parenting aboriginal people. *Advances in Nursing Science, 29*(2), E27–E44.

Speziale, H., & Carpenter, D. (2007). *Qualitative research in nursing: Advancing the humanistic imperative* (4th ed.). Philadelphia: Lippincott.

Spiegelberg, H. (1976). *The phenomenological movement* (Vols. 1–2). The Hague: Martinus Nijhoff.

Spradley, J. P. (1979). *The ethnographic interview.* New York: Holt, Rinehart, and Winston.

Stake, R. E. (1995). *The art of case study research.* Thousand Oaks, CA: Sage.

Stake, R. E. (2003). Case studies. In N. K. Denzin & Y. S. Lincoln (Eds.), *Strategies of qualitative inquiry* (2nd ed., pp. 134–164). Thousand Oaks, CA: Sage.

Strauss, A.L. (1987). *Qualitative analysis for social scientists.* New York: Cambridge University Press.

Strauss, A., & Corbin, J. (1990). *Basics of qualitative research: Grounded theory procedures and techniques.* Newbury Park, CA: Sage.

Strauss, A., & Corbin, J. (1994). Grounded theory methodology: An overview. In N. K. Denzin & Y. S.

Lincoln (Eds.), *Handbook of qualitative research* (pp. 273–285). Thousand Oaks, CA, Sage.

Strauss, A., & Corbin, J. (Eds.). (1997). *Grounded theory in practice.* Thousand Oaks, CA: Sage.

Stringer, E. T., & Genat, W. J. (2004). *Action research in health.* Thousand Oaks, CA: Sage.

Tedlock, B. (2000). Ethnography and ethnographic representation. In N. K. Denzin & Y. S. Lincoln (Eds.), *Handbook of qualitative research* (2nd ed., p. 455–486). Thousand Oaks, CA: Sage.

van Kaam, A. (1969). *Existential foundations in psychology.* New York: Doubleday.

Varcoe, C. (2001). Abuse obscured: An ethnographic account of emergency nursing in relation to violence against women. *Canadian Journal of Nursing Research, 32,* 95–115.

Vidick, A. J., & Lyman, S. M. (1998). Qualitative methods: Their history in sociology and anthropology. In N. K.

Denzin & Y. S. Lincoln (Eds.), *The landscape of qualitative research: Theories and issues* (pp. 55–130). Thousand Oaks, CA: Sage.

Walker, D., & Myrick, D. (2006). Grounded theory: An exploration of process and procedure. *Qualitative Health Research, 16,* 547–559.

Wang, C. (2005). Photovoice: Social change through photography. Retrieved August 3, 2007, from http://www.photovoice.com/

Worthington, C., & Myers, T. (2003). Factors underlying anxiety in HIV testing: Risk perceptions, stigma, and the patient-provider power dynamic. *Qualitative Health Research, 13,* 636–655.

Wuest, J., & Merritt-Gray, M. (2001). Beyond survival: Reclaiming self after leaving an abusive male partner. *Canadian Journal of Nursing Research, 32,* 79–94.

Yin, R. K. (1994). *Case study research: Design and methods.* Thousand Oaks, CA: Sage.

PART THREE

Quantitative Research

Tackling the Prevention of Falls Among Seniors

In the late 1980s, while working as a clinical nurse consultant at the Ottawa Public Health Department, I was asked to assist with a needs assessment of seniors living in low-income apartment buildings in Ottawa. The survey covered a wide range of topics, and, at the last minute, the public health nurses decided to add a few questions about seniors' experiences with falls. The findings were startling, revealing a high incidence of falls and injuries. Published epidemiological studies indicated that our findings were not spurious. Indeed, one-third of all seniors fall annually, and approximately 25% of falls result in some sort of injury.

Soon after this survey was conducted, our then medical officer of health, Dr. Steve Corber, spoke to me about the possibility of setting up and evaluating a fall prevention initiative. Dr. Corber suggested that preventing falls should become a program focus within the health department. I was working with a senior nursing manager (Maureen Murphy) at the time, and we were interested in a more theoretical question: the relative contribution of self-care versus collective action initiatives to promote health. However, we

decided to meld these two interests, and a randomized controlled trial was born!

With funding from the Ontario Ministry of Health and Long-Term Care, we compared the impact of fall prevention clinics and a community action strategy on the incidence of falls among seniors living in 48 apartment buildings. I worked closely with the fall prevention team as we piloted and implemented the two interventions. Although we did not detect a change in the rate of falls, we did note improvements in some behavioural outcomes for fall prevention among seniors in the community action buildings, compared with the control buildings.

Many important issues surfaced during this trial and have become the basis for nearly a decade of research. In particular, we became interested in the role of the built environment in falls. In some of our study buildings, seniors who had difficulties getting into and out of the bathtub described their failed efforts to convince landlords to have grab bars installed. Landlords were refusing them permission because the installation of grab bars was thought to "lower property values." In essence, aesthetics trumped safety.

Several qualitative and quantitative studies ensued. Seniors described the stigma of using grab bars and other assistive devices. A survey of seniors in apartment buildings with and without universally installed grab bars identified barriers to grab bar access. A comparison of low-income and public apartment buildings versus private apartment buildings indicated that seniors living in low-income buildings were much more likely to have access to grab bars than seniors living in private buildings.

Concerns about bathroom grab bars and safe stairs became a focus for our regional fall prevention coalition. We began to consider what research was required to inform changes to building codes in Canada. It became apparent that, to complement our community-based studies, we needed the expertise of researchers who were able to design and conduct laboratory studies to determine what grab bar configurations are optimal to assist transfers into and out of a bathtub.

From both the laboratory and the community studies, we were able to identify the configuration of grab bars that seniors find easiest to use. We determined that seniors are 2.8 times more likely to use universally installed grab bars consistently, in comparison with grab bars they had installed themselves, after adjusting for other factors. We also documented both the high proportion of falls in bathrooms and on stairs and the high injury rates that result from these falls relative to falls occurring in other locations.

In a subsequent community study funded by the Canadian Institutes of Health Research, we identified prevalent stair hazards in private homes and public buildings. Seniors were asked to identify the most common locations of hazardous stairs. Churches and community centres were among the locations most frequently identified. Independent raters also assessed indoor and outdoor stairs, both those identified by seniors as hazardous in the community and the stairs they used in their own homes or apartment buildings. The most common hazards were the lack of contrast marking on the edge of the stairs, inadequate tread length, risers that were too high, and nonuniform risers. Although seniors were able to identify hazardous stairs that they had difficulty navigating, less than one-quarter of them had specific suggestions for ways to improve stair safety.

We are now using our research findings on bathroom and stair falls to inform policy change. Specifically, I submitted a request to the National Research Council (NRC) for an additional requirement to the building codes for the universal installation of grab bars in showers and bathtubs in all residential homes. Our research provides strong support for this request. I am also a member of the NRC task group for stairs, handrails, ramps, and guards. Our research on stair falls is being reviewed as part of the evidence for changes to the building codes. I am hopeful that in the current cycle of building code changes, we will see a change in code requirements to improve stair and bathtub safety in homes and residential buildings.

Bridging the interface between research and policy is a critical knowledge translation strategy. Informing and influencing policy change require the engagement of an informed public which led us to establish a networking infrastructure called CHNET-Works (http://www.chnet-works.ca). Using teleconference lines, Bridgit (i.e., conferencing software), and the support of a network animateur, we host weekly "fireside chats" for nine months of the year. Our aim is to bring together academic researchers, front-line practitioners and managers, policymakers, and colleagues from the volunteer sector to address common issues. Participants consider how evidence might inform intersectoral practices and policies and how activities in the field and in policy arenas might inform research. We have held a series of fireside chats on changes to the building codes in an effort to provide timely input on the building code revisions. The outcome of these chats includes a photo gallery of stair hazards and preparation of a series of resolutions for submission to various professional associations. These resolutions concern support for evidence-based changes to the national building codes as they relate to bathtub grab bars and safe stairs.

Our work on preventing falls has reinforced the critical role interdisciplinary research plays in the design of community health interventions. Substantial health changes in populations such as senior citizens will come about only through long-term research and policy change efforts. "Quick fixes" are rare. As a researcher, I need to be prepared to work actively with colleagues at the local, provincial, and national levels and to use a wide repertoire of knowledge translation strategies.

Nancy C. Edwards
Full Professor, School of Nursing
Department of Epidemiology and Community Medicine
University of Ottawa
Ottawa, Ontario

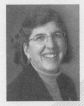

Geri Lobiondo-Wood
Mina D. Singh

CHAPTER 9

Introduction to Quantitative Research

LEARNING OUTCOMES

After reading this chapter, the student should be able to do the following:

- Define research design.
- Identify the purpose of the research design.
- Define control as it affects the research design.
- Compare the elements that affect control.
- Begin to evaluate the degree of control that should be exercised in the design.
- Define internal validity.
- Identify the threats to internal validity.
- Define external validity.
- Identify the conditions that affect external validity.
- Identify the links between study design and evidence-based practice.
- Evaluate the design using the critiquing questions.

STUDY RESOURCES

evolve Go to Evolve at
http://evolve.elsevier.com/Canada/LoBiondo/Research/
for Weblinks, content updates, and additional
research articles for practice in reviewing
and critiquing.

KEY TERMS

accuracy
bias
constancy
control
control group
experimental group
external validity
extraneous or mediating variable
feasibility
Hawthorne effect
history
homogeneity
instrumentation
internal validity
maturation
measurement effects
mortality
objectivity
pilot study
randomization
reactivity
selection
selection bias
testing

The word *design* implies the organization of elements into a masterful work of art. In the world of art and fashion, the word conjures up images of processes and techniques that are used to express a total concept. When an individual creates, process and form are employed. The form, process, and degree of adherence to structure depend on the aims of the creator.

The same can be said of the research process. The research process does not need to be a sterile procedure but rather it should be one in which the researcher develops a masterful work within the limits of a problem and the related theoretical basis. The framework that the researcher creates is the design. When reading a study, the research consumer should be able to recognize that the research problem, purpose, literature review, theoretical framework, and hypothesis all interrelate with, complement, and assist in the operationalization of the design (see Figure 9–1). The degree to which a fit exists between these design elements strengthens the study and the consumer's confidence in the evidence provided by the findings and their potential applicability to practice.

Nursing practice is concerned with a variety of structures that require varying degrees of process and form, such as the provision of quality care, cost-effective client care, responses of clients to disease, and factors that affect caregivers. When nurses administer client care, they draw on the nursing process. Previous chapters stressed the importance of theory and knowledge of subject matter to research. How a researcher structures, implements, or designs a study affects the results of a research project.

For the consumer to understand the implications and the use of research, the central issues in the design of a research project should be understood. This chapter provides an overview of the meaning, purpose, and issues related to quantitative research design. Chapters 10 and 11 discuss specific types of quantitative designs.

PURPOSE OF THE RESEARCH DESIGN

The purpose of the research design is to provide the plan for answering research questions. These questions can result in research driven by a researcher's *curiosity* or interest in a *theoretical* question. This process is called basic research, and its motivation is to expand nursing knowledge. In contrast, applied research is designed to solve *clinical problems* rather than to acquire knowledge for knowledge's sake; thus, the goal is to improve the client's health care condition.

The design in quantitative research then becomes the vehicle for hypothesis testing or answering research questions, whether they are basic or applied. The design involves a *plan*, a *structure*, and a *strategy*. These three design concepts guide a researcher in writing the hypothesis or research questions, conducting the project, and analyzing and evaluating the data. The overall purpose of the research design is two-fold: to aid in the solution of research problems and to maintain control. All research attempts to answer questions. The design,

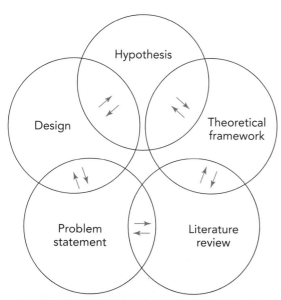

Figure 9–1 Interrelationships of design, problem statement, literature review, theoretical framework, and hypothesis

coupled with the methods and analysis, is the mechanism for finding solutions to research questions. **Control** is defined as the measures that the researcher uses to hold the conditions of the study uniform and avoid possible impingement of **bias** on the dependent variable or outcome.

A research example that demonstrates how the design can aid in answering a research question and maintain control is the study by Harkness, Morrow, Smith, Kiczula, and Arthur (2003). The main purpose of their study was to examine the effect of specialized early education on client anxiety while waiting for elective cardiac catheterization. To maintain control, the researchers had strict sample characteristics. Inclusion citeria were as follows: (1) referral for first-time, elective cardiac catheterization; (2) anticipated wait of between six weeks and six months; (3) ability to speak and read English; and (4) geographical accessibility to the hospital. Exclusion critera were as follows: (1) inability to provide written informed consent; (2) previous consultation with a surgeon for possible open heart surgery; (3) previous cardiac catheterization; and (4) current involvement in a cardiac rehabilitation program. By establishing the specific sample criteria and subject eligibility, the researchers were able to maintain control over the study's conditions and suggest an extension of the study's outcome with further research.

A variety of considerations, including the type of design, affect the accomplishment of the study. These considerations include **objectivity** in the conceptualization of the problem, accuracy, feasibility, control of the experiment, internal validity, and external validity. Statistical principles exist behind the many forms of control, but it is more important that the research consumer have a clear conceptual understanding of statistics and how they inform the research questions.

The type of design used in a study also affects its application to practice. Chapters 10 and 11 present a number of experimental, quasiexperimental, and nonexperimental designs. The type of design used in a study is linked to the level of evidence and, in turn, the contribution of a study's findings

to evidence-based practice. As you critically appraise the design, you must also take into account other aspects of a study's design, which are reviewed in this chapter.

OBJECTIVITY IN THE PROBLEM CONCEPTUALIZATION

Objectivity in the conceptualization of the problem is derived from a review of the literature and development of a theoretical framework (see Figure 9–1). Using the literature, the researcher assesses the depth and breadth of available knowledge on the problem. The literature review and theoretical framework should demonstrate to the reader that the researcher reviewed the literature with a critical and objective eye (see Chapters 2 and 5) because this conceptualization of the problem affects the type of design chosen. For example, a question about the relationship of the length of a breastfeeding education program may suggest either a correlational or an experimental design (see Chapters 10 and 11), whereas a question regarding the physical changes in a woman's body during pregnancy and the maternal perception of the unborn child may suggest a survey or correlation study (see Chapter 11). Therefore, the literature review should reflect the following:

- When the problem was studied
- The aspects of the problem that were studied
- Where the problem was investigated
- By whom the problem was investigated
- The gaps or inconsistencies in the literature

Helpful 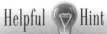 Hint

A review that incorporates the aspects presented here allows the consumer to judge the objectivity of the problem area and therefore whether the design chosen matches the problem.

ACCURACY

Accuracy in determining the appropriate design is also accomplished through the theoretical framework and review of the literature (see Chapters 2 and 5). Accuracy means that all aspects of a study systematically and logically follow from the research problem. The beginning researcher is wise to answer a question involving few variables that will not require the use of sophisticated designs. The simplicity of a research project does not render it useless or of a lesser value for practice. However, although the project is simple, the researcher should not forego accuracy. The consumer should feel that the researcher chose a design that was consistent with the research problem and offered the maximum amount of control.

Many clinical problems have not yet been researched, so a preliminary or **pilot study** is a wise approach to test the accuracy of a study design before beginning a larger study. The key is the accuracy, validity, and objectivity used by the researcher in attempting to answer the question. Accordingly, when reading research, you should read various types of studies and assess whether and how the criteria for each step of the research process were followed. Research consumers will find that many nursing journals publish not only sophisticated clinical research projects but also smaller clinical studies that can be applied to practice.

FEASIBILITY

When critiquing the study design, consumers of research must also be aware of the pragmatic consideration of feasibility. **Feasibility** refers to the capability of the study to be successfully completed. Sometimes, the reality of feasibility does not truly sink in until one carries out research. When reviewing a study, research consumers should consider feasibility, including availability of the subjects, timing of the research, time required for the subjects to participate, costs, and analysis of the data (see Table 9–1).

Bissonette, Logan, Davies, and Graham (2005) conducted a study in which they investigated the feasibility of providing a tailored education program to clients diagnosed with chronic obstructive pulmonary disease (COPD). This pilot study was conducted to determine the feasibility of providing such a program prior to full implementation or conducting a randomized controlled trial. The authors found two methodological issues: recruitment and retention of clients with chronic illness for research and choosing an outcome measure that would not obtain such high "not applicable" response rates.

A major objective of this Bissonette et al. (2005) study was to determine the feasibility of providing a tailored education program for clients diagnosed with COPD to avoid potentially costly and inappropriate resource expenditure. Before conducting a large experimental study, such as a randomized clinical trial, it is helpful to first conduct a pilot study with a small number of subjects to determine the feasibility of subject recruitment, the intervention, the data collection protocol, the likelihood that subjects will complete the study, the reliability and validity of new measurement tools, and the costs of the study.

These pragmatic considerations are not presented as a step in the research process, as are the theoretical framework and methods, but they do affect every step of the process and therefore should be considered when assessing a study. For example, the student researcher may or may not have monies or accessible services. When critiquing a study, note the credentials of the author(s) and whether the investigation was part of either a student project or a fully funded grant project. If the project was a student project, the standards of critiquing are applied more liberally than for an experienced researcher or clinician with a doctoral degree. Finally, the pragmatic issues raised affect the scope and breadth of an investigation and therefore its generalizability.

CONTROL

A researcher attempts to use a design to maximize the degree of control over the tested variables. Control involves holding the conditions of the study constant and establishing specific sampling criteria, as described by Samuels-Dennis (2006) (see Appendix C). An efficient design can maximize results, decrease errors, and control pre-existing

Factor	Pragmatic Consideration
Time	The research problem must be able to be studied within a realistic period of time. All researchers have deadlines for completion of a project. The scope of the problem must be circumscribed enough to provide ample time for the completion of the entire project. Research studies generally take longer than anticipated to complete.
Subject availability	The researcher must determine whether a sufficient number of eligible subjects will be available and willing to participate in the study. If a researcher has a captive audience (e.g., students in a classroom), it may be relatively easy to enlist their cooperation. When a study involves the subjects' independent time and effort, they may be unwilling to participate when they will receive no apparent reward for doing so. Other potential subjects may have fears about harm or confidentiality and be suspicious of the research process in general. Subjects with unusual characteristics, such as rare conditions, are often difficult to locate. People are generally cooperative about participating, but a researcher must consider needing a larger subject pool than will actually participate. At times, when reading a research report, the researcher may note how the procedures were liberalized or the number of subjects was altered—probably as a result of some unforeseen pragmatic consideration.
Facility and equipment availability	All research projects require some kind of equipment, such as questionnaires, telephones, stationery, stamps, technical equipment, or another apparatus. Most research projects also require the availability of a facility for the work, such as a hospital site for data collection, a laboratory space, or a computer centre for data analysis.
Money	Many research projects require some expenditure of money. Before embarking on a study, the researcher probably itemized the expenses and estimated the total cost of the project. This estimation of cost provides a clear picture of the budgetary needs for items such as books, stationery, postage, printing, technical equipment, telephone and computer charges, and salaries. These expenses can range from about $200 for a small-scale student project to hundreds of thousands of dollars for a large-scale federally funded project.
Researcher experience	The selection of the research problem should be based on the nurse's experience and interest. It is much easier to develop a research study related to a topic that is either theoretically or experientially familiar. Selecting a problem that is of interest to the researcher is essential for maintaining enthusiasm when the project has its inevitable successes and failures.
Ethics	Research problems that place unethical demands on subjects will not be feasible for study. Researchers must take ethical considerations seriously. The consideration of ethics may affect the choice of the design and the methodology.

conditions that may affect outcome. To accomplish these tasks, the research design and methods should demonstrate the researcher's efforts at control.

For example, in their study, Forchuk et al. (2004) examined the usefulness of arm massage from a significant other following lymph node dissection surgery. It was hypothesized that individuals receiving arm massage would have greater immediate comfort (less pain, higher perceived control) and fewer functional constraints (decreased swelling, increased range of motion, increased shoulder function, and decreased costs) compared with women receiving the standard postoperative treatment. To test their hypothesis and apply control, the investigators calculated a sample size (see Chapter 12) of a minimum of 25 participants per group. Thirty participants were recruited to compensate for dropouts. The intervention was controlled by asking the participants to demonstrate their massage technique to ensure proper administration. A registered nurse, with a master's degree, performed all of the teaching and demonstrations to avoid variance in the intervention from multiple teachers.

The Forchuk et al. (2004) study illustrated how the investigators in one study planned the design to apply controls. An efficient design can maximize results, decrease errors, and control pre-existing conditions that may affect outcomes. To accomplish these tasks, the research design and methods should demonstrate the researcher's efforts at control, such as in the Forchuk et al. (2004) study. Control is important in all designs. When various research designs are critiqued, the issue of control is always raised, but with varying levels of flexibility. The issues discussed here will become clearer as you review the various types of designs.

Control is accomplished by ruling out extraneous or mediating variables that compete with the independent variables as an explanation for a study's outcome. An **extraneous or mediating variable** interferes with the operations of the phenomena being studied (e.g., age and gender). Means of controlling extraneous variables include the following:

- Use of a homogeneous sample
- Use of consistent data collection procedures
- Manipulation of the independent variable
- Randomization

An investigator might be interested in how a new smoking cessation program (independent variable) affects smoking behaviour (dependent variable). The independent variable is assumed to affect the outcome or dependent variable. An investigator needs to be relatively sure that the decrease in smoking is truly related to the smoking cessation program rather than to another variable, such as motivation.

The following example illustrates and defines these concepts further. Singh and Cameron (2005) investigated the psychosocial aspects of caregiving to clients who have had a stroke. These factors (independent variables) were caregiver burden, caregiver self-efficacy, caregiver mastery, caregiver support, and the impact on the caregiver's life. To rule out the effects of extraneous variables on the emotional well-being of the caregiver (dependent variable), demographic information on the caregivers was collected, including age, length of care, number of children, pre-existing medical conditions, and level of education. Although the design of the research study alone does not inherently provide control, an appropriately designed study with the necessary controls can increase an investigator's ability to answer a research question.

Evidence-Based Practice Tip

As you read studies, assess whether the study includes a tested intervention and whether the report contains a clear description of the intervention and how it was controlled. If the details are not clear, the intervention may have been administered differently among the subjects, therefore affecting the interpretation of the results.

Homogeneous Sampling

In the smoking cessation example, extraneous variables may affect the dependent variable. The characteristics of a study's subjects are common extraneous variables. Age, gender, length of time smoked, amount smoked, and even smoking rules may affect the outcome in the smoking cessation example, even though they are extraneous or outside the study's design. As a control for these and other similar problems, the researcher's subjects should demonstrate **homogeneity** or similarity with respect to the extraneous variables relevant to the particular study (see Chapter 13). Extraneous variables are not fixed but must be reviewed and decided on, based on the study's purpose and theoretical base. By using a sample of homogeneous subjects, the researcher has used a straightforward step of control.

For example, in the study described earlier by Bissonette et al. (2005), the researchers ensured the homogeneity of the sample by having the following sampling criteria: primary or secondary admission diagnosis of COPD or COPD exacerbation, chronic bronchitis, bronchiectasis, emphysema, COPD with asthma, or COPD with pneumonia; male or female; and age 45 years or older. The sample was homogeneous based on age and diagnosis. This control step limits the generalizability or application of the outcomes to other populations when analyzing and discussing the outcomes (see Chapter 17). The results can then be generalized only to a similar population of individuals. Homogeneity could be considered limiting, but not necessarily because no treatment or program is applicable to all populations, and educated consumers of research must take into consideration the differences in populations. In the case of the Bissonette et al. (2005) study, the findings provided information for researchers in the recruitment and retention of clients with chronic illness and in deciding on a more efficient outcome measure.

Helpful Hint

When reviewing studies, remember that it is better to have a "clean" study, which can be used to make generalizations about a specific population, than a "messy" study, which can generalize little or nothing.

If the researcher feels that one of the extraneous variables is important, it may be included in the design. In the smoking cessation example, if individuals are working in an area where smoking is not allowed and this condition is considered to be important to the study, the researcher could build it into the design and set up a control for it. This control can be established by comparing two different work areas: one where smoking is allowed and one where it is not. The important idea to keep in mind is that before the data are collected, the researcher should have identified, planned for, and controlled the important extraneous variables.

Constancy in Data Collection

Another basic, yet critical, component of control is constancy in data collection procedures. **Constancy** refers to the ability of the data collection design to hold the conditions of the study to a cookbook-like recipe. In other words, for the purpose of collecting data for the study, each subject is exposed to the same environmental conditions, timing of data collection, data collection instruments, and data collection procedures (see Chapter 13).

An example of constancy in data collection is illustrated in the study by Doran et al. (2006). The objective of this study was to explore which nursing interventions provided during hospitalization are associated with clients' therapeutic self-care

and functional health outcomes. Nurses collected data on client outcomes using the Minimum Data Set and the Therapeutic Self-Care Scale. Chart audits were conducted by research assistants (RAs). Constancy was attained by training the RAs in a half-day session with a prescribed protocol, which included an introduction to the nursing intervention audit tool, instruction in the operational definition of each nursing intervention item, and the opportunity to conduct a chart audit with feedback. The audit of a research team member was used as the standard against which the RAs' chart audits were compared. This type of control aided the investigators' ability to draw conclusions, discuss the findings, and cite the need for further research in this area. For the consumer, constancy demonstrates a clear, consistent, and specific means of data collection.

When psychosocial interventions are implemented, researchers will often describe the training of interventionists or data collectors that took place to ensure constancy. They might also indicate that an intervention manual was used to script a standardized approach to intervention or data collection. For example, in the study by Ratner et al. (2004) on a smoking cessation intervention for clients who had undergone elective surgery, the researchers had strict intervention protocols for each component of the interventions and provided detailed descriptions of the preadmission clinic intervention, the in-hospital intervention, and the telephone counselling intervention.

Manipulation of the Independent Variable

A third means of control is manipulation of the independent variable. Manipulation refers to the administration of a program, treatment, or intervention to only one group within the study but not to the other subjects in the study. The first group is known as the **experimental group**, and the other group is known as the **control group**. In a control group, the variables under study are held at a constant or comparison level. For example,

Allard (2006) studied whether a psychoeducational nursing intervention could help women who underwent day surgery for breast cancer achieve better pain management and decrease emotional distress. The experimental group received the intervention, whereas the control group received the standard hospital teaching.

Experimental and quasiexperimental designs use manipulation, whereas nonexperimental designs do not manipulate the independent variable. This lack of manipulation does not decrease the usefulness of a nonexperimental design, but the use of a control group in an experimental or quasiexperimental design is related to the research question and, again, its theoretical framework.

Blinding is a technique used in experimental and quasiexperimental research in which the participants are not aware whether they are receiving the intervention. Double blinding is a technique in which both the researchers and the participants are not aware who is receiving the intervention and who is in the control group. For example, Forchuk, Martin, Chan, and Jensen (2005) (see Appendix A) used a technique called blinding randomization in which the individuals engaged in data collection were blind to which ward was receiving the transitional discharge model of care intervention.

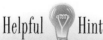

Helpful Hint

Be aware that the lack of manipulation of the independent variable does not mean a weaker study. The level of the problem, the amount of theoretical work, and the research that has preceded the project affect the researcher's choice of the design. If the problem is amenable to a design that manipulates the independent variable, the power of a researcher to draw conclusions will increase, provided that all of the considerations of control are equally addressed.

Randomization

Researchers may also choose other forms of control, such as randomization. **Randomization** is used when the required number of subjects from the population is obtained in such a manner that

each subject in a population has an equal chance of being selected. Randomization eliminates bias, aids in the attainment of a representative sample, and can be used in various designs. In their study, Harkness et al. (2003) randomly assigned participants to either the experimental group, which received nurse-delivered detailed information or an education session within two weeks of being placed on a waiting list for elective catheterization, or the control group, which received the usual care, consisting of no regular contact from any health care professional.

Randomization can also be done with paper-and-pencil-type instruments. By randomly ordering items on the instruments, the investigator can assess whether a difference in responses correlates to the order of the items. Randomization may be especially important in longitudinal studies, in which bias from giving the same instrument to the same subjects on a number of occasions can be a problem (see Chapter 12).

QUANTITATIVE CONTROL AND FLEXIBILITY

The same level of control cannot be exercised in all types of designs. At times, when a researcher wants to explore an area in which little or no literature on the concept exists, the researcher will probably use an exploratory design. In this type of study, the researcher is interested in describing or categorizing a phenomenon in a group of individuals. Estabrooks, O'Leary, Ricker, and Humphrey's (2003) study of the frequency and location from which nurses accessed the Internet is an example of exploratory research. In this research, the authors obtained data on the type of information nurses were seeking and how their use of this information differed from that of physicians and the public. In critiquing this type of study, the issue of control should be applied in a highly flexible manner because of the preliminary nature of the work.

If it is determined from a review of a study that the researcher intended to conduct a correlational study (a study that looks at the relationship between or among the variables), then the issue of control takes on more importance. Control must be exercised as strictly as possible. At this intermediate level of design, it should be clear to the reviewer that the researcher considered the extraneous variables that may affect the outcomes.

All aspects of control are strictly applied to studies that use an experimental design. The reader should be able to locate in the research report how the researcher met these criteria; in other words, the conditions of the research were constant throughout the study, the assignment of subjects was random, and experimental and control groups were used. Because of the control exercised in the study, the reader can see that all issues related to control were considered and the extraneous variables were addressed.

Evidence-Based Practice Tip

Remember that establishing evidence for practice is determined by assessing the validity of each step of the study, assessing whether the evidence assists in planning client care, and assessing whether clients respond to the evidence-based care.

INTERNAL AND EXTERNAL VALIDITY

Consumers of research must believe that the results of a study are valid, based on precision, and faithful to what the researcher wanted to measure. To form the basis of further research, practice, and theory development, a study must be credible and dependable. The two important criteria for evaluating the credibility and dependability of the results are **internal validity** and **external validity**. Threats to validity are listed in Box 9–1, and a discussion of each threat follows.

Internal Validity

Internal validity asks whether the difference or the change in the dependent variable is a result of

BOX 9–1 Threats to Validity
INTERNAL VALIDITY
History
Maturation
Testing
Instrumentation
Mortality
Selection bias
EXTERNAL VALIDITY
Selection effects
Reactive effects
Measurement effects

the independent variable. To establish internal validity, the researcher rules out other factors or threats as rival explanations of the relationship between the variables. A number of threats to internal validity exist and are considered by researchers in planning a study and by consumers before implementing the results in practice (Campbell & Stanley, 1996). Research consumers should note that the threats to internal validity are most clearly applicable to experimental designs, but attention to factors that can compromise outcomes should be considered to some degree in all quantitative designs. If these threats are not considered, they could negate the results of the research by affecting the design. Threats to internal validity include history, maturation, testing, instrumentation, mortality, and selection bias. Table 9–2 provides examples of these threats.

History

Not only the independent variable but also another specific event may affect the dependent variable, either inside or outside the experimental setting. This threat to internal validity is referred to as **history**. In a study of the effects of a breastfeeding education program on the length of time of breastfeeding, government-sponsored breastfeeding promotions on television and in newspapers could affect the length of time of breastfeeding and would

TABLE 9-2	Examples of Internal Validity Threats
Threat	**Example**
History	Bull, Hansen, and Gross (2000) tested a teaching intervention in one hospital and compared the outcomes with those of another hospital in which the usual care was given. During the final months of data collection, the control hospital implemented a congestive heart failure critical pathway; as a result, data from the control hospital (cohort 4) were not included in the analysis.
Maturation	Wikblad and Anderson (1995) controlled for the possibility of maturation in a study of wound-healing processes. Normal wound healing could have been a threat to the findings, but the researchers developed a careful data collection plan to control for the threat of maturation.
Testing	A researcher measured acute pain with a repeated measures design during a lengthy procedure. The researcher would have to consider the results in light of the possible bias of repeating the pain measurements over a short period of time. The measurements may have primed the clients' responses, and the practice of reporting pain repeatedly on the same instrument during a procedure may have influenced the results.
Instrumentation	Inoue, Kakehashi, Oomori, and Koizumi (2004) studied biochemical hypoglycemia in female nurses during shift work in Japan. The nurses determined their own blood glucose levels 12 times, at four points during three shifts. The researchers noted that the study depended on self-testing and self-reporting of blood glucose levels; thus, documenting the validity of the data was difficult. Even though the study was well developed and subjects were ensured confidentiality, the researchers still were concerned with this threat to the study's validity. Holditch-Davis, Brandon, and Schwartz (2003) examined the development of eight infant behaviours in preterm infants. Data collectors were trained and assessed for interrater reliability, thus avoiding the threat of instrumentation.
Mortality	Tranmer, Minard, Fox, and Rebelo (2003) described and compared the sleep experience of medical and surgical clients during a hospital stay over three consecutive nights. Of the 110 clients who consented, 97 (88%) clients remained on the second night and 86 (78%) clients on the third night. Clients were lost to follow-up because of early or unexpected discharge, an unexpected change in status, or transfer to the intensive care unit. A sample size of 100 clients was calculated prior to the start of the study. The effect of this sample loss was not discussed in relation to the findings.
Selection bias	Forchuk et al. (2004) controlled for selection bias by establishing selection criteria and having an experimental group and a control group.

be considered a threat of history. A published example of history affecting research findings is the Bull, Hansen, and Gross (2000) study (see Table 9–2).

Maturation

Maturation refers to the developmental, biological, or psychological processes that operate within an individual as a function of time and are external to the events of the investigation. For example, suppose that a researcher wished to evaluate the effect of a specific teaching method on the achievements of baccalaureate students on a skills test. The investigator would record the students' abilities before and after the teaching method. Between the pretest and the post-test, the students would have grown older and wiser. The growth or

change is unrelated to the investigation and may explain the differences between the two testing periods rather than the experimental treatment.

Maturation could also occur in a study focused on investigating the relationship between two methods of teaching about children's knowledge of self-care measures. Post-tests of student learning must be conducted in a relatively short time period after the teaching sessions are completed. A relatively short interval allows the investigator to conclude that the results were the result of the design of the study and not maturation in a population of children who are learning new skills rapidly. Maturation is more than change owing to an age-related developmental process; maturation can also be related to physical changes (see Table 9–2).

Testing

Taking the same test repeatedly could influence subjects' responses the next time a measure is completed. For example, the effect on the subject's post-test score as the result of having taken a pre-test is known as **testing**. The effect of taking a pretest may sensitize an individual and improve the score of the post-test. Individuals generally score higher when they take a test a second time, regardless of the treatment. The differences between post-test and pretest scores may not be a result of the independent variable but rather of the experience gained through the testing. For example, in a pilot study investigating the effect of a video and telephone counselling intervention for women with breast cancer and their partners (Hoskins et al., 2001), pretests and post-tests assessing the increase in health-relevant information were administered before and after the video intervention. Whether the significant increase in knowledge was due to the video or the effect of taking the test more than once was difficult to determine. Table 9–2 provides another example.

Instrumentation

Instrumentation threats are changes in the measurement of the variables or observational techniques that may account for changes in the obtained measurement. For example, a researcher may wish to study various types of thermometers (e.g., tympanic, digital, electronic, chemical indicator, plastic strip, and mercury) to compare the accuracy of the mercury thermometer with the other temperature-taking methods. To prevent instrumentation, a researcher must check the calibration of the thermometers according to the manufacturer's specifications before and after data collection.

Another example relates to techniques of observation or data collection. If a researcher has several raters collecting observational data, all must be trained in a similar manner. If they are not similarly trained, or even if they are similarly trained but unable to conduct the study as planned, a lack of consistency may occur in their ratings; therefore, a threat to internal validity will occur.

Boechler, Harrison, and Magill-Evans (2003) conducted a study examining whether the amount of caregiving is related to the behaviour of a father and his child during a structured teaching interaction. The father was observed teaching his child to use a standardized teaching item, such as grabbing a ring or taking the lid off a container. Two trained female observers watched the father and scored the interaction on the Nursing Child Assessment Teaching Scale; only consensus scores from both observers were used in the data analysis. (For another example, see Table 9–2.) Although the researcher takes steps to prevent problems of instrumentation, the threat of instrumentation may still occur. When a critiquer finds such a threat, it must be evaluated within the total context of the study, as, in fact, the researchers did in the Marsh, Prochoda, Pritchett, and Vojir (2000) study.

Mortality

Mortality is the loss of study subjects from the first data collection point (pretest) to the second data collection point (post-test). If the subjects who remain in the study are not similar to those who dropped out, the results could be affected. The loss of subjects may be from the sample as a whole; or, in a study that has both an experimental group and a control group, more of the subjects may drop out from one group than from the other group, an effect known as differential loss of subjects. In a study of the ways in which a media campaign affects the incidence of breastfeeding, if most dropouts were nonbreastfeeding women, the perception given could be that exposure to the media campaign increased the number of breastfeeding women, whereas the effect of experimental mortality led to the observed results. See Table 9–2 for an example of a study in which mortality may have influenced the results.

Selection Bias

If precautions are not used to gain a representative sample, **selection bias** could result from the way the subjects were chosen. Selection effects are a problem in studies in which the individuals themselves decide whether to participate in a study. Suppose an investigator wishes to assess whether a new smoking cessation program contributes to smoking cessation. If the new program is offered to all, chances are that only individuals who are more motivated to learn how to stop smoking will take part in the program. Assessment of the effectiveness of the program is problematic because the investigator cannot know for certain whether the new program encouraged smoking cessation behaviours or whether only highly motivated individuals joined the program. To avoid selection bias, the researcher could randomly assign subjects to either the new teaching method group or a control group that receives a different type of instruction. Table 9–2 provides another example of selection bias.

Helpful Hint

The list of internal validity threats is not exhaustive. More than one threat can be found in a study, depending on the type of study design. Finding a threat to internal validity in a study does not invalidate the results and is usually acknowledged by the investigator in the "Results" or "Discussion" section of the study.

Evidence-Based Practice Tip

Avoiding threats to internal validity when conducting clinical research can be difficult. Yet this reality does not render studies that have threats useless. Take the threats into consideration and weigh the total evidence of a study for not only its statistical meaningfulness but also its clinical meaningfulness.

External Validity

External validity deals with possible problems of generalizability of the investigation's findings to additional populations and to other environmental conditions. External validity questions the conditions and the types of subjects that can be expected to lead to the same results. The goal of the researcher is to select a design that maximizes both internal and external validity, but attaining this goal is not always possible. If it is not possible, the researcher must establish a minimum requirement of meeting the criteria of external validity.

The factors that may affect external validity are related to the selection of subjects, study conditions, and type of observations. These factors are termed effects of selection, reactive effects, and effects of testing. The reader will notice the similarity in the names of the factors of selection and testing and those of the threats to internal validity. When considering factors as internal threats, the reader assesses them as they relate to the *independent* and *dependent* variables within the study; when assessing them as external threats, the reader considers them in terms of the generalizability or use outside the study to other populations and settings.

The Critical Thinking Decision Path for threats to validity displays the way threats to internal and external validity can interact. This path is not, however, exhaustive of the type of threats and their interaction. Compared with problems of internal validity, generalizability issues are typically more difficult to deal with because they mean that the researcher is assuming that other populations are similar to the one being tested.

Selection Effects

Selection refers to the generalizability of the results to other populations. An example of the effects of selection occurs when the researcher cannot attain the ideal sample population. At times, the number of available subjects may be low or not accessible to the researcher. The researcher may then need to choose a nonprobability method of sampling, not a probability method. Therefore, the type of sampling method used and how subjects are assigned to research conditions will affect the generalizability to other groups or the external

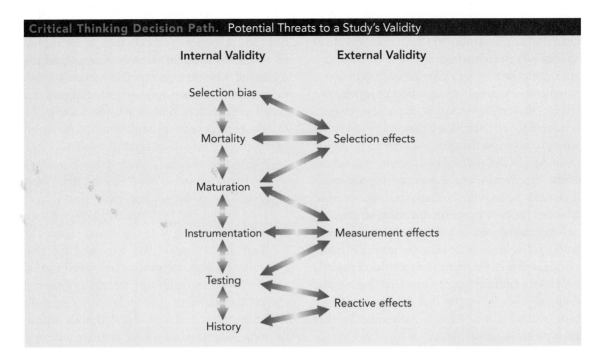

Critical Thinking Decision Path. Potential Threats to a Study's Validity

Internal Validity

External Validity

Selection bias

Mortality → Selection effects

Maturation

Instrumentation ↔ Measurement effects

Testing

History → Reactive effects

validity. Examples of selection effects are depicted when researchers note any of the following:

- "The wide age range may also have had an influence on the pilot study results, as well as the length of caregiving and the relationship of the caregiver to the terminally ill family member" (Duggleby et al., 2007, p. 30).

- "The cultural diversity of the sample (Caucasian 36.8%, Afro-Canadian 40%, Aboriginal 1.1%, South Asian 10.5%, Asian 5.3%, Latino 4.2%, Arabic 1.1%) may limit the generalizability of its findings to less culturally diverse populations" (Samuels-Dennis, 2006, p. 76) (see Appendix C).

- "Although participants comprised 82.6% of the sample population of nurses at the Health Department, these participants were not representative of nurses in other Public Health Departments" (Brathwaite & Majumdar, 2005, p. 477).

These remarks caution the reader but also point out the usefulness of the findings for practice and future research aimed at building the data in these areas.

Reactive Effects

Reactivity is defined as the subjects' responses to being studied. Subjects may respond to the investigator not because of the study procedures but merely as an independent response to being studied. This response is also known as the **Hawthorne effect**, named after Western Electric Corporation's Hawthorne plant, where a study of working conditions was conducted in the 1930s. The researchers developed several different working conditions, such as turning up the lights, piping in music loudly or softly, and changing work hours. They found that no matter what was done, the workers' productivity increased. They concluded that production increased as a result of the workers' knowing that they were being studied rather than because of the experimental conditions.

In the study by Ratner et al. (2004), an intervention was tested to help smokers abstain from smoking before and after surgery. Smokers were randomized to a counselling intervention and nicotine replacement program, and the control group received the usual hospital care. At the end of the study, the researchers found that the control group had a relatively high abstinence rate. They concluded that because the control group was aware of the group assignment, the participants tried to demonstrate that they could do as well as the treatment group, even though they did not receive the intervention.

Measurement Effects

Administration of a pretest in a study affects the generalizability of the findings to other populations and is known as **measurement effects**. Just as pretesting affects the post-test results within a study, pretesting affects the post-test results and generalizability outside the study. For example, suppose a researcher wants to conduct a study with the aim of changing attitudes toward acquired immune deficiency syndrome (AIDS). To accomplish this task, an education program on the risk factors for AIDS is incorporated. To test whether the education program changes attitudes toward AIDS, tests are given before and after the teaching intervention. The pretest on attitudes allows the subjects to examine their attitudes regarding AIDS.

The subjects' responses on follow-up testing may differ from those of individuals who were given the education program and did not see the pretest. Therefore, when a study is conducted and a pretest is given, it may prime the subjects and affect their ability to generalize to other situations.

Helpful Hint

When reviewing a study, be aware of the internal and external threats to validity. These threats do not make a study useless but instead make it more useful to you. Recognition of the threats allows researchers to build on data and allows consumers to think through what part of the study can be applied to practice. Specific threats to validity depend on the type of design and generalizations the researcher hopes to make.

Other threats to external validity depend on the type of design and methods of sampling used by the researcher but are beyond the scope of this text. Campbell and Stanley (1996) offered detailed coverage of the issues related to internal and external validity.

Critiquing Quantitative Research

Critiquing the design of a study requires knowledge of the overall implications of a particular design for the study as a whole (see the Critiquing Criteria box). Researchers want to consider the level of evidence provided by the design and how the study can be used to improve or change practice. Minimizing threats to internal and external validity enhances the strength of evidence for any quantitative design. The concept of the research design is all-inclusive and parallels the concept of the theoretical framework. The research design is similar to the theoretical framework in that it deals with a piece of the research study that affects the whole. To knowledgeably critique the design in light of the entire study requires understanding the factors that influence the choice and the implications of the design.

This chapter has introduced the meaning, purpose, and important factors of design choice, as well as the vocabulary that accompanies these factors.

Several criteria for evaluating the design can be drawn from this chapter. Remember that the criteria are applied differently with various designs. Different application does not mean that the consumer will find a haphazard approach to design but rather that each design has particular criteria that allow the consumer to classify the design by type (e.g., experimental or nonexperimental). These criteria must be met and addressed in conducting an experiment. The particulars of specific designs are addressed in Chapters 10 and 11. The following discussion primarily pertains to the overall evaluation of a quantitative research design.

The research design should demonstrate that an objective review of the literature and the establishment of a theoretical framework guided the choice of the design. No explicit statement regarding these areas is made in a research study. A consumer can evaluate the design by critiquing the theoretical framework (see Chapter 2) and literature review (see Chapter 5). Is the question new and not extensively researched? Has a great deal been done on the question, or is it a new or different way of looking at an old question? Depending on the level of the question, the investigators make certain choices. This choice allows researchers to look for differences in a controlled, comparative manner.

The consumer should be alert for the methods investigators use to maintain control (e.g., homogeneity in the sample, consistent data collection procedures, manipulation of the independent variable, and randomization). As you will see in Chapter 10, all of these criteria must be met for an experimental design. As you begin to understand the types of designs (i.e., experimental, quasiexperimental, and nonexperimental designs such as survey and relationship designs), you will find that control is applied in varying degrees, or—as in the case of a survey study—the independent variable is not manipulated (see Chapter 11). The level of control and its applications presented in Chapters 10 and 11 provide the remaining knowledge to fully critique the aspects of a study's design.

Once it has been established whether the necessary control or uniformity of conditions has been maintained, the consumer must determine whether the study is believable or valid. The consumer should ask whether the findings are the result of the variables tested—and thus internally valid—or whether another explanation is possible. To assess this aspect, the threats to internal validity should be reviewed. If the investigator's study was systematic, well grounded in theory, and followed the criteria for each of the processes, the consumer will probably conclude that the study is internally valid.

In addition, the consumer must know whether a study has external validity or generalizability to other populations or environmental conditions. External validity can be claimed only after internal validity has been established. If the credibility of a study (internal validity) has not been established, a study cannot be generalized (external validity) to other populations. Determination of external validity goes hand in hand with the sampling frame (see Chapter 12). If the study is not representative of any one group or phenomena of interest, external validity may be limited or not present. The establishment of internal and external validity requires not only knowledge of the threats to internal and external validity but also knowledge of the phenomena being studied, which allows critical judgements to be made about the linkage of theories and variables for testing. The consumer should find that the design follows from the theoretical framework, literature review, research question, and hypotheses. The consumer should feel, on the basis of clinical knowledge and knowledge of the research process, that the investigators are not comparing apples with oranges.

CRITIQUING CRITERIA

1. Is the type of study design employed appropriate?

2. Does the researcher use the various concepts of control that are consistent with the type of design chosen?

3. Does the design seem to reflect the issues of feasibility?

4. Does the design flow from the proposed research question, theoretical framework, literature review, and hypothesis?

5. What are the threats to internal validity?

6. What are the controls for the threats to internal validity?

7. What are the threats to external validity?

8. What are the controls for the threats to external validity?

9. Is the design appropriately linked to the levels of evidence hierarchy?

Critical Thinking Challenges

- Would you support or refute the following statement: "All research attempts to solve problems"?

- As a consumer of research, you recognize that control is an important concept in the issue of research design. You are critiquing an assigned experimental study as part of your "open book" midterm examination. From what is written, you cannot determine how the researchers kept the conditions of the study constant. How does this characteristic affect the study's use in an evidence-based practice model?

- Box 9–1 lists six major threats to the internal validity of an experimental study. Prioritize them and defend the one that you have made the essential, or number one, threat to address in a study.

- You will be critiquing the research design of an assigned study as a consumer of research. How does the research design influence the findings of evidence in the study?

- How do threats to external validity contribute to the strength and quality of evidence provided by the findings of a research study?

- No matter which design the researcher chooses, it should be evident to the reader that the choice was based on a thorough examination of the research question within a theoretical framework.

- The design, research question, literature review, theoretical framework, and hypothesis should all interrelate to demonstrate a woven pattern.

- The choice of the design is affected by pragmatic issues. At times, two different designs may be equally valid for the same question.

- The choice of design affects the study's level of evidence.

REFERENCES

Allard, N. (2006). Day surgery and recovery in women with a suspicious breast lesion: Evaluation of a psychoeducational nursing intervention. *Canadian Oncology Nursing Journal, 16*, 137–144.

Bissonette, J., Logan, J., Davies, B., & Graham, I. D. (2005). Methodological issues encountered in a study of hospitalized COPD patients. *Clinical Nursing Research, 14*, 81–97.

Boechler, V., Harrison, M. J., & Magill-Evans, J. (2003). Father-child teaching interventions: The relationship to father involvement in caregiving. *Journal of Pediatric Nursing, 18*, 46–51.

Brathwaite, A. C., & Majumdar, B. (2005). Evaluation of a cultural competence educational programme. *Issues and Innovations in Nursing Education, 53*(4), 470–479.

Bull, M. J., Hansen, H. E., & Gross, C. R. (2000). A professional–patient partnership model of discharge planning with elders hospitalized with heart failure. *Applied Nursing Research, 13*, 19–28.

Campbell, D., & Stanley, J. (1996). *Experimental and quasi-experimental designs for research.* Chicago: Rand-McNally.

Doran, D., Harrison, M. B., Laschinger, H., Hirdes, J., Rukholm, E., Sidani, S., et al. (2006). Relationship between nursing interventions and outcome achievement in acute care settings. *Research in Nursing & Health, 29*, 61–70.

Duggleby, W., Wright, K., Williams, A., Degner, L., Cammer, A., & Holtslander, L. (2007). Developing a Living with Hope Program for caregivers of family members with advanced cancer. *Journal of Palliative Care, 23*, 25–64.

Estabrooks, C. A., O'Leary, K. A., Ricker, K. L., & Humphrey, C. K. (2003). The Internet and access to evidence: How are nurses positioned? *Journal of Advanced Nursing, 42*, 73–81.

KEY POINTS

- The purpose of the design is to provide the format of masterful and accurate research.

- Many types of designs exist. No matter which type of design the researcher uses, the purpose remains the same.

- The research consumer should be able to locate within the study a sense of the question that the researcher wished to answer. The question should be proposed with a plan or scheme for the accomplishment of the investigation. Depending on the question, the consumer should be able to recognize the steps taken by the investigator to ensure control.

- The choice of the specific design depends on the nature of the question. Specification of the nature of the research question requires that the design reflects the investigator's attempts to maintain objectivity, accuracy, pragmatic considerations, and, most important, control.

- Control affects not only the outcome of a study but also its future use. The design should also reflect how the investigator attempted to control threats to both internal and external validity.

- Internal validity must be established before external validity can be established. Both are considered within the sampling structure.

Forchuk, C., Baruth, P., Prendergast, M., Holliday, R., Bareham, R., Brimner, S., et al. (2004). Postoperative arm massage: A support for women with lymph node dissection. *Cancer Nursing, 27,* 264–273.

Forchuk, C., Martin, M. L., Chan, Y. L., & Jensen, E. (2005). Therapeutic relationships: From psychiatric hospital to community. *Journal of Psychiatric and Mental Health Nursing, 12,* 556–564.

Harkness, K., Morrow, L., Smith, K., Kiczula, M., & Arthur, H. M. (2003). The effect of early education on patient while waiting for elective cardiac catheterization. *European Journal of Cardiovascular Nursing, 2,* 113–121.

Holditch-Davis, D., Brandon, D. H., & Schwartz, T. (2003). Development of behaviours in preterm infants: Relation to sleeping and waking. *Nursing Research, 52,* 3007–317.

Hoskins, C. N., Haber, J., Budin, W. C., Cartwright-Alcarase, F., Kowalski, M. O., Panke, J., et al. (2001). Breast cancer: Education, counseling and adjustment. A pilot study. *Psychological Reports, 8,* 677–704.

Inoue, K., Kakehashi, Y., Oomori, S., & Koizumi, A. (2004). Endemic hypoglycemia among female nurses. *Research in Nursing and Health, 27,* 87–96.

Marsh, G. W., Prochoda, K. P., Pritchett, E., & Vojir, C. P. (2000). Predicting hospice appropriateness for patients with dementia of the Alzheimer's type. *Applied Nursing Research, 13,* 187–196.

Ratner, P. A., Johnson, J. L., Richardson, C. G., Bottorff, J. L., Moffat, B., Mackay, M., et al. (2004). Efficacy of a smoking cessation intervention for elective surgical patients. *Research in Nursing & Health, 27,* 148–161.

Samuels-Dennis, J. (2006). Relationship among employment status, stressful life events, and depression in single mothers. *Canadian Journal of Nursing Research, 38,* 59–80.

Singh, M., & Cameron, J. (2005). Psychosocial aspects of caregiving to stroke patients. *AXON, 27,* 18–25.

Tranmer, J. E., Minard, J., Fox, L. E., & Rebelo, L. (2003). The sleep experiences of medical and surgical patients. *Clinical Nursing Research, 12,* 159–173.

Wikblad, K., & Anderson, B. (1995). Comparison of three wound dressings in patients undergoing heart surgery. *Nursing Research, 44,* 312–316.

Robin Whittemore
Margaret Grey
Mina D. Singh

CHAPTER 10

Experimental and

Quasiexperimental Designs

LEARNING OUTCOMES

After reading this chapter, the student should be able to do the following:

- List the criteria necessary for inferring cause-and-effect relationships.
- Distinguish the differences between experimental and quasiexperimental designs.
- Define internal validity problems associated with experimental and quasiexperimental designs.
- Describe the use of experimental and quasi-experimental designs for evaluation research.
- Critically evaluate the findings of selected studies that test cause-and-effect relationships.
- Apply levels of evidence to experimental and quasiexperimental designs.

STUDY RESOURCES

evolve Go to Evolve at
http://evolve.elsevier.com/Canada/LoBiondo/Research/
for Weblinks, content updates, and additional
research articles for practice in reviewing
and critiquing.

KEY TERMS

a priori
after-only design
after-only nonequivalent control
    group design
antecedent variable
control
dependent variable
designs
evaluation research
experiment
experimental design
formative evaluation
independent variable
intervening variable
manipulation
mortality
nonequivalent control group design
one group (pretest–post-test) design
post-test-only control group design
quasiexperiment
quasiexperimental design
randomization
Solomon four-group design
summative evaluation
testing
time series design
true experiment

RESEARCH PROCESS

One of the fundamental purposes of scientific research in any profession is to determine cause-and-effect relationships. In nursing, for example, we are concerned with developing effective approaches to maintaining and restoring wellness. Testing such nursing interventions to determine how well they actually work—that is, evaluating the outcomes in terms of efficacy and cost-effectiveness—is accomplished by using *experimental* and *quasiexperimental designs*. These **designs** differ from nonexperimental designs in one important way: the researcher actively seeks to bring about the desired effect and does not passively observe behaviours or actions. In other words, the researcher is interested in making something happen, not merely in observing customary client care. Experimental and quasiexperimental studies are also important to consider in relation to evidence-based practice because they provide Level II and Level III evidence. The findings of such studies provide the validation of clinical practice and the rationale for changing specific aspects of practice (see Chapters 20 and 21).

Experimental designs are particularly suitable for testing cause-and-effect relationships because they help eliminate potential alternative explanations (threats to validity) for the findings. Infering causality requires that the following three criteria be met:

1. The causal variable and effect variable must be associated with each other.

2. The cause must precede the effect.

3. The relationship must not be explainable by another variable.

When you critique studies that use experimental and quasiexperimental designs, the primary focus is on the validity of the conclusion that the experimental treatment, or the **independent variable**, caused the desired effect on the outcome, or **dependent variable**. The validity of the conclusion depends on how well the researcher controlled the other variables that may explain the relationship

studied. Thus, the focus of this chapter is to explain how various types of experimental and quasiexperimental designs control extraneous variables.

It should be made clear, however, that most research in nursing is not experimental. Considerable preliminary research is required to test the complex cause-and-effect relationships of nursing interventions (Whittemore & Grey, 2002). For example, an experimental design requires that all of the relevant variables have been previously defined so that they can be manipulated and studied. In most problem areas in nursing, this requirement has not been met. Therefore, nonexperimental designs used in identifying variables and determining their relationship to each other often need to be developed before experimental studies are performed.

The purpose of this chapter is to acquaint you with the issues involved in interpreting studies that use **experimental design** and **quasiexperimental design**. These designs are listed in Box 10–1. The Critical Thinking Decision Path shows an algorithm that influences a researcher's choice of experimental or quasiexperimental design.

TRUE EXPERIMENTAL DESIGN

An **experiment** is a scientific investigation that makes observations and collects data according to explicit criteria. A **true experiment**, or classic experiment,

---

BOX 10–1   Summary of Experimental and Quasiexperimental Research Designs

EXPERIMENTAL DESIGNS

1. True experimental (pretest–post-test control group) design
2. Solomon four-group design
3. After-only design

QUASIEXPERIMENTAL DESIGNS

1. Nonequivalent control group design
2. After-only nonequivalent control group design
3. One group (pretest–post-test) design
4. Time series design

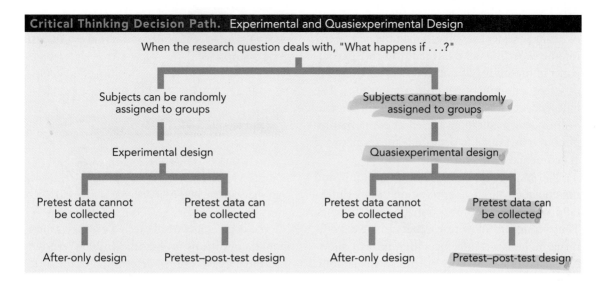

Critical Thinking Decision Path. Experimental and Quasiexperimental Design

When the research question deals with, "What happens if . . .?"

- Subjects can be randomly assigned to groups
  - Experimental design
    - Pretest data cannot be collected
      - After-only design
    - Pretest data can be collected
      - Pretest–post-test design
- Subjects cannot be randomly assigned to groups
  - Quasiexperimental design
    - Pretest data cannot be collected
      - After-only design
    - Pretest data can be collected
      - Pretest–post-test design

has three identifying properties: randomization, control, and manipulation. These properties allow for other explanations of the phenomenon to be ruled out and thereby provide the strength of the design for testing cause-and-effect relationships.

A research study using an experimental design is commonly called a *randomized clinical trial* (RCT). An RCT or experimental design is considered to be the best research design, "the gold standard," for providing information about cause-and-effect relationships. An individual RCT generates Level II evidence in the hierarchy of evidence because of the minimal bias introduced by this design. The higher a design on the evidence hierarchy, the more likely the results offer an unbiased estimate of the effect of an intervention and the more confident you are that the intervention will be effective and produce the same results over and over again.

Randomization

Randomization, or random assignment to a group, involves the distribution of subjects to either the experimental or the control group on a purely random basis. In other words, each subject has an equal and known probability of being assigned to any group. Random assignment may be done individually or by groups (Allard, 2006; Harkness, Morrow,

Smith, Kiczula, & Arthur, 2003; Tranmer & Parry, 2004). Random assignment to experimental or control groups allows for the elimination of any systematic bias in the groups with respect to attributes that may affect the dependent variable being studied. The procedure for randomization minimizes variance (as discussed in Chapter 12) and assumes that any important intervening variables will be equally distributed between the groups. Note that random assignment to groups is different from the random sampling discussed in Chapter 12.

Control

Control refers to the introduction of one or more constants into the experimental situation. Control is acquired by manipulating the causal or independent variable, randomly assigning subjects to a group, carefully preparing experimental protocols, and using comparison groups. In experimental research, the comparison group is the control group, or the group that receives the usual treatment rather than the innovative, experimental treatment.

Manipulation

As discussed previously, experimental designs are characterized by the researcher "doing something" to at least some of the subjects. This "something," or the independent variable, is manipulated by giving the experimental treatment to some participants in the study but not to others, or by giving different amounts of it to different groups. The independent variable might be a treatment, a teaching plan, or a medication. The effect of this **manipulation** is measured to determine the result of the experimental treatment.

The concepts of control, randomization, and manipulation and their application to experimental design are sometimes confusing for students. These concepts allow researchers to have confidence in the causal inferences they make by allowing them to rule out other potential explanations. Consider the use of control, randomization, and manipulation in the following example. Allard (2006) used a prospective, randomized clinical trial (RCT) to examine the effect of the Attentional Focus and Symptom Management Intervention (AFSMI) on symptom experience, emotional distress, and functional status for women who had surgery for breast cancer. The AFSMI, based on self-regulation theory, encourages clients to focus on the symptoms they are experiencing and to make decisions for managing these symptoms. The women were recruited from four regional cancer centres (one centre had two sites).

Randomization to the control and experimental groups was done within each site using a table of random numbers to minimize the influence of site. The clients were randomly assigned to usual care (control group) or the experimental group, which received the intervention in two sessions, 3 to 4 days and 10 to 11 days after surgery. The use of random assignment meant that all clients who met the study criteria had an equal and known chance of being assigned to the control group or the experimental group. The use of random assignment to groups helps ensure that the two study groups are comparable on pre-existing factors that might affect the outcome of interest, such as gender, age, length of stay in the hospital, and stage of cancer. Note that the researchers in this example checked statistically whether the procedure of random assignment did, in fact, produce groups that were similar at baseline. This check is called *analysis of covariance.*

Evidence-Based Practice Tip

In health care research, the term *randomized clinical trial* (RCT) often refers to a true experimental design. These designs are being used more frequently in nursing research, which is critical to evidence-based practice initiatives.

The degree of control exerted over the experimental conditions in the Allard (2006) study is illustrated by its detailed description of the intervention. This control helps ensure that all members of the experimental group receive similar treatment and assists the reader in understanding the nature of the experimental treatment. The control group provides a comparison against which the experimental group can be judged.

In the Allard (2006) study, receiving the AFSMI intervention was the manipulated treatment. Client outcomes were measured for all participants, including physical fatigue and insomnia, pain, functional status, and emotional distress. By controlling the experimental intervention by the use of standard protocol, Allard was able to make the assertion that the AFSMI intervention was effective in improving functional status, overall emotional distress, and confusion.

The use of the experimental design allows researchers to rule out many of the potential threats to internal validity of the findings, such as selection, history, and maturation (see Chapter 9). The strength of the true experimental design lies in its ability to help the researcher control the effects of any extraneous variables that might constitute threats to internal validity. Such extraneous variables can be either *antecedent* or *intervening.*

The **antecedent variable** occurs before the study but may affect the dependent variable and confuse the results. Factors such as age, gender, socioeconomic status, and health status might be important antecedent variables in nursing research because they may affect dependent variables, such as recovery time and ability to integrate health care behaviours. Antecedent variables that might affect the dependent variables in the study by Allard (2006) include age, employment history, education, and stage of cancer. Random assignment to groups helps ensure that the groups will be similar on these variables so that differences in the dependent variable may be attributed to the experimental treatment. It should be noted, however, that the researcher should check and report how the groups actually compared on such variables. An **intervening variable** occurs during the course of the study and is not part of the study; however, the intervening variable affects the dependent variable and can affect the study outcomes. An example of an intervening variable that might affect the outcomes of Allard's (2006) study is a change in health care status in any of the participants, such as a newly diagnosed medical condition or mental illness. Thus, if the care provided to clients changed in any major way while the study was being implemented, the study also would be affected.

Types of Experimental Designs

Several different experimental designs exist (Campbell & Stanley, 1966). Each is based on the classic design called the true experiment, diagrammed in Figure 10–1A. Above the description diagram, symbolic notations are routinely used:

- **R** represents random assignment (for both the experimental group and the control group).
- **O** signifies observation via data collection on the dependent variable.
- O_1 signifies pretest data collection.
- O_2 represents post-test data collection.
- **X** represents the group exposure to the intervention.

Therefore, in Figure 10–1, note that the subjects were assigned randomly (**R**) to the experimental or the control group. The experimental treatment (**X**) was given only to those in the experimental group,

and the pretests (O_1) and post-tests (O_2) are those measurements of the dependent variables that were made before and after the experimental treatment was performed. All true experimental designs have subjects randomly assigned to groups, an experimental treatment introduced to some of the subjects, and observation of the effects of the treatment. Designs vary primarily in the number of observations that are made.

As shown in Figure 10–1A, subjects are randomly assigned to the two groups, experimental and control, so that antecedent variables are controlled. Then pretest measures or observations are made so that the researcher has a baseline for determining the effect of the independent variable. The researcher then introduces the experimental variable to one of the groups and measures the dependent variable again to see whether it has changed. The control group receives no experimental treatment but also is measured later for comparison with the experimental group. The degree of difference between the two groups at the end of the study indicates the confidence the researcher has that a causal link exists between the independent and dependent variables. Because random assignment and the control inherent in this design minimize the effects of many threats to internal validity, the true experimental design is a strong design for testing cause-and-effect relationships.

However, the design is not perfect. Some threats cannot be controlled in true experimental studies (see Chapter 9). People tend to drop out of studies that require their participation over an extended period. The influence over the outcome of an experiment of people dropping out or dying is commonly known as **mortality** effects. If the number or type of people who drop out of the experimental group differs from that of the control group, a mortality effect might explain the findings. When reading such a work, examine the sample and the results carefully to see whether dropouts or deaths occurred.

Testing also can be a problem in these studies because the researcher is usually giving the same measurement twice, and subjects tend to score

A. True or classic experiment

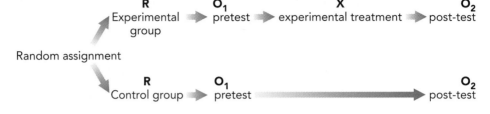

B. Solomon four-group design

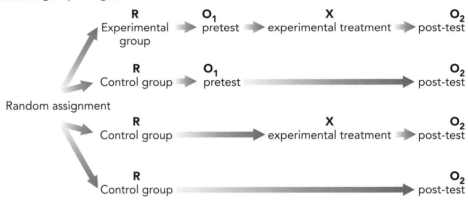

C. After-only experimental design

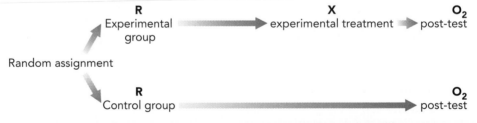

Figure 10–1 Comparison of experimental designs. A, True or classic experiment. B, Solomon four-group design. C, After-only experimental design.

better the second time just by learning the test. Researchers can get around this problem in one of two ways: they might use different forms of the same test for the two measurements, or they might use a more complex experimental design called the Solomon four-group design. Swanson (1999) used a Solomon four-group design to test the effects of caring-based counselling, measurement, and time on the integration of loss (from miscarriage) and women's emotional well-being in the first year after

miscarrying. She studied four groups: two treatment groups and two control groups.

The **Solomon four-group design**, shown in Figure 10–1B, has two groups that are identical to those used in the classic experimental design, plus two additional groups, an experimental after-group and a control after-group. As the diagram shows, all four groups have randomly assigned (R) subjects, as in all experimental studies. However, the addition of these last two groups helps rule out testing threats to internal validity that the before- and after-groups may experience. For example, suppose a researcher is interested in the effects of counselling on the self-esteem of clients with chronic illness. Just taking a measure of self-esteem (O_1) may influence how the subjects report themselves. The items might make the subjects think more about how they view themselves so that the next time they fill out the questionnaire (O_2), their self-esteem might appear to have improved. In reality, however, their self-esteem may be the same as it was before—it just looks different because the subjects had previously taken the test. The use of this design with the two groups that do not receive the pretest allows for evaluating the effect of the pretest on the post-test in the first two groups.

Although this design helps evaluate the effects of testing, the threat of mortality remains a problem, as with the classic experimental design. Aschen (2004) used the Solomon four-group design to develop a clinical procedure to decrease the anxiety and increase the responsiveness (assertion) of inpatients of a psychiatric ward of both sexes in mixed diagnostic categories and to evaluate the effectiveness of the procedure. Clients, matched on age, sex, and diagnosis, were assigned to one of the following conditions: (1) pretest, treatment, post-test; (2) pretest, no treatment, post-test; (3) treatment, post-test; or (4) no treatment, post-test. The results indicated that (1) clients receiving assertion training therapy were less anxious and more responsive after treatment than before; (2) clients receiving assertion training therapy were less anxious and more responsive than were matched control subjects; (3) control subjects who received no assertion training therapy and were pretested showed moderate significant gains on the post-test measure; (4) clients reported a greater reduction of anxiety than they did an increase in responsiveness; and (5) pretesting did not significantly influence post-test scores.

A less frequently used experimental design is the **after-only design**, shown in Figure 10–1C. This design, which is sometimes called the **post-test-only control group design**, is composed of two randomly assigned groups (**R**), but unlike the true experimental design, neither group is pretested or measured. Again, the independent variable is introduced to the experimental group (**X**) and not to the control group. The process of randomly assigning the subjects to groups is assumed to be sufficient to ensure a lack of bias so that the researcher can still determine whether the treatment (**X**) created significant differences between the two groups (**O**). This design is particularly useful when testing effects are expected to be a major problem and the number of available subjects is too limited to use a Solomon four-group design.

O'Sullivan and Jacobson (1992) used this design in their study of the impact of a program for adolescent mothers because it was impossible to measure infant outcomes before the birth of the infant. They carefully examined the two groups to ensure that the groups were equivalent at baseline so that they could be assured that random assignment had yielded equivalent groups. Other interventions, such as postoperative pain management, cannot be measured before surgery and require an after-only design.

Helpful Hint

Remember that mortality is a problem in most experimental studies because data are usually collected more than once. The researcher should demonstrate that the groups are equivalent both when they enter the study and at the final analysis.

Field and Laboratory Experiments

Experiments also can be classified by setting. Field experiments and laboratory experiments share the properties of control, randomization, and manipulation and use the same design characteristics but are conducted in different environments. Laboratory experiments take place in an artificial setting created specifically for the purpose of research. In the laboratory, the researcher has almost total control over the features of the environment, such as temperature, humidity, noise level, and subject conditions. Conversely, field experiments are exactly what the name implies—

experiments that take place in a real, pre-existing social setting, such as a hospital or clinic, where the phenomenon of interest usually occurs.

Because most experiments in the nursing literature are field experiments and control is such an important element in the conduct of experiments, studies conducted in the field are subject to treatment contamination by factors specific to the setting that the researcher cannot control. However, studies conducted in the laboratory are by nature "artificial" because the setting is created for the purpose of research. Thus, laboratory experiments, although stronger with respect to internal validity questions than fieldwork studies, suffer more from problems with external validity. For example, a subject's behaviour in the laboratory may be quite different from the person's behaviour in the real world—a dichotomy that presents problems in generalizing findings from the laboratory to the real world. When research reports are read, then, research consumers need to consider the experiment's setting and the impact it might have on the findings of the study.

Consider the study comparing a wound treatment gel with a placebo gel for the management of pressure sores (Hirshberg, Coleman, Marchant, & Rees, 2001). This study could have been done in a laboratory using animals, which would have allowed complete control over the external environment of the study—a variable that might be important in studying wound healing. However, researchers have no guarantee that the results found in a study in a laboratory would be applicable to clients in hospital settings, resulting in the loss of some external validity.

Advantages and Disadvantages of the Experimental Design

As previously discussed, experimental designs are the most appropriate for testing cause-and-effect relationship because of the design's ability to control the experimental situation. Therefore, experimental designs offer better corroboration than if the independent variable is manipulated in such a way that certain consequences can be expected.

Such studies are important because one of nursing's major research priorities is documenting outcomes to provide a basis for changing or supporting current nursing practice. For example, in the study by Allard (2006), the author was able to conclude that increased functional status, lower emotional distress, and less confusion in the experimental group were important at this point in the women's illness trajectory.

Similarly, Ratner et al. (2004) conducted a randomized experiment to test an intervention to assist smokers to abstain from smoking "before surgery, maintain abstinence postoperatively, and achieve long-term cessation" (p. 148). These researchers used many control measures (including randomization, a control group, inclusion criteria, and a rigid intervention protocol) that enhanced the validity of the results. Ratner et al. were able to conclude that participants in the treatment group were more likely to fast than participants in the control group and more likely to be abstinent six months after surgery. Studies such as Allard's (2006) and Ratner et al.'s (2004), as well as others like them, allow nurses to anticipate the outcomes of their actions in a scientific manner and provide the basis for effective, high-quality care strategies.

Still, experimental designs are not the study designs most commonly used in nursing research, for several reasons. First, experimentation assumes that all of the relevant variables involved in a phenomenon have been identified. For many areas of nursing research, this is simply not the case, and descriptive studies need to be completed before experimental interventions can be applied. Second, these designs have some significant disadvantages.

One problem with an experimental design is that many variables important in predicting outcomes of nursing care are not amenable to experimental manipulation. It is well known that health status varies with age and socioeconomic status. No matter how careful a researcher is, no one can assign subjects randomly by age or a certain level of income. In addition, some variables may be technically manipulable, but their nature may preclude actually doing so.

For example, if a researcher tried to randomly assign groups to study the effects of cigarette smoking and asked the experimental group to smoke two packs of cigarettes a day, that researcher's ethics would be seriously questioned. It is also potentially true that such a study would not work because nonsmokers randomly assigned to the smoking group would be unlikely to comply with the research task. Thus, sometimes even when a researcher plans to conduct a true experiment, subjects dropping out of the study or other factors may, in effect, make the study a quasiexperiment.

Quasiexperimental designs are considered when it is not possible to randomly assign subjects. For example, in a study by McGilton et al. (2003), researchers found that health care professionals in long-term care facilities can be taught how to enhance their care without adding staff. To conduct the study, randomly assigning residents to nursing staff was not feasible; therefore, two separate units were used for the control and the intervention.

Another problem with experimental designs is that they may be difficult or impractical to perform in field settings. It may be quite difficult to randomly assign clients on a hospital floor to different groups when they might talk to each other about the different treatments. Experimental procedures also may be disruptive to the usual routine of the setting. If several nurses are involved in administering the experimental program, it may be impossible to ensure that the program is administered in the same way to each subject.

Because of these problems in carrying out true experiments, researchers frequently turn to another type of research design to evaluate cause-and-effect relationships. Such designs, because they look like experiments but lack some of the control of the true experimental design, are called quasiexperiments.

QUASIEXPERIMENTAL DESIGNS

Quasiexperimental designs are intended to test cause-and-effect relationships; however, in a quasiexperimental design, full experimental control is not possible. A **quasiexperiment** is a research design in which the researcher initiates an experimental treatment, but some characteristic of a true experiment is lacking. Control may not be possible because of the nature of the independent variable or the nature of the available subjects. Usually, in a quasiexperimental design, the element of randomization is lacking, as described earlier with the McGilton et al. (2003) study. In other cases, the control group may be missing. However, like experiments, quasiexperiments involve the introduction of an experimental treatment.

Compared with the true experimental design, quasiexperiments are similar in their use. Both types of designs are used when the researcher is interested in testing cause-and-effect relationships. However, the basic problem with the quasiexperimental approach is a weakened confidence in making causal assertions. Because of the lack of some controls in the research situation, quasiexperimental designs are subject to contamination by many, if not all, of the threats to internal validity discussed in Chapter 9.

Types of Quasiexperimental Designs

Many different quasiexperimental designs exist. Only the ones most commonly used in nursing research are discussed in this book. To illustrate, the symbols and notations introduced earlier in the chapter are used. Refer back to the true experimental design shown in Figure 10–1A and compare it with the **nonequivalent control group design** shown in Figure 10–2A. Note that this design looks exactly like the true experiment except that subjects are not randomly assigned to groups.

For example, suppose a researcher is interested in the effects of a new diabetes education program on the physical and psychosocial outcomes of clients newly diagnosed with diabetes. If the conditions were right, the researcher might be able to randomly assign subjects to either the group receiving the new program or the group receiving the usual program, but for any number of reasons, that design might not be possible (e.g., nurses on the unit where clients are admitted might be so excited about the new program that they cannot help

A. Nonequivalent control group design

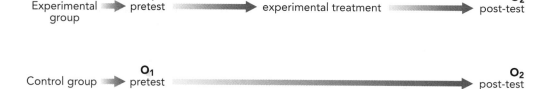

B. After-only nonequivalent control group design

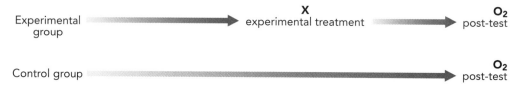

C. One group (pretest–post-test) design

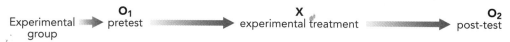

D. Time series design

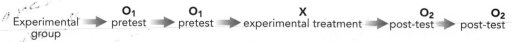

Figure 10–2 Comparison of quasiexperimental designs. A, Nonequivalent control group design. B, After-only nonequivalent control group design. C, One group (pretest–post-test) design. D, Time series design.

but include the new information for all clients). So, the researcher has two choices: to abandon the experiment or to conduct a quasiexperiment. To conduct a quasiexperiment, the researcher might find a similar unit that has not been introduced to the new program and study the newly diagnosed clients with diabetes who are admitted to that unit as a comparison group. The study would then involve the quasiexperimental type of design.

Studies that utilize both quantitative and qualitative methods are called mixed methods studies. Ducharme, Lebel, Lachance, and Trudeau (2006) conducted a mixed method design study to evaluate the implementation of a stress management intervention for family members of elderly persons. The quantitative study used was a quasi-experimental pretest–post-test design. The experimental group was compared with the control group, which received the usual services under a home support program. The pretest measures were taken prior to the start of the study, and two post-tests were done, one at the end of the program and the other three months later. The measures included caregiver burden, caregiver stress, caregiver coping, psychological distress, caregiver health, and goal attainment. Significant differences were found between the two groups on perceived challenge, control by self of the situation, perceived control by others, and the use of problem solving as a coping strategy.

The nonequivalent control group design is commonly used in nursing research studies conducted in field settings. The basic problem with the design is the weakened confidence the researcher can have in assuming that the experimental and comparison groups are similar at the beginning of the study. Threats to internal validity, such as selection, maturation, testing, and mortality, are possible with this design. However, the design is relatively strong because the gathering of the data at the time of the pretest allows the researcher to compare the equivalence of the two groups on important antecedent variables before the independent variable is introduced.

In the previous example (Ducharme et al., 2006), the motivation of the caregivers to learn about stress management might be important in determining the effect of this program. In the measures taken at the outset of the study, the researcher could include a measure of motivation to learn. Then the differences between the two groups on this variable could be tested, and if significant differences existed, they could be controlled statistically in the analysis. Nonetheless, the strength of the causal assertions that can be made on the basis of such designs depends on the ability of the researcher to identify and measure or control possible threats to internal validity.

Suppose that the researcher did not measure the subjects before the introduction of the new treatment (or the researcher was hired after the new program began) but later decided that it would be useful to have data demonstrating the effect of the program. Perhaps, for example, a third party asks for such data to determine whether it should pay the extra cost of the new teaching program.

Sometimes, the outcomes simply cannot be measured before the intervention, as with prenatal interventions that are expected to impact birth outcomes. The study that could be conducted would look like the **after-only nonequivalent control group design**, shown in Figure 10–2B.

This design is similar to the after-only experimental design, but randomization is not used to assign subjects to groups. This design makes the assumption that the two groups are equivalent and comparable before the introduction of the independent variable (**X**). Thus, the soundness of the design and the confidence that we can have in the findings depend on the soundness of this assumption of preintervention comparability. Often, the assertion that the two nonrandomly assigned groups are comparable at the outset of the study is difficult to assert because the validity of the statement cannot be assessed.

In the example of the teaching program for clients with newly diagnosed diabetes, measuring the subjects' motivation after the teaching program would not tell us whether their motivations differed before they received the program, and it is possible that the teaching program would motivate individuals to learn more about their health problem. Therefore, the researcher's conclusion that the teaching program improved physical status and psychosocial outcome would be subject to the alternative conclusion that the results were an effect of preexisting motivations (selection effect) in combination with greater learning in those so motivated (selection–maturation interaction). Nonetheless, this design is frequently used in nursing research because opportunities for data collection are often limited and because this design is particularly useful when testing effects may be problematic.

Consider again the example of the experiment conducted by Allard (2006). Suppose that Allard had not randomly assigned the clients to the preoperative intervention but rather took all clients before a certain point and assigned them to the control group and then assigned all new clients to the experimental treatment. The study would then be an example of an after-only nonequivalent control group design. If Allard had chosen to conduct the study with this design and had found the same results, she would have been less confident of the results because the selection and effects may have been more problematic.

A study by Tranmer and Parry (2004) used an after-only design to test the effects of an advanced practice nursing intervention and clients' health-related quality of life, symptom distress, and satisfaction with care among cardiac surgery clients. The intervention was telephone support for four weeks following hospital discharge.

Another quasiexperimental design is a **one-group (pretest–post-test) design** (Figure 10–2C), which is used by researchers when only one group is available for study. Data are collected before and after an experimental treatment on one group of subjects. In this type of design, the subjects act as their own controls and no randomization occurs. Because controls and randomization are important characteristics that enhance the internal validity of the study, the evidence generated by the findings of this type of quasiexperimental design needs to be interpreted with careful consideration of the design limitations.

Lavoie-Tremblay et al. (2005) conducted a one-group (pretest–post-test) pilot design study to determine the effectiveness of a participatory organizational intervention to improve the psycho-social work environment on a long-term unit in Quebec. The results indicated that a significant decrease in reward and a decrease in the Effort–Reward Imbalance scale occurred following the intervention. Also, the absenteeism rates on this unit decreased compared with the rest of the institution. The researchers clearly identified the limitations of the study design, including that a reciprocal or cause-and-effect relationship was impossible to confirm.

An approach used by researchers when only one group is available is to study that group over a longer period. This quasiexperimental design is called a **time series design** and is illustrated in Figure 10–2D. Time series designs are useful for determining trends, as in a study examining the impact of adult

day programs on family caregivers of elderly relatives (Warren, Ross-Kerr, Smith, & Godkin, 2003). The caregivers were measured on burden, quality of life, perceived health, and opinion on institutionalization at four time points (just prior to client admission and two weeks, two months, and six months after admission to the day program).

To rule out some alternative explanations for the findings of a one-group pretest–post-test design, researchers typically measure the phenomenon of interest over a longer period and introduce the experimental treatment sometime during the course of the data collection period. Even with the absence of a control group, the broader range of data collection points helps rule out threats to validity such as history effects. Obviously, our problem related to the earlier example of teaching clients with diabetes does not lend itself to this design because we do not have access to the clients before the diagnosis.

Helpful 💡 Hint

One of the reasons replication is so important in nursing research is that many problems cannot be subjected to experimental methods. Therefore, the consistency of findings across many client populations helps support a cause-and-effect relationship even when an experiment cannot be conducted.

Advantages and Disadvantages of Quasiexperimental Designs

Because of the problems inherent in interpreting the results of studies using quasiexperimental designs, you may wonder why anyone would use them. Quasiexperimental designs are used frequently because they are practical, feasible, and generalizable. These designs are more adaptable to the real-world practice setting than controlled experimental designs. In addition, for some hypotheses, these designs may be the only way to evaluate the effect of the independent variable of interest.

The weaknesses of the quasiexperimental approach involve mainly the inability to make clear cause-and-effect statements. However, if the researcher can rule out any plausible alternative explanations for the findings, such studies can lead to increased knowledge about causal relationships. Researchers have several options for ruling out these alternative explanations. They may control extraneous variables (alternative events that could explain the findings) **a priori** (before initiating the intervention) by design. For example, Allard (2006) could have requested written assurance from the hospital administration that no new programs would be started during the course of the study that could affect the intervention findings. Such an assurance would have made the introduction of the critical pathway that the control group received less likely.

Researchers can also use methods to control extraneous variables statistically. In some cases, common sense knowledge of the problem and the population can suggest that a particular explanation is not plausible. Nonetheless, replicating such studies is important to support the causal assertions developed through the use of quasi-experimental designs.

The literature on cigarette smoking is an excellent example of how findings from many studies, experimental and quasiexperimental, can be linked to establish a causal relationship. A large number of well-controlled experiments with laboratory animals randomly assigned to smoking and non-smoking conditions have documented that lung disease will develop in smoking animals. Although such evidence is suggestive of a link between smoking and lung disease in humans, it is not directly transferable because animals and humans are different. Because we cannot randomly assign humans to smoking and nonsmoking groups for ethical and other reasons, researchers interested in this problem must use quasiexperimental data to test their hypotheses about smoking and lung disease.

Several different quasiexperimental designs have been used to study this problem, and all had similar results—a causal relationship does exist between cigarette smoking and lung disease. Note that the combination of results from both experimental and quasiexperimental studies led to the conclusion that smoking causes cancer because the studies together meet the causal criteria of relationship, timing, and lack of an alternative explanation.

The tobacco industry has argued that because the studies on humans are not true experiments, another explanation is possible for the relationships that have been found. For example, these relationships suggest that the tendency to smoke is linked to the tendency for lung disease to develop, and smoking is merely an unimportant intervening variable. The reader needs to review the evidence from studies to determine whether the cause-and-effect relationship postulated is believable.

Evidence-Based Practice Tip

Experimental designs are considered Level II evidence, and quasiexperimental designs are considered Level III evidence. Quasiexperimental designs are lower on the hierarchy of evidence owing to a lack of a research control, which limits the ability to make confident cause-and-effect statements that influence clinical decision making.

EVALUATION RESEARCH AND EXPERIMENTATION

As the science of nursing expands and the cost of health care rises, nurses and others have become increasingly concerned with the ability to document the costs and the benefits of nursing care (see Chapter 1). This task is a complex process, but at its heart is the ability to evaluate or measure the outcomes of nursing care to inform health care decision making. Such studies usually are associated with quality assurance, quality improvement, and evaluation. Studies of evaluation or quality assurance do exactly what the name implies; they are concerned with the determination of the quality of nursing and health care and with the assurance that the public is receiving high-quality care.

Quality assurance and quality improvement in nursing are a current and important topics for nursing care. Many early quality assurance studies documented whether nursing care met predetermined standards. The goal of quality improvement studies is to evaluate the effectiveness of nursing interventions and to provide direction for further improvement in the achievement of quality clinical outcomes and cost-effectiveness.

Evaluation research is the utilization of scientific research methods and procedures to evaluate a program, treatment, practice, or policy. Evaluation research uses analytical means to document the worth of an activity such as an intervention, but such research is not a different design. Both experimental and quasiexperimental designs (as well as nonexperimental designs) are used to determine the effect or outcomes of a program. When these designs are used in evaluating a program, the term *evaluation research* is used. Bigman (1961) listed the following purposes and uses of evaluation research:

1. To discover whether and how well the objectives are being fulfilled
2. To determine the reasons for specific successes and failures
3. To direct the course of the experiment with techniques for its effectiveness
4. To uncover principles underlying a successful program
5. To base further research on the reasons for the relative success of alternative techniques
6. To redefine the means to be used for attaining objectives and to redefine subgoals in light of research findings

According to Clarke (2001), the following four levels of evaluation research are being highlighted in health care, especially nursing research: evaluation of the effectiveness of clinical interventions; evaluation of the impact of new ways of health care delivery; evaluation of structured programs to specific client groups; and evaluation of the quality of service. Many evaluation research studies use mixed methods, as in the case of the Ducharme et al. (2006) study, which used a participatory action research design with a quasi-experimental methodology.

Evaluation studies may be either formative or summative. **Formative evaluation** refers to

assessment of a program as it is being implemented; usually, the focus is on evaluation of the process of a program rather than the outcomes. **Summative evaluation** refers to the assessment of the outcomes of a program that is conducted after completion of the initial program.

Majumdar, Browne, Roberts, and Carpio (2004) used a summative evaluation with an experimental design to evaluate the effectiveness of a cultural sensitivity training program (delivered to health care professionals) on the knowledge and attitudes of health care professionals and on the satisfaction and health outcomes of clients from different minority groups whose health care professionals received the training. In contrast, Marshall, Mead, Jones, Kaba, and Roberts (2001) used formative evaluation to describe the process of care associated with implementing venous leg ulcer guidelines in primary health care. Knowledge related to summative (outcomes) and formative (process) evaluation of programs is important in translating research into clinical practice.

The use of experimental and quasiexperimental designs in quality improvement and evaluation studies allows for the determination of not only whether care is adequate but also which method of care is best under certain conditions. Furthermore, such studies can be used to determine whether a particular type of nursing care or intervention is cost-effective—that is, that the care or intervention does what it is intended to do but at less or equivalent cost. Cost studies are usually incorporated into the evaluation of an intervention. For example, Steel-O'Connor et al. (2003) evaluated the effects of public health nurse follow-up programs in terms of infant health problems, breastfeeding rates, and the use of postpartum health services in Ontario. The authors studied the costs associated with routine home visiting by a public health nurse after early obstetrical discharge versus a screening telephone call. Steel-O'Connor et al. found that the direct, indirect, and total costs of health services per 100 infants were greater for the home visit group and concluded that a routine home visit is not always necessary to identify women who need that service. In an era of health care reform and cost containment for health expenditures, evaluating the relative costs and benefits of new programs of care is increasingly important. Relatively few studies in nursing and medicine have done so, but in terms of outcomes, nursing costs and cost savings will be important to future studies.

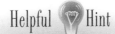

Helpful Hint

Think of quality assurance and quality improvement projects as research-related activities that enhance the ability of nurses to generate cost and quality outcome data. These outcome data contribute to documenting the way nursing practice makes a difference.

Critiquing Experimental and Quasiexperimental Designs

As discussed earlier in the chapter, various designs for research studies differ in the amount of control the researcher has over the antecedent and intervening variables that may affect the results of the study. True experimental designs, which provide Level II evidence, offer the most possibility for control, whereas pre-experimental designs, which provide Level IV, V, or VI evidence, offer the least. Quasiexperimental designs, which provide Level III evidence, fall somewhere in between. Research designs must balance the needs for internal validity and external validity to produce useful results. In addition, judicious use of design requires that the chosen design be appropriate to the problem, free of bias, and capable of answering the research question.

Questions that the reader should pose when reading studies that test cause-and-effect relationships are listed in the Critiquing Criteria box. All of these questions should help the reader judge, with confidence, whether a causal relationship exists.

For studies in which either experimental or quasi-experimental designs are used, first try to determine the type of design that was used. Often, a statement describing the design of the study appears in the abstract and in the methods section of the article. If such a statement is not present, the reader should examine the study for evidence of the following three characteristics: control, randomization, and manipulation. If all are discussed, the design is probably experimental. Conversely, if the study involves the administration of an experimental treatment but does not involve the random assignment of subjects to groups, the design is quasiexperimental. Next, try to identify which of the various designs within these two types of designs was used. Determining the answer to these questions gives you a head start because each design has its inherent threats to validity, and this step makes it easier to critically evaluate the study. The next question to ask is whether the researcher required a solution to a cause-and-effect problem. If so, the study is suited to these designs. Finally, think about the conduct of the study in the setting. Is it realistic to think that the study could be conducted in a clinical setting without some contamination?

The most important question to ask as you read experimental studies is, "What else could have happened to explain the findings?" Thus, the author must provide adequate accounts of how the procedures for randomization, control, and manipulation were carried out. The study should include a description of the procedures for random assignment to such a degree that the reader can determine the likelihood for any one subject to be assigned to a particular group. The description of the independent variable also should be detailed. The inclusion of this information helps the reader decide whether the treatment given to some subjects in the experimental group might differ from what was given to others in the same group. In addition, threats to validity, such as testing and mortality, should be addressed. Otherwise, the potential exists for the findings of the study to be in error and less believable to the reader.

CRITIQUING CRITERIA

1. What design is used in the study?

2. Is the design experimental or quasiexperimental?

3. Is the problem one of a cause-and-effect relationship?

4. Is the method used appropriate to the problem?

5. Is the design suited to the setting of the study?

EXPERIMENTAL DESIGNS

1. What experimental design is used in the study, and is it appropriate?

2. How are randomization, control, and manipulation applied?

3. Are there reasons to believe that alternative explanations exist for the findings?

4. Are all threats to validity, including mortality, addressed in the report?

5. Whether the experiment was conducted in the laboratory or a clinical setting, are the findings generalizable to the larger population of interest?

QUASIEXPERIMENTAL DESIGNS

1. What quasiexperimental design is used in the study, and is it appropriate?

2. What are the most common threats to the validity of the findings of this design?

3. What are the plausible alternative explanations, and have they been addressed?

4. Are the author's explanations of threats to validity acceptable?

5. What does the author say about the limitations of the study?

6. Do other limitations related to the design exist but are not mentioned?

EVALUATION RESEARCH

1. Does the study identify a specific problem, practice, policy, or treatment that it will evaluate?

2. Does the study identify the outcomes to be evaluated?

3. Is the problem analyzed and described?

4. Is the program to be analyzed described and standardized?

5. Does the study identify the measurement of the degree of change (outcome) that occurs?

6. Does the author determine whether the observed outcome is related to the activity or to another cause(s)?

This question of potential alternative explanations or threats to internal validity for the findings is even more important when critically evaluating a quasi-experimental study because these study designs cannot possibly control many plausible alternative explanations. A well-written report of a quasiexperimental study systematically reviews potential threats to the validity of the findings. Then the reader's work is to decide whether the author's explanations make sense.

When critiquing evaluation research, the reader should look for a careful description of the program, policy, procedure, or treatment being evaluated. In addition, the reader may need to determine the design used to evaluate the program and assess the appropriateness of the design for the evaluation. Once the design has been determined, the reader assesses threats to validity for the appropriate design in determining the appropriateness of the author's conclusions related to the outcomes. As with all research, studies using these designs need to be generalizable to a larger population of people than was actually studied. Thus, researchers need to decide whether the experimental protocol eliminated some potential subjects and whether this weakness affected not only internal validity but also external validity.

Critical Thinking Challenges

- Discuss the barriers to nurse researchers meeting the three criteria of a true experimental design.
- How is it possible to have a research design that includes an experimental treatment intervention and a control group yet is not considered a true experimental study? How does this affect the usefulness of the findings in an evidence-based practice?
- Argue your case for supporting or not supporting the following claim: "A study that does not use true experimental design does not decrease the value of the study even though it may decrease the utility of the findings in practice." Include examples with your rationale.
- Respond to the following question: Why are experimental studies considered the best evidence for an evidence-based practice model? Justify your answer.

KEY POINTS

- Experimental designs or randomized clinical trials provide the strongest evidence (Level II) in terms of whether an intervention or treatment impacts client outcomes.
- Two types of design commonly used in nursing research to test hypotheses about cause-and-effect relationships are experimental and quasiexperimental designs. Both are useful for the development of nursing knowledge because they test the effects of nursing actions and lead to the development of prescriptive theory.
- True experiments are characterized by the ability of the researcher to control extraneous variation, manipulate the independent variable, and randomly assign subjects to research groups.
- Experiments conducted in clinical settings or in the laboratory provide the best evidence in support of a causal relationship because the following three criteria can be met: (1) the independent and dependent variables are related to each other; (2) the independent variable chronologically precedes the dependent variable; and (3) the relationship cannot be explained by the presence of a third variable.
- Researchers frequently turn to quasiexperimental designs to test cause-and-effect relationships because experimental designs are often impractical or unethical.

- Quasiexperiments may lack either the randomization or the comparison group characteristics of true experiments or both of these factors. Their usefulness in studying causal relationships depends on the ability of the researcher to rule out plausible threats to the validity of the findings, such as history, selection, maturation, and testing effects.
- The level of evidence (Level III) provided by quasiexperimental designs weakens confidence that the findings were the result of the intervention rather than extraneous variables.
- The overall purpose of critiquing such studies is to assess the validity of the findings and to determine whether these findings are worth incorporating into the nurse's personal practice.

REFERENCES

Allard, N. (2006). Day surgery and recovery in women with a suspicious breast lesion: Evaluation of a psychoeducational nursing intervention. *Canadian Oncology Nursing Journal, 16,* 137–144.

Aschen, S. R. (2004.) Assertion training in psychiatric milieus. *Archives of Psychiatric Nursing, 11,* 46–51.

Bigman, S. K. (1961). Evaluating the effectiveness of religious programs. *Review of Religious Research, 2,* 99–110.

Campbell, D., & Stanley, J. (1966). *Experimental and quasiexperimental designs for research.* Chicago: Rand-McNally.

Clarke, A. (2001). Evaluation research in nursing and health care. *Nurse Researcher, 8* (3), 4–14.

Ducharme, F., Lebel, P., Lachance, L., & Trudeau, D. (2006). Implementation and effects of an individual stress management intervention for family caregivers of an elderly relative living at home: A mixed research design. *Research in Nursing & Health, 29,* 427–441.

Harkness, K., Morrow, L., Smith, K., Kiczula, M. & Arthur, H. M. (2003). The effect of early education on patient anxiety while waiting for elective cardiac catheterization. *European Journal of Cardiovascular Nursing, 2,* 113–121.

Hirshberg, J., Coleman, J., Marchant, B., & Rees, R. S. (2001). TGF-β3 in the treatment of pressure ulcers: A preliminary report. *Advances in Skin and Wound Care, 14,* 91–95.

Lavoie-Tremblay, M., Bourbonnais, R., Viens, C., Vezina, M., Durand, P. J., & Rochette, L. (2005). Improving the psychosocial work environment. *Journal of Advanced Nursing, 49,* 655–664.

Majumdar, B., Browne, G., Roberts, J., & Carpio, B. (2004). Effects of cultural sensitivity training on health care provider attitudes and patient outcomes. *Journal of Nursing Scholarship, 36,* 161–166.

Marshall, J. L., Mead, P., Jones, K., Kaba, E., & Roberts, A. P. (2001). The implementation of venous leg ulcer guidelines: Process analysis of the intervention used in a multi-centre, pragmatic, randomized, controlled trial. *Journal of Clinical Nursing, 10,* 758–766.

McGilton, K. S., O'Brien-Pallas, L. L., Darlington, G., Evans, M., Wynn, F., & Pringle, D. M. (2003). Effects of a relationship-enhancing program of care on outcomes. *Journal of Nursing Scholarship, 35,* 151–156.

O'Sullivan, A. O., & Jacobson, B. J. (1992). A randomized trial of a health care program for first-time adolescent mothers and their infants. *Nursing Research, 41,* 210–215.

Ratner, P. A., Johnson, J. L., Richardson, C. G., Bottorff, J. L., Moffatt, B., Mackay, M., et al. (2004). Efficacy of a smoking-cessation intervention for elective-surgical patients. *Research in Nursing & Health, 27,* 148–161.

Steel-O'Connor, K. O., Mowat, D. L., Scott, H. M., Carr, P. A., Dorland, J. L., & Young-Tai, K. F. (2003). A randomized trial of two public health nurse follow-up programs after early discharge. *Canadian Journal of Public Health, 94,* 98–103.

Swanson, K. (1999). Effects of caring, measurement, and time on miscarriage impact and women's well-being. *Nursing Research, 48,* 288–298.

Tranmer, J. E., & Parry, M. J. E. (2004). Enhancing postoperative recovery of cardiac surgery patients: A randomized clinical trial of an advanced practice nursing intervention. *Western Journal of Nursing Research, 26,* 515–532.

Warren, S., Ross-Kerr, J., Smith, D., & Godkin, D. (2003). The impact of adult day programs on family caregivers of elderly relatives. *Journal of Community Health Nursing, 20*(4), 209–221.

Whittemore, R., & Grey, M. (2002). The systematic development of nursing interventions. *Journal of Nursing Scholarship, 34,* 115–120.

Geri LoBiondo-Wood

Judith Haber

Mina D. Singh

CHAPTER 11

Nonexperimental Designs

LEARNING OUTCOMES

After reading this chapter, the student should be able to do the following:
- Describe the overall purpose of nonexperimental designs.
- Describe the characteristics of survey and relationship or difference designs.
- Define the differences between survey and relationship or difference designs.
- List the advantages and disadvantages of surveys and each type of relationship or difference design.
- Identify methodological, secondary analysis, and meta-analysis research.
- Identify the purposes of methodological, secondary analysis, and meta-analysis research.
- Discuss relational inferences versus causal inferences as they relate to nonexperimental designs.
- Identify the criteria used to critique nonexperimental research designs.
- Apply the critiquing criteria to the evaluation of nonexperimental research designs as they appear in research reports.
- Apply levels of evidence to nonexperimental designs.

STUDY RESOURCES

KEY TERMS

cohort
correlational study
cross-sectional study
developmental study
descriptive or exploratory survey
epidemiological study
ex post facto study
hierarchical linear modelling (HLM)
incidence
longitudinal study
meta-analysis
methodological research
nonexperimental research designs
prediction study
prevalence
prospective study
psychometrics
relationship or difference study
retrospective data
retrospective study
secondary analysis
survey study

Many phenomena of interest and relevance to nursing do not lend themselves to an experimental design. For example, nurses studying pain may be interested in the amount of pain, variations in the amount of pain, and client responses to postoperative pain. The investigator would not design an experimental study that would potentially intensify a client's pain just to study the pain experience. Instead, the researcher would examine the factors that contribute to the variability in a client's postoperative pain experience using a nonexperimental design. **Nonexperimental research designs** are used in studies when the researcher wishes to construct a picture of a phenomenon; explore events, people, or situations as they naturally occur; or test relationships and differences among variables. Nonexperimental designs may construct a picture of a phenomenon at one point or over a period of time.

In experimental research, the independent variable is manipulated; in nonexperimental research, the independent variable is not manipulated. In nonexperimental research, the independent variables have occurred naturally, so to speak, and the investigator cannot directly control them by manipulation. In contrast, in an experimental design, the researcher actively manipulates one or more variables. The researcher in a nonexperimental design explores relationships or differences among the variables. Nonexperimental research requires a clear, concise research problem or hypothesis that is based on a theoretical framework. Even though the researcher does not actively manipulate the variables, the concepts of control (see Chapter 9) should be considered as much as possible.

Researchers do not agree on how to classify nonexperimental studies. A continuum of quantitative research design is presented in Figure 11–1. Nonexperimental studies explore the relationships or the differences among variables. This chapter

BOX 11–1	**Summary of Nonexperimental Research Designs**

I. Survey studies
  A. Descriptive
  B. Exploratory
  C. Comparative
II. Relationship or difference studies
  A. Correlational
  B. Developmental
    1. Cross-sectional
    2. Longitudinal or prospective
    3. Retrospective or ex post facto

divides nonexperimental designs into *survey studies* and *relationship or difference studies*, as illustrated in Box 11–1. These categories are flexible, and other sources may classify nonexperimental studies in a different way. Some studies fall exclusively within one of these categories, whereas other studies have the characteristics of more than one category (see Table 11–1). As you read the research literature, you will often find that researchers who are conducting a nonexperimental study use several design classifications. This chapter introduces the various types of nonexperimental designs, their advantages and disadvantages, the use of nonexperimental research, the issues of causality, and the critiquing process as it relates to nonexperimental research. The Critical Thinking Decision Path outlines the path to the choice of a nonexperimental design.

Evidence-Based ◯ Practice Tip

When critically appraising nonexperimental studies, be aware of possible sources of bias that can be introduced at any point in the study.

Nonexperimental ➡ Quasiexperimental ➡ Experimental

Figure 11–1 Continuum of quantitative research design

TABLE 11–1 Examples of Studies with More Than One Design Label

Design Type	Study's Purpose
Descriptive with repeated measures	To evaluate the impact of intervention dosage on client outcomes over time in different case management models within substance abuse (Huber, Vaughan-Sarrazin, Vaughn, & Hall, 2003)
Descriptive, correlational	To examine relationships among mothers' resilience, family health-promoting activity, and mothers' health-promoting lifestyle practices in families with preschool-aged children (Monteith & Ford-Gilboe, 2002)
Correlational, cross-sectional	To examine the influence of motor function, memory, and behaviour changes of survivors of stroke, as well as family conflict surrounding stroke recovery, on the mental and physical health of caregivers during the subacute recovery period (Clark et al., 2004).
Comparative, longitudinal	To determine differences in health behaviours between two groups of university students over a three-year period (Clement, Jankowski, Bouchard, Perreault, & Lepage, 2002)
Prospective, descriptive	To examine the effect of gender (female) on early recovery from cardiac surgery at 1, 6, and 12 months (King, 2000)
Correlational, predictive	To identify factors that predict caregiving experiences to clients who have had a stroke and who are living at home (Singh & Cameron, 2005)

SURVEY STUDIES

The broadest category of nonexperimental designs is the survey study. A **survey study** is further classified as *descriptive*, *exploratory*, or *comparative*. Descriptive, exploratory, or comparative surveys collect detailed descriptions of existing variables and use the data to justify and assess current conditions and practices or to make more plans for improving health care practices. The reader of research will find that the terms *exploratory*, *descriptive*, *comparative*, and *survey* may be used either

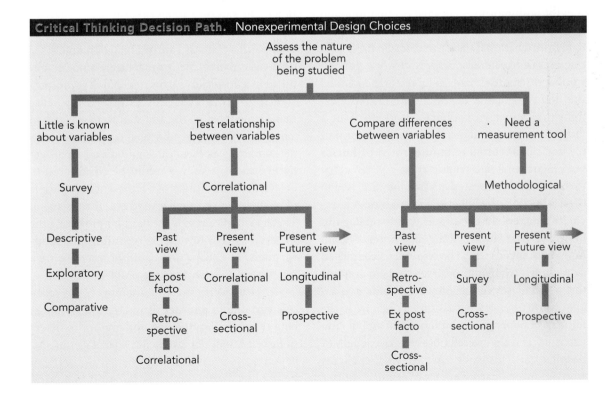

Critical Thinking Decision Path. Nonexperimental Design Choices

alone, interchangeably, or together to describe the design of a study (see Table 11–1). For example, investigators may use a **descriptive or exploratory survey** design to search for accurate information about the characteristics of particular subjects, groups, institutions, or situations or about the frequency of a phenomenon's occurrence, particularly when little is known about the phenomenon.

In survey studies, the types of variables of interest can be classified as opinions, attitudes, or facts. For example, Bowman and Epp (2005) conducted a cross-sectional study using mailed surveys to evaluate the outcomes of diabetes education, care, and support provided at two clinics in rural Manitoba. The results of this study would inform a more standardized approach to diabetes education and care. In another example, to understand the reasons for absenteeism among nurses, Zboril-Benson (2002) conducted a survey by mailing out questionnaires to 2000 registered nurses.

Fact variables include attributes of individuals that are a function of their membership in society, such as gender, income level, political and religious affiliations, ethnicity, occupation, and educational level. Andrews et al. (2005) used the data from a national survey to describe the demographics of registered nurses who work alone in rural and remote Canada. The researchers noted that the significance of this study was to determine the issues surrounding the worklife of these nurses because this information is critical for policy decisions related to employment of nurses working in rural and remote areas.

Surveys are comparative when they are used to determine differences between variables. A comparative survey by Anderson, Higgins, and Rozmus (1999) addressed an important dimension of health care: cost containment. The researchers conducted a descriptive comparative survey study to examine the length of stay in the intensive care unit (ICU) after coronary artery bypass surgery relative to the number of hours postoperation, when ambulation occurred, and the overall postoperative length of hospital stay. This study assessed whether clients who ambulated earlier after surgery had shorter

stays in the ICU. The study did find a significant difference between length of stay in the ICU and the time when ambulation began. This study, like the two previously discussed, did not manipulate variables but assessed data to provide evidence for future nursing intervention studies.

Data in survey research can be collected through a questionnaire or an interview (see Chapter 14). For example, in the study by Andrews et al. (2005), the researchers administered a mailed questionnaire. Another example is the study by Estabrooks, O'Leary, Ricker, and Humphrey (2003), who were interested in obtaining more information on the use of the Internet by nurses because the Internet is now a common workplace tool, but was underused by nurses. These authors used survey research to facilitate data collection. They administered questionnaires to nurses in Alberta in 1996 and 1998. Data were collected on how often nurses used the Internet, the location of Internet access, and the type of information sought.

Survey researchers study either small or large samples of subjects drawn from defined populations. The sample can be either broad or narrow and can be made up of people or institutions. For example, if a primary care rehabilitation unit based on a case management model were to be established in a hospital, a survey might look at prospective applicants' attitudes with regard to case management before the unit staff were selected. In a broader example, if a hospital were contemplating converting all client care units to a case management model, a survey might be conducted to determine the attitudes of a representative sample of nurses in the hospital toward case management. The data might provide the basis for projecting the in-service needs of nursing regarding case management. The scope and depth of a survey are a function of the nature of the problem.

In surveys, investigators attempt only to relate one variable to another or to assess differences between variables; they do not attempt to determine causation. The two major advantages of surveys are the great deal of information that can be obtained from a large population in a fairly economical manner and the surprisingly accurate survey research information that can be gleaned. If a sample is representative of the population (see Chapter 12), a relatively small number of subjects can provide an accurate picture of the population.

However, survey studies have several disadvantages. First, the information obtained in a survey tends to be superficial. The breadth rather than the depth of the information is emphasized. Second, conducting a survey requires a great deal of expertise in various research areas. The survey investigator must have skills in sampling techniques, questionnaire construction, interviewing, and data analysis to produce a reliable and valid study. Third, large-scale surveys can be time-consuming and costly, although the use of on-site personnel can reduce costs.

Helpful Hint

Research consumers should recognize that a well-constructed survey can provide a wealth of data about a particular phenomenon of interest, even though causation is not being examined.

Evidence-Based Practice Tip

Evidence gained from a survey may be coupled with clinical expertise and applied to a similar population to develop an educational program to enhance knowledge and skills in a particular clinical area (e.g., a survey designed to measure nursing staff's knowledge and attitudes about evidence-based practice in which the data are used to develop an evidence-based practice staff development course).

RELATIONSHIP OR DIFFERENCE STUDIES

Investigators endeavour to trace the relationships or differences between variables that can provide a deeper insight into a phenomenon. This type of study can be classified as a **relationship or difference study**. The following types of relationship or difference studies are discussed: *correlational studies* and *developmental studies*.

Correlational Studies

In a **correlational study**, an investigator examines the relationship between two or more variables. The researcher is not testing whether one variable causes another variable or how different one variable is from another variable. Instead, the researcher is testing whether the variables covary; in other words, as one variable changes, does a related change occur in the other variable? The researcher using this design is interested in quantifying the strength of the relationship between the variables or in testing a hypothesis about a specific relationship. The positive or negative direction of the relationship is also a central concern (see Chapter 17 for an explanation of the correlation between variables).

In their correlational study, Harrisson, Loiselle, Duquette, and Semenic (2002) explored relationships among hardiness, psychological distress, and work support in nursing assistants and compared the results with those from a previous study of a sample of registered nurses. The researchers noted that nursing assistants represent a large segment of Canadian health care professionals, but little is known about the psychological well-being of nursing assistants and how it compares with that of registered nurses. Each step of this study was consistent with the aims of exploring a relationship among the variables.

Harrisson et al. (2002) were not testing a cause-and-effect relationship. The researchers found a relationship and determined that one variable (hardiness) was negatively correlated with another variable (psychological distress) for the particular sample studied, nurses and nursing assistants in Quebec. Another finding was that hardiness was positively correlated with work support. When reviewing a correlational study, remember the relationship the researcher tested and notice whether the researcher implied a relationship consistent with the theoretical framework and hypothesis being tested.

Another example of correlational research is provided by Forchuk et al. (2002), who explored the relationship between schizophrenia and the motivation to smoke. They were interested in the relationships among psychiatric symptoms, medication side effects, and the reasons for smoking.

Correlational studies offer researchers and research consumers the following advantages:

- An increased flexibility when investigating complex relationships among variables
- An efficient and effective method of collecting a large amount of data about a problem
- A potential for practical application in clinical settings
- A potential foundation for future experimental research studies
- A framework for exploring the relationship between variables that cannot be inherently manipulated

The reader will find that the correlational design has a quality of realism and is particularly appealing because it suggests the potential for practical solutions to clinical problems. The following are the disadvantages of correlational studies:

- The researcher is unable to manipulate the variables of interest.
- The researcher does not employ randomization in the sampling procedures because the study deals with pre-existing groups; therefore, generalizability is decreased.
- The researcher is unable to determine a causal relationship between the variables because of the lack of manipulation, control, and randomization.

One of the most common misuses of a correlational design is the researcher's conclusion that a causal relationship exists between the variables. In their study, Harrisson et al. (2002) appropriately concluded that hardiness is related to lower psychological distress and a more negative appraisal of the work environment. The investigators also appropriately concluded that the ability to generalize from this study is limited by the lack of background variables. The study concludes with some very thoughtful recommendations for future studies in this area.

Correlational studies may be further labelled as *descriptive correlational* or *predictive correlational*. A study by McGillis-Hall, Doran, and Pink (2004) is an example of a descriptive correlational study because the goal was to describe the relationship of variables. The objective of the study was to evaluate the effect of different staffing models on costs and client outcomes, such as falls, medication errors, wound infections, and urinary tract infections. A study by Singh and Cameron (2005) that examined the factors associated with caregiving to clients who had had a stroke is classified as a predictive correlational study. The factors examined were the characteristics of self-efficacy, mastery, burden, impact, and support of the caregivers. This study tested multiple variables to assess the relationships among the variables and the ability of the chosen variables to predict caregiver emotional well-being. The researchers concluded that several of the variables were able to predict (not cause) caregiver outcomes.

The Harrisson et al. (2002) study is a good example of a study that uses a correlational design well. The inability to draw causal statements should not lead the research consumer to conclude that a nonexperimental correlational study is a weak design. In terms of evidence for practice, researchers, based on the literature review and their findings, frame the utility of the results in light of previous research and therefore help establish supportive evidence of the study's applicability to a specific client population. A correlational design is a very useful design for clinical research studies because many of the phenomena of clinical interest are beyond the researcher's ability to manipulate, control, and randomize.

Developmental Studies

Nonexperimental designs that use a time perspective can be further classified. Investigators who use a **developmental study** design are concerned not only with the existing status and the relationship and differences among phenomena at one point in time but also with changes that result from elapsed time. The following three types of developmental study designs are discussed here: *cross-sectional*, *longitudinal* or *prospective*, and *retrospective* or *ex post facto*. Remember that, in the literature, studies may be designated by more than one design name. This practice is accepted because many studies have elements of several nonexperimental designs. Table 11–1 provides examples of studies classified with more than one design label.

CROSS-SECTIONAL STUDIES

A **cross-sectional study** examines data at one point in time; in other words, the data are collected on only one occasion with the same subjects rather than with the same subjects at several time points. For example, Chalmers, Sequire, and Brown (2002) studied attitudes, beliefs, and behaviours regarding tobacco use among undergraduate nursing students. The data were collected from 272 nursing students through a self-administered questionnaire. Chalmers et al. believe that nurses have the potential to influence clients' behaviours and that the nursing curriculum is a forum to emphasize the knowledge and skills to realize this goal.

Another cross-sectional study approach is to simultaneously collect data on the study's variables from different **cohort** (subjects) groups. An example of a cross-sectional study with different cohort groups was conducted by Goodridge et al. (1998), who investigated the association among pressure ulcer incidence, prevention strategies, and risk assessment scores. The cohorts were clients over the age of 65 years from two Canadian tertiary care teaching hospitals and two long-term care facilities. Research assistants completed the study's instruments on one occasion, and responses from the different types of institutions were compared.

Cross-sectional studies can explore relationships and correlations, differences and comparisons, or both. For instance, the Goodridge et al. (1998) study posed research questions that allowed the researchers to explore both differences and relationships among and between variables.

Evidence-Based Practice Tip

Replication of significant findings in nonexperimental studies, using similar or different populations or both, increases your confidence in the conclusions offered by the researcher and the strength of evidence generated by consistent findings from more than one study.

LONGITUDINAL OR PROSPECTIVE STUDIES

In contrast to the cross-sectional design, the **longitudinal study** or **prospective study** (also referred to as *repeated measures* studies) collects data from the same group at different points in time. Longitudinal studies also explore differences and relationships. For example, the investigator conducting a study with children with diabetes could elect to use a longitudinal design. In that case, the investigator could collect yearly data or follow the same children over a number of years to compare changes in the variables at different ages. By collecting data from each subject at yearly intervals, a longitudinal perspective of the diabetic process is accomplished.

In another example of a longitudinal study, Voyer, Cappeliez, Pérodeau, and Préville (2005) collected data from a sample of 138 older adults. The purpose of the study was to describe the mental health status of long-term users of benzodiazepines (BZDs) and to compare their status with the mental health of seniors who have either begun or stopped consuming BZDs over a one-year period. Clement et al. (2002) also conducted a comparative longitudinal study, the purpose of which was to determine the degree to which a health science curriculum might affect health-related behaviours among students. Data were collected for three consecutive years to compare differences between a comparable group of students registered in that time period.

Cross-sectional and longitudinal designs have many advantages and disadvantages. When assessing the appropriateness of a cross-sectional study versus a longitudinal study, the research consumer should first assess the researcher's goal in light of the theoretical framework. For example, in a hypothetical study of infant colic, the researchers are exploring a developmental process; therefore, a longitudinal design seems more appropriate. However, the disadvantages inherent in a longitudinal design also must be considered. The period of data collection may be long because of the time the subjects take to progress to each data collection point. In the infant colic study, it might take the researchers between 12 and 18 months to collect the data from the total sample. Internal validity threats, such as testing and mortality, also are ever present and unavoidable in a longitudinal study (see Chapter 15). These realities make a longitudinal design costly in terms of time, effort, and money. Moreover, a possibility exists that confounding variables can affect the interpretation of the results. Subjects in these studies may respond in a socially desirable way that they believe is congruent with the investigators' expectations (see the discussion of the Hawthorne effect in Chapter 9).

Despite the pragmatic constraints imposed by a longitudinal study, the researcher should proceed with this design if the theoretical framework supports a longitudinal developmental perspective. The advantages of a longitudinal study are that subjects are followed separately and thereby serve as their own controls, an increased depth of responses can be obtained, and early trends in the data can be analyzed. The researcher can assess changes in the variables of interest over time and explore both relationships and differences between variables.

Cross-sectional studies, when compared with longitudinal studies, are less time-consuming and less expensive and are thus more manageable for the researcher. Because large amounts of data can be collected at one point, the results are more readily available. In addition, the confounding variable of maturation, resulting from the elapsed time, is not present. However, the investigator's ability to establish an in-depth developmental assessment of the interrelationships of the phenomena being studied is reduced. Thus, the researcher is unable to determine whether the change that occurred is related to the change that was predicted because

the same subjects were not followed over a period of time. In other words, the subjects are unable to serve as their own controls (see Chapter 9).

In summary, longitudinal studies begin in the present and end in the future, and cross-sectional studies look at a broader perspective of a cross-section of the population at a specific point in time.

Evidence-Based Practice Tip

The quality of evidence provided by a longitudinal cohort study is stronger than that from other nonexperimental designs because the researcher can determine the incidence of a problem and its possible causes.

RETROSPECTIVE OR EX POST FACTO STUDIES

A **retrospective study** is essentially the same as an **ex post facto study**. Epidemiologists primarily use the term *retrospective*, whereas social scientists prefer the term *ex post facto*. In either case, the dependent variable has already been affected by the independent variable, and the investigator attempts to link present events to events that have occurred in the past.

When scientists wish to explain causality or the factors that determine the occurrence of events or conditions, they prefer to employ an experimental design. However, they cannot always manipulate the independent variable X or use random assignments. In cases in which experimental designs cannot be employed, ex post facto studies may be used. Ex post facto literally means "from after the fact." Ex post facto or retrospective studies also are known as *causal-comparative* studies or *comparative* studies. As this design is discussed further, you will see that ex post facto research is similar to quasiexperimental research because both explore differences between variables (Campbell & Stanley, 1963).

In retrospective or ex post facto studies, a researcher hypothesizes, for example, that X (cigarette smoking) is related to and a determinant of Y (lung cancer), but X, the presumed cause, is not manipulated, and subjects are not randomly assigned to groups. Instead, the researcher chooses a group of subjects who have experienced X (cigarette smoking) in a normal situation and a control group of subjects who have not experienced X. The behaviour, performance, or condition (lung tissue) of the two groups is compared to determine whether the exposure to X had the effect predicted by the hypothesis. Table 11–2 illustrates this example and reveals that although cigarette smoking appears to be a determinant of lung cancer, the researcher is still not able to conclude that a causal relationship exists between the variables because the independent variable has not been manipulated and the subjects were not randomly assigned to groups.

Dahinten (2003) conducted a retrospective study in which she described the sexual harassment experiences of high school students and discussed the influence of the social construction of gender on those experiences. She administered self-report questionnaires to 565 students from 12 schools in two Canadian provinces. From the results, she offered recommendations for school health programming and discussed the role of the school nurse.

A study by Tourangeau et al. (2006) is another example of a retrospective study. The researchers were interested in the impact of the structures and processes of hospital nursing care on 30-day mortality for acute medical clients. They collected **retrospective data** from several clinical and administrative secondary databases, which included the Ontario Hospital Insurance Plan, the Ontario Registered Persons Database, and the Ontario Hospital Reporting System, file 2002–2003. Self-reports, via the Ontario Nurses Survey 2003, were collected from nurses on the type of clinical unit in which they worked, their evaluation of client care quality, their career intentions, their feelings of burnout, and many other work-related variables. The study found that lower 30-day mortality rates were associated with hospitals that had a higher percentage of registered nurse staff, a higher percentage of nurses with bachelor's degrees, higher use of care maps or protocols to guide client care, and higher nurse burnout.

The advantages of the retrospective or ex post facto design are similar to those of the correlational design. The additional benefit of the ex post facto design is that it offers a higher level of control than a correlational study. For example, in a cigarette smoking study, the lung tissue samples of nonsmokers and smokers could be compared. This comparison would enable the researcher to establish the existence of a differential effect of cigarette smoking on lung tissue. However, the researcher would remain unable to draw a causal link between the two variables. This inability is the major disadvantage of the retrospective or ex post facto design.

Another disadvantage of retrospective research is the problem of an alternative hypothesis as the reason for the documented relationship. If the researcher obtains data from two existing groups of subjects, such as one that has been exposed to X and one that has not, and the data support the hypothesis that X is related to Y, the researcher cannot be sure whether X or an extraneous variable is the cause of the occurrence of Y. Finding naturally occurring groups of subjects who are similar in all respects except for their exposure to the variable of interest is very difficult. The possibility always exists that the groups differ in another way (e.g., in exposure to another lung irritant, such as asbestos), which can affect the findings of the study

TABLE 11–2 **Paradigm for the Ex Post Facto Design**		
Groups (Not Randomly Assigned)	Independent Variable (Not Manipulated by Investigator)	Dependent Variable
Exposed group: cigarette smokers	X Cigarette smoking	Y_e Lung cancer
Control group: nonsmokers		Y_c No lung cancer

and produce spurious results. Consequently, the reader of such a study needs to cautiously evaluate the conclusions drawn by the investigator.

Helpful 💡 Hint

When reading research reports, the reader will note that, at times, researchers classify a study's design with more than one design label. This classification is correct because research studies often reflect aspects of more than one design.

Longitudinal or prospective (cohort) studies are less common than retrospective studies because it can take a long time for the phenomenon of interest to become evident in a prospective study. For example, if researchers were studying pregnant women who regularly consume alcohol, it would take nine months for the effect of low birth weight in the subjects' infants to become evident. The problems inherent in a prospective study are therefore similar to those of a longitudinal study. However, longitudinal or prospective studies are considered stronger than retrospective studies because of the degree of control that can be imposed on extraneous variables that might confound the data.

Helpful 💡 Hint

Remember that nonexperimental designs can test relationships, differences, comparisons, or predictions, depending on the purpose of the study.

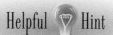

PREDICTION AND CAUSALITY IN NONEXPERIMENTAL RESEARCH

Researchers and research consumers are concerned with the issues of prediction and causality in explaining cause-and-effect relationships. Historically, researchers have said that only experimental research can support the concept of causality. For example, nurses are interested in discovering what causes anxiety in many settings. If we can uncover the causes, we could perhaps develop interventions that would prevent or decrease the anxiety.

Causality makes it necessary to order events chronologically, so if we find in a randomly assigned experiment that event 1 (stress) occurs before event 2 (anxiety) and that subjects in the stressed group were anxious, whereas those in the unstressed group were not, then the hypothesis of stress causing anxiety is supported by these empirical observations. If these results were found in a nonexperimental study in which some subjects underwent the stress of surgery and were anxious, whereas others did not have surgery and were not anxious, we would say that an association or relationship exists between stress (surgery) and anxiety. But on the basis of the results of a nonexperimental study, we could not say that the stress of surgery caused the anxiety.

Many variables (e.g., anxiety) that nurse researchers wish to study to explore causation cannot be manipulated, nor would it be wise to try to manipulate the variables. Yet, studies that can assert a predictive or causal sequence are needed. In light of this need, many nurse researchers use several analytical techniques that can explain the relationships among variables to establish predictive or causal links. These techniques are called *causal modelling*, *model testing*, and *associated causal analysis* (Hoyle, 1995; Kaplan, 2000; Schumacker & Lomax, 1996). The reader of research also will find the terms *path analysis, LISREL, analysis of covariance structures, structural equation modelling (SEM)*, and **hierarchical linear modelling** *(HLM)* used to describe the statistical techniques (see Chapter 16) used in these studies.

Cummings, Estabrooks, Midodzi, Wallin, and Hayduk (2007) used causal modelling to test a theoretical model of organizational influences that predict research utilization by nurses and to assess varying degrees of context, based on the Promoting Action on Research Implementation in Health Services (PARIHS) framework. The results revealed that the hospital characteristics of staff development, opportunity for nurse-to-nurse collaboration, and staffing and support services influenced research utilization by nurses. Nurses working in contexts with more positive culture, leadership, and evaluation also report more research utilization.

An example of HLM appears in a study by Estabrooks, Midodzi, Cummings, & Wallin (2007), who examined how the individual characteristics of nurses (i.e., gender, amount of Internet use, emotional exhaustion, and age) within a specialty and within the group characteristics of hospitals (i.e., responsive administration, staff development, staffing and support services, and innovative organization) can affect research use among nurses. The authors found that research utilization was explained mainly by individual characteristics and that hospital size was the only significant determinant among the hospital-level variables.

At times, researchers want to make a forecast or prediction about, for example, how clients will respond to an intervention or a disease process or the likelihood of success for individuals in a particular setting or field of specialty. In a **prediction study**, a model may be tested to assess which independent variables can best explain the dependent variable(s). For example, Poss (2000) wanted to analyze the relationship between participation by Mexican migrant workers in a tuberculosis (TB) screening program and variables such as susceptibility, severity, and barriers, among others, of the Health Belief Model and the Theory of Reasoned Action. Poss recruited subjects who had participated in a TB screening program and interviewed them to assess which of the independent variables predicted their behaviour and intention to participate in the TB screening program.

In another example, Singh and Cameron (2005) tested a model for predicting the psychosocial impact of caregiving to clients who had experienced a stroke. The variables of the model were developed from a previous systematic study and further tested in this study. The researchers explained the development of the model and the premise of the study. The explanation enables the reader of the study to clearly understand the purpose and aim of the research and the test of the model using regression analyses. Although the research does not test a cause-and-effect relationship between the

chosen independent predictor variables and the dependent criterion variable, the study does demonstrate a theoretically meaningful model of how variables work together in a group in a particular situation.

As nurse researchers develop their programs of research in a specific area, more studies that test models will be available. The statistics used in model-testing studies are advanced, but the beginning reader should be able to read the article, understand the purpose of the study, and determine whether the model generated was logical and developed with a solid basis from the literature and past research. This section cites several studies that conducted sound tests of theoretical models.

A full description of the techniques and principles of causal modelling is beyond the scope of this text.

Helpful Hint

Nonexperimental clinical research studies have progressed to the point where prediction models are used to explore or test relationships between independent variables and dependent variables.

Evidence-Based Practice Tip

Research studies that use nonexperimental designs and provide Level IV evidence can build the foundation for a program of research leading to experimental designs that test the effectiveness of nursing interventions.

ADDITIONAL TYPES OF QUANTITATIVE STUDIES

Other types of quantitative studies complement the science of research. These additional designs provide a means of viewing and interpreting phenomena that gives further breadth and knowledge to nursing science and practice. These types of quantitative studies are *methodological research*, *meta-analysis*, *secondary analysis*, and *epidemiological studies*.

Methodological Research

Methodological research is the development and evaluation of data collection instruments, scales, and techniques. As you will find in succeeding chapters (see Chapters 13 and 14), methodology has a strong influence on research. The most significant and critically important aspect of methodological research addressed in measurement development is psychometrics. **Psychometrics** deals with the theory and development of measurement instruments (such as questionnaires) and measurement techniques (such as observational techniques) through the research process. Thus, psychometrics deals with the measurement of a concept, such as anxiety or interpersonal conflict, with reliable and valid tools. (See Chapter 14 for a discussion of reliability and validity.)

Psychometrics is a critical issue for nurse researchers, who have used the principles of psychometrics to develop and test measurement instruments that focus on nursing phenomena. Nurse researchers also use instruments developed by other disciplines, such as psychology and sociology, which have been psychometrically tested. Sound measurement tools are critical to the reliability and validity of a study. Although a study's purpose, problems, and procedures may be clear, and the data analysis may be correct and consistent, if the measurement tool has inherent psychometric problems, the findings will be rendered questionable or limited.

The main problem for nurse researchers is locating appropriate measurement tools. Many of the phenomena of interest to nursing practice and research are intangible, such as interpersonal conflict, caring, coping, and maternal–fetal attachment. The intangible nature of various phenomena, yet the need to measure them, places methodological research in an important position in research. Methodological research differs from other designs of research. First, it does not include all of the research process steps discussed in Chapter 2. Second, to implement methodical research techniques, the researcher must have a sound knowledge of psychometrics or must consult with a researcher knowledgeable in psychometric techniques. The methodological researcher is not interested in the relationship of the independent variable and dependent variable or in the effect of an independent variable on a dependent variable. Instead, the methodological researcher is interested in identifying an intangible construct (concept) and making it tangible with a paper-and-pencil instrument or observation protocol.

A methodological study includes the following steps:

- Defining the construct, or concept, or behaviour to be measured
- Formulating the tool's items
- Developing instructions for users and respondents
- Testing the tool's reliability and validity

These steps require a sound, specific, and exhaustive literature review to identify the theories underlying the construct. The literature review provides the basis of item formulation. Once the items have been developed, the researcher assesses the tool's reliability and validity (see Chapter 14). Various aspects of these procedures may differ according to the tool's use, purpose, and stage of development.

In an example of methodological research, Estabrooks et al. (2002) documented the psychometric properties of the revised Nursing Work Index (NWI-R) in a sample of Canadian nurses. This study was part of an international study to investigate the organization of nursing care on hospital outcomes and to determine whether the psychometric properties of the NWI-R differed across countries.

Common considerations that researchers incorporate into methodological research are outlined in Table 11–3. Many more examples of methodological research can be found in the nursing research literature (Bottorff et al., 2003; Goodyear-Whiteley, Kristjanson, Degner, Yanofsky, & Mueller, 1999) and many nursing journals (Lockett, Aminzadeh, & Edwards, 2002). Psychometric or methodological studies are found primarily in journals that report research. The *Journal of Nursing Measurement* is devoted to the publication of information on instruments, tools, and approaches for measurement of variables.

The specific procedures of methodological research are beyond the scope of this book, but the reader is urged to look closely at the tools used in studies.

TABLE 11–3 Common Considerations in the Development of Measurement Tools	
Consideration	Example
The well-constructed scale, test, interview schedule, or other form of index should consist of an objective, standardized measure of samples of a behaviour that has been clearly defined. Observations should be made on a small but carefully chosen sampling of the behaviour of interest, thus creating confidence that the samples are representative.	A new tool should be based on a thorough review of previous theoretical and research literature to ensure validity.
The tool should be standardized, that is, a set of uniform items and response possibilities are uniformly administered and scored.	Without specific criteria and rating procedures, the evaluations of the items would be based on the subjective impressions, which may have varied significantly between observers and conditions.
The items of a measurement tool should be unambiguous; they should be clear-cut, concise, exact statements with only one idea per item. Negative stems or items with negatively phrased response possibilities result in a double negative and ambiguity in meaning and scoring.	In constructing a tool to measure job satisfaction, a nurse scientist writes the following item: "I never feel that I don't have time to provide good nursing care." The response format consists of "Agree," "Undecided," and "Disagree." A response of "Disagree" will likely not reflect the respondent's true intention because of the confusion that is created by the double negatives.
The type of items used in any one test or scale should be restricted to a limited number of variations. Subjects who are expected to shift from one kind of item to another may fail to provide a true response as a result of the distraction of making such a change.	Mixing true-or-false items with questions that require a yes-or-no response and items that provide a response format of five possible answers can lead to a high level of measurement error.
Items should not provide irrelevant clues. Unless carefully constructed, an item may furnish an indication of the expected response or answer. Furthermore, the correct answer or expected response to one item should not be given by another item.	An item that provides a clue to the expected answer may contain value words that convey cultural expectations, such as "A good wife enjoys caring for her home and family."
The items of a measurement tool should not be made difficult by requiring unnecessarily complex or exact operations. Furthermore, the difficulty of an item should be appropriate to the level of the subjects being assessed. Limiting each item to one concept or idea helps accomplish this objective.	A test constructed to evaluate learning in an introductory course in research methods may contain an item that is inappropriate for the designated group, such as "A nonlinear transformation of data to linear data is a useful procedure before testing a hypothesis of curvilinearity."
The diagnostic, predictive, or measurement value of a tool depends on the degree to which it serves as an indicator of a relatively broad and significant area of behaviour known as the universe of content for the behaviour. As already emphasized, a behaviour must be clearly defined before it can be measured. The definition is developed from the universe of content, that is, the information and research findings that are available for the behaviour of interest. The items should reflect that definition. The extent to which the test items appear to accomplish this objective is an indication of the validity of the instrument.	Two nurse researchers, A and B, are studying the construct of quality of life. Each nurse has defined this construct in a different way. Consequently, the measurement tool that each nurse devises will include different questions. The questions on each tool will reflect the universe of content for quality of life as defined by each researcher.

TABLE 11–3 **Common Considerations in the Development of Measurement Tools (cont'd)**	
Consideration	Example
The instrument also should adequately cover the defined behaviour. The primary consideration is whether the number and nature of items in the sample are adequate. If the sample has too few items, the accuracy or reliability of the measure must be questioned. In general, the sample should have a minimum of 10 items for each independent aspect of the behaviour of interest.	Few people would be satisfied with an assessment of traits such as intelligence if the scales were limited to three items.
The measure must prove its worth empirically through tests of reliability and validity.	The researcher should demonstrate to the reader that the scale is accurate and measures what it purports to measure (see Chapter 14).

Meta-analysis

Meta-analysis is not a design per se but a research method based on a strict scientific approach that takes the results of many studies in a specific area, synthesizes their findings, and statistically summarizes the data to obtain a precise estimate of the effect (impact) of the results of the studies (Whittemore, 2005). Each study is a unit of analysis. The goal is to bring together all of the studies concerning a particular clinical question and, using rigorous inclusion and exclusion criteria, to analyze those studies that are similar and to analyze the results to quantify the effectiveness of the intervention under study. This method is more powerful because it is a rigorous process of summarizing evidence rather than estimating the effect of the results derived from single studies alone. Johnston (2005) noted that the meta-analysis of a number of randomized clinical trials (RCTs) gives due weight to the sample size of the studies included and provides an estimate of treatment effect; in other words, a meta-analysis asks whether the intervention makes a difference. Meta-analysis is a type of systematic review that provides the most powerful and useful evidence available to guide practice, Level I evidence (see Chapter 3).

When the research consumer critically appraises a meta-analysis, some of the questions to consider are the following:

- Does the meta-analysis address a focused research question?

- Does the meta-analysis include specific inclusion and exclusion criteria for judging the studies?
- Does a publication bias exist?
- Are the studies included homogeneous?
- Are the designs of the studies similar?
- Are the interventions similar?
- Are the outcome measures similar?

Think about the meta-analysis method as progressively sifting and sorting data until the highest quality of evidence is used to arrive at the conclusions. First, the researcher combines the results of all of the studies that focus on a specific question. The studies considered of lowest quality are then excluded, and the data are reanalyzed. This process is repeated sequentially, excluding studies until only the studies of highest quality available are included in the analysis. An alteration in the overall results as an outcome of this sifting and sorting process suggests the sensitivity of the conclusions to the quality of the studies included in the meta-analysis (Johnston, 2005; Stevens, 2001).

Such considerations determine whether it is reasonable to combine the studies for analysis. The consumer of research should note that a researcher who conducts a meta-analysis does not conduct the original analysis of data in the area but instead takes the data from already published studies and synthesizes the information by following a set of controlled and systematic steps. Meta-analysis can be used to synthesize both nonexperimental and experimental research studies.

Finally, evidence-based practice requires that you, the research consumer, determine, based on the strength and quality of the evidence provided by the meta-analysis, coupled with your clinical expertise and client values, whether you would consider a change in practice. For example, a meta-analysis by Edwards, Hailey, and Maxwell (2004) addressed the clinical question, "Do psychological interventions (education, individual cognitive behavioural or psychotherapeutic programs, or group support) improve survival and psychological outcomes in women with metastatic breast cancer?" The results of the meta-analysis were reported as follows:

A search was conducted of published and unpublished RCTs in any language that assessed the effectiveness of psychological or psychosocial interventions in women with breast cancer. Data sources included the following: Cochrane Breast Cancer Group Trials Register, Cochrane Central Register of Controlled Trials, Medline, CINAHL, PsychINFO, and SIGLE; references of relevant studies and reviews; hand searches of relevant journals; and known authors in the field. Two reviewers assessed the quality of individual RCTs using the Jadad scale and another method score that was more relevant for trials of psychological interventions.

The main results of the meta-analysis indicate that five studies ($N = 636$) met the selection criteria; two studies assessed cognitive behavioural group interventions, and three studies assessed supportive-expressive group therapy. Meta-analysis using a fixed effects model showed that group psychological interventions did not differ from usual care for survival at 1, 5, or 10 years. Cognitive behavioural therapy did not differ from the usual care for anxiety (one trial), self-esteem (one trial), or mood state (one trial) at six months. Supportive-expressive group therapy improved scores on the Courtauld Emotional Control scale at eight months (one trial) and reduced reported pain assessed using a 10-point visual analogue scale (meta-analysis of two trials; weighted mean difference 0.75 reduction; 95% confidence interval 0.63 to 0.86) compared with the usual care. The groups did not differ in mood states at 10 to 12 months (two trials) or quality of life at 1 year (one trial). The authors concluded that existing evidence did not support a survival benefit for women with metastatic breast cancer who received group psychological interventions compared with those who received the usual care. Evidence on the effects on various aspects of psychological functioning is mixed.

A commentary by Haber (2004) noted that because of the diverse nature of the RCTs and the participants, Edwards et al. (2004) used a rigorous approach to data analysis that considered the heterogeneity and scarcity of data in the field as potential factors that could affect the meta-analysis. Potential modifiers, such as a family history of breast cancer, age, time of diagnosis of metastasis, variation in the length of follow-up, and failure to follow up, were also considered. Although the evidence suggests some short-term psychosocial benefits, these benefits were not maintained in the longer term. Haber concluded by commenting on the disappointing results, especially considering the conceptually logical and anecdotal evidence of the benefits of such psychosocial interventions. Because of the human and financial resource commitment of breast cancer services to psychosocial interventions, the lack of evidence supporting the efficacy of this approach justifies evaluation of traditional programming and resource allocation for this client population.

Systematic reviews that use multiple RCTs to combine study results offer stronger evidence (Level I) in estimating the magnitude of an effect for an intervention (see Chapter 3, Table 3-3). The strength of evidence provided by systematic reviews has become the "heart and soul" of evidence-based practice (Stevens, 2001).

Evidence-Based ⊘ Practice Tip

Evidence-based practice methods, such as meta-analysis, increase a nurse's ability to manage the ever-increasing volume of information produced to develop the best practices that are evidence based.

Secondary Analysis

Secondary analysis also is not a design but a form of research in which the researcher takes previously collected and analyzed data from one study and reanalyzes the data for a secondary purpose. The original study may be either an experimental or a nonexperimental design. For example, Hollingsworth and Ford-Gilboe (2006) conducted a secondary analysis of data from the Violence against Women: Health Care Provider Survey to examine the self-efficacy of registered nurses with respect to assessing and responding to woman abuse in the emergency department. The original study collected data from health care professionals practising in Ontario in 2005. In another study, Robinson and Molzahn (2007) conducted a secondary analysis of Canadian data from a larger international study designed to develop and test a new module for the measurement of quality of life of older adults. Data were available from a convenience sample of 426 older adults in British Columbia. The purpose of the study was to explore the relationships between sexual activity and intimacy and the quality of life of older adults.

EPIDEMIOLOGICAL STUDIES

An **epidemiological study** examines factors affecting the health and illness of populations in relation to the environment. The purview of public health for many years, epidemiological studies investigate the distribution, determinants, and dynamics of health and disease. Although these studies attempt to link effects with cause, a clear understanding of the causes is often not possible, especially when the illness or problem has already occurred and the method is to look retrospectively at the evidence.

Some of the questions epidemiological studies attempt to answer are "Did exposure to a certain environment affect health?" and "Does staff shortage or organizational issues affect burnout?" Research cannot answer such questions directly but can establish a statistically significant association between exposure to causative factors and disease or the effects of ill health.

Two frequently conducted types of epidemiological studies are **prevalence** and **incidence** studies. An example of prevalence is illustrated by Adlaf, Gliksman, Demers, and Newton-Taylor (2003), who examined the rates and patterns of illicit drug use among Canadian university undergraduates. They also compared these rates with those of nonuniversity students and described drug-use trends among university graduates.

Helpful 💡 Hint

As you read the literature, you will find labels such as *outcomes research, needs assessments, evaluation research, and quality assurance*. These studies are not designs per se. Instead, these studies use either experimental or nonexperimental designs. Studies with these labels are designed to test the effectiveness of health care techniques, programs, or interventions. When reading such a research study, the reader should assess which design was used and whether the principles of the design, sampling strategy, and analysis are consistent with the study's purpose.

Critiquing Nonexperimental Designs

The criteria for critiquing nonexperimental designs are presented in the Critiquing Criteria box. When critiquing nonexperimental research designs, the research consumer should keep in mind that such designs offer the researcher the least amount of control. The first step in critiquing nonexperimental research is to determine which type of design was used in the study. Often, a statement describing the design of the study appears in the abstract and in the methods section of the report. If such a statement is not present, the reader should closely examine the study for evidence of which type of design was employed. The reader should be able to discern that either a survey or a relationship design was used, as well as the specific subtype. For example, the reader would expect an investigation of self-concept development in children from birth to 5 years of age to be a relationship study using a longitudinal design.

CRITIQUING CRITERIA

1. Which nonexperimental design is used in the study?

2. Based on the theoretical framework, is the rationale for the type of design evident?

3. How is the design congruent with the purpose of the study?

4. Is the design appropriate for the research problem?

5. Is the design suited to the data collection methods?

6. Does the researcher present the findings in a manner congruent with the design used?

7. Does the research go beyond the relational parameters of the findings and erroneously infer cause-and-effect relationships between the variables?

8. Are alternative explanations for the findings possible?

9. How does the researcher discuss the threats to internal and external validity?

10. How does the author deal with the limitations of the study?

Next, the reader should evaluate the theoretical framework and underpinnings of the study to determine whether a nonexperimental design was the most appropriate approach to the problem. For example, many of the studies on pain discussed throughout this text are suggestive of a nonmanipulable relationship between pain and any of the independent variables under consideration. As such, these studies suggest a nonexperimental correlational, longitudinal, or cross-sectional design. Investigators will use one of these designs to examine the relationship between the variables in naturally occurring groups. Sometimes, the reader may think that it would have been more appropriate for the investigators to use an experimental or a quasi-experimental design. However, the reader must recognize that pragmatic or ethical considerations also may have guided the researchers in their choice of design (see Chapters 6 and 10).

The evaluator should assess whether the problem is at a level of experimental manipulation. Often, researchers merely wish to examine whether relationships exist between variables. Therefore, when critiquing such studies, the purpose of the study should be determined. If the purpose of the study does not include the expectation of a cause-and-effect relationship, the researcher should not be criticized for not looking for one. However, the evaluator should be wary of a nonexperimental study when the researcher suggests a cause-and-effect relationship in the findings.

Finally, the factor or factors that influence changes in the dependent variable are often ambiguous in nonexperimental designs. As with all complex phenomena, multiple factors can contribute to variability in the subjects' responses. When an experimental design is not used for controlling some of these extraneous variables that can influence results, the researcher must strive to provide as much control of these variables as possible within the context of a nonexperimental design.

When it has not been possible to randomly assign subjects to treatment groups as an approach to controlling an independent variable, the researcher may use a strategy of matching subjects for identified variables. For example, in a study of infant birth weight, pregnant women could be matched on variables such as weight, height, smoking habits, drug use, and other factors that might influence birth weight. The independent variable of interest, such as the type of prenatal care, would then be the major difference in the groups. The reader would then feel more confident that the only difference between the two groups was the differential effect of the independent variable because the other factors in the two groups were theoretically the same. However, the research consumer should also remember that other influential variables might exist that were not matched, such as income, education, and diet. Threats to internal and external validity represent a major influence on the interpretation of a nonexperimental study because they impose limitations on the generalizability of the results.

If the research consumer is critiquing one of the additional types of research discussed, the type of research used must be identified first. Once the type of research is identified, its specific purpose and format need to be understood. The format and methods of secondary analysis, methodological research, and meta-analysis vary; knowing how they vary allows a research consumer to assess whether the process was applied appropriately. Some of the basic principles of these methods were presented in this chapter. The specific criteria for evaluating these designs are beyond the scope of this text, but the references provided will assist in this process. Even though the format and methods vary, all research has a central goal: to answer questions scientifically.

Critical Thinking Challenges

- Discuss which type of nonexperimental design might help validate the defining characteristics of a particular nursing diagnosis you use in practice. Do you think it is possible to use nurses and clients as the subjects in this type of study?

- The midterm group (five students) assignment for your research class is to critique an assigned quantitative study. To proceed, you must first decide the study's overall type. You think it is an ex post facto nonexperimental design, whereas the other students think it is an experimental design because the study has several explicit hypotheses. How would you convince the other students that you are correct?

- You are completing your senior practicum on a surgical step-down unit. The nurses completed an evidence-based practice protocol for client-controlled analgesics. Some of the nurses want to implement it immediately, whereas others want to implement it with only some clients. You think that it should be implemented as a research study. Could either of the ways the nurses want to implement the protocol be considered a research study?

- You are part of a journal club at your hospital. Your group has been looking at a phenomenon specific to your client population and noticed that 20 correlational studies on the topic have been published. Your group decides to do a meta-analysis of the data. What steps need to be considered in doing the meta-analysis? What level of evidence would you expect to obtain with this method? Explain your answer.

KEY POINTS

- Nonexperimental research designs are used in studies that construct a picture or make an account of events as they naturally occur. The major difference between nonexperimental and experimental research is that in nonexperimental designs, the independent variable is not actively manipulated by the investigator.

- Nonexperimental designs can be classified either as survey studies or as relationship or difference studies.

- Survey studies and relationship or difference studies are both descriptive and exploratory in nature.

- Survey research collects detailed descriptions of existing phenomena and uses the data either to justify current conditions and practices or to make more intelligent plans for improving them.

- Relationship or difference studies endeavour to explore the relationships or differences between variables to provide deeper insight into the phenomena of interest.

- Correlational studies examine relationships.

- Developmental studies are further divided into categories of cross-sectional, longitudinal, prospective, retrospective, and ex post facto studies.

- Methodological research, secondary analysis, and meta-analysis are examples of other means of adding to the body of nursing research. Both the researcher and the reader must consider the advantages and disadvantages of each design.

- Nonexperimental research designs do not enable the investigator to establish cause-and-effect relationships between the variables. Consumers must be wary of nonexperimental studies that make causal claims about the findings unless a causal modelling technique is used.

- Nonexperimental designs offer the researcher the least amount of control. Threats to validity represent a major influence on the interpretation of a non-experimental study because they impose limitations on the generalizability of the results and, as such, should be fully assessed by the critical reader.

- The critiquing process is directed toward evaluating the appropriateness of the selected nonexperimental design in relation to factors such as the research problem, the theoretical framework, the hypothesis, the methodology, and the data analysis and interpretation.

- Although nonexperimental designs do not provide the highest level of evidence (Level I), they do provide a wealth of data that become useful for formulating both Level I and Level II studies that are aimed at developing and testing nursing interventions.

REFERENCES

Adlaf, E. M., Gliksman, L., Demers, A., & Newton-Taylor, B. (2003). Illicit drug use among Canadian university indergraduates. *Canadian Journal of Nursing Research, 35*, 24–43.

Anderson, B., Higgins, L., & Rozmus, C. (1999). Critical pathways: Application to selected patient outcomes following coronary bypass graft. *Applied Nursing Research, 12*, 168–174.

Andrews, M. E., Stewart, N. J., Pitblado, J. R., Morgan, D. G., Forbes, D., & D'Arcy, C. (2005). Registered nurses working alone in rural and remote Canada. *Canadian Journal of Nursing Research, 37*, 14–33.

Bottorff, J. L., Ratner, P. A., Richardson, C., Balneaves, L. G., McCullum, M., Hack, T., et al. (2003). The influence of wording on assessments of interest in genetic testing for breast cancer risk. *Psycho-Oncology, 12*, 720–728.

Bowman, A., & Epp, D. (2005). Rural diabetes education: Does it make a difference? *Canadian Journal of Nursing Research, 37*, 34–53.

Campbell, D. T., & Stanley, J. C. (1963). *Experimental and quasi-experimental designs for research.* Chicago: Rand-McNally.

Chalmers, K., Sequire, M., & Brown, J. (2002). Tobacco use and baccalaureate nursing students: A study of their attitudes, beliefs and personal behaviours. *Journal of Advanced Nursing, 40*, 17–24.

Clark, P. C., Dunbar, S. B., Shields, C. G., Viswanathan, B., Aycock, D. M., & Wolf, S. L. (2004). Influence of stroke survivor characteristics and family conflict surrounding recovery on caregivers' mental and physical health. *Nursing Research, 53*, 406–413.

Clement, M., Jankowski, L., Bouchard, L., Perreault, M., & Lepage, Y. (2002). Health behaviours of nursing students: A longitudinal study. *Journal of Nursing Education, 41*, 257–265.

Cummings, G. G., Estabrooks, C. A., Midodzi, W. K., Wallin, L., & Hayduk, L. (2007). *Nursing Research, 56*(45), S24–S39.

Dahinten, V. S. (2003). Peer sexual harassment in adolescence: The function of gender. *Canadian Journal of Nursing Research, 35*, 56–73.

Edwards, A. G., Hailey, S., & Maxwell, M. (2004). Psychological interventions for women with metastatic breast cancer. *Cochrane Database Systematic Review, 2*, CD004253.

Estabrooks, C. A., Midodzi, W. K., Cummings, G. G., & Wallin, L. (2007). Predicting research use in nursing organizations: A multilevel analysis. *Nursing Research, 56*(4S), S7–S23.

Estabrooks, C. A., O'Leary, K. A., Ricker, K. L., & Humphrey, C. K. (2003). The Internet and access to evidence: How are nurses positioned? *Journal of Advanced Nursing, 42*, 73–81.

Estabrooks, C. A., Tourangeau, A. E., Humphrey, C. K., Hesketh, K. L., Giovannetti, P., Thomson, D., et al. (2002). Measuring the hospital practice environment: A Canadian context. *Research in Nursing and Health, 25*, 256–268.

Forchuk, C., Norma, R., Malla, A., Martin, M., McLean, T., Cheng, S., et al. (2002). Schizophrenia and the motivation for smoking. *Perspectives in Psychiatric Care, 38*(2), 41–49.

Goodridge, D., Sloan, J., LeDoyen, Y., McKenzie, J., Knight, W., & Gayari, M. (1998). Risk-assessment scores, prevention strategies, and the incidence of pressure ulcers among the elderly in four Canadian health-care facilities. *Canadian Journal of Nursing Research, 30*(2), 23–44.

Goodyear-Whiteley, E. M., Kristjanson, L. J., Degner, L. F., Yanofsky, R., & Mueller, B. (1999). Measuring the care needs of mothers of children with cancer: Development of the FIN-PED. *Canadian Journal of Nursing Research, 31*, 103–123.

Haber, J. (2004). Commentary: Psychological interventions for women with metastatic breast cancer. *Evidence-Based Nursing, 7*, 111.

Harrisson, M., Loiselle, C., Duquette, A., & Semenic, S. (2002). Hardiness, work support and psychological distress among nursing assistants and registered nurses in Quebec. *Journal of Advanced Nursing, 38*, 584–591.

Hollingsworth, E., & Ford-Gilboe, M. (2006). Registered nurses' self-efficacy for assessing and responding to woman abuse in emergency department settings. *Canadian Journal of Nursing Research, 38*, 54–77.

Hoyle, R. (Ed.). (1995). *Structural equation modeling.* Newbury Park, CA: Sage.

Huber, D. L., Vaughan-Sarrazin, M., Vaughn, T., & Hall, J. A. (2003). Evaluating the impact of case management dosage. *Nursing Research 52*, 276–288.

Johnston, L. (2005). Critically appraising quantitative evidence. In B. M. Melnyk & E. Fineout-Overholt (Eds.), *Evidence-based practice in nursing and healthcare* (pp. 79–126). Philadelphia: Lippincott Williams & Wilkins.

Kaplan, D. (2000). *Structure equation modeling: Foundations and extensions.* Thousand Oaks, CA: Sage.

King, K. K. (2000). Gender and short-term recovery from cardiac surgery. *Applied Nursing Research, 49*(6), 29–36.

Lockett, D., Aminzadeh, F., & Edwards, N. (2002). Development and evaluation of an instrument to measure seniors' attitudes toward the use of bathroom grab bars. *Public Health Nursing, 19*, 390–397.

McGillis-Hall, L., Doran, D., & Pink, G. H. (2004). Nurse staffing models, nursing hours, and patient safety outcomes. *The Journal of Nursing Administration, 34*(1), 41–45.

Monteith, B., & Ford-Gilboe, M. (2002). The relationships among mother's resilience, family health work, and mother's health promoting lifestyle practices in families with preschool children. *Journal of Family Nursing, 8*, 383–407.

Poss, J. E. (2000). Factors associated with participation by Mexican migrant farmworkers in a tuberculosis screening program. *Nursing Research, 49*, 20–28.

Robinson, J. G., & Molzahn, A. E. (2007, March). Sexuality and quality of life. *Journal of Gerontological Nursing, 33*(3),19–27.

Schumacker, R. E., & Lomax, R. C. (1996). *A beginner's guide to structural equation modeling.* Hillsdale, NJ: Lawrence Erlbaum Associates.

Singh, M., & Cameron, J. (2005). Psychosocial aspects of caregiving to stroke patients. *AXON, 27*, 18–25.

Stevens, K. R. (2001) Systematic reviews: The heart of evidence-based practice. *AACN Clinical Issues: Advanced Practice in Acute and Critical Care, 12*, 529–538.

Tourangeau, A. E., Doran, D. M., McGillis-Hall, L., O'Brien-Pallas, L., Pringle, D., Tu, J. V., et al. (2006). Impact of hospital nursing care on 30-day mortality for acute medical patients. *Journal of Advanced Nursing, 57*, 32–44.

Voyer, P., Cappeliez, P., Pérodeau, G., & Préville, M. (2005). Mental health for older adults and benzodiazepine. *Journal of Community Health Nursing, 22*, 213–229.

Whittemore, R. (2005). Combing evidence in nursing research. *Nursing Research, 54*, 56–62.

Zboril-Benson, L. (2002). Why nurses are calling in sick: The impact of health-care restructuring. *Canadian Journal of Nursing Research, 33*, 89–107.

PART FOUR

Processes Related to Research

Interprofessional Learning: Impetus for Collaborative Nursing Practice

As a teacher at George Brown College since 2002, I have always been interested in educational research. When I was recently asked to participate in the creation of interprofessional education (IPE) curricula in health sciences at the College, I jumped at the opportunity to get involved because of my belief that interdisciplinary collaboration is key to achieving high-quality client care.

Through my work on this project, I discovered that although the concept of "learning in an interdisciplinary context" as a preparatory step for "real world" practice makes sense to everyone, students generally lack the understanding of each member's role on a health care team and have limited opportunities to interact with students from other health care professions while in their respective programs. Moreover, at times, professional boundary issues are misinterpreted as barriers to learning collaboratively. Although a growing body of evidence exists on the short-term student outcomes of IPE focused on knowledge and skills related to collaboration, less is known about the long-term impact of IPE on student behaviour, postregistration collaborative practice, and client care (Hammick, Freeth, Koppel, Reeves, & Barr, 2007).

In my former role as a mental health clinical nurse, it was natural for me to work collaboratively with multidisciplinary staff, including nurses, psychiatrists, psychologists, dietitians, physiotherapists, occupational therapists, and a myriad of other consultants. From the outside looking in, one could say that this type of collaborative working scenario is not unique to the mental health setting but is true of all specialties. Conversely, those who work or spend a considerable amount of time in psychiatric settings would argue that clinical discussions, and those related to the therapeutic "milieu," decision making, and team dynamics have, at times, a different "feel" than within more traditional clinical settings.

Although reality in this context is highly subjective to the interpretation of the individuals involved, my curiosity related to the following research questions was, of course, expected and grounded in my past experience within a psychiatric interdisciplinary context:

> Does IPE, "when two or more professions learn with, from and about each other to improve collaboration and the quality of care" (Centre for the Advancement of Interprofessional Education,* 2002), result in the formation of a more collaborative nursing practitioner?

*The Centre for Health Sciences at George Brown College uses the term *interprofessional education* to include all such learning in academic and work-based settings before and after qualification, adopting an inclusive view of a professional.

Does IPE lead to nurses' adoption of an inclusive view of a health care professional?

The answers to these questions have since preoccupied my thoughts and those of many of my colleagues. As a beginning step to meeting the identified need for IPE, a team of committed leaders and faculty members embarked on a developmental journey that involved the creation of a curriculum framework for IPE and four key IPE learning outcomes (George Brown College, 2004) for all students attending programs in the Centre for Health Sciences. It is hoped that the four key IPE learning outcomes will enable students to do the following:

- Appraise the relationship between their own profession and the background, scope, and roles of other health care professionals
- Evaluate their ability to work in a team
- Participate collaboratively as a health team member to support clients' achievement of their expected health outcomes
- Assess the impact of the broader legislative and ethical framework on interprofessional practice

Although our team recognized that specific learning outcomes were paramount to the increased IPE focus, it also became clear that appropriate interprofessional learning spaces were needed for this type of education to take place. To this end, renovations were undertaken and resulted in the creation of interdisciplinary learning spaces, which included a clinical simulation practice environment. These spaces now enable a variety of opportunities for interprofessional learning among students of the disciplines who previously used this space in more "insular" ways.

Following the space renovations, a series of IPE programs and projects were piloted to expose both faculty and students to this form of learning. One project actively involved nursing and dental health students learning from each other blood pressure monitoring skills and oral cleaning techniques. Another project involved nursing students collaborating with students from the dental hygiene, fitness and lifestyle management, health information management, and health informatics programs to develop a common client assessment tool. These pilot projects provided a unique opportunity to gather insight into the perspectives of students who participated in these IPE learning activities.

My participation in evaluating these projects was as a co-investigator with Scott Reeves, a sociologist and an expert in the evaluation of IPE and interprofessional practice. We used a multiple case study design and a mixed approach to collecting data in the form of questionnaires and semi-structured interviews. A total of 141 students participated in the study, 76 of whom were nursing students.

The preliminary results indicated that students showed an overall strong positive attitude toward IPE, people from other professions, and one another. The narratives of students on the benefits of learning with others reflected these positive feelings. As one student said, "I have gained a positive attitude about IPE and see the important positive implications that collaborative teamwork has on improving patient outcomes." Another nursing student added: "I would like to collaborate with other health care professionals to see what kind of roles they play on the team. I hope that we can learn from one another to maximize our knowledge in being able to provide the best care possible." However, the following comment from this student also reflected concerns that many share, related to nursing's professional identity: "I fear that in engaging in IPE, I may move away from the scope of nursing."

Although some of these early findings are encouraging and thought provoking, much research is needed to determine whether learning in interprofessional contexts will result in nursing students being able to practise in more collaborative ways in the future and whether it will ultimately lead to safer client outcomes or to more holistic care. Given that nurses make up the bulk of practitioners on a health care team in acute and chronic care settings, it is imperative that we determine whether the health outcomes and well-being of clients can be improved as a result of nurses being trained in this interdisciplinary team-based approach.

Engaging in IPE curriculum development and research has been tremendously rewarding. I have witnessed at first-hand how willing and eager various students are to collaborate toward a common goal. Although learning what is unique to nursing is paramount for developing professional competence, optimal client-centred holistic care cannot be achieved independent of the contributions of other health care professionals. The pursuit of excellence in team-based collaborative practice will take time, but nursing can be a driving force toward achieving this goal!

Julie Gaudet
RN, MN (Admin.)
Professor, Ryerson,
  Centennial, George Brown
  Collaborative Nursing
  Degree Program
School of Nursing, Centre
  for Health Sciences
George Brown College
Toronto, Ontario

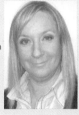

REFERENCES

Centre for the Advancement of Interprofessional Education. (2002). Retrieved from http://www.caipe.org.uk

George Brown College. (2004, December 7). *The future of health science education: Framework for inter-professional education.* Toronto: George Brown College.

Hammick, M., Freeth, D., Koppel, I., Reeves, S., & Barr, H. (2007). A best evidence systematic review of interprofessional education. *Medical Teacher, 22,* 461–467.

Judith Haber

Mina D. Singh

CHAPTER 12

Sampling

LEARNING OUTCOMES

After reading this chapter, the student should be able to do the following:

- Identify the purpose of sampling.
- Define population, sample, and sampling.
- Compare a population and a sample.
- Discuss the eligibility criteria for sample selection.
- Define nonprobability and probability sampling.
- Identify the types of nonprobability and probability sampling strategies.
- Identify the types of qualitative sampling.
- Compare the advantages and disadvantages of specific nonprobability and probability sampling strategies.
- Discuss the contribution of nonprobability and probability sampling strategies to the strength of evidence provided by study findings.
- Discuss the factors that influence determination of sample size.
- Discuss the procedure for drawing a sample.
- Identify the criteria for critiquing a sampling plan.
- Use the critiquing criteria to evaluate the "Sample" section of a research report.

STUDY RESOURCES

evolve Go to Evolve at
http://evolve.elsevier.com/Canada/LoBiondo/Research/
for Weblinks, content updates, and additional
research articles for practice in reviewing and critiquing.

KEY TERMS

accessible population
cluster sampling
convenience sampling
data saturation
delimitations
effect size
element
eligibility criteria
heterogeneity
homogeneous
matching
multistage sampling
network sampling
nonprobability sampling
pilot study
population
probability sampling
purposive sampling
quota sampling
random selection
representative sample
sample
sampling
sampling frame
sampling interval
sampling unit
simple random sampling
snowball effect sampling
stratified random sampling
systematic sampling
target population
theoretical sampling

ampling is the process of selecting representative units of a population for study in a research investigation. Although sampling is a complex process, it is a familiar one. In our daily lives, we gather knowledge, make decisions, and formulate predictions based on sampling procedures. For example, nursing students may make generalizations about the overall quality of nursing professors as a result of their exposure to a sample of nursing professors during their undergraduate programs. Clients may make generalizations about a hospital's food or quality of nursing care during a one-week hospital stay. Limited exposure to a limited portion of these phenomena forms the basis of our conclusions, so much of our knowledge and many of our decisions are based on our experience with samples.

Researchers also derive knowledge from samples. Many questions in scientific and naturalistic research cannot be answered without employing sampling procedures. For example, when the effectiveness of a medication for clients with cancer is tested, the drug is administered to a sample of the population for whom the drug is potentially appropriate. The researcher must come to some conclusions without administering the drug to every known client with cancer or every laboratory animal in the world. But because human lives are at stake, the researcher cannot afford to arrive casually at conclusions that are based on the first dozen clients available for study. The consequences of arriving at erroneous conclusions or making generalizations from a small, nonrepresentative sample are much more severe in scientific investigations than in everyday life. Consequently, research methodologists have expended considerable effort to develop sampling theories and procedures that produce accurate and meaningful information. Essentially, researchers sample representative segments of the population because sampling the entire population of interest to obtain relevant information is rarely feasible or necessary.

This chapter familiarizes the research consumer with the basic concepts of sampling as they pertain to the principles of quantitative and qualitative research designs, nonprobability and probability sampling, sample size, and the related critiquing process.

SAMPLING CONCEPTS

Population

A **population** is a well-defined set that has certain specified properties or characteristics from which data can be gathered and analyzed. A population can be composed of people, animals, objects, or events. For example, if a researcher is studying undergraduate nursing students, the type of educational preparation of the population must be specified. In this instance, the population consists of undergraduate students enrolled in a generic baccalaureate nursing program. Examples of other possible populations might be all of the female clients admitted to a certain hospital for lumpectomies for treatment of breast cancer during 2008, all of the children with asthma in the province of Alberta, or all of the men and women with a diagnosis of schizophrenia in North America. These examples illustrate that a population may be broadly defined and potentially involve millions of people or narrowly specified to include only several hundred people.

The reader of a research report should consider whether the researcher has identified the population descriptors that form the basis for the inclusion (eligibility) or exclusion (**delimitations**) criteria that are used to select the sample from the array of all possible units—whether people, objects, or events. These terms—inclusion or **eligibility criteria** and exclusion criteria or delimitations—are used synonymously when considering subject attributes that would lead a researcher to specify inclusion or exclusion criteria. Consider the population previously defined as undergraduate nursing students enrolled in a generic baccalaureate program. Would this population include both part-time and full-time students? Would it include students who had previously attended another nursing program? What about foreign students?

Would first-year students through seniors qualify? Insofar as it is possible, the researcher must demonstrate that the exact criteria used to decide whether an individual would be classified as a member of a given population have been specifically delineated. The population descriptors that provide the basis for inclusion (eligibility) criteria should be evident in the sample; in other words, the characteristics of the population and the sample should be congruent. The degree of congruence is evaluated to assess the representativeness of the sample. For example, if a population is defined as full-time, Canadian-born, senior nursing students enrolled in a generic baccalaureate nursing program, the sample would be expected to reflect these characteristics.

Think about the concept of inclusion or eligibility criteria applied to a research study in which the subjects are clients. For example, in a study investigating the effects of music on dyspnea during exercise in individuals with chronic obstructive pulmonary disease (COPD), the participants had to meet all of the the following inclusion (eligibility) criteria:

1. A confirmed medical diagnosis of COPD (i.e., chronic bronchitis, emphysema, or both)
2. Can speak and read English
3. Can ambulate independently
4. Experience dyspnea at least once a week
5. An increase in the level of dyspnea of at least two points on the Borg scale after a six-minute walk

Examples of exclusion criteria or delimitations include the following: gender, age, marital status, socioeconomic status, religion, ethnicity, level of education, age of children, health status, and diagnosis. In a study exploring loss of self in early schizophrenia and chronic kidney disease, Beanlands, McCay, and Landeen (2006) established the following exclusion criteria: participants must have no drug-related psychosis, significant medical illness, or organic brain syndrome because these characteristics will confound the findings owing to the severity of these conditions.

In a study evaluating the usefulness of arm massage from a significant other following lymph node dissection surgery, the researcher established the following exclusion criteria: participants must have been diagnosed with an organic brain disease and a pre-existing disorder affecting the functional ability of the affected arm or lymphatic system (Forchuk et al., 2004). These exclusion criteria or delimitations were selected because of their potential effect on the accurate evaluation of the effect of massage intervention.

The **heterogeneity**, or dissimilarities, of a sample group inhibit the researchers' ability to interpret the findings meaningfully and make generalizations. It is much wiser to study only one **homogeneous** group, that is, a group with limited variation in attributes or characteristics, as in the above-mentioned study, or include specific groups as distinct subsets of the sample and study the groups comparatively, as was the case in the Armstrong-Stassen and Cameron (2005) study. These researchers explored the work-related concerns, job satisfaction, and factors influencing the retention of community health nurses. They sampled 1044 nurses working in Ontario and divided the sample into three groups: public health, home care, and community care access centre nurses and studied these groups comparatively.

Remember that exclusion criteria or delimitations are not established in a casual or meaningless way but are established to control for extraneous variability or bias. Each exclusion criterion should have a rationale, presumably related to a potential contaminating effect on the dependent variable. The careful establishment of sample exclusion criteria, or delimitations, will increase the precision of the study and contribute to accuracy while constraining the generalizability of the findings (see Chapter 9).

The population criteria establish the **target population**, that is, the entire set of cases about which the researcher would like to make generalizations. A target population might include all undergraduate nursing students enrolled in generic baccalaureate programs in Canada. Because of time, money, and personnel, however, using a target population is often not feasible. An **accessible population**, one that meets the population criteria and is available, is used instead. For example, an accessible population might include all full-time generic baccalaureate students attending school in Manitoba. Pragmatic factors must also be considered when identifying a potential population of interest.

A population is not restricted to human subjects. The population may consist of hospital records; blood, urine, or other specimens taken from clients at a clinic; historical documents; or laboratory animals. For example, a population might consist of all urine specimens collected from clients in the Mount Sinai Hospital antepartum clinic or all client charts on file at a day surgery centre. A population can be defined in a variety of ways. The important point to remember is that the basic unit of the population must be clearly defined because the generalizability of the findings will be a function of the population criteria.

Helpful Hint

Often, researchers do not clearly identify the population under study, or the population is not clarified until the "Discussion" section, when an effort is made to discuss the group (population) to which the study findings can be generalized.

Evidence-Based Practice Tip

Consider whether the choice of participants was biased, thereby influencing the strength of evidence provided by the outcomes of the study.

Samples and Sampling

Sampling is a process of selecting a portion or subset of the designated population to represent the entire population. A **sample** is a set of elements that make up the population; an **element** is the most basic unit about which information is collected. The most common element in nursing research is individuals, but other elements (e.g., places or objects) can form the basis of a sample

or population. For example, a researcher was planning a study to compare the effectiveness of different nursing interventions on reducing falls in older adults in long-term care facilities. Four facilities, each using a different treatment protocol, were identified as the sampling units, not the nurses themselves or the treatment alone.

The purpose of sampling is to increase the efficiency of a research study. The novice reviewer of research reports must realize that examining every element or unit in the population would not be feasible. When sampling is done properly, the researcher can draw inferences and make generalizations about the population without examining each unit in the population.

In qualitative research, the results can have good transferability to the population under study. Sampling procedures that entail the formulation of specific criteria for selection ensure that the characteristics of the phenomena of interest will be, or are likely to be, present in all of the units being studied. The researcher's efforts to ensure that the sample is representative of the target population provide a stronger position from which to draw conclusions from the sample findings that are generalizable or transferable to the population (see Chapter 9).

After having reviewed a number of research studies, you will recognize that samples and sampling procedures vary in terms of merit. The foremost criterion in evaluating a sample is its representativeness. A **representative sample** has key characteristics that closely approximate those of the population. If 70% of the population in a study of child-rearing practices consisted of women and 40% were full-time employees, a representative sample should reflect these characteristics in the same proportions.

The representativeness of a sample cannot be guaranteed without obtaining a database about the entire population. Because it is difficult and inefficient to assess a population, the researcher must employ sampling strategies that minimize or control for sample bias. If an appropriate sampling strategy is used, obtaining a reasonably accurate understanding of the phenomena under investigation is almost always possible from the sample data.

TYPES OF SAMPLES

Sampling strategies are generally grouped into two categories: *nonprobability sampling* and *probability sampling*. In **nonprobability sampling**, elements are chosen by nonrandom methods. The drawback of this strategy is that each element's probability of being included in the samples cannot be estimated. In other words, ensuring that every element has a chance for inclusion in the nonprobability sample is not possible. **Probability sampling** uses some form of random selection when the sample units are chosen. This type of sample enables the researcher to estimate the probability that each element of the population will be included in the sample. Probability sampling is the more rigorous sampling strategy and is more likely to result in a representative sample. Nonprobability sampling is useful and appropriate in applied research, and the validity of the research findings are discussed in terms of the sampling strategy.

The remainder of this section is devoted to a discussion of different types of nonprobability and probability sampling strategies. A summary of sampling strategies appears in Table 12–1. You may wish to refer to this table as the various nonprobability and probability strategies are discussed in the following sections.

Nonprobability Sampling

Owing to a lack of random selection, the nonprobability sampling strategy is less generalizable than the probability sampling strategy because it tends to produce less representative samples. Such samples are more feasible for the researcher to obtain, however, and most samples—in nursing research and the research of other disciplines—are nonprobability samples. When a nonprobability sample reflects the target population through the careful use of inclusion and exclusion criteria, the research consumer can have more confidence in the representativeness of the sample and the external validity of the findings. The major types of nonprobability sampling are: *convenience*, *quota*, *network*, and *purposive sampling strategies*. Convenience and quota sampling can be used in both quantitative and qualitative research, whereas network and purposive sampling are mostly used in qualitative research and are discussed later in this chapter.

CONVENIENCE SAMPLING

Convenience sampling is the use of the most readily accessible persons or objects as subjects in a study. The subjects may include volunteers, the first 25 clients admitted to hospital X with a particular diagnosis, all of the people who enrolled in program Y during the month of September, or all of the students enrolled in course Z at a particular university during 2005. The subjects are convenient and accessible to the researcher and are thus called a convenience sample.

A researcher studying health promotion and cardiovascular health in adult monozygotic twins used a convenience sample of 77 monozygotic twins ranging in age from 20 to 60 years who had attended a special conference, met the eligibility criteria, and volunteered to participate in the study (Wynd, Murrock, & Zeller, 2004). Another researcher, studying the effect of a nursing intervention that sought to determine whether providing individualized information to men who are newly diagnosed with prostate cancer and their partners would lower their levels of psychological distress and enable them

TABLE 12–1 **Summary of Sampling Strategies**			
Sampling Strategy	Ease of Drawing a Representative Sample	Risk of Bias	Representativeness of the Sample
Nonprobability *non random*			
Convenience	Very easy	Greater than any other sampling strategy	Because samples tend to be self-selecting, representativeness is questionable
Quota	Relatively easy	Contains an unknown source of bias that affects external validity	Builds in some representativeness by using knowledge about the population of interest
Purposive	Relatively easy	Bias increases with greater heterogeneity of the population; conscious bias is also a danger but is offset with maximum variation	Very limited ability to generalize because the sample is hand-picked from a quantitative view, but this approach is necessary for the qualitative researcher to choose participants based on the phenomenon of study
Network	Can be easy if the network is accessible	Minimal if a thorough sampling plan is developed	Represents the event, incident, or experience being studied
Theoretical	Requires a two-stage process; can be prolonged	Minimal if a thorough sampling plan is developed	Typically begins with another type of sampling, such as convenience or criterion sampling aimed at variation in the phenomenon, and thus represents aspects of the theory being constructed
Probability *some form of random selection*			
Simple random	Laborious	Low	Maximized; the probability of non-representativeness decreases with increased sample size
Stratified random	Time-consuming	Low	Enhanced
Cluster	Less time-consuming than simple or stratified sampling	Subject to more sampling errors than simple or stratified sampling	Less representative than simple or stratified sampling
Systematic	More convenient and efficient than simple, stratified, or cluster sampling	Bias in the form of non-randomness can be inadvertently introduced	Less representative if bias occurs as a result of coincidental non-randomness

to become more active participants in treatment decision making, used a sample of 80 couples referred to the Prostate Centre at Hospital X in British Columbia who met the eligibility criteria (Davison, Goldenberg, Gleave, & Degner, 2003). The advantage of a convenience sample is that it is easier for the researcher to obtain subjects. The researcher may only need to be concerned with obtaining a sufficient number of subjects who meet the same criteria.

Singh and Cameron (2005) used a convenience sample obtained from The Toronto Hospital Stroke Registry database and a community support group for their study investigating the psychosocial aspects of caregiving to clients who have had a stroke. An example of using convenience sampling as a first stage of sampling in a qualitative, grounded theory study was provided by Chiovitti (2006), who explored nurses' meaning of caring with clients in acute psychiatric hospital settings. Convenience sampling was used because no data were available to guide gathering information from the nurses.

The major disadvantage of a convenience sample is that the risk of bias is greater than in any other type of sample (see Table 12–1). Because convenience samples use voluntary participation, the probability of researchers recruiting those people who feel strongly about the issue being studied is increased, which may favour certain outcomes (Sousa, Zauszniewski, & Musil, 2004). The problem of bias is related to the tendency of convenience samples to be self-selecting; in other words, the researcher obtains information only from the people who volunteer to participate. In this case, the following questions must be raised:

- What motivated some of the people to participate and others not to participate?
- What kind of data would have been obtained if nonparticipants had also responded?
- How representative are the people who did participate in relation to the population?

For example, a researcher may stop people on a street corner to ask their opinion on an issue; place advertisements in the newspaper; or put signs in local churches, community centres, or supermarkets indicating that volunteers are needed for a particular study. A study examining the prevention or treatment of osteoporosis in women post-menopause who had completed treatment (except for tamoxifen) for breast cancer, and for whom hormone replacement therapy was contraindicated, recruited subjects from breast cancer support groups, physician referrals, and local television and radio announcements (Waltman et al., 2003). To assess the degree to which a convenience sample approximates a random sample, a researcher can compare the convenience sample data with the known demographics and by examining variability around the mean. In this manner, the researcher checks for the representativeness of the convenience sample and the extent to which bias is or is not evident (Cochran, 1977; Sousa et al., 2004).

Because acquiring research subjects is a problem that confronts many nurse researchers, innovative recruitment strategies are sometimes used. For example, a researcher may offer to pay the participants for their time. A unique method of accessing and recruiting subjects is through online computer networks (e.g., disease-specific chat rooms and bulletin boards). In the evidence hierarchy in Table 3–3 (see page 52), nonprobability sampling is most commonly associated with quantitative nonexperimental or qualitative studies that contribute Level IV through Level VI evidence.

The evaluator of a research report should recognize that the convenience sample strategy, although the most common, is the weakest form of sampling strategy in quantitative research in terms of generalizability. When a convenience sample is used, caution should be exercised in analyzing and interpreting the data. When critiquing a research study that has employed this sampling strategy, the reviewer will be justifiably skeptical about the external validity of the findings (see Chapter 9).

QUOTA SAMPLING

Quota sampling refers to a form of nonprobability sampling in which knowledge about the population of interest is used to build some representativeness into the sample (see Table 12–1). A quota sample identifies the strata of the population and proportionally represents the strata in the sample. For example, the data in Table 12–2 reveal that 20% of the 5000 nurses in city X are diploma graduates, 40% are post–Registered Nurse (R.N.) students, and 40% are baccalaureate graduates. Each stratum of the population should be proportionately represented in the sample. In this case, the researcher used a proportional quota sampling strategy and decided to sample 10% of a population of 5000 (i.e., 500 nurses). Based on the proportion of each stratum in the population, 100 diploma

TABLE 12–2	**Numbers and Percentages of Students in Strata of a Quota Sample of 5000 Graduates of Nursing Programs in City X**		
	Diploma Graduates	Associate Degree Graduates	Baccalaureate Graduates
Population	1000 (20%)	2000 (40%)	2000 (40%)
Strata	100	200	200

graduates, 200 post-R.N. graduates, and 200 baccalaureate graduates were the quotas established for the three strata. The researcher recruited subjects who met the eligibility criteria of the study until the quota for each stratum was filled. In other words, once the researcher obtained the necessary 100 diploma graduates, 200 post-R.N. graduates, and 200 baccalaureate graduates, the sample was complete in light of both the research design and other pragmatic matters, such as economy.

The researcher systematically ensures that proportional segments of the population are included in the sample. An example is illustrated by Kaasalainen and Crook (2004), who conducted a study to evaluate the ability of elderly residents of a long-term care facility to report their pain. The researchers stratified a sample of 130 residents according to their level of cognitive impairment: cognitively intact, mild impairment, moderate impairment, and extreme impairment. The quota sample is not randomly selected (i.e., once the proportional strata have been identified, the researcher obtains subjects until the quota for each stratum has been filled), but it does increase the representativeness of the sample. This sampling strategy addresses the problem of overrepresentation or underrepresentation of certain segments of a population in a sample.

The characteristics chosen to form the strata are selected according to a researcher's judgement based on knowledge of the population and the literature review. The criterion for selection should be a variable that reflects important differences in the dependent variables under investigation. Age, gender, religion, ethnicity, medical diagnosis, socioeconomic status, level of completed education, and occupation are among the variables that are likely to be important stratifying variables in nursing research investigations.

The critiquer of a research strategy seeks to determine whether the sample strata appropriately reflect the population under consideration and whether the variables used are homogeneous enough to ensure a meaningful comparison. Even when the researcher has addressed these factors, the critiquer must remember that a quota strategy is a nonprobability sample and thus includes an unknown source of bias that affects the external validity. Those who choose to participate may not be typical of the population in terms of the variables being measured, and assessing the possible biases that may be operating is not possible. When the phenomena being investigated are relatively similar within the population, the risk of bias may be minimal; however, in heterogeneous populations, the risk of bias is greater.

Evidence-Based Practice Tip

When thinking about applying study findings to your clinical practice, consider whether the participants comprising the sample are similar to your own clients.

Probability Sampling

The primary characteristic of probability sampling is the random selection of elements from the population. **Random selection** occurs when each element of the population has an equal and independent chance of being included in the sample. In the hierarchy of evidence, probability sampling represents the strongest type of sampling strategy. The research consumer has greater confidence that the sample is representative rather than biased and that it more closely reflects the characteristics of the population of interest. Four commonly used probability sampling strategies are *simple random sampling, stratified random sampling, cluster sampling,* and *systematic sampling.*

Random selection of sample subjects should not be confused with random assignment of subjects. As discussed in Chapter 10, *randomization* refers to the assignment of subjects to either an experimental or a control group on a purely random basis.

SIMPLE RANDOM SAMPLING

Simple random sampling is a laborious and carefully controlled process. Because more complex probability designs incorporate the principles of simple random sampling in their procedures, the principles of this strategy are presented.

The researcher defines the population (a set), lists all units of the population (a **sampling frame**), and selects a sample of units (a subset) from which the sample will be chosen. For example, if Canadian hospitals specializing in the treatment of cancer were the sampling unit, a list of all such hospitals would be the sampling frame. If certified adult nurse practitioners constituted the accessible population, a list of those nurses would be the sampling frame.

Once a list of the population elements has been developed, the best method of selecting a sample is to employ a table of random numbers containing columns of digits, as shown in Figure 12–1. Such tables can be generated by computer programs. After assigning consecutive numbers to units of the population, the researcher starts at any point on the table of random numbers and reads consecutive numbers in any direction (i.e., horizontally, vertically, or diagonally). When a number is read that corresponds with the written unit on a card, that unit is chosen for the sample. The investigator continues to read until a sample of the desired size is drawn. The advantages of simple random sampling are as follows:

- The sample selection is not subject to the conscious biases of the researcher.
- The representativeness of the sample is maximized in relation to the population characteristics.
- The differences in the characteristics of the sample and the population are purely a function of chance.
- The probability of choosing a nonrepresentative sample decreases as the size of the sample increases.

Armstrong-Stassen and Cameron (2005) used simple random sampling to select 3000 community health nurses from the College of Nurses of Ontario. Research consumers must remember that despite using a carefully controlled sampling procedure that minimizes error, no guarantee exists that the sample will be representative. Factors such as sample heterogeneity and subject dropout may jeopardize the representativeness of the sample despite the most stringent random sampling procedure. In a study examining stress and the effects of hospital restructuring in nurses, Greenglass and Burke (2001) engaged in simple random sampling using a computer-generated randomized program. A sample of 3892 hospital nurses in Ontario was chosen from among the nursing union's 45,000 members. A total of 1363 questionnaires were returned, yielding a response rate of 35%, which is considered adequate.

No simple answer exists as to an acceptable response rate of surveys, but researchers will consider the accuracy of their results, whether the population is heterogeneous, and the sorts of biases introduced by the number of responses received. A smaller sample may mean less statistical power. An assessment of the differences between responders and nonresponders can also provide valuable information, such as length of survey, degree of responder fatigue, and relevance of questions (Berk, 2003).

The major disadvantage of simple random sampling is that it is a time-consuming and inefficient method of obtaining a random sample. (Consider the task of listing all baccalaureate nursing students in Canada.) With random sampling, it may also be impossible to obtain an accurate or complete listing of every element in the population. Imagine trying to obtain a list of all completed suicides in Toronto for 2001. Although suicide may have been the cause of death, another cause (e.g., cardiac failure) often appears on the death certificate. It would be difficult to estimate how many elements of the target population would be eliminated from consideration. Bias would definitely be an issue, despite the researcher's best efforts. Thus, the evaluator of a research article must exercise caution in generalizing from reported findings, even when random sampling is the stated strategy, if the target population has been difficult or impossible to list completely.

STRATIFIED RANDOM SAMPLING

Stratified random sampling requires that the population be divided into strata or subgroups. The

| 1000 random integers between 0 and 99 |

```
40  23   0  29  10  94  17  58  12  85  13  25  80  84  72  74  54  63  55  31
32  98  49  23  74  97  51  42  21  87  48  64  54  38  84  68  14  17  35  48
84  34  84  14  53  65  67  37   2  45  84  21  71  34  10  80  72  27  11  13
86  37  24  89  23   4  44  40  72  81  44  69  25  44  34  34  34  75  50  50
50  58  85   8  22  24  73  20  63  35  60  87  91  92  96  80  19  22  87  24
 1  87  43  82   9  31  40  88  33  28  82  73  18   6  48  64  59  45  34   3
21  19  42  76  84  67  29  68   8  66  93  89  96  28  12  14  38  47  52  65
32  66  33  21  81  97  39  76  67  27  97  22  76  89  41  11  91  29   6  66
16  82  42  75  35  42  92  90  77  24  21   8  36  16   5  54  89  51  57  85
74  32  63  65  93  96  18  36  82  72  39  69  37  97  51  17  36  71  38  30
50  94   4  66  17  37  10  53   8  29  67  74  88  38  11  59  60  91  56  17
71  47  81  18  53  98   7  87  29  37  22  93  13   6  95   7  95  71  14   6
71  93  48  16  33  19  46  21  60  44  52  91  52  58  10   9  41  31  35  18
20  94  13  99  45   6  53  54   1  25  79  28   1  48  36  26  68  37  59   7
75  22  69  56  62  40  64  45  40  99  94  14  98  84  22  38  24  87  43  71
16  87  41   0  88  83  11  37  71  78  22  39  43  37  75  84  84  11  55  58
92  90  80   2  30  37  85  55  56  50   3  71  24  13  62  74  82  44  90  32
96  89  31  32  37  45  70  67  80  55  58   9  55  60  61  55  86  44  27  77
38  29  36  94  65  39  56  29  29  65  88  13  71  38  71   8  81  66  31  44
20   6  61  66  90  13  70  60  92  53  87  49  34  42  14  47  75  33  26   9
63  44  94  21  14  13  41  80  39  72  29   3  25  89  44  88  13  49  18  58
13  32  93  90  31  75  86  95  18  51  61  59  84  95  67  54  40  30  29  63
26  35  48  81  19  24  36  36  76  16  46   5  93  41  97  46  79  54  95  49
89  74  96  95  94  69  31  60  16  69  76  42  28  71  69  34  46  55  20  42
50  39  28  64  20  68  60  33  92  82  61  70   5  68  95  88  12  85  18  94
55  86   5  96  87  69  75  93  54  79   0  57  45   8  86  59  25  21   9  29
75  35   1   2  86  62  70  83  85  13  97  37  13  73  16  38  36  23  54  11
74  50   1  77  87  92  68  87  57  36  17  47   0  97  78  72  72  45  54  51
34  24  35  13  26  42  22  75  47   2  34  87  15  50  65  27   5  72  28  68
73  33  42  65  91  24  44  84  71  55  70   1  27  30   8  61  65  61  18  92
 7  55  12   6  61  17  23  95  91  58  60  30  35  61  34  27  75  44  35  64
10  94  18   4   3  19  21  37  28  55  76  25  10  29  80  64   8  81  20  32
20  48  92  87  95  58  57  73  42   1  12  81  94  85  63  97  24  19  93  51
81  10  92  49  70  15  76   4  36  92  62  99  78  32  86  74  43  22  98  46
66  67  82  94  67  75  16  88  84  98   0  52  37   0  43   9   0  51   2  62
64  92  36  11   3  52  44  65  45  67  97  86  92   2  50   5  93  66  73  40
36  29  98  46  88  23  28  44   8  71  69  43  53  16  87  21  56  23  37  24
15  11  82  30  59  94  23  30  40  25  87  26  24  30  44  53  33  65  72  55
89  57  49  79  83  88  42  45  41  93  38  24  15  80  97  18  61  12  13  42
23  36  65   9  64  26  93  37  26  44  42  17  45  68  27  77  74  56  49  34
 9  93  90  61  45  40  75  85  64  66  36  89  72  43  99  90  92  10  10  85
53  94  30  31  62  92  82  30  94  56  40   4  50  53   9  74  87   2  36  36
18  69  77  38  89  78  30  68  71  92  22  93  91  74  52   1  97  69  71  42
50  20  76  36   6  20  75  56  36   5  14  70   9  78  23  33  91  33  25  72
30  46   1  10  16  72  69  26  94  39  80  36  36  68  92  74  22  74  41  42
59  47   7  92  77  55   2  12   5  24   0  30  25  62  83  36  92  96  36  75
93  22   3  20  82  44  16  69  98  72  30  57  77  15  90  29  32  38   3  48
 9  55  27  41  40  94  77  14  54  10  25  75   1  74  72  15  69  80  33  58
70   8   3   5  46  89  28  86  40   6  25  40  81  26  63  97  87  48  26  41
19   6  89  31  80  60  13  89  17  69  38  93  58  55  54  69  74  33   8  55
```

Figure 12–1 A table of random numbers

subgroups or subsets that the population is divided into are homogeneous. An appropriate number of elements from each subset is randomly selected on the basis of the proportion in the population. The goal of this strategy is to achieve a greater degree of representativeness. Stratified random sampling is similar to the proportional stratified quota sampling strategy discussed earlier in the chapter. The major difference is that stratified random sampling uses a random selection procedure for obtaining sample subjects. Figure 12–2 illustrates the use of stratified random sampling.

The population is stratified according to any number of attributes, such as age, gender, ethnicity, religion, socioeconomic status, or level of education completed. The variables selected to make up the strata lead to subgroups that share one or more of the attributes being studied. The following questions can be asked in the selection of a stratified sample:

- Does a critical variable or attribute exist that provides a logical basis for stratifying the sample?

- Does the population list contain sufficient information about the attributes that will be used to divide the sample into subsets?

- Is it appropriate for each subset to be equal in size, or is it more appropriate for each subset to be proportionally stratified based on the proportion of each subset in the population?

- If proportional sampling is being used, is the number of subjects in each subset sufficient as a base for meaningful comparisons?

- Once the subset comparison has been determined, are random procedures used for selection of the sample?

A stratified random sampling plan was used to study the sociodemographic correlates of cigarette smoking among high school students (Johnson et al., 2004). The British Columbia Youth Survey on Smoking and Health was administered to 3280 students enrolled in Grades 10 to 11 in 13 schools in two school districts. For Vancouver, another stratum was used, that of the west side and east side of the city. As illustrated in Table 12–1, a stratified

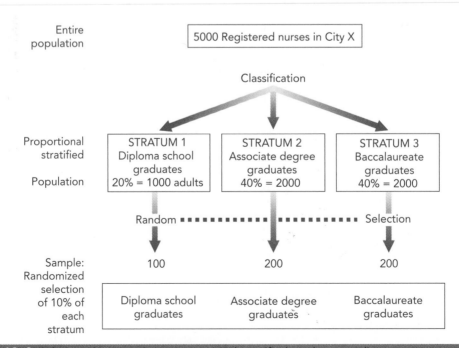

Figure 12–2 Subject selection using a proportional stratified random sampling strategy

ADVahtages [handwritten]

sampling strategy has the following advantages: (1) the representativeness of the sample is enhanced; and (2) the risk of bias is low (i.e., the researcher has a valid basis for making comparisons among subsets if information on the critical variables has been available. A third advantage is that the researcher is able to oversample a disproportionately small stratum to adjust for the researchers' underrepresentation, statistically weigh the data accordingly, and continue to make legitimate comparisons. *disAdvaH* [handwritten]

The obstacles encountered by a researcher using this strategy include the following: (1) the difficulty of obtaining a population list containing complete critical variable information; (2) the time-consuming effort of obtaining multiple enumerated lists; (3) the challenge of enrolling proportional strata; and (4) the time and money involved in carrying out a large-scale study using a stratified sampling strategy. The critiquer must question the appropriateness of this sampling strategy to the problem under investigation.

In a study investigating data collection of nursing-sensitive outcomes in acute care and long-term care settings, Doran et al. (2006) used stratified sampling to ensure that each type of agency was represented. They created a list of hospitals and long-term care facilities that included large teaching facilities, moderate-size nonteaching facilities, and small facilities from rural and urban settings in Ontario. Stratification of the sample by the type, size, and location of the facility was conducted to achieve equal distribution of health care settings. It is appropriate for the researcher to strive to represent all strata proportionally in the study sample.

Minore, Boone, and Hill (2004) used a stratified random sample to survey nurses to determine the viability of creating a relief pool to serve the Aboriginal communities of Northwestern Ontario. The database from the College of Nurses of Ontario was used to select the sample. A stratified random sample was drawn of 1126 registrants living in the northern part of the province. The key stratum was the type of nursing preparation: diploma or B.Sc.N. A proportionate sample of 622 nurses was drawn, with 170 B.Sc.N. and 452 diploma R.N.s, reflecting the levels of preparation found in the region's nurses.

MULTISTAGE SAMPLING (CLUSTER SAMPLING)

Multistage sampling or **cluster sampling** involves a successive random sampling of units (clusters) that progress from large to small and meet sample eligibility criteria. The first-stage **sampling unit** consists of large units or clusters. The second-stage sampling unit consists of smaller units or clusters. Third-stage sampling units are even smaller.

Consider an example in which a sample of nurse practitioners is desired. The first sampling unit is a random sample of hospitals, obtained from a provincial nurses association list, that meet the eligibility criteria (e.g., size, type). The second-stage sampling unit consists of a list of acute care nurse practitioners (ACNPs) practising at each hospital selected in the first stage (i.e., the list obtained from the vice president for nursing at each hospital). The criteria for inclusion in the list of ACNPs are as follows: (1) participants must be certified ACNPs with at least two years' experience as an ACNP; (2) at least 75% of the ACNPs' time must be spent in providing direct client care in acute or critical care practices; and (3) the participants must be in full-time employment at the hospital. The second-stage sampling strategy calls for random selection of two ACNPs from each hospital who meet the eligibility criteria.

Smaller set [handwritten] *tiny sAmple set* [handwritten]

When multistage sampling is used in relation to large national surveys, provinces are used as the first-stage sampling unit, followed by successively smaller units, such as counties, cities, districts, and blocks, as the second-stage sampling unit and then households as the third-stage sampling unit.

Sampling units or clusters can be selected by simple random or stratified random sampling methods. Suppose that the hospitals described in the example above are grouped into four strata according to size (i.e., number of beds) as follows: (1) 200 to 299; (2) 300 to 399; (3) 400 to 499; and (4) 500 or more. Stratum 1 comprises 25% of the population; stratum 2 comprises 30%

of the population; stratum 3 comprises 20% of the population; and stratum 4 comprises 25% of the population. Thus, either a simple random or a proportional stratified sampling strategy can be used to randomly select hospitals that would proportionately represent the population of hospitals in the provincial nurses association list.

Goulet, Lampron, Marcil, and Ross (2003) used a cluster sampling plan to study the attitudes of Quebec's adolescents about breastfeeding. Four high schools were randomly selected among those offering the equivalent of Grades 7 to 11. One class from each grade was chosen, and all students in that class were sampled.

adv — The main advantage of cluster sampling, as illustrated in Table 12–1, is that it is considerably more economical in terms of time and money than other types of probability sampling, particularly when the population is large and geographically dispersed or a sampling frame of the elements is not available. However, cluster sampling has the *dis adv* following two major disadvantages: (1) more sampling errors tend to occur than with simple random or stratified random sampling and (2) the appropriate handling of the statistical data from cluster samples is very complex.

The critiquer of a research report will need to consider whether the use of cluster sampling is justified in light of the research design, as well as other pragmatic matters, such as economy. Durbin, Goering, Streiner, and Pink (2004) examined the relationship between program structure and continuity of mental health care. A cluster or multistage sampling strategy was used. First, a random sample of 2293 clients, stratified by type of program, was drawn for the staff assessment. From this staff assessment sample, a subset of individuals was randomly selected to complete a self-report survey ($n = 432$).

Systematic Sampling

Systematic sampling refers to a sampling strategy that involves the selection of every "kth" case drawn from a population list at fixed intervals, such as every tenth member listed in the directory of the Alberta Association of Registered Nurses. Systematic sampling might be used to sample every "kth" person to enter a hospital lobby or be hospitalized with a diagnosis of acquired immune deficiency syndrome (AIDS) in 2005. When systematic sampling is used, the population must be narrowly defined (e.g., as consisting of all people entering or leaving the hospital lobby) for the sample to be considered a probability sample. If senior citizens were sampled systematically on entering a hospital lobby, the resulting sample would not be called a probability sample because not every senior citizen would have a chance of being selected. As such, systematic sampling can sometimes represent a nonprobability sampling strategy.

Systematic sampling strategies can be designed, however, to fulfill the requirements of a probability sample. First, the listing of the population (sampling frame) must be random in relation to the variable of interest. For example, subjects were being selected from every tenth hospital room for a study on client satisfaction with nursing care. In the hospital where the study was being conducted, every tenth room happened to be a private room. Clients in private rooms might respond differently regarding their satisfaction than clients in semiprivate rooms. Because of the nonrandom arrangement of the rooms, bias may have been introduced.

Second, the first element or member of the sample must be selected randomly. In this case, the researcher—who has a population list or sampling frame—first divides the population (N) by the size of the desired sample (n) to obtain the sampling interval width (k). The **sampling interval** is the standard distance between the elements chosen for the sample. For example, to select a sample of 50 family nurse practitioners from a population of 500 family nurse practitioners, the sampling interval would be as follows:

$$k = \frac{500}{50} = 10$$

Essentially, every tenth case on the family nurse practitioner list would be sampled.

Once the sampling interval has been determined, the researcher uses a table of random numbers (see Figure 12–1) to obtain a starting point for the selection of the 50 subjects. If the population size is 500 and a sample size of 50 is desired, a number between 1 and 500 is randomly selected as the starting point. In this instance, if the first number is 51, the family nurse practitioners corresponding to numbers 51, 61, 71, and so forth would be included in the sample of 50.

Another procedure recommended in many texts is to randomly select the first element from within the first sampling interval. If the sampling interval is 5, a number between 1 and 5 is selected as the random starting point. For example, the number 3 is randomly chosen. Keeping in mind the sampling interval of 5, the next elements selected would correspond to the numbers 8, 13, 18, and so on, until the sample was obtained. Although this procedure is technically correct, choosing a random starting point from across the total population of elements is more attractive because every element has a chance to be chosen for the sample during the first selection step. Systematic sampling and simple random sampling are essentially the same type of procedure. The advantage of systematic sampling is that the results are obtained in a more convenient and efficient manner (see Table 12–1). The disadvantage of systematic sampling is that bias in the form of nonrandomness can inadvertently be introduced into the procedure. This problem may occur if the population list is arranged so that a certain type of element is listed at intervals that coincide with the sampling interval. For example, if every tenth nursing student on a population list of all types of nursing students in Ontario was a baccalaureate student and the sampling interval was 10, baccalaureate students would be overrepresented in the sample.

Cyclical fluctuations are also a factor in systematic sampling. For example, if a list is kept of nursing students using the college library each day to do computer literature searches, a biased sample would probably be obtained if every seventh day is chosen as the sampling interval because probably fewer and perhaps different nursing students use the library on Sundays than on weekdays. Therefore, caution must be exercised about departures from randomness because they affect the representativeness of the sample and, as a result, the external validity of the study.

The critiquer will want to note whether a satisfactory random selection procedure was carried out. If randomization was not used, the systematic sampling may have become a nonprobability quota sample. Critiquers need to be cognizant of this issue because the implications related to interpretation and generalizability are drastically altered when dealing with a nonprobability sample.

For example, in their study, Cho, Ketefian, Barkauskas, and Smith (2003) sought to determine the effects of nurse staffing on adverse events, including morbidity, mortality, and medical costs. The study used two existing databases: California Hospital Financial Data and 1997 data for the state of California released by the Agency for Healthcare Research and Quality (AHRQ). In the selection of hospitals and clients, the researchers strived to create a sample that included homogeneous hospital and client groups while representing the majority of the target population. Hospitals were stratified by ownership, hospital size, teaching affiliation, and location; nurse staffing was stratified by type of care unit (e.g., medical–surgical acute care, medical–surgical intensive care, and coronary care). Client characteristics were stratified by "Diagnostic Related Group" and selected demographic variables. Because randomization was not used at any phase of this multilevel sampling procedure, the evaluator would consider this study to be a nonprobability stratified sample with the external validity limitations of that sampling strategy (see Chapter 9).

In contrast, in a study comparing the clinical manifestations of first-time myocardial infarction in three groups of men and women, the researchers used a retrospective review of a systematic sample of 153 clients (Then, Rankin, & Fofonoff, 2001). Because random selection was used in this example of systematic sampling, the critiquer would have more confidence in the generalizability of the findings to a similar target population.

Special Sampling Strategies

Several special sampling strategies are used in non-probability sampling. **Matching** is a special strategy used to construct an equivalent comparison sample group by filling it with subjects who are similar to each subject in another sample group in terms of pre-established variables, such as age, gender, level of education, medical diagnosis, or socioeconomic status. Theoretically, any variable other than the independent variable that could affect the dependent variable should be matched. In reality, the more variables matched, the more difficult it is to obtain an adequate sample size.

Matching was used in a study that sought to determine whether unmarried adolescent mothers and married adult mothers differ in terms of satisfaction with inpatient postpartum nursing care. In this sample, adolescent and adult postpartum mothers were matched in terms of parity, mode of delivery, infant health status, and infant feeding method (Peterson & DiCenso, 2002). When an organization or institution composes the sampling unit, matching may also be an important consideration. For example, in a study examining the effect of an ankle-strengthening and walking exercise program on improving fall-related outcomes in older adults, Schoenfelder and Rubenstein (2004) recruited participants from 10 private, urban nursing homes in eastern Iowa. Participants were matched in pairs by Risk Assessment for Falls Scale II scores and then randomly assigned within each pair to the intervention or control group.

Nonprobability Sampling Strategies Used in Qualitative Research

Because nonprobability sampling is the best method to obtain individuals who are key informants of a phenomenon these sampling methods are widely used in qualitative research. As you will recall from Chapter 6, qualitative research methods are conducted to gain both insights into and in-depth meaning about experiences, incidents, or events. In qualitative research, the sampling procedure is governed by the methodology used. Many sampling strategies are used in qualitative sampling, but the most common approaches are *network sampling, purposive sampling,* and *theoretical sampling.*

Network sampling, sometimes referred to as **snowball effect sampling** or snowballing, is a strategy used for locating samples that are difficult or impossible to locate in other ways. This sampling strategy takes advantage of social networks and the tendency of friends to share characteristics. When a few subjects with the necessary eligibility criteria are found, the researcher asks for their assistance in getting in touch with others with similar criteria.

Smith, Edwards, Varcoe, Martens, and Davies (2006) (see Appendix B) used network sampling in their study on bringing safety and responsiveness into the forefront of care for pregnant and parenting Aboriginal people. They interviewed 16 key informants working in policy, leadership, and provider positions in mother–child health.

Today, online computer networks, as described in the section on purposive sampling, can be used to assist researchers in acquiring otherwise difficult to locate subjects, thereby taking advantage of the networking or snowball effect. The Critical Thinking Decision Path illustrates the relationship between the type of sampling strategy and the appropriate generalizability.

PURPOSIVE SAMPLING

Purposive sampling is an increasingly common strategy in which the researcher's knowledge of the population and its elements is used to handpick the cases to be included in the sample. The researcher usually selects subjects who are considered typical of the population.

For example, in a qualitative study, King, LeBlanc, Sanguins, and Mather (2006) investigated the gender-based challenges of older Sikh women

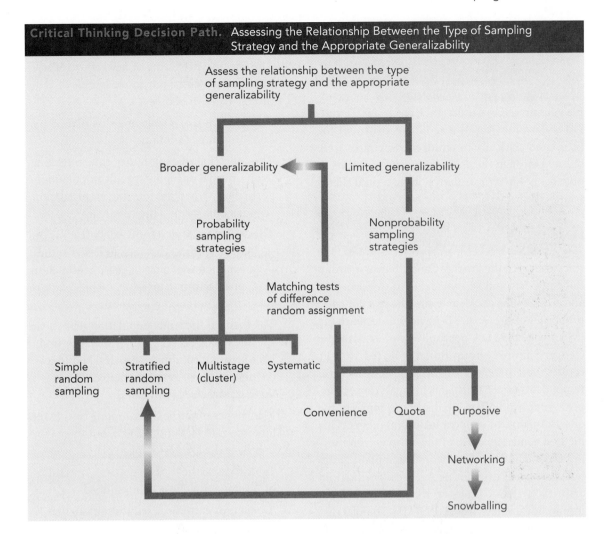

Critical Thinking Decision Path. Assessing the Relationship Between the Type of Sampling Strategy and the Appropriate Generalizability

when faced with the need to make behavioural changes to reduce the risk of coronary artery disease. A purposive sample was used to obtain participants from this very specific cultural group. The researchers tried for maximum variation by recruiting, from the two Gurdwaras (Sikh place of worship), a group of participants with variability in ages, time since coronary artery disease diagnosis, and time since immigration to Canada. A subset of purposive sampling, maximum variation purposive sampling is the "process of deliberately selecting a hetero-geneous sample and observing commonalities in their experiences" (Morse, 1994, p. 229).

A purposive sample is also used when a highly unusual group is being studied, such as a population with a rare genetic disease (e.g., Tay-Sachs disease). In this case, the researcher would describe the sample characteristics precisely to ensure that the reader will have an accurate picture of the subjects in the sample. This type of sample can also be used to study the differential effect of risk factors in a specific population longitudinally. For example, in the longitudinal Delaware Valley Twin Study examining the differential effect of cardiovascular risk factors that have the potential to respond to environmental and lifestyle modification, participant families were recruited from Mothers of Twins clubs and schools in the Philadelphia metropolitan area. Same-sex monozygotic and dizygotic twin pairs who met the eligibility criteria were recruited into this study (Meininger Hayman, Coates, & Gallagher 1998).

In another situation, the researcher may wish to interview individuals who reflect different ends of the range of a particular characteristic. For example, Alexander, Carnevale, and Razack (2002) studied the evaluation of a sedation protocol for intubated critically ill children. Ten cases were selected through the use of purposive sampling to obtain a group representative of the typical clients seen in the pediatric intensive care unit.

Today, computer networks (e.g., online services) can be of great value in helping researchers access and recruit subjects for purposive samples. One researcher used the Prodigy Cancer Support Group Bulletin Board and personal mailbox to help access and acquire subjects when testing the psychometric properties of the Sexual Behaviors Questionnaire (Wilmoth, 1995). A posting was placed on the Cancer Support Group Bulletin Board, and 11 replies were received within 24 hours. Several respondents were participants in breast cancer support groups and offered to distribute copies of the questionnaires to support group members. This method contributed 4% of the sample in an inexpensive and timely way. Other online support group bulletin boards exist for people with rheumatoid arthritis, systemic lupus erythematosus, human immunodeficiency virus (HIV)/AIDS, bipolar disorder, Lyme disease, and many other diseases.

The researcher who uses a purposive sample assumes that errors of judgement in overrepresenting or underrepresenting elements of the population in the sample will tend to balance each other. No objective method exists, however, for determining the validity of this assumption. The evaluator must be aware that the more heterogeneous the population, the greater the chance of bias being introduced in the selection of a purposive sample. As indicated in Table 12–1, conscious bias in the selection of subjects remains a constant danger. Therefore, the findings from a study using a purposive sample should be regarded with caution. As with any nonprobability sample, the ability to generalize is very limited. The following are several instances when a purposive sample may be appropriate:

- The effective pretesting of newly developed instruments with a purposive sample of diverse types of people
- The validation of a scale or test with a known-groups technique
- The collection of exploratory data in relation to an unusual or highly specific population, particularly when the total target population remains unknown to the researcher
- The collection of descriptive data (e.g., as in qualitative studies) that seek to describe the lived experience of a particular phenomenon (e.g., postpartum depression, caring, hope, or surviving childhood sexual abuse)
- The focus of the study population relates to a specific diagnosis (e.g., type 1 diabetes, multiple sclerosis), condition (e.g., legal blindness, terminal illness), or demographic characteristic (e.g., same-sex twin pairs)

Many types of purposive sampling exist (Miles & Huberman, 1994; Patton, 2003), but three types of cases have the greatest impact:

1. Typical cases: those cases that are "normal" or "average" for those being studied

2. Deviant or extreme cases: those cases that represent unusual manifestations of the phenomenon of interest

3. Confirming or disconfirming cases: those cases that are exceptions, that seek variation, or that require an initial elaborate analysis

In any type of purposive sampling, sampling is stopped when data saturation occurs, that is, when the information being shared with the researcher becomes repetitive.

THEORETICAL SAMPLING

Theoretical sampling is associated with grounded theory research. As you learned in Chapter 7, the goal of grounded research is theory generation; thus, a **theoretical sampling** strategy is used to fully elaborate and validate variations in the data by finding examples of a theoretical construct (Sandelowski, 1995). Sampling is stopped when theory saturation or redundancy occurs.

Theoretical sampling was used in the study by Young, Siden, and Tredwell (2007), which evaluated the relative effectiveness of telephone and videophone follow-up for children and families after a child's surgery for scoliosis. The researchers used memo writing to guide the initial coding of concepts and the theoretical sampling process. Different family members were compared for their views, situations, and experiences; and data from the same individuals were gathered at different points in time. The researchers engaged in constant comparative analyses as new categories arose.

Helpful Hint

Look for a brief discussion of a study's sampling strategy in the "Methods" section of a research article. Sometimes, the article has a separate subsection with the heading "Sample, Subjects, or Study Participants." A statistical description of the characteristics of the actual sample often does not appear until the "Results" section of a research article.

SAMPLE SIZE: Quantitative

No single rule can be applied to the determination of a sample's size. When arriving at an estimate of sample size, many factors, such as the following, must be considered:

- The type of design used
- The type of sampling procedure used
- The type of formula used for estimating the optimum sample size
- The degree of precision required
- The heterogeneity of the attributes under investigation
- The relative frequency at which the phenomenon of interest occurs in the population (i.e., a common versus a rare health problem)
- The projected cost of using a particular sampling strategy

The sample size should be determined before the study is conducted. A general rule of thumb is always to use the largest sample possible. The larger the sample, the more likely it is to be representative of the population; smaller samples produce less accurate results.

An exception to the rule about sample size is the **pilot study**, which is defined as a small sample study conducted as a prelude to a larger-scale study. The pilot study is typically a smaller scale of the "parent study," with similar methods and procedures that both yield preliminary data for determining the feasibility of conducting a larger-scale study and establish that sufficient scientific evidence exists to justify subsequent, more extensive research (Jaireth, Hogerney, & Parsons, 2000).

For example, Hoskins et al. (2001) conducted a pilot study, "Breast Cancer: Education, Counseling and Adjustment," using a small sample ($n = 12$). The researchers sought to determine the feasibility of and to analyze preliminary data about the differential effect of a standardized phase-specific educational and telephone counselling intervention for women with breast cancer and their partners prior to conducting the parent study, a randomized clinical trial that would have a sample size of 240.

The principle of "larger is better" holds true for both probability and nonprobability samples. Results based on small samples (fewer than 10) tend to be unstable; the values fluctuate from one sample to the next. Small samples tend to increase the probability of obtaining a markedly nonrepresentative sample. As the sample size increases, the mean more closely approximates the population values, thus introducing fewer sampling errors.

An example of this concept is illustrated by a study in which the average monthly consumption of sleeping pills was investigated for clients on a rehabilitation unit after a cerebrovascular accident. The data in Table 12–3 indicate that the population consisted of 20 clients whose average consumption of sleeping pills was 15.15 per month.

Two simple random samples with sizes of two, four, six, and ten have been drawn from the population of 20 clients. Each sample average in the

TABLE 12–3 **Comparison of Population and Sample Values and Averages in Study of Sleeping Pill Consumption**

Number in Group	Group	Number of Sleeping Pills Consumed (Values Expressed Monthly)	Average
20	Population	1, 3, 4, 5, 6, 7, 9, 11, 13, 15, 16, 17, 19, 21, 22, 23, 25, 27, 29, 30	15.1
2	Sample 1A	6, 9	7.5
2	Sample 1B	21, 25	23.0
4	Sample 2A	1, 7, 15, 25	12.0
4	Sample 2B	5, 13, 23, 29	17.5
6	Sample 3A	3, 4, 11, 15, 21, 25	13.3
6	Sample 3B	5, 7, 11, 19, 27, 30	16.5
10	Sample 4A	3, 4, 7, 9, 11, 13, 17, 21, 23, 30	13.8
10	Sample 4B	1, 4, 6, 11, 15, 17, 19, 23, 25, 27	14.8

right-hand column represents an estimate of the population average, which is known to be 15.15. In most cases, the population value is unknown to the researchers, but because the population is so small, it could be calculated. In Table 12–3, note that with a sample size of two, the estimate might have been wrong by as much as eight sleeping pills in sample 1B. As the sample size increases, the averages get closer to the population value, and the differences in the estimates between samples A and B also get smaller. Large samples permit the principles of randomization to work effectively (i.e., to counterbalance atypical values in the long run).

The sample size can be estimated with the use of a statistical procedure known as power analysis (see Chapter 16). A simple example will illustrate this concept. A researcher wants to determine the effect of nurse preoperative teaching on client postoperative anxiety. Clients are randomly assigned to an experimental group or a control group. How many clients should be used in the study? When using power analysis, the researcher must estimate how large of a difference will be observed between the groups (i.e., the difference in the mean amount of postoperative anxiety after the experimental preoperative teaching program). This difference is called the **effect size**. If a small difference is expected, the sample must be large (in this case, 196 clients in each group) to ensure that the differences will be revealed in a statistical analysis. If a medium-size difference is expected, the total sample size would be 128 (64 in each group). When expected

differences are large, it does not take a very large sample to ensure that differences will be revealed through statistical analysis.

An example is illustrated by Harkness, Morrow, Smith, Kiczula, and Arthur (2003) in their study on the effect of early education on client anxiety while awaiting elective cardiac catheterization. The study included two groups of participants: a control group and an experimental group. The authors conducted a power analysis and concluded that to detect a 15% reduction in anxiety as a result of the intervention, a sample size of 104 subjects per group was required at alpha 0.05 and 90% power. To account for a 10% dropout rate, the researchers enrolled 114 subjects per group, for a total sample size of 228.

Power analysis is an advanced statistical technique that is commonly used by researchers and is a requirement for external funding. When power analysis is not used, research studies may be based on samples that are too small, which may lead to the researcher having unsupported hypotheses and committing a type I error of rejecting a null hypothesis when it should have been accepted; in other words, the researcher finds significant results when none exist (see Chapter 16). A researcher may also commit a type II error of accepting a null hypothesis when it should have been rejected if the sample is too small; in other words, the sample is too small to detect treatment effects (see Chapter 16).

Despite the principles related to determining sample size that have been identified in this chapter, the research consumer should be aware that large samples do not ensure representativeness or accuracy. A large sample cannot compensate for faulty research design. The proportion of the population that is sampled does not provide a guarantee of accurate results. Accurate results can be obtained from only a small fraction of a large population. For example, a 10% probability sample of a population containing 1500 elements will yield more precise results than a nonprobability 0.01% sample of a population with 100,000 elements.

The critiquer should evaluate the sample size in terms of the following: (1) how representative the sample is relative to the target population and (2) to whom the researcher wishes to generalize the results of the study. The goal of sampling is to gather a sample as representative as possible with as few sampling errors as possible.

SAMPLE SIZES: Qualitative

In qualitative research, no power analyses are conducted a priori to determine sample size requirements. According to Sandelowski (1995), sample size is determined by the purpose and type of the sampling and the research method to be used. Morse (1994) recommended about six participants for phenomenological studies and about 30 to 50 cases for ethnographies and grounded theory studies. These suggestions are not a hard and fast rule because a one-person case study may be sufficient for a phenomenological study. When critiquing a study, the reader must note how the researcher has explained the sampling plan and what limitations have been noted. Subjects are added to the sample until **data saturation** is reached (i.e., new data no longer emerge during the data collection process). The fittingness of the data is a more important concern than the representativeness of subjects (see Chapter 14).

Helpful Hint

Remember to look for some rationale about the sample size and those strategies the researcher has used (e.g., matching, test of differences on demographic variables) to ascertain or build in sample representativeness.

Evidence-Based Practice Tip

Research designs and types of samples are often linked. The research consumer would expect to see experimental designs using probability sampling strategies; if a nonprobability purposive sampling strategy is used to recruit participants to such a study, the research consumer would expect random assignment to intervention and control groups to follow.

SAMPLING PROCEDURES

The criteria for drawing a sample vary according to the sampling strategy. Regardless of which strategy is used, the procedure must be systematically organized. This organization will eliminate the bias that occurs when sample selection is carried out inconsistently. Bias in sample representativeness and generalizability of findings are important sampling issues that have generated national concern.

For example, many of the landmark adult health studies (e.g., the Framingham Heart Study and the Baltimore Longitudinal Study of Aging) historically excluded women as subjects. The findings of these studies were generalized from males to all adults despite the lack of female representation in the samples. Similarly, the use of largely Euro-American subjects in medication clinical trials limits the identification of variant responses to drugs in ethnic or racially distinct groups (Campinha-Bacote, 1997). Findings based on Euro-American data cannot be generalized to Punjabis, Chinese, West Indians, or any other cultural group. Consequently, careful identification of the target population is a crucial step in the process.

If a researcher wants to be able to draw conclusions about psychosocial stressors related to all clients with a first-time myocardial infarction, then both males and females must be included in the target population. When a researcher wants to be able to draw conclusions about the incidence of extrapyramidal side effects of haloperidol (Haldol) in Chinese clients in a psychiatric ward compared with Euro-Americans, the target population must be diverse. Sometimes, however, the target population must be gender specific, as when breast or prostate cancer or aspects of pregnancy or menopause are studied.

Several general steps (illustrated in Figure 12–3) will ensure the identification of a consistent approach by the researcher. Initially, the target population (i.e., the entire group of people or objects about whom the researcher wants to draw conclusions or make generalizations) must be identified. The target population may consist of all female clients with a first-time diagnosis of breast cancer, all children with asthma, all pregnant teenagers, or all doctoral students in Canada.

Next, the accessible portion of the target population must be delineated. An accessible population might consist of all nurse practitioners in the province of New Brunswick, all male clients with AIDS admitted to hospital X during 2001, all pregnant teenagers in a specific prenatal clinic, or all children with rheumatoid arthritis under care at a specific hospital specializing in the treatment of autoimmune diseases.

Then a sampling plan or a protocol for actually selecting the sample from the accessible population is formulated. The researcher makes decisions about how subjects will be approached, how the study will be explained, and who will select the sample—the researcher or a research assistant. Regardless of who implements the sampling plan, consistency in how it is done is paramount. The reader of a research study will want to find a description of the sample, as well as the sampling procedure, in the report. On the basis of the appropriateness of what has been reported, the critiquer can make judgements about the soundness of the sampling protocol, which, of course, will affect the interpretations of the findings.

Finally, once the accessible population and sampling plan have been established, permission is obtained from the institution's research board, which is commonly referred to as the research ethics board. This permission provides free access to the desired population.

Step 1

Identify target population

Step 2

Delineate the accessible population

Step 3

Develop a sampling plan

Step 4

Obtain approval from research ethics board

Figure 12-3   Summary of the general sampling procedure

When an appropriate sample size and sampling strategy have been used, the researcher can feel more confident that the sample is representative of the accessible population; however, it is more difficult to feel confident that the accessible population is representative of the target population. Are nurse practitioners in New Brunswick representative of all nurse practitioners in Canada? It is impossible to know for sure. Researchers must exercise judgement when assessing typicality. Unfortunately, no guidelines for making such judgements exist, and critiquers have even less basis to make such decisions. The best rule of thumb to use when evaluating the representativeness of a sample and its generalizability to the target population is to be realistic and conservative about making sweeping claims relative to the findings.

Helpful Hint

Remember to evaluate the appropriateness of the generalizations made about the study findings in light of the target population, the accessible population, the type of sampling strategy, and the sample size.

Critiquing the Sample

The criteria for critiquing the sampling technique of a study are presented in the Critiquing Criteria box. The research consumer approaches the "Sample" section of a research report with a different perspective from the researcher. The consumer must raise the following two questions:

1. If this study were to be replicated, does it present enough information about the nature of the population, the sample, the sampling strategy, and the sample size for another investigator to carry out the study?

2. Are the previously mentioned factors appropriate in light of the particular research design, and, if not, which factors require modification, especially if the study is to be replicated?

Sampling is considered to be one important aspect of the methodology of a research study. As such, data pertaining to the sample usually appear in the "Methodology" section of the research report. The sampling content presented should reflect the outcome of a series of decisions based on sampling criteria appropriate to the design of the study, as

CRITIQUING CRITERIA

1. Have the sample characteristics been completely described?

2. Can the parameters of the study population be inferred from the description of the sample?

3. To what extent is the sample representative of the population as defined?

4. Are criteria for eligibility in the sample specifically identified?

5. Have sample delimitations been established?

6. Would it be possible to replicate the study population?

7. How was the sample selected? Is the method of sample selection appropriate?

8. What kind of bias, if any, is introduced by this method?

9. Is the sample size appropriate? How is it substantiated?

10. Does the researcher indicate that the rights of subjects have been ensured?

11. Does the researcher identify the limitations in generalizability of the findings from the sample to the population? Are they appropriate?

12. Is the sampling strategy appropriate for the design of the study and level of evidence provided by the design?

13. Does the researcher indicate how replication of the study with other samples would provide increased support for the findings?

well as the options and limitations inherent in the context of the investigation. The following discussion highlights several sampling criteria that the research consumer will want to consider when evaluating the merit of a sampling strategy as it relates to a specific research study.

Initially, the parameters or attributes of the study population should clearly specify to what population the findings may be generalized. In general, the target population of the study is not specifically identified by the researcher, but the nature of it is implied in the description of the accessible population, the sample, or both. For example, if a researcher states

that 100 subjects were randomly drawn from a population of men and women over 65 years of age diagnosed with COPD who were treated in a respiratory rehabilitation program at hospital X during 2001, the critiquer can specifically evaluate the parameters of the population. The demographic characteristics of the sample (e.g., age, gender, diagnosis, ethnicity, religion, and marital status) should also be presented in either a tabled or a narrative summary because they provide further explication about the nature of the sample and enable the critiquer to evaluate the sampling procedure more accurately. For example, in their study titled "Nursing-Related Determinants of 30-Day Mortality for Hospitalized Patients," Tourangeau, Giovannetti, Tu, and Wood (2002) present detailed data summarizing demographic variables of importance. These data are reproduced as follows:

> *The mean risk-adjusted mortality rate for the 75 sample hospitals was 15.03 (SD = 2.28) and ranged from 10.53 to 21.53. Teaching hospitals on average had the lowest risk-adjusted mortality rate, 14.02 (SD = 1.29). Urban community hospitals had a mean risk-adjusted mortality rate of 15.05 (SD = 2.21). On average, non-urban community hospitals had the highest risk-adjusted mortality rate, 15.27 (SD = 2.48). (Tourangeau et al., 2002, p. 80)*

This example illustrates how a detailed description of the sample both provides the critiquer with a frame of reference for the study population and sample and generates questions to be raised. For example, the critiquer will note the variability in the range of mean risk-adjusted mortality rate. The evaluator who has this demographic sample information available is able to question a sampling strategy that does not also consider the differential effect on the mortality rate of the size or type of hospital, which are factors that might affect the difference in the mortality rate. Also helpful for the critiquer is the researcher's rationale for having elected to study one type of population versus another. For example, why did the Tourangeau et al. (2002) study use only teaching and urban and nonurban community hospitals?

In a research study that uses a nonprobability sampling strategy, it is particularly important to fully describe the population and the sample in terms of who the study subjects were, the way they were chosen, and the reason they were chosen. If these criteria are adhered to, the degree of heterogeneity or homogeneity of the sample can be determined. The use of a homogeneous sample minimizes the amount of sampling error introduced, a problem particularly common in nonprobability sampling.

Next, the defined representativeness of the population should be examined. Probability sampling is clearly the ideal sampling procedure for ensuring the representativeness of a study population. Use of random selection procedures (e.g., simple random, stratified, cluster, or systematic sampling strategies) minimizes the occurrence of conscious and unconscious biases that affect the researcher's ability to generalize about the findings from the sample to the population. The critiquer should be able to identify the type of probability strategy used and determine whether the researcher adhered to the criteria for a particular sampling plan. In experimental and quasi-experimental studies, the evaluator must also know whether or how the subjects were assigned to groups. If the criteria have not been followed, the reader has a valid basis for being cautious about the proposed conclusions of the study.

Although random selection is the ideal in establishing the representativeness of a study population, more often, realistic barriers (e.g., institutional policy, inaccessibility of subjects, lack of time or money, and current state of knowledge in the field) necessitate the use of nonprobability sampling strategies. Many important research problems that are of interest to nursing do not lend themselves to experimental design and probability sampling, particularly qualitative research designs. A well-designed, carefully controlled study using a nonprobability sampling strategy can yield accurate and meaningful findings that make a significant contribution to nursing's scientific body of knowledge. As the critiquer, you must ask a philosophical question: "If it is not possible or appropriate to conduct an experimental or quasiexperimental investigation that uses probability sampling, should the study be abandoned?" The answer usually suggests that it is better to carry out the investigation and be fully aware of the limitations of the methodology than to lose the knowledge that can be gained. The researcher is always able to move on to subsequent studies that either replicate the study or use more stringent design and sampling strategies to refine the knowledge derived from a nonexperimental study.

The greatest difficulty in nonprobability sampling stems from the fact that not every element in the population has an equal chance of being represented in the sample. Therefore, some segment of the population will likely be systematically underrepresented. If the population is homogeneous on critical characteristics, systematic bias will not be very important. Few of the attributes that researchers are interested in, however, are sufficiently homogeneous to render sampling bias an irrelevant consideration.

Next, the sampling plan's suitability to the research design should be evaluated. Experimental and quasiexperimental designs use some form of random selection or random assignment of subjects to groups (see Chapter 10). The critiquer evaluates whether the researcher adhered to the principles of random selection and assignment. Lack of adherence to such principles compromises the representativeness of the sample and the external validity of the study. The following are questions the evaluator might pose relative to this issue:

- Has a random selection procedure (e.g., a table of random numbers) been identified?

- Has the appropriate random sampling plan been selected; in other words, has a proportional stratified sampling plan been selected instead of a simple random sampling plan in a study in which three distinct occupational levels appear to be critical variables for stratification?

- Has the particular random sampling plan been carried out appropriately; in other words, if a cluster sampling strategy was used, did the sampling units logically progress from the largest to the smallest?

Random sampling should not be regarded as a perfect method of obtaining a representative sample. Sometimes, bias is inadvertently introduced even when the principle of random selection is used. Nonexperimental designs often use nonprobability sampling strategies. In this instance, the critiquer can ask whether a nonexperimental design and a related nonprobability sampling plan were most appropriate for this study. Sometimes, if the researchers had used another type of design or sampling plan, they could have constructed a stronger study that would have allowed more generalizability and greater confidence to be placed in the findings. The critiquer, however, is rarely in a position to know what factors entered into the decision to plan one type of study rather than another.

When critiquing qualitative research designs, the evaluator applies criteria related to sampling strategies that are relevant for a particular type of qualitative study. In general, sampling strategies are purposive because the study of specific phenomena in their natural setting is emphasized; any subject belonging to a specified group is considered to represent that group. For example, in the qualitative study "Beyond Survival: Reclaiming Self after Leaving an Abusive Partner" (Wuest & Merritt-Gray, 2001), the specified group is women who have left abusive partners. The researcher's goal was to establish the experiences of their lives, that is, the typicality or atypicality of the observed events, behaviours, or responses in the lives of the survivors abuse, to better understand the effect of these events on peoples' lives and how nursing can best meet their needs.

The evaluator should then determine whether the sample size is appropriate and its size is justifiable. The researcher usually indicates in a research article how the sample size was determined; a similar indication is also seen commonly in doctoral dissertations. The method of arriving at the sample size and the rationale should be briefly mentioned. For example, a researcher may state the following:

> *Based on a power analysis, it was estimated that the sample size needs to be 120 for a 95% chance of detecting a treatment effect. (King, 2000 p. 31)*

The importance of such examples lies in understanding that this type of statement meets the criteria stated at the beginning of the paragraph and should be evident on the research report. Other considerations with respect to sample size, especially when the sample size appears to be small or inadequate and no rationale is stated for the size, are as follows:

- How will the sample size affect the accuracy of the results?

- Are any subsets or cells of the sample overrepresented or underrepresented?

- Are any of the subsets so small as to limit meaningful comparisons?
- Has the researcher examined the effect of attrition or dropouts on the results?
- Has the researcher recognized and identified any limitations posed by the size of the sample?

Essentially, these criteria demand that the critiquer carefully scrutinize several important elements pertaining to sample size that have implications for the generalizability of the findings. Keep in mind that qualitative studies will not discuss predetermining the sample size or the method of arriving at the sample size. Rather, the sample size will tend to be small and a function of data saturation (see Chapter 8).

Finally, evidence that the rights of human subjects have been protected should appear in the "Sample" section of the research report. The critiquer will evaluate whether permission was obtained from an institutional research ethics board that reviewed the study relative to the maintenance of ethical research standards (see Chapter 6). For example, the research ethics board examines the research proposal to determine whether the introduction of an experimental procedure may be potentially harmful and therefore undesirable. The critiquer also examines the report for evidence of the subjects' informed consent, as well as protection of their confidentiality or anonymity. Research studies that do not demonstrate evidence of having met these criteria are highly unusual. Nevertheless, the careful critiquer will want to be certain that ethical standards that protect sample subjects have been maintained.

Many factors must be considered when critiquing the "Sample" section of a research report. The type and appropriateness of the sampling strategy become crucial elements in the analysis and interpretation of data, in the conclusions derived from the findings, and in the generalizability of the findings from the sample to the population. As stated earlier in this chapter, the major purpose of sampling is to increase the efficiency of a research study by using a sample that is representative of the particular population so that every element need not be studied,

while generalizing the findings from the sample to the population. The critiquer must justify that the sampling strategy used provided a valid basis for the findings and their generalizability.

Critical Thinking Challenges

- A research classmate asks the instructor the following question: "Why isn't it better to study an entire population of clients with lung cancer instead of using the research technique of sampling?" How would you answer this question? Include examples that will help the student see your point of view.
- A quasiexperimental study indicated that it used a convenience sample with random assignment. How is this possible? Would the study have used a nonprobability or a probability sample? If you agree that this is a legitimate sampling technique, present both the advantages and the disadvantages; if you disagree, indicate your rationale.
- Your research class is having a debate on probability versus nonprobability sampling with regard to desirability and feasibility. You are assigned to present the pros of nonprobability sampling in nursing research. What arguments would you use?
- Discuss the principle of "larger is better" and its relationship to "networking" sampling and the sample size of qualitative studies. Include in your discussion the concept of data saturation and the use of computer technology.
- Your research classmate is arguing that a random sample is always better, even if it is small and represents only one site. Another student is arguing that a very large convenience sample representing multiple sites can be very significant. Which classmate would you defend and why?

KEY POINTS

- Sampling is a process that selects representative units of a population for study. Researchers sample representative segments of the population because sampling entire populations of interest to obtain accurate and meaningful information is rarely feasible or necessary.
- Researchers establish eligibility criteria; these are descriptors of the population and provide the basis for selection into a sample. Eligibility criteria, also referred to as delimitations, include age, gender, socioeconomic status, level of education, religion, and ethnicity.

- The researcher must identify the target population (i.e., the entire set of cases about which the researcher would like to make generalizations). Because of pragmatic constraints, however, the researcher usually uses an accessible population (i.e., one that meets the population criteria and is available).

- A sample is a set of elements that make up the population.

- A sampling unit is the element or set of elements used for selecting the sample. The foremost criterion in evaluating a sample is the representativeness or congruence of characteristics with the population.

- Sampling strategies consist of nonprobability and probability sampling.

- In nonprobability sampling, the elements are chosen by nonrandom methods. Types of nonprobability sampling include convenience, quota, and purposive sampling.

- Probability sampling is characterized by the random selection of elements from the population. In random selection, each element in the population has an equal and independent chance of being included in the sample. Types of probability sampling include simple random, stratified random, cluster, and systematic sampling.

- Sample size is a function of the type of sampling procedure being used, the degree of precision required, the type of sample estimation formula being used, the heterogeneity of the study attributes, the relative frequency of occurrence of the phenomena under consideration, and the cost.

- Criteria for drawing a sample vary according to the sampling strategy. Systematic organization of the sampling procedure minimizes bias. The target population is identified, the accessible portion of the target population is delineated, permission to conduct the research study is obtained, and a sampling plan is formulated.

- The critiquer of a research report evaluates the sampling plan for its appropriateness in relation to the particular research design.

- The completeness of the sampling plan is examined in light of the potential replicability of the study. The critiquer evaluates whether the sampling strategy is the strongest plan for the particular study under consideration.

- An appropriate systematic sampling plan will maximize the efficiency of a research study. It will increase the accuracy and meaningfulness of the findings and enhance the generalizability of the findings from the sample to the population.

REFERENCES

Alexander, E., Carnevale, F., & Razack, S. (2002). Evaluation of a sedation protocol for intubated critically ill children. *Intensive and Critical Care Nursing, 18*, 292–301.

Armstrong-Stassen, M., & Cameron, S. (2005). Concerns, satisfaction, and retention of Canadian community health nurses. *Journal of Community Health Nursing, 22*, 181–194.

Beanlands, H., McCay, E., & Landeen, J. (2006). Strategies for moving beyond the illness in early schizophrenia and in chronic kidney disease. *Canadian Journal of Nursing Research, 38*, 10–30.

Berk, R. (2003). *Regression analysis: A constructive critique.* Thousand Oaks, CA: Sage.

Campinha-Bacote, J. (1997). Understanding the influence of culture. In J. Haber, B. Krainovich-Miller, A. L. McMahon, & P. Price-Hoskins (Eds.), *Comprehensive psychiatric nursing* (5th ed., pp. 70–95). St. Louis, MO: Mosby.

Chiovitti, R. F. (2006, October 14). Nurses' meaning of caring with patients in acute psychiatric hospital settings: A grounded theory study. *International Journal of Nursing Studies, 45*(2), 203–223.

Cho, S. H., Ketefian, S., Barkauskas, V. H., & Smith, D. G. (2003). The effects of nurse staffing on adverse events, morbidity, mortality, and medical costs. *Nursing Research, 52*, 71–79.

Cochran, W. G. (1977). *Sampling technique* (3rd ed.). New York: Wiley.

Davison, B. J., Goldenberg, S. L., Gleave, M. E., & Degner, L. F. (2003). Provision of individualized information to men and their partners to facilitate treatment decision making in prostate cancer. *Oncology Forum, 30*, 107–114.

Doran, D. M., Harrison, M. B., Laschinger, H. S., Hirdes, J. P., Rukholm, E., Sidani, S., et al. (2006). Nursing-sensitive outcomes data collection in acute care and long-term-care settings. *Nursing Research, 55*(2S), S75–S81.

Durbin, J., Goering, P., Streiner, D. L., & Pink, G. (2004). Program structure and continuity of mental health care. *Canadian Journal of Nursing Research, 36*, 12–37.

Forchuk, C., Baruth, P., Prendergast, M., Holliday, R., Bareham, R., Brimner, S., et al. (2004). Postoperative arm massage: A support for women with lymph node dissection. *Cancer Nursing, 27*(1), 25–33.

Goulet, C., Lampron, A., Marcil, I., & Ross, L. (2003). Attitudes and subjective norms of male and female adolescents toward breastfeeding. *Journal of Human Lactation, 19*, 402–410.

Greenglass, E., & Burke, R. (2001). Stress and the effects of hospital restructuring in nurses. *Canadian Journal of Nursing Research, 33*, 93–108.

Harkness, K. Morrow, L., Smith, K., Kiczula, M., & Arthur, H. M. (2003). The effect of early education on patient anxiety while waiting for elective cardiac catheterization. *European Journal of Cardiovascular Nursing, 2*, 113–121.

Hoskins, C. N., Haber, J., Budin, W. C., Cartwright, Alcarise, F., Kowalski, M. O., et al. (2001). Breast cancer: Education, counseling and adjustment—A pilot study. *Psychological Reports, 89*, 677–704.

Jaireth, N., Hogerney, M., & Parsons, C. (2000). The role of the pilot study: A case illustration from cardiac nursing research. *Applied Nursing Research, 13*, 92–96.

Johnson, J. L., Tucker, R. S., Ratner, P. A., Bottorff, J. L., Prkachin, K. M., Shoveller, J., et al. (2004). Socio-demographic correlates of cigarette smoking among high school students. *Canadian Journal of Public Health, 95*, 268–271.

Kaasalainen, S., & Crook, J. (2004). An exploration of seniors' ability to report pain. *Clinical Nursing Research, 13*, 199–215.

King, K. (2000). Gender and short-term recovery from cardiac surgery. *Nursing Research, 49*(1), 29–36.

King, K. M., LeBlanc, P. L., Sanguins, J., & Mather, C. (2006). Gender-based challenges faced by older Sikh women as immigrants: Recognizing and acting on the risk of coronary artery disease. *Canadian Journal of Nursing Research, 38*, 16–40.

Meininger, J. C., Hayman, L. L., Coates, P. M., & Gallagher, P. R. (1998). Genetic and environmental influences on cardiovascular disease risk factors in adolescents. *Nursing Research, 47*, 11–18.

Miles, M. B., & Huberman, A. M. (1994). *Qualitative data analysis: An expanded sourcebook* (2nd ed.). Thousand Oaks, CA: Sage.

Minore, B., Boone, M., & Hill, M. E. (2004). Finding temporary relief: Strategy for nursing recruitment in northern Aboriginal communities. *Canadian Journal of Nursing Research, 36*, 148–163.

Morse, J. M. (1994). Designing funded qualitative research. In N. K. Denzin & Y. S. Lincoln (Eds.), *Handbook of qualitative research* (pp. 220–235). Thousand Oaks, CA: Sage.

Patton, M. Q. (2003). *Qualitative evaluation checklist.* Retrieved September 24, 2007, from http://www.wmich.edu/evalctr/checklists/qec.pdf

Peterson, W., & DiCenso, A. (2002). A comparison of adolescent and adult mothers' satisfaction with their postpartum nursing care. *Canadian Journal of Nursing Research, 34*, 117–127.

Sandelowski, M. (1995). Sample size in qualitative research. *Research in Nursing & Health, 18*, 179–183.

Schoenfelder, D. P., & Rubenstein, L. M. (2004). An exercise program to improve fall-related outcomes in elderly nursing home residents. *Applied Nursing Research, 17*(1), 21–31.

Singh, M., & Cameron, J. (2005). Psychosocial aspects of caregiving to stroke patients. *AXON, 27*, 18–25.

Smith, D., Edwards, N., Varcoe, C., Martens, P. J., & Davies, B. (2006). Bringing safety and responsiveness into the forefront of care for pregnant and parenting Aboriginal people. *Advances in Nursing Science, 29*(2), E27–E44.

Sousa, V. D., Zauszniewski, J. A., & Musil, C. M. (2004). How to determine whether a convenience sample represents the population. *Applied Nursing Research, 17*, 130–133.

Then, K. L., Rankin, J. A., & Fofonoff, D. A. (2001). Atypical presentation of acute myocardial infarction in 3 age groups. *Heart & Lung, 30*, 285–293.

Tourangeau, A., Giovannetti, P., Tu, J., & Wood, M. (2002). Nursing-related determinants of 30-day mortality for hospitalized patients. *Canadian Journal of Nursing Research, 33*, 71–88.

Waltman, N. L., Twiss, J. J., Ott, C. D., Gross, G. J., Lindsey, A. M., Moore, T. E., et al. (2003). Testing an intervention for preventing osteoporosis in postmenopausal breast cancer survivors. *Journal of Nursing Scholarship, 35*, 333–338.

Wilmoth, M. C. (1995). Computer networks as a source of research subjects. *Western Journal of Nursing Research, 17*, 335–338.

Wuest, J., & Merritt-Gray, M. (2001). Beyond survival: Reclaiming self after leaving an abusive male partner. *Canadian Journal of Nursing Research, 32*(4), 79–94.

Wynd, C. A., Murrock, C. J., & Zeller, R. A. (2004). Health promotion and cardiovascular health in adult monozygotic twins. *Journal of Nursing Scholarship, 36*, 140–145.

Young, L., Siden, H., & Tredwell, S. (2007). Post-surgical telehealth support for children and family care-givers. *Journal of Telemedicine and Telecare, 13*, 15–19.

Robin Whittemore
Margaret Grey
Mina D. Singh

CHAPTER 13

Data Collection Methods

LEARNING OUTCOMES

After reading this chapter, the student should be able to do the following:

- Define the types of data collection methods used in nursing research.
- List the advantages and disadvantages of each of these methods.
- Compare how specific data collection methods contribute to the strength of evidence in a research study.
- Critically evaluate the data collection methods used in published nursing research studies.

STUDY RESOURCES

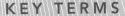 Go to Evolve at
http://evolve.elsevier.com/Canada/LoBiondo/Research/
for Weblinks, content updates, and additional
research articles for practice in reviewing
and critiquing.

KEY TERMS

biological measurement
close-ended item
concealment
consistency
content analysis
debriefing
external criticism
internal criticism
interrater reliability
intervention
intervention fidelity
interview
Likert-type scale
measurement
objective
open-ended item
operational definition
operationalization
physiological measurement
questionnaire
reactivity
records or available data
scale
scientific observation
social desirability
systematic

Nurses use all of their senses when collecting data from the clients to whom they provide care. Nurse researchers also have available many ways to collect information about their research subjects. Both the data collected when performing client care and the data collected for the purpose of research are objective and systematic. **Objective** means that the data must not be influenced by the person who collects the information. **Systematic** means that the data must be collected in the same way by each person involved in the collection procedure. The methods that researchers use to collect information about subjects are the identifiable and repeatable operations that define the major variables being studied.

Operationalization is the process of translating the concepts of interest to a researcher into observable and measurable phenomena. The same information may be collected in a number of ways. For example, a researcher interested in measuring blood pressure (BP) could measure it using an ambulatory BP monitor or an automated oscillometric BP monitor (Yucha, Yang, Tsai, & Calderon, 2003). The method chosen by the researcher would depend on a number of decisions regarding the problem being studied, the nature of the subjects, and the relative costs and benefits of each method.

This purpose of this chapter is to familiarize you with the various ways in which researchers collect information from and about subjects. The chapter provides nursing research consumers with the tools for evaluating the selection, utilization, and practicality of the various ways to collect data.

MEASURING VARIABLES OF INTEREST

To a large extent, the success of a study depends on the quality of the data collection methods chosen and employed. Researchers have many types of methods available for collecting information from subjects in research studies. Determining which **measurement** to use in a particular investigation may be the most difficult and time-consuming step in the study design. In addition, as nursing research develops, researchers are beginning to have available an array of quality instruments with adequate reliability and validity (see Chapter 14). This aspect of the research process demands painstaking effort from the researcher. Thus, the process of evaluating and selecting the available tools to measure variables of interest is of critical importance to the potential success of the study. In this section, the selection of measures and the implementation of the data collection process are discussed. An algorithm that influences a researcher's choice of data collection methods is diagrammed in the Critical Thinking Decision Path.

Information about phenomena of interest to nurses can be collected in many different ways. Nurses are interested in the biological and physical indicators of health (e.g., BP and heart rates), but they are also interested in complex psychosocial questions presented by clients. Psychosocial variables, such as anxiety, hope, social support, and self-concept, may be measured by several different techniques, such as observation of behaviour or self-reports of feelings or attitudes by means of interviews or questionnaires. To study variables of interest, researchers also may use data that have already been collected for another purpose, such as records, diaries, or other media.

The data collection method must be appropriate to the problem, the hypothesis, the setting, and the population. For example, Van Cleve et al. (2004) were interested in studying the pain experiences of children across multiple age groups. Because they were measuring children from ages 4 to 17 years, the same type of instrument could not be used. To deal with the reading and development levels of the children, they used tested age-appropriate instruments. For example, the children who were 4 to 13 years of age used the poker chip tool, in which the child chooses from one to four red chips to represent "a little bit" to "the most pain" the child can experience. The older children, however, used the adolescent pediatric pain tool, which uses words and graphics to rate the pain experience.

Selection of the data collection method begins during the literature review. As noted in Chapter 5,

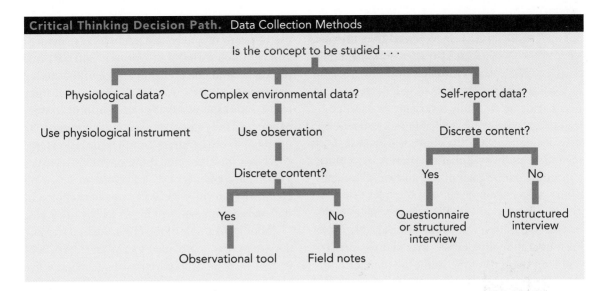

Critical Thinking Decision Path. Data Collection Methods

Is the concept to be studied . . .

- Physiological data?
  - Use physiological instrument
- Complex environmental data?
  - Use observation
    - Discrete content?
      - Yes
        - Observational tool
      - No
        - Field notes
- Self-report data?
  - Discrete content?
    - Yes
      - Questionnaire or structured interview
    - No
      - Unstructured interview

one purpose of the literature review is to provide clues to instrumentation. As the literature review is conducted, the researcher begins to explore how previous investigators defined and operationalized variables similar to those of interest in the current study. The researcher uses this information to define conceptually the variables to be studied. Once a variable has been defined conceptually, the researcher returns to the literature to define the variable operationally. This **operational definition** translates the conceptual definition into behaviours or verbalizations that can be measured for the study. In this second literature review, the researcher searches for measurement instruments that might be used "as is" or adapted for use in the study. If instruments are available, the researcher must obtain permission for their use from the author.

The following examples will illustrate the relationship of conceptual and operational definitions. Stress research is of interest to researchers from many disciplines, including nursing. Definitions of stressors may be psychological, social, or physiological. If a researcher is interested in studying stressors, the researcher must first define what he or she means by the concept of stressor, both conceptually and operationally. Quality of life research is popular with researchers from many disciplines,

including nursing. Definitions of quality of life may be related to health functioning, life satisfaction, or well-being.

Quality of life may also be interpreted in a general way (well-being) or be related specifically to a type of illness. Therefore, if a researcher is interested in studying quality of life, the researcher needs first to define what he or she means by the concept of quality of life. For example, Molzahn (2007) was interested in quality of life as it relates to spirituality in later life. The author wrote that this concept has many definitions but chose the World Health Organization's definition: "quality of life is the individuals' perception of their position in life in the context of the culture and value systems in which they live and in relation to their goals, expectations, standards and concerns" (as cited in Molzahn, 2007, p. 35). According to this conceptual definition, the researcher would use a quality of life instrument specifically for spirituality to determine the perceived quality of life of participants in the study. If another researcher disagreed with this definition or was more interested in the quality of life of people with a specific illness or the quality of life of children, a different instrument may be more appropriate.

Sometimes, no suitable measuring device exists, so the researcher must then decide how important the variable is to the study and whether a new device should be constructed. The construction of new instruments for data collection that have reasonable reliability and validity (see Chapter 14) is a difficult task. Sometimes, the researcher may decide not to study a variable if no suitable measuring device exists; at other times, the researcher may decide to invest time and energy in instrument development. Either decision is acceptable, depending on the goals of the study and the goals of the researcher.

Whether the researcher uses available methods or creates new ones, once the variables have been operationally defined in a manner consistent with the aims of the study, the population to be studied, and the setting, the researcher will decide how the data collection phase of the study will be implemented. This decision deals with how the instruments for data collection will be given to the subjects. Consistency is the most important issue in this phase.

Consistency refers to the state of data that are collected from each subject in the study in exactly the same way or as close to the same way as possible. Consistency can minimize the bias introduced when more than one person collects the data. Data collectors must be carefully trained and supervised. To ensure consistency in data collection, sometimes referred to as **intervention fidelity** (Santacroce, Maccarelli, & Grey, 2004), researchers must train data collectors in the methods to be used in the study so that each person collects the information in the same way. Information about how to observe, ask questions, and collect data often is included in a kind of "cookbook" protocol or manual for the research project. A researcher needs to spend time developing the protocol and training research assistants to collect data systematically and reliably. If data collectors are used, comments about their training and the consistency with which they collected data for the study should be provided by the researcher.

An example of intervention fidelity is provided by Ratner et al. (2004) in their study on the efficacy of a smoking cessation intervention for clients about to undergo elective surgery. The researchers used several ways to ensure fidelity: (a) structured and rigorous training of research staff; (b) role playing to evaluate the competence of the study's Registered Nurses (R.N.s); (c) checkouts every three to six months to assess the extent of drift in role-playing; (d) regular staff meetings to review the protocol and to address complex situations; (e) checklists for every timed intervention to ensure that all components of the intervention were covered; and (f) a video recording of an enactment of the intervention protocol for review by the R.N.s.

Another example of the importance of training data collectors is provided by Doran et al. (2006) in their study on data collection of nursing-sensitive outcomes in acute care and long-term care settings. These researchers needed to be accurate in their assessment of nursing-sensitive outcomes. Staff nurses were trained on how to collect data on client outcomes by research assistants using didactic content and case studies. Interrater reliability was assessed by having the research assistants conduct an independent assessment of three to five clients for each nurse over the six-month period of data collection. Agreement between raters was calculated using the kappa statistic. The index of agreement in this study ranged from .64 to .93, and the average percent agreement between rates was 86%, demonstrating a high level of interrater agreement between the two observers, nurses and research assistants. **Interrater reliability** (see Chapter 14) is the consistency of observations between two or more observers. It is often expressed as a percentage of agreement among raters or observers or as a coefficient of agreement that considers the element of chance (coefficient kappa).

Helpful Hint

Remember that the researcher may not always present complete information about the way the data were collected, especially when established tools were used. To learn about the tool that was used, the reader may need to consult the article that originally used the tool.

TYPES OF DATA COLLECTION METHODS

In general, data collection methods can be divided into the following five types: *physiological measurements, observational methods, interviews, questionnaires,* and *records* or *available data*. Each method has a specific purpose, as well as certain advantages and disadvantages inherent in its use. In the following sections, these data collection methods are discussed, as well as their respective uses and problems.

Physiological or Biological Measurements

In everyday practice, nurses collect physiological data about clients, such as their temperature, pulse rate, BP, blood glucose, urine-specific gravity, and pH of bodily fluids. Such data are frequently useful to nurse researchers. For example, Bryanton, Walsh, Barrett, and Gaudet (2004) compared the effects of tub bathing versus traditional sponge bathing in healthy, term newborns and their mothers' ratings in pleasure and confidence. The physiological variable of newborn temperature was one of the outcome variables and was measured by one route, the axillary route, for standardization. In studies that use physiological variables, such as cardiac output and BP, which can be measured in several different ways, researchers need to measure these outcomes at similar intervals and in similar ways for all participants of the study.

Physiological measurement and **biological measurement** involve the use of specialized equipment to determine the physical and biological status of subjects. Frequently, such measures also require specialized training. These measures can be *physical,* such as weight or temperature; *chemical,* such as blood glucose level; *microbiological,* as with cultures; or *anatomical,* as in radiological examinations. What separates these measurements from others used in research is that they require special equipment to make the observation. We can say, "This subject feels warm," but to determine how warm the subject is requires the use of a sensitive instrument, a thermometer.

Physiological or biological measurement is particularly suited to the study of several types of nursing problems. The Bryanton et al. (2004) example is typical of studies dealing with ways to improve the performance of certain nursing actions, such as the measuring and recording of clients' physiological data. Physiological measures may yield important criteria for determining the effectiveness of certain nursing interventions. In the study of the effect of types of bathing and newborns' temperatures, Bryanton et al. (2004) reported that tub-bathed infants had significantly less temperature loss than sponge-bathed infants.

The advantages of using physiological data collection methods include their objectivity, precision, and sensitivity. Such methods are generally considered to be objective because unless a technical malfunction occurs, two readings of the same instrument taken at the same time by two different nurses are likely to yield the same result. Because such instruments are intended to measure the variable being studied, they offer the advantage of being precise and sensitive enough to pick up subtle variations in the variable of interest. Also, the deliberate distortion of physiological information by a subject in a study is highly unlikely.

Physiological measurements are not without inherent disadvantages, however. Some instruments, if not available through a hospital, may be quite expensive to obtain and use. In addition, such instruments often require specialized knowledge and training to be used accurately. Another problem with physiological measurements is that simply by using them, the variable of interest may be changed. Although some researchers think of these instruments as being nonintrusive, the presence of some types of devices might change the measurement. For example, the presence of a heart rate monitoring device might make some clients anxious and increase their heart rate. In addition, nearly all types of measuring devices are affected in some way by the environment. Even a simple thermometer can be affected by the subject drinking something hot immediately before the temperature is taken. Thus, research consumers need to consider whether the researcher controlled such environmental variables in the study. Finally, a physiological way to measure the variable of interest may not exist. Occasionally, researchers try to force a physiological parameter into a study in an effort to increase the precision of measurement. If the device does not measure the variable of interest, however, the validity of the device's use is suspect.

Observational Methods

Sometimes, nurse researchers are interested in determining how subjects behave under specific conditions. For example, the researcher might be interested in how children respond to painful situations. We might ask children how painful an experience was, but they may not be able to answer the question or to quantify the amount of pain, or they may distort their responses to please the researcher. Therefore, sometimes observing the subject may give a more accurate picture of the behaviour in question than asking the client.

Although observing the environment is a normal part of living, scientific observation places a great deal of emphasis on the objective and systematic nature of the observation. The researcher is not merely watching what is happening but is watching with a trained eye for certain specific events. To be scientific, observations must fulfill the following four conditions:

1. The observations undertaken are consistent with the study's specific objectives.

2. A standardized and systematic plan exists for the observation and the recording of data.

3. All of the observations are checked and controlled.

4. The observations are related to scientific concepts and theories.

Observation is particularly suitable as a data collection method in complex research situations that are best viewed as total entities and that are difficult to measure in parts, such as studies dealing with the nursing process, parent–child interactions, or group processes. In addition, observational methods can be the best way to operationalize some variables of interest in nursing research studies, particularly individual characteristics and conditions, such as traits and symptoms; verbal and nonverbal communication behaviours, activities and skill attainment; and environmental characteristics.

For example, Billinghurst, Morgan, and Arthur (2003) conducted a prospective, observational study to explore the client- and nurse-related implications of remote cardiac telemetry. Research assistants arrived unannounced at the coronary respiratory care unit to observe and document the actual number of arrhythmia events during each study block of time. In addition, the telemetry nurses' responses to the alarms were observed and documented. Remote telemetry data were collected by two experienced coronary care nurses. The findings revealed that nurses detected 60% to 100% of valid warning arrhythmias and that approximately 80% of the remote telemetry warning arrhythmias were artifact. The researchers suggested that remote cardiac telemetry without a dedicated monitor watcher places an unnecessary demand on the unit nurses' time because of the large percentage of inconsequential alarms.

Observational methods can also be distinguished by the role of the observer. This role is determined by the amount of interaction between the observer and those being observed. Each of the following four basic types of observational roles is distinguishable by the amount of concealment or intervention implemented by the observer:

1. Concealment without intervention

2. Concealment with intervention

3. No concealment without intervention

4. No concealment with intervention

These methods are illustrated in Figure 13–1; examples are given later. Concealment refers to

		Concealment	
		Yes	No
Intervention	Yes	Researcher hidden An intervention	Researcher open An intervention
	No	Researcher hidden No intervention	Researcher open No intervention

Figure 13–1 Types of observational roles in research

whether the subjects know they are being observed, and **intervention** deals with whether the observer provokes actions from those who are being observed.

The study by Bryan (2000) of the effect on parent–child interactions of an education program to promote expectant couples' transition to parenthood is an excellent example of no concealment with intervention. The researcher was not concealed in postnatal observations of parent–child teaching interactions and, if necessary, provided information on how the parents could improve their interactions with their infants after the observations.

When a researcher is concerned that the subjects' behaviour will change as a result of being observed (reactivity), the type of observation most commonly employed is that of concealment without intervention. In this case, the researcher watches the subjects without their knowledge of the observation and does not provoke them into action. Often, such concealed observations use hidden television cameras, audiotapes, or one-way mirrors. Concealment without intervention is often used in observational studies of children. You may be familiar with rooms with one-way mirrors through which a researcher can observe the behaviour of the occupants of the room without being observed by them. Such studies allow the observation of children's natural behaviour and are often used in developmental research.

No concealment without intervention also is commonly used for observational studies. In this case, the researcher obtains informed consent from the subject to be observed and then simply observes the subject's behaviour. Steele (2002) used

this type of observation in her study, in which she observed the interactions of families with a child who had a neurodegenerative, life-threatening illness.

Observing subjects without their knowledge may violate assumptions of informed consent; therefore, researchers face ethical problems with this type of approach. However, sometimes, researchers have no other way to collect such data, and the data collected are unlikely to have negative consequences for the subject. In these cases, the disadvantages of the study are outweighed by the advantages. Further, the problem of consent is often handled by informing subjects after the observation and allowing them the opportunity to refuse to have their data included in the study and to discuss any questions they might have. This process is called **debriefing**.

When the observer is neither concealed nor intervening, the ethical question is not a problem. Here, the observer makes no attempt to change the subjects' behaviour and informs them that they are to be observed. Because the observer is present, this type of observation allows a greater depth of material to be studied than if the observer is separated from the subjects by an artificial barrier, such as a one-way mirror. Participant observation is a commonly used observational technique in which the researcher functions as part of a social group to study the group in question. The problem with this type of observation is **reactivity** (also referred to as the Hawthorne effect; see Chapter 9), or the distortion created when the subjects change behaviour because they are being observed.

In her study, Steele (2002) used unconcealed observation because the parents had given full consent for participation in the study. No concealment with intervention is employed when the researcher is observing the effects of an intervention introduced for scientific purposes. Because the subjects know they are participating in a research study, few problems with ethical concerns occur, but reactivity is a problem with this type of study.

Concealed observation with intervention involves staging a situation and observing the behaviours that are evoked in the subjects as a result of the intervention. Because the subjects are unaware of their participation in a research study, this type of observation has fallen into disfavour and is rarely used in nursing research.

Observational methods may be structured or unstructured. Unstructured observational methods, such as those suggested by West, Bondy, and Hutchinson (1991) for working with older adults, are not characterized by a total absence of structure but usually involve collecting descriptive information about the topic of interest. In unstructured observations, the observer keeps field notes that record the activities, as well as the observer's interpretations of these activities. Field notes are usually not restricted to any particular type of action or behaviour; rather, they intend to paint a picture of a social situation in a more general sense.

Another type of unstructured observation is the use of anecdotes. Despite popular usage of the term, anecdotes are not necessarily funny but usually focus on the behaviours of interest and frequently add to the richness of research reports by illustrating a particular point. In the study by Smith, Edwards, Varcoe, Martens, and Davies (2006) (see Appendix B), interviews were conducted, and field notes were made and incorporated into the data set of this very innovative exploration of the topic.

In contrast, structured observations, such as the standardized tools used to evaluate mother–infant interaction in the Koniak-Griffin et al. (2003) study, require formal training and the competence of the evaluators. The use of structured observations without a standardized tool involves specifying in advance what behaviours or events are to be observed and preparing forms for record keeping, such as categorization systems, checklists, and rating scales. Whichever system is employed, the observer watches the subject and then marks on the recording form what was seen. In both cases, the observations must be similar among the observers (see the earlier discussion and Chapter 14 for an explanation of interrater reliability). Thus, observers need to be trained to be consistent in their observations and ratings of behaviour.

Evidence-Based Practice Tip

When reading a research report that uses observation as a data collection method, the research consumer wants to note evidence of consistency across data collectors through use of internal consistency reliability data. When that evidence is present, the research consumer has greater confidence that the data were collected systematically.

Scientific observation has several advantages as a data collection method. The main advantage is that observation may be the only way for the researcher to study the variable of interest. For example, what people say they do often is not what they really do. Therefore, if the study is designed to obtain substantive findings about human behaviour, observation may be the only way to ensure the validity of the findings. In addition, no other data collection method can match the depth and variety of information that can be collected when using the techniques of scientific observation. Such techniques also are flexible so that they may be used in both experimental and nonexperimental designs and in laboratory and field studies.

Helpful Hint

Sometimes, a researcher may carefully train observers or data collectors, but the research report does not address this training. Often, the length of research reports dictates that certain information cannot be included. Readers can often assume that if reliability data are provided, then appropriate training occurred.

As with all data collection methods, observation also has its disadvantages. Earlier in this chapter, the problems of reactivity and ethical concerns were mentioned with respect to the dimensions of concealment and intervention. In addition to these problems, data obtained by observational techniques are vulnerable to the bias of the observer. Emotions, prejudices, and values can influence the way that behaviours and events are observed. In general, the more the observer needs to make inferences and judgements about what is being observed, the more likely it is that distortions will occur. Thus, in judging the adequacy of observational methods, the research consumer needs to consider how observational tools were constructed and how observers were trained and evaluated.

Interviews and Questionnaires

Subjects in a research study often have information that is important to the study and that can be obtained only by asking the subjects. Such questions may be asked through the use of interviews and questionnaires. Both have the purpose of asking subjects to report data for themselves, but each method has unique advantages and disadvantages. The **interview** is a method of data collection in which a data collector questions a subject verbally. Interviews may be face to face or performed over the telephone and may consist of open-ended or close-ended questions. In contrast, the **questionnaire** is a paper-and-pencil instrument designed to gather data from individuals about knowledge, attitudes, beliefs, and feelings. Survey research relies almost entirely on questioning subjects with either interviews or questionnaires, but these methods of data collection also can be used in other types of research.

No matter what type of study is conducted, the purpose of questioning subjects is to seek information. This information may be of either direct interest, such as the subject's age, or indirect interest, such as when the researcher uses a combination of items to estimate the degree to which the respondent has a particular trait or characteristic. An intelligence test is an example of how individual items are combined with several others to develop an overall scale of intelligence. When items of indirect interest are combined to obtain an overall score, the measurement tool is called a **scale**.

The investigator determines the content of an interview or questionnaire from the literature review (see Chapter 5). When evaluating interviews and questionnaires, the reader should consider the content of the scale, the individual items, and the order of the items. The basic standard for evaluating the individual items in an interview or questionnaire is that the item must be clearly written so that the intention of the question and the nature of the information sought are clear to the respondent. The only way to know whether the questions are understandable to the respondents is to pilot-test them in a similar population. It is also critical not to rely on only the instrument developer's reports of reliability and validity (see Chapter 14). A pilot test allows researchers to test the reliability and validity for their unique sample rather than relying only on previously reported results.

Although items must ask only one question, be free of suggestions, and use correct grammar, they may be either open-ended or close-ended. An **open-ended item** is used when the researcher wants the subjects to respond in their own words or when the researcher does not know all of the possible alternative responses. A **close-ended item** is used with a fixed number of alternative responses. Many scales use a fixed-response format called a Likert-type scale. A **Likert-type scale** is a list of statements on which respondents indicate, for example, whether they "strongly agree," "agree," "disagree," or "strongly disagree." Sometimes, finer distinctions are given, or a neutral category may be provided. The use of the neutral category, however, sometimes creates problems because it is often the most frequent response and is difficult to interpret. Fixed-response items also can be used for questions requiring a "yes" or "no" response or when the interview or questionnaire has categories, as with income.

Structured, fixed-response items are best used when the question has a finite number of responses and the respondent is to choose the option closest to the right response. Fixed-response items have the advantage of simplifying the respondent's task and the researcher's analysis, but they may miss some important information about the subject. Sword, Watt, and Kreuger (2006) used self-reported fixed-response items via a structured telephone interview in their study on postpartum health, service needs, and access to care experiences of immigrant and Canadian-born women. Unstructured response formats allow such information to be included but require a special technique to analyze the responses. This technique, called **content analysis**, is a method for the objective, systematic, and quantitative description of communications and documentary evidence.

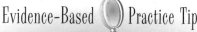

Evidence-Based Practice Tip

Scales used in nursing research should have evidence of adequate reliability and validity so that research consumers feel confident that the findings reflect what the researcher intended to measure
(see Chapter 14).

Figure 13–2 shows a few items from a fictional survey of pediatric nurse practitioners. The first items are taken from a list of similar items, and they are both closed and of a Likert-type format. Note that respondents are asked to choose how strongly they agree with each item. In using these questions in the survey, respondents are forced to choose from only these answers because it is thought that these will be the only responses. The only possible alternative response is to skip the item, leaving it blank.

Sometimes, researchers have no idea or have only a limited idea of what the respondent will say, or researchers want the answer in the respondent's own words, as with the second (open-ended) set of items. Here, respondents may also leave the item blank but are not forced to make a particular response.

Interviews and questionnaires are commonly used in nursing research. Both are strong approaches to gathering information for research because they approach the task directly. In addition, both have the ability to obtain certain kinds of information, such as the subjects' attitudes and beliefs, which would be difficult to obtain without asking the subject directly.

All methods that involve verbal reports, however, share a problem with accuracy. Often, it is impossible to know whether what the researcher is told is indeed true. For example, people are known to respond to questions in a way that makes a favourable impression. This response style is

known as **social desirability**, which can be regarded as resulting from two factors: self-deception and other-deception.

Neyerhof (2006) discussed the two main modes of coping with social desirability bias. The first mode consists of two methods aimed at the detection and measurement of social desirability bias: the use of social desirability scales and the rating of item desirability. The second mode consists of the following methods to prevent or reduce social desirability bias: forced-choice items, the randomized response technique, the bogus pipeline, self-administration of the questionnaire, the selection of interviewers, and the use of proxy subjects. Neyerhof found that no one method excelled completely and suggested that a combination of prevention and detection methods is the best strategy to reduce social desirability bias.

Questionnaires and interviews also have some specific purposes, advantages, and disadvantages. Questionnaires are useful tools when the purpose is to collect information. If questionnaires are too long, however, they are not likely to be completed. Questionnaires and paper-and-pencil tests are most useful when the set of questions to be asked is finite and the researcher can be assured of the clarity and specificity of the items. Face-to-face techniques or interviews are best used when the researcher may need to clarify the task for the respondent or is interested in obtaining more personal information from the respondent. Telephone interviews allow the researcher to reach more respondents than face-to-face interviews and provide more clarity than questionnaires.

Helpful Hint

Remember, sometimes researchers make trade-offs when determining the measures to be used. For example, if a researcher wants to learn about an individual's attitudes regarding practice, and practicalities preclude using an interview, a questionnaire may be used instead.

Koniak-Griffin et al. (2003) used a combination of interview, questionnaire, and observational

Close-Ended (Likert-Type Scale)

A. How satisfied are you with your current position?

  1. Very satisfied
  2. Moderately satisfied
  3. Undecided
  4. Moderately dissatisfied
  5. Very dissatisfied

B. To what extent do the following factors contribute to your current level of positive satisfaction?

	Not at all	Very little	Somewhat	Moderate amount	A great deal
1. % of time in client care	1	2	3	4	5
2. Types of clients	1	2	3	4	5
3. % of time in educational activity	1	2	3	4	5
4. % of time in administration	1	2	3	4	5

Close-Ended

A. On average, how many clients do you see in one day?

  1. 1 to 3
  2. 4 to 6
  3. 7 to 9
  4. 10 to 12
  5. 13 to 15
  6. 16 to 18
  7. 19 to 20
  8. More than 20

B. How would you characterize your practice?

  1. Too slow
  2. Slow
  3. About right
  4. Busy
  5. Too busy

Open-Ended

A. Are there incentives that the National Association of Pediatric Nurse Associates and Practitioners ought to provide for members that are currently not being provided?

_____

_____

_____

_____

Figure 13–2 Examples of close-ended and open-ended questions

data collection methods to study the effects of an early intervention program for pregnant adolescents on infant and mother outcomes. Interviews by trained public health nurses assessed maternal health behaviours, complications of pregnancy, substance use, community resource use, employment status, and infant health status. In addition, questionnaires were administered to participants to evaluate social competence. Lastly, mother–infant interactions during a play episode were videotaped and evaluated using a structured observation method. Thus, the researchers were able to evaluate both infant and mother outcomes. This use of multiple measures gives a more complete picture than the use of just one measure.

When determining whether to use interviews or questionnaires, researchers face difficult choices. The final decision is often based on the instruments available and their relative costs and benefits.

Both face-to-face and telephone interviews offer some advantages over questionnaires. All things being equal, interviews are better than questionnaires because the response rate is almost always higher, which helps eliminate bias in the sample (see Chapter 12). Respondents seem to be less likely to hang up the telephone or to close the door in an interviewer's face than to throw away a questionnaire. Another advantage of the interview is that some people, such as children, people with visual impairments, and people who are illiterate, cannot fill out a questionnaire but can participate in an interview. With an interview, the data collector knows who is giving the answers. When questionnaires are mailed, for example, anyone in the household could be the person who supplies the answers.

Interviews also allow for some safeguards to be built into the interview situation. Interviewers can clarify misunderstood questions and observe the level of the respondent's understanding and co-operativeness. In addition, the researcher has strict control over the order of the questions. With questionnaires, the respondent can answer questions in any order. Sometimes, changing the order of the questions can change the response.

Finally, interviews allow for richer and more complex data to be collected, particularly when open-ended responses are sought. Vallianatos et al. (2006) used open-ended questions in their audio-taped interviews to study the beliefs and practices of First Nations women regarding weight gain during pregnancy. The interviews were done on an individual basis in the participants' homes and in community centres.

Even when close-ended response items are used, interviews can probe to understand why a respondent answered in a particular way. Interviews can also be conducted in a group setting, which is called a focus group interview. Beanlands, McCay, and Landeen (2006) used semi-structured interview schedules to guide focus group discussions to explore loss of self between individuals with early schizophrenia and individuals with chronic kidney disease. These small-group interviews allow the participants to freely explain and share information individually and collectively. Agreement and disagreement among participants may be elicited, which allows the researchers to obtain specific information from a number of subjects efficiently and simultaneously.

Questionnaires are much less expensive to administer than interviews because interviews may require the hiring and training of interviewers. Thus, if a researcher has a fixed amount of time and money, a larger and more diverse sample can be obtained with questionnaires. Questionnaires also provide complete anonymity, which may be important if the study deals with sensitive issues. Finally, the fact that no interviewer is present assures the researcher and the reader that no interviewer bias will occur. Interviewer bias occurs when the interviewer unwittingly leads the respondent to answer in a certain way. This problem is especially pronounced in studies that use unstructured interview formats. A subtle nod of the head, for example, could lead a respondent to change an answer to correspond with what the researcher wants to hear.

Questionnaires were employed by Starzomski and Hilton (2000) to collect data on client and family adjustment to kidney transplantation with and without an interim period of dialysis. To reach a large sample, questionnaires are mailed to save on time and the labour costs of interviewing. Armstrong-Stassen and Cameron (2005) mailed questionnaires to 3000 community health nurses randomly selected from the College of Nurses of Ontario to investigate the work-related concerns, job satisfaction, and factors influencing the retention of community health nurses. The questionnaire packets contained a cover letter from the researchers, an informed consent form, a questionnaire booklet, and a reply envelope.

Records or Available Data

All of the data collection methods discussed thus far concern the ways that nurse researchers gather new data to study phenomena of interest. Not all studies, however, require a researcher to acquire new information. Sometimes, existing information can be examined in a new way to study a problem. The use of records and available data is sometimes considered to be primarily the concern of historical research, but hospital records, care plans, and existing data sources (e.g., the census) are frequently used for collecting information. What sets these studies apart from a literature review is that these available data are examined in a new way and not merely summarized; they also answer specific research questions.

Records or available data, then, are forms of information that are collected from existing materials, such as hospital records, historical documents, or videotapes, and are used to answer research questions in a new manner. For example, most of the data analyzed in a study by Rhèaume (2003) on the changing division of labour between nurses and nursing assistants in New Brunswick consisted of archival material from three nursing organizations: the Canadian Nurses Association, the Nurses Association of New Brunswick, and the New Brunswick Nurses Union. These data covered the years 1978 to 1990 and consisted of minutes from meetings, internal memos and notes, internal reports, speeches from the leaders of these organizations, and correspondence.

The use of available data has certain advantages. Because the data collection step of the research process is often the most difficult and time-consuming, the use of available records often means a significant saving of time. If the records have been kept in a similar manner over time, analysis of these records allows examination of trends over time. In addition, the use of available data decreases problems of reactivity and response set bias. The researcher also does not have to ask individuals to participate in the study.

However, institutions are sometimes reluctant to allow researchers access to their records. If the records are kept so that an individual cannot be identified, access for research purposes is usually not a problem. Also, the *Privacy Act*, a federal law, protects the rights of individuals who may be identified in records, thus anonymity would be violated.

One problem that affects the quality of available data occurs when the researcher has access to only the records that have survived. If the records available are not representative of all of the possible records, the researcher may have a problem with bias. Often, because researchers have no way to tell whether the records have been saved in a biased manner, they need to make an intelligent guess as to their accuracy. For example, a researcher might be interested in studying socioeconomic factors associated with the suicide rate. These data frequently are underreported because of the stigma attached to suicide, so the records would be biased. Recent interest in computerization of health records has led to an increase in the discussion about the desirability of access to such records for research. At this point, how much of such data will continue to be readily available for research without consent is unclear.

Another problem is related to the authenticity of the records. The distinction of primary and secondary sources is as relevant here as it was in the discussion of the literature review to determine the source of the work (see Chapter 5). A book, for example, may have been ghost-written, but all credit was accorded to the known author. The researcher may have a difficult time ferreting out these subtle types of biases.

Lastly, existing records may have a significant amount of missing data. For example, years of education may be recorded on only a portion of the sample records.

Nonetheless, records and available data constitute a rich source of data for study. Schnelle et al.

(2003), in their study to evaluate a standardized protocol to assess and score urinary incontinence in nursing homes, used available data in the form of existing medical records, which contained histories of the clients' illnesses.

ONLINE AND COMPUTERIZED METHODS OF DATA COLLECTION

With the fast-paced progression of the Internet and computer technology, many researchers are using computerized data collection. The information obtained can be quantitative or qualitative, close-ended or open-ended. This method of data collection can be in the form of Web-based surveys or the use of microcomputers directly inputting the data.

Many online survey tools, such as Survey Monkey® or QuestionPro®, are available; a survey can be loaded quickly and the results obtained for a small fee. The advantages of this method are that it is anonymous and low cost; respondents can do the survey in their own time; a large number of participants can be accessed; respondent time is reduced; data collection time is reduced; duplicate responses can be identified; and, for the researcher, implementation is time efficient. The disadvantages are that not everyone has access to a computer or is computer literate, the response rates may be low, and a high amount of data may be missing.

Computerized data collection can be accomplished through the use of personal digital assistants (PDAs). Researchers can input their data directly into these hand-held microcomputers. The data can then be transferred to a larger computer for analysis.

Evidence-Based Practice Tip

A critical evaluation of any data collection method includes evaluating the appropriateness, objectivity, and consistency of the method employed.

CONSTRUCTION OF NEW INSTRUMENTS

As already mentioned in this chapter, researchers sometimes cannot locate an existing instrument or method with acceptable reliability and validity to measure the variable of interest. This situation is often the case when testing part of a nursing theory or when evaluating the effect of a clinical intervention. An example is provided by Gillis (1997), who developed and tested an instrument to measure adolescent lifestyle. The instrument was used to assess lifestyle patterns for identification of health education and counselling priorities (see Chapter 14).

Instrument development is complex and time-consuming, however. It consists of the following steps:

- Defining the construct to be measured
- Formulating the items (questions)
- Assessing the items for content validity
- Developing instructions for respondents and users
- Pretesting and pilot testing the items
- Estimating reliability and validity

To define the construct (concepts at a higher level of abstraction) to be measured requires that the researcher develop an expertise in the construct, which requires an extensive review of the literature and of all tests and measurements that deal with related constructs. The researcher will use all of this information to synthesize the available knowledge so that the construct can be defined.

Once defined, the individual items measuring the construct can be developed. The researcher will develop many more items than are needed to address each aspect of the construct or subconstruct. A panel of experts in the field evaluates the items so that the researcher is assured that the items measure what they are intended to measure (content validity; see Chapter 14). Eventually, the number of items will be decreased because some items will not work as intended and will be dropped. In this phase, the researcher needs to ensure consistency both among the items and in testing and scoring procedures.

Finally, the researcher administers or pilot-tests the new instrument by giving it to a group of people who are similar to those who will be studied in the larger investigation. The purpose of this analysis is to determine the quality of the instrument as a whole (reliability and validity) and the ability of each item to discriminate individual respondents (variance in item response). The researcher also may administer a related instrument to see whether the new instrument is sufficiently different from the older one.

It is important that researchers who invest significant time in tool development publish their results. For example, Goulet, Lampron, Marcil, and Ross (2003) were interested in understanding the attitudes of Quebec's adolescents about breastfeeding and how others influence their opinions. From their literature review, the researchers determined that no suitable instrument was available to measure this concept. The authors devised their own instru-

ment based on the Theory of Reasoned Action. To ensure reliability and validity, they engaged in the following steps: (a) a panel composed of lactation consultants and nurse researchers reviewed the items for content validity; (b) pilot testing was done prior to the full study to ensure ease of administration, clarity, and precision of the instrument; (c) a factor analysis was done to determine clusters of variables linked to form a construct; and (d) reliability analysis produced Cronbach's alpha between .71 and .70 for different parts of the instrument. This type of research serves not only to introduce other researchers to the tool but also to ultimately enhance the field because our ability to conduct meaningful research is limited only by our ability to measure important phenomena.

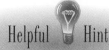

Helpful Hint

Determine whether a newly developed paper-and-pencil test was pilot-tested to obtain preliminary evidence of reliability and validity.

Critiquing Data Collection Methods

Evaluating the adequacy of data collection methods from written research reports is often problematic for new nursing research consumers. Because the tool itself is not available for inspection, the reader may not feel comfortable judging the adequacy of the method without seeing it. However, the reader can ask questions to judge the method chosen by the researcher. These questions are listed in the Critiquing Criteria box.

All studies should have clearly identified data collection methods. The conceptual and operational definitions of each important variable should be present in the report. Sometimes, it is useful for the researcher to explain why a particular method was chosen. For example, if the study dealt with young children, the researcher may explain that a questionnaire was deemed to be an unreasonable task, so an interview was chosen.

Once you have identified the method chosen to measure each variable of interest, you should decide whether the method used was the best way to measure the variable. If a questionnaire was used, for example, you might wonder why the decision was made not to use an interview. In addition, consider whether the method was appropriate to the clinical situation. Does it make sense to interview clients in the recovery room, for example?

Once you have decided whether all relevant variables are operationalized appropriately, you can begin to determine how well the method was carried out. For studies using physiological measurement, determine whether the instrument was appropriate to the problem and not forced to fit it. The rationale for selecting a particular instrument should be given. For example, it may be important to know that the study was conducted under the auspices of a manufacturing

CRITIQUING CRITERIA

1. Is the framework for research clearly identified?

DATA COLLECTION METHODS

1. Are all of the data collection instruments clearly identified and described?
2. Is the rationale for their selection given?
3. Is the method used appropriate to the problem being studied?
4. Were the methods used appropriate to the clinical situation?
5. Are the data collection procedures similar for all subjects?
6. Were efforts made to ensure intervention fidelity through the data collection protocol?

PHYSIOLOGICAL MEASUREMENT

1. Is the instrument used appropriate to the research problem and not forced to fit it?
2. Is a rationale given for why a particular instrument was selected?
3. Is there a provision for evaluating the accuracy of the instrument and the skill of those who used it?

OBSERVATIONAL METHODS

1. Who did the observing?
2. Were the observers trained to minimize any bias?
3. Was an observational guide provided?
4. Were the observers required to make inferences about what they saw?
5. Is there any reason to believe that the presence of the observers affected the behaviour of the subjects?
6. Were the observations performed using the principles of informed consent?

INTERVIEWS

1. Is the interview schedule described adequately enough to know whether it covers the subject?
2. Is it clear that the subjects understood the task and the questions?
3. Who were the interviewers, and how were they trained?
4. Is any interviewer bias evident?

QUESTIONNAIRES

1. Is the questionnaire described well enough to know whether it covers the subject?
2. Is evidence provided that subjects were able to perform the task?
3. Is it clear that the subjects understood the questionnaire?
4. Are the majority of the items appropriately close- or open-ended?

AVAILABLE DATA AND RECORDS

1. Are the records used appropriate to the problem being studied?
2. Are the data examined in such a way as to provide new information and not summarize the records?
3. Has the author addressed questions of internal and external criticism?
4. Is there any indication of selection bias in the available records?

firm that provided the measuring instrument. In addition, provision should be made to evaluate the accuracy of the instrument and the skill level of those who used it.

Several considerations are important when reading studies that use observational methods. Who were the observers, and how were they trained? Is there any reason to believe that different observers saw events or behaviours differently? Remember that the more inferences the observers are required to make, the more likely it is that problems with biased observations will occur. Also, consider the problem of reactivity: in any observational situation, the possibility exists that the mere presence of the observer will change the behaviour in question. What is important here is not that reactivity could occur but the extent to which reactivity could affect the data. Finally, consider whether the observational procedure was ethical. You need to consider whether the subjects were informed that they were being observed, whether any intervention was performed, and whether the subjects had agreed to be observed.

Interviews and questionnaires should be clearly described to allow the reader to decide whether the variables were adequately operationalized. Sometimes, the researcher will reference the original report about the tool, and you may wish to read this study before deciding whether the method was appropriate for the present study. Also, the respondents' task should be clear. Thus, provision should have been made for the subjects to understand both their overall responsibilities and the individual items of the interview or questionnaire. The following questions must be considered: Who were the interviewers in the interview situation? Does the researcher explain how they were trained to decrease any interviewer bias?

Available data, such as medical records, are subject to internal and external criticism. **Internal criticism deals with the evaluation of the worth of the records and primarily refers to the accuracy of the data.** The researcher should present evidence that the records are genuine. **External criticism** is concerned with the authenticity of the records. Are the records really written by the first author? The researcher may not have an unbiased sample of all of the possible records in the problem area, which may have a profound effect on the validity of the results.

Once you have decided that the data collection method used was appropriate to the problem and the procedures were appropriate to the population studied, the reliability and validity of the instruments themselves need to be considered. These characteristics are discussed in Chapter 14.

Critical Thinking Challenges

- Physiological measurements are objective, precise, and sensitive. Discuss factors that might influence their validity and feasibility.
- A student in research class asks why nurses who participate in a clinical research study in the role of a data collector or who perform a "treatment intervention" need to be trained. What important factors or rationale would you offer to support the establishment of interrater reliability?
- Observational methods are a frequent data collection method in nursing research. Discuss the factors that make nurses perfect potential candidates for this role and the disadvantages of using this method.
- Studies often use a survey to collect data. How can researchers increase their return rate for the survey, and how do they determine whether the survey return is adequate?

KEY POINTS

- Data collection methods are described as being both objective and systematic. The data collection methods of a study provide the operational definitions of the relevant variables.

- Types of data collection methods include physiological measurements, observational methods, interviews, questionnaires, and available data or records. Each method has advantages and disadvantages.

- Physiological measurements are those methods that use technical instruments to collect data about clients' physical, chemical, microbiological, or anatomical status. These methods are suited to studying how to improve the effectiveness of nursing care. Physiological measurements are objective, precise, and sensitive, but they may be very expensive and may distort the variable of interest.

- Observational methods are used in nursing research when the variables of interest deal with events or behaviours. Scientific observation requires preplanning, systematic recording, controlling the observations, and determing the relationship to scientific theory. This method is best suited to research problems that are difficult to view as part of a whole. Observers may be passive or active and concealed or obvious.

- Observational methods have several advantages: (1) they provide flexibility to measure many types of situations and (2) they enable a great depth and breadth of information to be collected.

- Observation has disadvantages as well: (1) data may be distorted as a result of the observer's presence (reactivity), (2) concealment requires the consideration of ethical issues, and (3) observations may be biased by the person who is doing the observing.

- Interviews are commonly used data collection methods in nursing research. Items on interview schedules may be of direct or indirect interest. Either open-ended or close-ended questions may be used when asking subjects questions. The form of the question should be clear to the respondent, free of suggestion, and grammatically correct.

- Questionnaires, or paper-and-pencil tests, are useful when a finite number of questions will be asked. The questions need to be clear and specific. Questionnaires are less costly in time and money to administer to large groups of subjects, particularly if the subjects are geographically widespread. Questionnaires also can be completely anonymous and prevent interviewer bias.

- Interviews are best used when a large response rate and an unbiased sample are important because the refusal rate for interviews is much less than that for questionnaires. Interviews allow for the participation of portions of the population, such as children and people who are illiterate, for whom the use of a questionnaire would otherwise prevent their involvment. An interviewer can clarify and maintain the order of the questions for all participants.

- Records and available data also are an important source of research data. The use of available data may save the researcher considerable time and money when conducting a study. This method reduces problems with both reactivity and ethical concerns. However, records and available data are subject to problems of availability, authenticity, and accuracy.

- A critical evaluation of data collection methods should emphasize the appropriateness, objectivity, and consistency of the method employed.

REFERENCES

Armstrong-Stassen, M., & Cameron, S. (2005). Concerns, satisfaction, and retention of Canadian community health nurses. *Journal of Community Health Nursing, 22*, 181–194.

Beanlands, H., McCay, E., & Landeen, J. (2006). Strategies for moving beyond the illness in early schizophrenia and in chronic kidney disease. *Canadian Journal of Nursing Research, 38*, 10–30.

Billinghurst, F., Morgan, B., & Arthur, H. M. (2003). Patient and nurse-related implications of remote cardiac telemetry. *Clinical Nursing Research, 12*, 356–370.

Bryan, A. A. (2000). Enhancing parent-child interaction with a prenatal couple intervention. *MCN: The American Journal of Maternal/Child Nursing, 25*, 139–144.

Bryanton, J., Walsh, D., Barrett, M., & Gaudet, D. (2004). Tub bathing versus traditional sponge bathing for the newborn. *Journal of Obstetric, Gynecologic, and Neonatal Nursing, 33*, 704–712.

Doran, D. M., Harrison, M. B., Laschinger, H. S., Hirdes, J. P., Rukholm, E., Sidani, S., et al. (2006). Nursing-sensitive outcomes data collection in acute care and long-term-care settings. *Nursing Research, 55*(2S), S75–S81.

Gillis, A. J. (1997). The adolescent lifestyle questionnaire: Development and psychometric testing. *Canadian Journal of Nursing Research, 29*, 29–46.

Goulet, C., Lampron, A., Marcil, I., & Ross, L. (2003). Attitudes and subjective norms of male and female adolescents toward breastfeeding. *Journal of Human Lactation, 19*, 402–410.

Koniak-Griffin, D., Verzemnieks, I. L., Anderson, N. L. R., Brecht, M., Lesser, J., Kim, S. et al. (2003). Nurse visitation for adolescent mothers. *Nursing Research, 52*, 127–136.

Molzahn, A. E. (January 2007). Spirituality in later life: Effect on quality of life. *Journal of Gerontological Nursing, 15*(1), 32–39.

Neyerhof, A. J. (2006). Methods of coping with social desirability bias: A review. *European Journal of Psychology, 15*, 263–280.

Ratner, P. A., Johnson, J. L., Richardson, C. G., Bottorff, J. L., Moffatt, B., Mackay, M., et al. (2004). Efficacy of a smoking-cessation intervention for elective-surgical patients. *Research in Nursing & Health, 27*, 148–161.

Rhèaume, A. (2003). The changing division of labour between nurses and nursing assistants in New Brunswick. *Journal of Advanced Nursing, 41*, 435–443.

Santacroce, S. J., Maccarelli, L. M., & Grey, M. (2004). Intervention fidelity. *Nursing Research 53*, 63–66.

Schnelle, J. F., Cadogan, M. P., Grbic, D., Bates-Jensen, B. M., Osterweil, D., Yoshii, J., et al. (2003). A standardized quality assessment system to evaluate incontinence in the nursing home. *Journal of American Geriatric Society, 51*, 1754–1761.

Smith, D., Edwards, N., Varcoe, C., Martens, P. J., & Davies, B. (2006). Bringing safety and responsiveness into the forefront of care for pregnant and parenting Aboriginal people. *Advances in Nursing Science, 29*(2), E27–E44.

Starzomski, R., & Hilton, A. (2000). Patient and family adjustment to kidney transplantation with and without an interim period of dialysis. *Nephrology Nursing Journal, 27*(1), 17–32.

Steele, R. (2002). Experiences of families in which a child has a prolonged terminal illness: Modifying factors. *International Journal of Palliative Nursing, 8*, 418–433.

Sword, W., Watt, S., & Kreuger, P. (2006). Postpartum health, service needs, and access to care experiences of immigrant and Canadian-born women. *JOGNN, 35*(6), 717–727.

Vallianatos, H., Brennand, E. A., Raine, K., Stephen, Q., Petawabano, B., Dannenbaum, D., et al. (2006). Beliefs and practices of First Nation women about weight gain during pregnancy and lactation: Implications for women's health. *Canadian Journal of Nursing Research, 38*, 102–119.

Van Cleve, L., Bossert, E., Beecroft, P., Adlard, K., Alvarez, O., & Savedra, M. C. (2004). The pain experience of children with leukemia during the first year after diagnosis. *Nursing Research, 53*, 1–10.

West, M., Bondy, E., & Hutchinson, S. (1991). Interviewing institutionalized elders: Threats to validity. *Image, 23*, 171–176.

Yucha, C. B., Yang, M. C. K., Tsai, P. S., & Calderon, K. S. (2003). Comparison of blood pressure measurement consistency using tonometric and oscillometric instruments. *Journal of Nursing Measurement, 11*, 73–86.

Geri LoBiondo-Wood

Judith Haber

Mina D. Singh

CHAPTER 14

Rigour in Research

LEARNING OUTCOMES

After reading this chapter, the student should be able to do the following:

- Discuss the purposes of reliability and validity.
- Define reliability.
- Discuss the concepts of stability, equivalence, and homogeneity as they relate to reliability.
- Compare the estimates of reliability.
- Define validity.
- Compare content, criterion-related, and construct validity.
- Discuss how measurement error can affect the outcomes of a research study.
- Discuss the purpose of credibility, auditability, and fittingness.
- Identify the criteria for critiquing the reliability and validity of measurement tools.
- Use the critiquing criteria to evaluate the reliability and validity of measurement tools.
- Discuss how evidence related to research rigour contributes to clinical decision making.

STUDY RESOURCES

KEY TERMS

alpha coefficient

alternate form reliability

auditability

chance error

concurrent validity

constant error

construct validity

content validity

contrasted-groups approach

convergent validity

credibility

criterion-related validity

Cronbach's alpha

divergent validity

equivalence

error variance

face validity

factor analysis

fittingness

homogeneity

hypothesis-testing approach

internal consistency

interrater reliability

item-to-total correlation

kappa

known-groups approach

Kuder–Richardson (KR-20) coefficient

multitrait–multi-method approach

observed test score

parallel form reliability

predictive validity

random error

reliability

reliability coefficient

rigour

split-half reliability

stability

systematic error

test–retest reliability

validation sample

validity

In both quantitative and qualitative research, the purpose is to collect trustworthy data that can be used for analyses to make generalizations about the population and that are transferable to other groups. Because findings need to be generalizable and transferable, measurement of nursing phenomena is a major concern of nursing researchers, and **rigour** is strived for. Rigour refers to the quality, believability, or trustworthiness of the study findings. Rigour in quantitative research is determined by measurement instruments that validly and reliably reflect the concepts of the theory being tested, so that conclusions drawn from a study will be valid and will advance the development of nursing theory and evidence-based practice. Thus, psychometric assessments are designed to obtain evidence of the quality of these instruments, that is, their reliability and validity.

Issues of reliability and validity are of central concern to the researcher, as well as the critiquer of research. From either perspective, the measurement instruments that are used in a research study must be evaluated. Many new constructs are relevant to nursing theory, and a growing number of established measurement instruments are available to researchers. However, researchers often face the challenge of developing new instruments and, as part of that process, establishing the reliability and validity of those tools.

In qualitative research, rigour is ascertained by credibility, auditability, and fittingness. The growing importance of measurement issues, tool development, and related issues (e.g., reliability and validity, qualitative rigour) is evident in issues of the *Journal of Nursing Measurement*, *Canadian Journal of Nursing Research*, *International Journal of Qualitative Methods*, and other nursing research journals. In this chapter, concepts related to quantitative rigour are discussed first, followed by factors that contribute to the trustworthiness of qualitative research.

When reading quantitative research studies and reports, the critiquer of research must assess the reliability and validity of the instruments used in each study to determine the soundness of the selection of these instruments in relation to the concepts or variables under investigation. The appropriateness of the instruments and the extent to which reliability and validity are demonstrated have a profound influence on the findings and the internal and external validity of the study. Invalid measures produce invalid estimates of the relationships between variables, thus affecting internal validity. The use of invalid measures also produces inaccurate generalizations to the populations being studied, thus affecting external validity and the ability to apply or not apply research findings in clinical practice. As such, the assessment of reliability and validity is an extremely important skill for critiquers of nursing research to develop.

Regardless of whether a new or already developed measurement tool is used in a research study, evidence of reliability and validity is of crucial importance. Box 14–1 identifies several computer resources that research consumers can use to access and evaluate the reliability and validity of the measurement instruments used in research studies.

RELIABILITY, VALIDITY, AND MEASUREMENT ERROR

Reliability

Reliable people are those whose behaviour is consistent and predictable. Likewise, the **reliability** of a research instrument is defined as the extent to which the instrument yields the same results on repeated measures. Reliability, then, is concerned with consistency, accuracy, precision, stability, equivalence, and homogeneity. Concurrent with questions of validity, or after these questions are answered, the researcher and the critiquer ask how reliable the instrument is.

A reliable measure can produce the same results if the behaviour is measured again by the same scale. Reliability, then, refers to the proportion of accuracy to inaccuracy in measurement. In other words, if we use the same or comparable instruments on more than one occasion to measure behaviours that ordinarily remain relatively constant, we would expect similar results if the tools are reliable.

The three main attributes of a reliable scale are stability, homogeneity, and equivalence. The stability of an instrument refers to the instrument's ability to produce the same results with repeated testing. The homogeneity of an instrument means that all of the items in a tool measure the same concept or characteristic. An instrument is said to exhibit equivalence if the tool produces the same results when equivalent or parallel instruments or procedures are used. Each of these attributes and the means to estimate them are discussed here. Before these are discussed, however, an understanding of how to interpret reliability is essential.

Interpretation of the Reliability Coefficient

Because all of the attributes of reliability are concerned with the degree of consistency between scores that is obtained at two or more independent times of testing, these attributes often are expressed in terms of a correlation coefficient. The **reliability coefficient**, which expresses the relationship between the error variance, true variance, and the observed score, ranges from 0 to 1. A zero correlation indicates no relationship. When the error variance in a measurement instrument is low, the reliability coefficient will be closer to 1. The closer to 1 the coefficient is, the more reliable the tool is. For example, a reliability coefficient of a tool is reported to be .89. This number indicates that the error variance is small and the tool has little measurement error. But if the reliability coefficient of a measure is reported to be .49, the error variance is high, and the tool has a problem with measurement error. For a tool to be considered reliable, a level of .70 or higher should be reported, although the intended purpose of the instrument needs to be considered if lower levels are accepted.

The interpretation of the reliability coefficient (also called the **alpha coefficient**) depends on the proposed purpose of the measure. Seven major tests of reliability can be used to calculate a reliability coefficient, depending on the nature of the tool. They are known as *test–retest reliability, parallel or alternate form reliability, item-to-total correlation, split-half reliability, Kuder–Richardson (KR-20) coefficient, Cronbach's alpha,* and *interrater reliability.*

These tests are discussed as they relate to the attributes of stability, homogeneity, and equivalence (see Box 14–2). The critiquer should be aware that no single best way exists to assess reliability in relation to these attributes and that the researcher's method should be consistent with the aim of the research.

Stability

An instrument is thought to be stable or to exhibit **stability** when the same results are obtained on repeated administration of the instrument. Researchers are concerned with an instrument's stability because they expect the instrument to measure a concept consistently over a period of time. Measurement over time is important when an instrument is used in a longitudinal study and therefore will be used on several occasions. Stability is also a consideration when a researcher is conducting an intervention study that is designed to effect a change in a specific variable. In this case, the instrument is administered once and then again after the alteration or change intervention has been completed. The tests that are used to estimate stability are test–retest and parallel or alternate form reliability.

TEST–RETEST RELIABILITY

Test–retest reliability is the administration of the same instrument to the same subjects under similar conditions on two or more occasions. Scores from repeated testing are compared. This comparison is expressed by a correlation coefficient, usually a Pearson r (see Chapter 16). The interval between repeated administrations varies and depends on the concept or variable being measured. For example, if the variable that the test measures is related to developmental stages in children, the interval between tests should be short. The amount of time over which the variable was measured should also be recorded in the report.

An example of an instrument that was assessed for test–retest reliability is the Multidimensional Fatigue Inventory (MFI) (Filion, Gélinas, Simard, Savard, & Gagnon, 2003). The MFI had been previously developed and tested for reliability and validity in various languages, including English and Dutch. Filion et al. conducted a study to examine the reliability and validity of the French Canadian adaptation of the MFI for clients undergoing therapy for breast or prostate cancer. The concept of test–retest reliability is illustrated by the researchers calculating test–retest coefficients to estimate temporal stability on two occasions: week 2 and week 4 of radiation treatment. The correlations were .51 for mental fatigue, .63 for reduced activity, .68 for reduced motivation, .78 for general and physical fatigue, and .83 for the total MFI score. In this case, the interval was adequate (two weeks between testing), and some of the coefficients were under .70 to be adequate (Nunnally & Bernstein, 1994). The researchers explained their results by stating, "considering both that the MFI is a situational measure in which a certain amount of individual variation is to be expected . . . and that a normal increase of fatigue for most patients during the course of radiation treatment also can be expected, these are strong results" (p. 149).

PARALLEL OR ALTERNATE FORM RELIABILITY

Parallel form reliability, or **alternate form reliability**, is applicable and can be tested only if two comparable forms of the same instrument exist. Parallel form reliability is like test–retest reliability in that the same individuals are tested within a specific

---

BOX 14–2   Measures Used to Test Reliability

STABILITY

Test–retest reliability
Parallel or alternate form reliability

HOMOGENEITY

Item-to-total correlation
Split-half reliability
Kuder–Richardson coefficient
Cronbach's alpha

EQUIVALENCE

Parallel or alternate form reliability
Interrater reliability

interval, but in parallel form reliability, a different form of the same test is given to the subjects on the second testing. Parallel forms or tests contain the same types of items that are based on the same domain or concept, but the wording of the items is different. The development of parallel forms is desired if the instrument is intended to measure a variable for which a researcher believes that "test-wiseness" will be a problem.

For example, the pilot study "Breast Cancer: Education, Counseling, and Adjustment" (Hoskins et al., 2001) examined the differential effect of a phase-specific standardized educational video intervention in comparison with a telephone counselling intervention on the physical, emotional, and social adjustment of women with breast cancer and their partners. The use of repeated measures over the four data collection points—coping with the diagnosis, recovering from surgery, understanding adjuvant therapy, and ongoing recovery—made it appropriate to use two alternate forms of the Partner Relationship Inventory (Hoskins, 1988) to measure emotional adjustment in partners. An item on one scale ("I am able to tell my partner how I feel") is consistent with the paired item on the second form ("My partner tries to understand my feelings").

Practically speaking, developing alternate forms of an instrument is difficult because of the many issues of reliability and validity. If alternate forms of a test exist, they should be highly correlated if the measures are to be considered reliable.

Helpful Hint

When a longitudinal design with multiple data collection points is being conducted, look for evidence of test–retest or parallel form reliability.

Homogeneity or Internal Consistency

Another attribute related to reliability of an instrument is the **homogeneity** or **internal consistency** with which the items within the scale reflect or measure the same concept. In other words, the items within the scale correlate or are complementary to each other, and the scale is *unidimensional*. A unidimensional scale measures one concept, such as exercise self-efficacy. A total score is then used in the analysis of data.

When the California Critical Thinking Disposition Inventory (Profetto-McGrath, 2003) was tested for homogeneity, the testing of the instrument revealed an alpha coefficient of .91. Because the alpha was above .70, it provided sufficient evidence for supporting the internal consistency of the instrument. Homogeneity can be assessed by using one of four methods: item-to-total correlations, split-half reliability, Kuder–Richardson (KR-20) coefficient, or Cronbach's alpha.

Helpful Hint

When the characteristics of a study sample differ significantly from the sample in the original study, check to see whether the researcher has re-established the reliability of the instrument with the current sample.

ITEM-TO-TOTAL CORRELATION

The **item-to-total correlation** measures the relationship between each of the items and the total scale. When item-to-total correlations are calculated, a correlation for each item on the scale is generated (see Table 14–1). Items that do not achieve a high correlation may be deleted from the instrument. Usually, in a research study, all of the item-to-total correlations are not reported unless the study is a report of a methodological study. The lowest and highest correlations are typically reported. An example of an item-to-total correlation report is illustrated in the study by McGilton et al. (2005). In that study, the item-to-total correlations ranged between .4 and .7, and the majority of items had interitem correlations above .50. According to Nunnally and Bernstein (1994), these results are acceptable because the criterion is greater than .3.

SPLIT-HALF RELIABILITY

Split-half reliability involves dividing a scale into two halves and making a comparison. The halves

TABLE 14–1	Examples of Item-to-Total Correlations from Computer-Generated Data
Item	**Item-to-Total Correlation**
1	.5069
2	.4355
3	.4479
4	.4369
5	.4213
6	.4216

may be odd-numbered and even-numbered items or a simple division of the first from the second half, or items may be randomly selected into halves that will be analyzed opposite one another. Split-half reliability provides a measure of consistency in terms of sampling the content. The two halves of the test or the contents in both halves are assumed to be comparable, and a reliability coefficient is calculated. If the scores for the two halves are approximately equal, the test may be considered reliable.

The Spearman–Brown formula is one method used to calculate the reliability coefficient. In a study testing the Worry Interference Scale (WIS), a seven-item self-report measure was developed to assess the degree to which thoughts about breast cancer are perceived as interfering with the respondent's daily functioning. The measure is embedded within a larger questionnaire that also assesses perceived risk, intention to undergo genetic testing, and frequency of worry about getting breast cancer. The WIS scale items assess disruptions in sleep, work, concentration, relationships, having fun, feeling sexually attractive, meeting family needs, and reproductive decisions. Ibrahim (2002) computed a Spearman–Brown split-half reliability and found a reliability coefficient that ranged from .83 to .92 for the first four items and from .75 to .83 for the other items. Split-half reliabilities of at least .75 are considered internally consistent.

KUDER–RICHARDSON (KR-20) COEFFICIENT

The **Kuder–Richardson (KR-20) coefficient** is the estimate of homogeneity used for instruments that have a *dichotomous response format*. A dichotomous response format is one in which the question asks for a "yes/no" or "true/false" response. The technique yields a correlation that is based on the consistency of responses to all items of a single form of a test that is administered once.

For example, in a study investigating the effectiveness of a randomized support group intervention for women with breast cancer, breast cancer knowledge was assessed with a 25-item true/false scale developed for the study. Items were obtained from the American Cancer Society's publication *Cancer Facts and Figures* and comprised the following categories: knowledge of risk factors for developing breast cancer (10 items, e.g., "Most women diagnosed with breast cancer have at least one known risk factor for the disease"); symptoms of breast cancer (5 items, e.g., "Women who have breast cancer never experience any symptoms of the disease"); side effects of treatment (3 items, e.g., "A common side effect of radiation is sunburn-like symptoms"); treatment efficacy (4 items, e.g., "For women with small tumors that may not have spread outside the breast, having either a mastectomy or lumpectomy with axillary lymph node dissection results in the same overall life expectancy"); and methods of treatment (3 items, e.g., "Hormone treatment is used only for premenopausal women"). Because the scale was a binary format (true/false), Kuder–Richardson reliability for the entire scale was calculated at .75, which is acceptable, having exceeded the minimum acceptable KR-20 score of .70; however, the magnitude of the correlation is not robust.

CRONBACH'S ALPHA

The fourth and most commonly used test of internal consistency is **Cronbach's alpha**. Many tools used to measure psychosocial variables and attitudes have a Likert scale response format, which is very suitable for testing internal consistency. A Likert scale format asks the subject to respond to a question on a scale of varying degrees of intensity between two extremes. The two extremes are anchored by responses ranging from "strongly agree" to "strongly disagree" or "most like me" to "least like me." The points between the two extremes

The health care professional takes your likes and dislikes into account when she/he is providing care.	Never 1	Seldom 2	Occasionally 3	Often 4	Always 5
The health care professional tries to meet your needs, for example, in such ways as listening to you if you need someone to talk to or comforting you when something bad or unexpected happens.	Never 1	Seldom 2	Occasionally 3	Often 4	Always 5
The health care professional knows you well enough to recognize when you are happy, sad, mad, or stressed about something.	Never 1	Seldom 2	Occasionally 3	Often 4	Always 5
You can depend on the health care professional when you ask for help and know that she/he will do what she/he promises to do.	Never 1	Seldom 2	Occasionally 3	Often 4	Always 5
The health care professional tries to make your day go the way you like and helps you with any unexpected changes.	Never 1	Seldom 2	Occasionally 3	Often 4	Always 5
The health care professional tolerates your being frustrated or irritable without responding negatively in return.	Never 1	Seldom 2	Occasionally 3	Often 4	Always 5

Figure 14–1 Examples of a Likert scale

Adapted from McGilton, K. S., Pringle, D. M., O'Brien-Pallas, L. L., Wynn, F., & Streiner, D. (2005). Development and psychometric testing of the Relational Care Scale. *Journal of Nursing Measurement, 13*(1), 51–57. Reprinted with permission.

may range from 1 to 5 or 1 to 7. Subjects are asked to circle the response closest to how they feel.

Figure 14–1 provides examples of items from a tool that uses a Likert scale format. Cronbach's alpha simultaneously compares each item in the scale with the others. A total score is then used in the analysis of data. The School-Age Temperament Inventory (SATI) (McClowry, Halverson, and Sanson, 2003) was tested for internal consistency and construct validity. The testing of the instrument revealed alpha coefficients that ranged from .80 to .92 for the four dimensions or constructs, which supported internal consistency data from the original SATI reliability studies, as illustrated in Table 14–2. Because the alphas were above .70, they provided sufficient evidence for supporting the internal consistency of the instrument. Examples of reported Cronbach's alpha are shown in Box 14–3.

Equivalence

Equivalence is either the consistency or agreement among observers using the same measurement tool or the consistency or agreement between alternate forms of a tool. An instrument is thought to

TABLE 14–2 Cronbach's Alpha of the SATI Dimensions				
Dimensions	**Original**	**Sample 1**	**Sample 2**	**Sample 3**
Negative reactivity	.90	.89	.90	.92
Task persistence	.90	.89	.91	.92
Approach/withdrawal	.88	.84	.86	.92
Activity	.85	.80	.86	.92

SATI: School-Age Temperament Inventory.

BOX 14–3   Examples of Reported Cronbach's Alpha

- "The 11-item scale yielded a Cronbach's alpha level of .64 for girls and .76 for boys" (Dahinten, 2003, p. 61).

- "The measure indicated good internal consistency ($\alpha = .86$) and moderate test–retest reliability two weeks apart ($r = .69$)" (McGilton et al., 2003, p. 153).

- "The Cronbach's alphas for the entire Relational Care Scale were .86 ($n = 50$) with residents from sample 2 and .88 ($n = 72$) with residents from sample 3" (McGilton, Pringle, O'Brien-Pallas, Wynn, & Streiner, 2005, p. 58).

- "The Cronbach's alpha coefficients of the MDS (Minimum Data Set) functional status scale indicated very good reliability at admission and discharge in acute care (.91 and .88, respectively) and long-term care (.94 and .92, respectively)" (Doran et al., 2006, p. S78).

Helpful Hint

If a research article provides information about the reliability of a measurement instrument but does not specify the type of reliability, it is probably safe to assume that internal consistency reliability was assessed using Cronbach's alpha.

demonstrate equivalence when two or more observers have a high percentage of agreement of an observed behaviour or when alternate forms of a test yield a high correlation. Two methods to test equivalence are interrater reliability and alternate or parallel form reliability.

INTERRATER RELIABILITY

Some measurement instruments are not self-administered questionnaires but are direct measurements of observed behaviour that must be systematically recorded. Such instruments must be tested for **interrater reliability**. To accomplish interrator reliability, either two or more individuals should make an observation or one observer should observe the behaviour on several occasions. The observers should be either trained in or oriented to the definition and operationalization of the behaviour to be observed.

When the research method of direct observation of a behaviour is required, consistency, or reliability, of the observations among all observers is extremely important. Interrater reliability tests the reliability, or consistency, of the observer, not the reliability of the instrument. Interrator reliability is expressed either as a percentage of agreement between scorers or as a correlation coefficient of the scores assigned to the observed behaviours.

In their study, Resnick, Nahm, Orwig, Zimmerman, and Magaziner (2001) established interrater reliability for the step activity monitor (SAM), a step counter developed for a wide variety of gait styles (ranging from a slow shuffle, such as a Parkinsonian-type gait, to a fast run) and used to measure activity in older adults. The authors noted that other tools available to assess activity or exercise in older adults are generally self-report instruments that provide researchers or nurses with the individual's perception of the amount of activity performed, not an objective accounting. In contrast, the SAM provides objective information about step activity (the total number of steps taken over a period of time).

Participants in the study ($N = 30$) were recruited from the outpatient office in a continuing care retirement community. They were asked to walk at their own speed on a carpeted level surface for one minute, rest for two minutes, and then ambulate over the same path for another minute. Two observers, observing at the same time, counted steps during both episodes of ambulation. The two observers, both advanced practice nurses, had prior experience in observational gait assessment of older adults and step counting.

Interrater reliability was based on intraclass correlations of the two separate one-minute readings of the SAM done two minutes apart. Statistically significant correlations of .80 or greater between the mean of the two observers and the results of the SAM at each testing interval (calculating the average deviation between the SAM and the mean of the two observers) produced an interrater reliability estimate of .98, indicating a high level of agreement between observers. According to Santacroce, Maccarelli, and Grey (2004), consistency in observation or intervention delivery is key to concluding that the evidence provided by the study findings is valid and reliable.

Another type of interrater reliability is Cohen's kappa, a coefficient of agreement between two raters that is considered to be a more precise estimate of interrater reliability. **Kappa** expresses the level of agreement that is observed beyond the level that would be expected by chance alone. A kappa of .08 or better is generally taken to indicate good interrater reliability. A kappa of .68 allows tentative conclusions to be drawn when lower levels are accepted (McDowell & Newell, 1996). McGilton, O'Brien-Pallas, Darlington, Evans, Wynn and Pringle (2003) evaluated interrater reliability and obtained coefficients of .80, .80, and .83, in the development of the Relational Behaviour Scale.

Evidence-Based ⊘ Practice Tip

Interrater reliability is an important approach to minimizing bias.

PARALLEL OR ALTERNATE FORM

Parallel or alternate form reliability was described in the discussion of stability (see pages 300–301). Use of parallel forms, then, is a measure of stability and equivalence. The procedures for assessing equivalence using parallel forms are the same.

VALIDITY

Validity refers to whether a measurement instrument accurately measures what it is intended to measure. To be valid, an instrument must first be reliable. Reliability is a necessary but not sufficient condition for validity. Without reliability, the instrument cannot have validity. Note that the study must also have validity, which is discussed in Chapter 9 under internal and external validity.

For example, a valid instrument that is intended to measure anxiety does so; it does not measure another construct, such as stress. A reliable measure can consistently rank participants on a given

construct (e.g., anxiety), but a valid measure correctly measures the construct of interest. A measure can be reliable but not valid. Let us say that a researcher wanted to measure anxiety in clients by measuring their body temperatures. The researcher could obtain highly accurate, consistent, and precise temperature recordings, but such a measure would not be a valid indicator of anxiety. Thus, the high reliability of an instrument is not necessarily congruent with evidence of validity. A valid instrument, however, is reliable. An instrument cannot validly measure the attribute of interest if it is erratic, inconsistent, and inaccurate.

The three major kinds of validity—content, criterion-related, and construct validity—vary according to the kind of information provided and the investigator's purpose. A critiquer of research articles will want to evaluate whether sufficient evidence of validity is present and whether the type of validity is appropriate to the design of the study and instruments used in the study. The sample that provides the initial data for determining the reliability and validity of a measurement tool is termed a **validation sample**.

Evidence-Based ⊘ Practice Tip

Selecting measurement instruments that have strong evidence of validity increases the reader's confidence in the study findings—that the researchers actually measured what they intended to measure.

Content Validity

Content validity represents the universe of content, or the domain of a given construct. The universe of content provides the framework and basis for formulating the items that will adequately represent the content. When an investigator is developing a tool and issues of content validity arise, the concern is whether the measurement tool and the items it contains are representative of the content domain that the researcher intends to measure. The researcher begins by defining the concept and identifying the dimensions that are the components of the concept. The items that reflect the concept and its dimensions are formulated.

When the researcher has completed this task, the items are submitted to a panel of judges considered to be experts on this concept. Researchers typically request that the judges indicate their agreement with the scope of the items and the extent to which the items reflect the concept under consideration.

For example, Gillis (1997) engaged in the development and psychometric testing of an instrument designed to measure healthy lifestyle in adolescents in eastern Canada, the Adolescent Lifestyle Questionnaire (ALQ). Two categories of healthy lifestyle were identified: health-promoting and health-protecting behaviours. Items were developed through a qualitative research study using an inductive approach and a review of the literature. The pilot questionnaire was composed of "66 items in seven categories: physical participation, nutrition, safety, social support, health awareness, stress management, and identity awareness" (Gillis, 1997, p. 34). Eight nurses who had specialized knowledge of adolescent health promotion assessed content validity. The items were rated by four of these nurses using four criteria: readability, cultural relevance, age appropriateness of behaviours, and conceptual congruence of the items with the concept of healthy lifestyle. The remaining four nurses classified the items according to seven categories, and if the agreement in the placement was 75% or greater, the items were kept. Items were added, deleted, and modified based on the review of the panel, resulting in 56 items.

A subtype of content validity is **face validity**, which is a rudimentary type of validity that verifies that the instrument gives the appearance of measuring the concept. It is an intuitive type of validity in which colleagues or subjects are asked to read the instrument and evaluate the content in terms of whether it appears to reflect the concept the researcher intends to measure. This procedure may be useful in the tool development process in terms of determining the readability and clarity of the content. Face validity should in no way, however, be considered a satisfactory alternative to other types of validity. In the development of the ALQ (Gillis, 1997), the concept of healthy lifestyle was derived from qualitative interviews with adolescents. The scale comprised two subscales: health-promoting and health-protecting behaviours. Face validity, in addition to content validity, was developed by having the panel of eight nurses review the items for clarity and relevance.

Evidence-Based 🔍 Practice Tip

When face validity and content validity, the most basic types of validity, are the only types of validity reported in a research article, the research consumer cannot appraise the measurement tools as having strong psychometric properties, indicating a lack of confidence about the study findings.

Criterion-Related Validity

Criterion-related validity indicates the degree of relationship between the subject's performance on the measurement tool and the subject's actual behaviour. The criterion is usually the second measure, which assesses the same concept under study.

Two forms of criterion-related validity are concurrent and predictive. **Concurrent validity** refers to the degree of correlation of two measures of the same construct administered at the same time. A high correlation coefficient indicates agreement between the two measures. **Predictive validity** refers to the degree of correlation between the measure of the concept and a future measure of the same concept. Because of the passage of time, the correlation coefficients are likely to be lower for predictive validity studies.

McGilton et al. (2005) evaluated the concurrent validity of the newly developed Relational Care Scale (RCS) with the Relational Behaviour Scale (RBS) because both scales are based on the empathic and reliable behaviours of care providers and on Winnicott's relational theory. In addition, the RCS was assessed with the Relationship Visual Analogue Scale (RVAS). The results indicated that the RCS was positively correlated with the RVAS, $r = .63$, $p < .0001$ ($n = 50$), and the RBS was positively moderately correlated with the RCS, $r = .42$, $p < .001$ ($n = 72$).

An example of predictive validity is provided by Dennis (2003), who developed a short form of the Breastfeeding Self-Efficacy Scale (BSES-SF), which measures the self-confidence of mothers in breastfeeding. The researcher assessed the predictive validity of this scale by correlating the mothers' scores with their method of infant feeding at four and eight months postpartum because infant feeding was determined to be a strong and objective comparison criterion.

Construct Validity

Construct validity refers to the extent to which a test measures a theoretical construct or trait. This type of validity attempts to validate a body of theory underlying the measurement and testing of the hypothesized relationships. Empirical testing confirms or fails to confirm the relationships that would be predicted among concepts and, as such, provides more or less support for the construct validity of the instruments measuring those concepts. Establishing construct validity is a complex process, often involving several studies and approaches. The following approaches are discussed in this section: hypothesis-testing, convergent and divergent, contrasted-groups, and factor analytical.

HYPOTHESIS-TESTING APPROACH

When the **hypothesis-testing approach** is used, the investigator uses the theory or concept underlying the measurement instrument to validate the instrument. The investigator accomplishes this task by first developing hypotheses regarding the behaviour of individuals with varying scores on the measure; then gathering data to test the hypotheses; and finally, on the basis of the findings, by making inferences about whether the rationale underlying the instrument's construction is adequate to explain the findings.

For example, Barnason, Zimmerman, Atwood, Nieveen, and Schmaderer (2002) used a hypothesis-testing approach to establish the construct validity of the Barnason Efficacy Expectation Scale

(BEES). Construct validity was tested based on the empirically supported hypothesis that individuals with better health status and functioning also would have higher levels of self-efficacy. To explore this hypothesis, correlations were made between the BEES total score and physiological behaviours of interest in a population of clients who had received a coronary artery bypass graft. Measures of physiological functioning used in this psychometric study were subscales of the Medical Outcomes Study Short-Form 36 (MOS SF-36), which has been used extensively in the literature as a measure of health status and functioning with established reliability and validity. The MOS SF-36 is a multidimensional scale measuring health concepts. However, in this study, the physiological functioning subscales of physical functioning, role-physical functioning (role limitations due to physical problems), and general health were specifically used because those aspects of functioning were more closely related to the behaviours measured by the BEES.

The BEES mean score was correlated with aspects of physiological functioning (physical, role-physical, and general health), with significant weak to moderate correlations ranging from $r = .25$ to .41. These findings provide support for the hypothesis and therefore preliminary support for the theoretical basis, conceptual accuracy, and construct validity of the BEES in the client population: individuals with better health status have higher levels of self-efficacy. The homogeneous nature of the sample and the use of a convenience sampling strategy, however, suggest the need for further testing of the BEES with adults from various age, gender, socioeconomic, and cultural groups.

CONVERGENT AND DIVERGENT APPROACHES

Two strategies for assessing construct validity are convergent and divergent approaches.

Convergent validity exists when two or more tools that are intended to measure the same construct are administered to subjects and are found to positively correlate. A correlational analysis (i.e., a test of relationship; see Chapters 11 and 16) determines whether the measures are positively correlated, in which case convergent validity is said to be supported.

Powers, Zentner, Nelson, and Bergstrom (2004) evaluated the convergent validity of one of the most widely used tools for predicting pressure sore risk, the Braden Scale's mobility subscale (Braden & Bergstrom, 1994). Client immobility had been identified as an important risk factor for the development of pressure sores, and the mobility subscale of the Braden Scale was designed to quantify levels of mobility, based on individual clinical observations.

To assess convergent validity, actigraphy (a noninvasive method of monitoring rest and activity cycles) was used to measure a client's frequency of movement. The researchers hypothesized that participants scoring low (i.e., a score of 1) on the mobility subscale would have a lower mean frequency of movement recorded by actigraphy than participants with higher scores. They further hypothesized that as the mobility subscale scores increased, the mean frequency of the movements recorded by actigraphy would also increase.

Two consecutive data collection periods, from 6 A.M. to 6 P.M. in a 48-hour interval, were chosen for analysis. The researchers found that only spontaneous client movement was noted in the data analysis of the actigraph recordings. The statistically significant difference in the mean activity by subscale groups $[F(3,15) = 31.69; p = .001]$ supported the hypothesis that as the mean activity in each group increased, the mean frequency of the movements recorded by actigraphy would also increase, and the greatest amount of activity occurred in the group with the highest scores. The researchers also found that the mean activity of participants assessed at mobility subscale level 4 (no mobility limitations) was significantly greater than the activity of participants in the other three levels, which supported the convergent validity of the mobility subscale of the Braden Scale.

More recently, causal modelling has been used to develop and test a hypothesized explanation of causes of a phenomenon, and to establish convergent validity, as in the development of the Caregiver Reciprocity Scale (CRS) by Carruth (1996). As illustrated in Table 14–3, several indicators have been recommended to assess convergent validity: standardized item loadings, item/composite reliability, examination of standard error (SE), and estimated average variance, as extracted by each construct.

The item loadings indicate the extent to which a single variable is related to the cluster of variables; for example, in Table 14–3, under the cluster of variables for *warmth and regard*, item #30 has a loading of .82, which is closer to the composite reliability of .89, and thus is more related to the cluster than item #2, which has a loading of .52. Item reliability is the reliability of that item within that subscale; for example, in Table 14–3, the reliability for item #4 on the subscale *love and affection* is .60, whereas the reliability for the subscale of *love and affection* with the four items is .88. Average variance is the amount of variance explained by a cluster of variables in that construct; for example, of the four subscales, *love and affection* has the highest estimate, .64. SE is the standard deviation divided by the sample size. Table 14–3 presents data indicating significant findings between the CRS factor structure and the relevant causal modelling indicators, thereby offering support for the convergent validity of the items in each factor of the CRS.

In contrast to convergent validity, **divergent validity** uses measurement approaches that differentiate one construct from others that may be similar. Sometimes, researchers search for instruments that measure the opposite of the construct. If the divergent measure is negatively related to other measures, the measure's validity is strengthened.

McGilton et al. (2003) assessed the divergent validity of the RBS, which consisted of three subscales related to the empathic and reliable relational behaviours of care providers to older adults. More positive care provider behaviour was illustrated by higher scores on the RBS. The researchers hypothesized that the scale would correlate negatively to a negative affect scale. This hypothesis was

TABLE 14–3 **Estimated LISREL Parameters of Construct Validity**				
Construct	Standardized Loadings	Item/Composite Reliability	2 × SE	Variance Extracted Estimate
Warmth and regard				
		.89*		.48
#2	.52	.27	—†	
#10	.70	.48	.40	
#12	.76	.58	.42	
#21	.60	.35	.37	
#22	.71	.51	.40	
#25	.67	.45	.39	
#28	.70	.49	.40	
#30	.82	.66	.43	
#33	.74	.54	.41	
Intrinsic rewards of giving				
		.83*		.49
#1	.62	.38	—†	
#13	.64	.40	.29	
#17	.74	.55	.30	
#29	.76	.60	.30	
#32	.74	.55	.30	
Love and affection				
		.88*		.64
#4	.77	.60	—†	
#5	.73	.53	.18	
#8	.90	.80	.18	
#15	.81	.65	.18	
Balance within family caregiving				
		.77*		.47
#6	.72	.51	—†	
#19	.69	.48	.24	
#20	.75	.56	.24	
#34	.56	.31	.23	

From Carruth, A. K. (1996). Development and testing of the Caregiver Reciprocity Scale. *Nursing Research, 45,* 92–97.
*Denotes composite reliabilities.
†Denotes that the value was not estimated (parameter constrained at 1.0 in LISREL).

supported by using the Philadelphia Center Affect Rating Scale, where the RBS was found to be negatively correlated with anxiety ($r = .59, p < .005$), sadness ($r = -.59, p < .005$), and agitation ($r = -.39, p < .05$), thus supporting the construct validity of the RBS in measuring empathy and reliable relational behaviours. More recently, the data from a factor analysis being conducted for other validity purposes has been used to determine divergent (sometimes called discriminant) validity. Carruth (1996) assessed the divergent validity of the four

factors (subscales) of the CRS by examining the correlations between each factor or subscale that appears in Table 14–3.

A specific method of assessing convergent and divergent validity is the **multitrait–multimethod approach**. Similar to the divergent validity approach just described, this method, proposed by Campbell and Fiske (1959), also involves examining the relationship between instruments that intend to measure the same construct and between those that intend to measure different constructs. A variety of measurement strategies, however, are used. For example, anxiety could be measured by the following:

- Administering the State-Trait Anxiety Inventory
- Recording blood pressure readings
- Asking the subject about anxious feelings
- Observing the subject's behaviour

The results of one of these measures should then be correlated with the results of each of the others in a multitrait–multimethod matrix (Waltz, Strickland, & Lenz, 1991).

In their classic study designed to develop, validate, and normalize a measure of dimensions of interpersonal relationships (including social support, reciprocity, and conflict), Tilden, Nelson, and May (1990) used the multitrait–multimethod approach to validity assessment. The two traits of social support and conflict of the Interpersonal Relationship Inventory (IPRI) were each measured with two different methods: a subject self-report tool and an investigator–observation visual analogue rating. Reciprocity was not included because of its high correlation with social support.

The use of multiple measures of a concept decreases systematic error. A variety of data collection methods (e.g., self-report, observation, interview, and collection of physiological data) will also diminish the effect of systematic error.

CONTRASTED-GROUPS APPROACH

When the **contrasted-groups approach** (sometimes called the **known-groups approach**) to the development of construct validity is used, the researcher identifies two groups of individuals expected to score extremely high or extremely low in the characteristic being measured by the instrument. The instrument is administered to the high-scoring and low-scoring groups, and the differences in scores are examined. If the instrument is sensitive to individual differences in the trait being measured, the mean performance of these two groups should differ significantly, and evidence of construct validity would be supported. A t test or analysis of variance is used to statistically test the difference between the two groups.

A study by Secco (2002) sought to develop and assess the psychometric properties of the Infant Care Questionnaire (ICQ), a self-report scale designed to measure a mother's perception of her abilities and competence as an infant care provider. The researcher used the contrasted-groups approach to provide evidence of construct validity for the Mom and Baby dimension of the ICQ.

The known groups were mothers of different parity (healthy low-risk primiparous versus multiparous mothers [$n = 164$] of term infants) and mothers with different amounts of past infant care experience. Multiparous mothers, those with higher ratings of past infant care experience, and those with greater time in the mothering role were expected to have significantly higher Mom and Baby scores than primiparous mothers with lower ratings of infant care experience.

As illustrated in Table 14–4, repeated measures analysis of variance demonstrated significantly higher Mom and Baby scores for the multiparous mothers compared with primiparous mothers by time [$F(2, n = 140) = 21.78, p = .000$] and parity [$F(1, n = 140) = 10.78, p = .001$]. Over time, trends were observed in the infant care provider role of lower scores for primiparous mothers at all three measurement times and diminished mean

TABLE 14–4	Repeated Measures Analysis of Variance for Mean Mom and Baby Dimension Scores by Time [F(2, n = 140) = 21.78, p <.001] and Parity [F(1, n = 140) = 10.78, p <.001]		
Week	**Primiparous (n = 97)**	**Multiparous (n = 43)**	**Mothers (n = 140)**
1	3.74	4.09	3.85
2	4.00	4.23	4.10
3	4.07	4.18	4.10

differences between parity groups. The author proposed that these findings are associated with the maternal role attainment theory, which states that knowledge, skill, and competence perceptions are acquired during the postnatal period and that experience is a key factor in attainment of competence. The significantly higher scores on the Mom and Baby means for the multiparous mothers suggest that the ICQ was sensitive enough to capture the differences between primiparous and multiparous mothers, thereby providing evidence of construct validity using the contrasted-groups approach.

FACTOR ANALYTICAL APPROACH

A final approach to assessing construct validity is **factor analysis**. This procedure gives the researcher information about the extent to which a set of items measures the same underlying construct or the same dimension of a construct. Factor analysis assesses the degree to which the individual items on a scale truly cluster around one or more dimensions. Items designed to measure the same dimension should load on the same factor; those designed to measure differing dimensions should load on different factors (Anastasi, 1988; Nunnally & Bernstein, 1994).

A factor analysis also indicates whether the items in the instrument reflect a single construct or several constructs. Several factors may be identified in a set of data. The study must have a large sample size to conduct a factor analysis. Nunnally and Bernstein (1994) recommended 10 observations for each variable. Thus, to develop the factor structure and reliability of the Brain Impairment Behavior Scale, Cameron et al. (2008) used data from several small studies that had used this scale to obtain a sample size of 300. Table 14–5 gives an example of how factor analysis can be used, as it was in causal modelling.

Gillis (1997) conducted a factor analysis during the initial assessment of the construct validity of the ALQ. A principal axis factor analysis with an oblique rotation was used to determine whether the hypothesis of seven subscales could be realized. The solution of seven factors explained 56% of the variance of the revised 43-item ALQ. The findings from the factor analysis are presented in Table 14–5.

Helpful Hint

When validity data about the study's measurement instruments are not included in a research article, you cannot determine whether the intended concept is being captured by the measurement tool. Before you use the results check the instrument's validity by reviewing the original source.

Evidence-Based Practice Tip

When the tools used in a study are presented, note whether the sample used to develop the measurement instruments is similar to your client population.

The Critical Thinking Decision Path will help you assess the appropriateness of the type of validity and reliability selected for use in a particular research study.

Researchers may be concerned about whether the scores that were obtained for a sample of subjects were consistent, true measures of the behaviours and thus an accurate reflection of the differences between individuals. The extent of variability in test scores that is attributable to error rather than a true measure of the behaviours is the **error variance**.

An **observed test score** that is derived from a set of items consists of the true score plus error (see Figure 14–2). The error may be either chance (random) error or systematic error.

A **chance error** or a **random error** is an error that is difficult to control (e.g., a respondent's anxiety at the time of testing). These errors are unsystematic and are not predictable; thus, they cannot be corrected. However, being aware of the sources of these errors may minimize their impact on measurement accuracy. These sources are (1) transient human conditions, such as hunger, fatigue, health, lack of motivation, and anxiety, which are often beyond the awareness and control of the examiner; (2) variations in the measurement procedure,

Items	Factors							
	1	2	3	4	5	6	7	Alpha
Subscale: Identity Awareness								.84
Like who I am	.65							
Know my strengths and weaknesses	.45							
Happy and content	.72							
Look forward to the future	.64							
Set goals for myself	.55							
Examine my beliefs	.46							
My life has purpose	.75							
Try to do my best	.59							
Confident about my beliefs	.71							
Subscale: Nutrition								.88
Read food labels		.46						
Follow a healthy diet		.46						
Limit foods high in fat		.81						
Limit foods high in salt		.76						
Limit foods high in sugar		.84						
Choose healthy snacks		.47						
Limit junk food		.60						
Choose foods without additives		.47						
Subscale: Physical Participation								.82
Run, take long walks, dance, or swim 3–4 times weekly			.71					
Participate in sports at school			.69					
Exercise vigorously for 30 min. 3 times weekly			.68					
Play sports 3 times a week			.81					
Subscale: Safety								.74
Wear seat belts in automobile				.47				
Avoid doing drugs				.60				
Refuse a ride if the driver is drinking				.47				
Avoid tobacco products				.60				
Avoid alcohol				.66				
Make informed choices regarding sexual relationships				.45				
Use protection if sexually active				.47				
Subscale: Health Awareness								.71
Report unusual body changes					.58			
Talk to teacher or nurse regarding ways to improve my health					.67			
Read magazines about health topics					.67			
Discuss health issues with others					.67			
Subscale: Social Support								.80
Discuss problems with people close to me						.65		
Enjoy spending time with my friends						.72		
Express my concerns to others						.68		
Have good friendships with girls and guys my age						.61		
If I had a problem, I would have people to turn to						.65		
Can express my feelings to others						.60		
If I needed help, I could turn to family and friends, teachers, and coaches						.65		.63
Subscale: Stress Management								.60
Exercise to control my stress							.45	
Use helpful strategies to deal with stress							.64	
Use spiritual beliefs to deal with stress							.49	
Talk to my friends about my stress							.57	.57

Adapted from Gillis, A. J. (1997). The Adolescent Lifestyle Questionnaire: Development and psychometric testing. *Canadian Journal of Nursing Research, 29,* 29–46.

Critical Thinking Decision Path. Determining the Appropriate Type of Validity and Reliability Selected for a Study

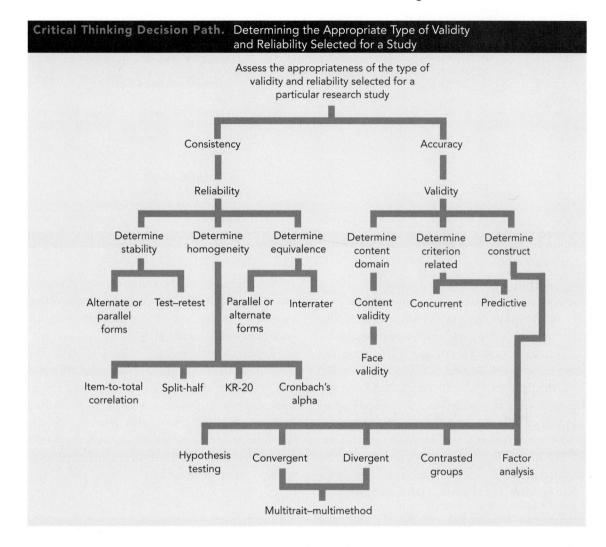

such as misplacement of the blood pressure cuff, not waiting for a specific time period before taking the blood pressure, or placing the arm randomly in relation to the heart while measuring blood pressure; changing the wording of interview questions between administrations; environmental factors, such as the presence of others while data are being obtained, a cold room, or discomfort with the researcher (who is part of the environment); and (3) errors in data processing, such as coding errors and incorrect inputting into the computer. Chance errors affect an individual's observed score, such that one person's observed score is higher than his or her true score, whereas another person's observed

score can be lower than his or her true score. Instruments that are free of chance errors are considered reliable (Nunnally, 1978).

A **systematic error** or a **constant error** is a measurement error that is attributable to relatively stable characteristics of the study population that may bias their behaviour, cause incorrect instrument calibration, or both. Such error has a systematic biasing influence on the subjects' responses and thereby influences the validity of the instruments. Level of education, socioeconomic status, social desirability, response pattern, or other characteristics may influence the validity of the instrument by altering the measurement of the "true"

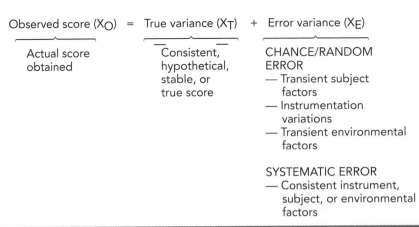

Observed score (X_O)   =   True variance (X_T)   +   Error variance (X_E)

| Actual score obtained | Consistent, hypothetical, stable, or true score | CHANCE/RANDOM ERROR
— Transient subject factors
— Instrumentation variations
— Transient environmental factors

SYSTEMATIC ERROR
— Consistent instrument, subject, or environmental factors |

Figure 14–2 Components of observed scores

responses in a systematic way. For example, a subject who wants to please the investigator may constantly answer items in a socially desirable way, thus making the estimate of validity inaccurate.

Systematic error also occurs when an instrument is improperly calibrated. Consider a scale that consistently gives a person's weight at 1 kilogram less than the actual body weight. The scale could be quite reliable (i.e., capable of reproducing the precise measurement), but the result is consistently invalid. Systematic error is considered part of the true score. The multimethod–multitrait technique is one method to decrease systematic error. The validity of an instrument is the extent to which it is free of both chance errors and systematic errors (Nunnally, 1978).

Research articles vary considerably in the amount of detail included about reliability and validity. When the focus of a study is tool development, psychometric evaluation—including extensive reliability and validity data—is carefully documented and appears throughout the article rather than briefly in the "Instruments" section, as in other research studies.

Critiquing Reliability and Validity

Reliability and validity are two crucial aspects in the critical appraisal of a measurement instrument. The reviewer evaluates an instrument's level of reliability and validity, as well as the manner in which these were established. In a research report, the reliability and validity for each measure should be presented. If these data have not been presented, the reviewer must seriously question the merit and use of the tool and the study's results. Criteria for critiquing reliability and validity are presented in the Critiquing Criteria box.

If a study does not use reliable and valid questionnaires, the results cannot be credible. The critiquer has an ethical responsibility to question the reliability and validity of instruments used in research studies and to examine the findings in light of the quality of the instruments used and the data presented. The following discussion highlights key areas related to reliability and validity that should be evident to the critiquer of a research article.

Appropriate reliability tests should have been performed by the developer of the measurement tool and should then have been included by the current user in the research report. If the initial standardization sample and the current sample have

CRITIQUING CRITERIA

1. Was an appropriate method used to test the reliability of the tool?

2. Is the reliability of the tool adequate?

3. Was an appropriate method used to test the validity of the instrument?

4. Is the validity of the measurement tool adequate?

5. If the sample from the developmental stage of the tool was different from the current sample, were the reliability and validity recalculated to determine whether the tool is still adequate?

6. Have the strengths and weaknesses of the reliability and validity of each instrument been presented?

7. Did the researcher paint a clear picture of the participant's reality?

8. Is evidence provided that the researcher's interpretation captured the participant's meaning?

9. Have other professionals confirmed the researcher's interpretation?

10. Are the strengths and weaknesses of the rigour of the research appropriately addressed in the "Discussion," "Limitations," or "Recommendations" sections of the report?

different characteristics, the reader would find either (1) that a pilot study for the present sample would have been conducted to determine whether the reliability was maintained or (2) that a reliability estimate was calculated on the current sample. For example, if the standardization sample for a tool that measures "satisfaction in an intimate heterosexual relationship" comprises undergraduate college students and if an investigator plans to use the tool with married couples, the reliability of the tool should be established with the latter group.

The investigator determines which type of reliability procedure is used in the study, depending on the nature of the measurement tool and how it will be used. For example, if the instrument is to be administered twice, the critiquer might determine that test–retest reliability should have been used to establish the stability of the tool. If an alternate form has been developed for use in a repeated measures design, evidence of alternate form reliability should be presented to determine the equivalence of the parallel forms.

If the degree of internal consistency among the items is relevant, an appropriate test of internal consistency should be presented. In some instances, more than one type of reliability will be presented, but the critiquer should determine whether all are

appropriate. For example, the Kuder–Richardson formula implies that a single right or wrong answer exists, making the coefficient inappropriate to use with scales that provide a format of three or more possible responses. In such cases, another formula is applied, such as Cronbach's coefficient alpha.

Another important consideration is the acceptable level of reliability, which varies according to the type of test. Coefficients of reliability of .70 or higher are desirable. The validity of an instrument is limited by its reliability; in other words, less confidence can be placed in scores from tests with low reliability coefficients.

Satisfactory evidence of validity is probably the most difficult item for the reviewer to determine. This aspect of measurement is most likely to fall short of meeting the required criteria. Validity studies are time-consuming and complex, and, sometimes, researchers will settle for presenting minimal validity data.

Therefore, the critiquer should closely examine the item content of a tool when evaluating its strengths and weaknesses and try to find conclusive evidence of content validity. In the body of a research article, however, it is unusual to have more than a few sample items available for review. Thus, the critiquer should determine whether the appropriate assessment of content validity was used to meet the researcher's goal.

Such procedures provide the critiquer with assurance that the tool is psychometrically sound and that the content of the items is consistent with the conceptual framework and the construct definitions. Construct validity and criterion-related validity are two of the more precise statistical tests of whether the tool measures what it is intended to measure. Ideally, an instrument should provide evidence of content validity, as well as criterion-related or construct validity, before a reviewer invests a high level of confidence in the tool.

The reader should also expect to see the strengths and weaknesses of instrument reliability and validity presented in the "Discussion," "Limitations," or "Recommendations" section, or in all of these sections, of a research article. In this context, the reliability and validity might be discussed in relation to other tools devised to measure the same variable. The relationship of the study's findings to the strengths and weaknesses in instrument reliability and validity is another important discussion point.

Finally, the researcher should propose recommendations for improving future studies in relation to instrument reliability and validity. For example, in the "Instruments" and "Discussion" sections of a study examining relationships among spirituality, perceived social support, death anxiety, and nurses' willingness to care for clients with acquired immune deficiency syndrome (AIDS), Sherman (1996) appropriately reported the weaknesses in the reliability of the Templer Death Anxiety Scale (TDAS). She stated that although the TDAS is often cited in the literature, the low internal consistency reliability of the scale (.76) supports the recommendation that the instrument be pilot-tested on the specific sample on which it will be administered. Because of the marginally acceptable reliability of the TDAS and because the study sample (i.e., registered nurses) differed from the original sample (i.e., college students) used for establishing reliability, Sherman conducted a pilot study using a sample of 30 nurses enrolled in a doctoral course. The pilot study yielded a marginally acceptable reliability coefficient of .78. However, in the actual study, the TDAS's reliability coefficient of .63 was lower than anticipated based on the results

of the pilot study. Although Sherman appropriately addressed the low reliability of TDAS in relation to the psychometric properties of the tool and made recommendations about revising the response format, she did not address this weakness in relation to the hypotheses and the findings of the study.

Reliability and validity in research reports can be evaluated to varying degrees. The research consumer should not feel inhibited by the complexity of these topics but may use the guidelines presented in this chapter to systematically assess the reliability and validity of a research study.

Collegial dialogue is also an approach to evaluating the merits and shortcomings of an existing, as well as a newly developed, instrument that is reported in the nursing literature. Such an exchange promotes the understanding of methodologies and techniques of reliability and validity, stimulates the acquisition of a basic knowledge of psychometrics, and encourages the exploration of alternative methods of observation and the use of reliable and valid tools in clinical practice.

RIGOUR IN QUALITATIVE RESEARCH: Credibility, Auditability, and Fittingness

As in quantitative research, the basic approach to ensure rigour in qualitative research is methodical research design, data collection, interpretation, and communication. Qualitative researchers seek to achieve two goals: (1) to account for the method and the data, which must stand independently so that another researcher can analyze the same data in the same way and make the same conclusions, and (2) to produce a credible and reasoned explanation of the phenomenon under study. Thus, this rigour in qualitative methodology is judged by unique criteria appropriate to the research approach. **Credibility**, **auditability**, and **fittingness** are the scientific criteria proposed for qualitative research studies by Guba (1981). Although these criteria were proposed two decades ago, they still capture the rigorous spirit of qualitative inquiry and persist as reasonable criteria for evaluation. The meanings of credibility, auditability, and fittingness are briefly explained in Table 14–6.

TABLE 14–6 Criteria for Judging Scientific Rigour: Credibility, Auditability, Fittingness	
Criteria	**Characteristics**
Credibility	Truth of findings as judged by participants and others within the discipline. For example, you may find the researcher returning to the participants to share interpretation of findings and query accuracy from the perspective of the persons living the experience.
Auditability	Accountability as judged by the adequacy of information leading the reader from the research question and raw data through various steps of analysis to the interpretation of findings. For example, you should be able to follow the reasoning of the researcher step by step through explicit examples of data, interpretations, and syntheses.
Fittingness	Faithfulness to the everyday reality of the participants, described in enough detail so that others in the discipline can evaluate importance for their own practice, research, and theory development. For example, you will know enough about the human experience being reported that you can decide whether it "rings true" and is useful for guiding your practice.

Credibility

Credibility is similar to internal validity in qualitative research. The methods to ensure credibility are prolonged engagement, persistent observation, peer debriefing, and member checks (Lincoln, 1995). In prolonged engagement and persistent observation, the researchers spend sufficient time with the study's participants to check for discrepancies in responses. Peer debriefing is conducted with experts in the field, whose probing questions and review about the research can assist the researchers to improve trustworthiness in the data. Member checking verifies the accuracy of participants' responses by asking the study participants to review the themes and narratives to determine whether the researchers captured their experiences (Lincoln & Guba, 1985).

Triangulation, crystallization, and searching for disconfirming evidence through negative case analyses are also used to ensure credibility and confirmability. Chapter 7 discusses triangulation and crystallization in both qualitative and mixed method research. To review, triangulation is the cross-checking and verification of data through the use of different information sources, such as a variety of data sources, investigators, theoretical models, and research methods. Triangulation is viewed as offering completeness to naturalistic inquiry (Tobin & Begley, 2004).

Auditability and Fittingness

Engaging in an inquiry audit establishes both the auditability and the fittingness of the data. The audit trail was proposed by Guba (1981) to allow external auditors to follow the trail of qualitative data gathering and has been described by Lincoln and Guba (1985) as "the most important trustworthiness technique available to the naturalistic" (p. 285). The audit trail involves reviewing all documents relating to the study, such as research protocol, memos and correspondences, research tools, and field notes.

To illustrate how rigour is ascertained, Webster, Bouck, Wright, and Dietrich (2006) conducted a qualitative study to describe the experiences of public health nurses who screen for woman abuse within their clinical practice. These researchers established trustworthiness in the data by engaging in a variety of methods: member checking, inviting participants to attend a presentation of the findings followed by open dialogue, and employing a team analysis approach to confirm that the findings were grounded in the participants' words and that the researchers attended to their biases.

Critical reflexivity, maintaining the integrity of participants' voices in context, taking direct action on the research problem, confirmability, credibility, and fittingness were aspects of rigour used by Smith, Edwards, Varcoe, Martens, and Davies (2006) (see Appendix B).

The study by Baker (2007) incorporated several strategies to ascertain rigour. This author explored the social health of a small immigrant community of Muslims in Canada following the terror attacks in September 2001. Prolonged engagement was fulfilled by having the research team conduct fieldwork for six months before recruiting participants; during this time, the team established trust and gathered contextual information about the Muslim communities in the region. Both people triangulation and place triangulation were strived for, that is, men and women, francophones and Anglophones, and the use of three different cities. Data source triangulation was accomplished through interviews with Arab Christians and African Muslims. A triangulation of investigators occurred via an advisory panel, who helped formulate the data collection instrument and the initial and final analyses. Negative case analyses involved cross-checking and refining data interpretations with ongoing analyses. Member checking was conducted by sending the research report to all participants for feedback. Having two trained interviewers enhanced dependability in the data. To ensure confirmability, an audit trail was made throughout data reduction.

An example of peer debriefing is offered by Jack, DiCenso, and Lohfeld (2005) in their study on developing a theory of maternal engagement with public health nurses and family. These authors engaged academic colleagues and practising public health nurses to give feedback on the emerging concepts and the relevance of the model to nursing practice.

Emden and Sandelowski (1999) inferred that one set of criteria cannot "fit the bill" for every research study. Thus, Chiovitti and Piran (2003, p. 427) developed a framework of rigour consisting of the following eight methods of research practice to enhance rigour during the research process and for critiquing published grounded theory research reports:

1. Let participants guide the inquiry process.
2. Check the theoretical construction generated against participants' meanings of the phenomenon.
3. Use participants' actual words in the theory.
4. Articulate the researcher's personal views and insights about the phenomenon explored.
5. Specify the criteria built into the researcher's thinking.
6. Specify how and why participants in the study were selected.
7. Delineate the scope of the research
8. Describe how the literature relates to each category that emerged in the theory.

Speziale and Carpenter (2007) commented that these criteria can provide a guide in critiquing grounded theory research.

Another concept to increase rigour that has not received much attention is goodness, represented as a "means of locating situatedness, trustworthiness and authenticity" (Tobin & Begley, 2004, p. 391). Tobin and Begley recommended that goodness be reflected by the entire study and discussed Arminio and Hultgren's (2002) six elements of goodness:

1. Foundation (epistemology and theory)
2. Approach (methodology)
3. Collection of data (method)
4. Representation of voice
5. The art of meaning making
6. Implication for professional practice

These six elements of goodness will help a research consumer greatly when critiquing a study for research utilization.

Critical Thinking Challenges

- Discuss the three types of validity that must be established before a reviewer invests a high level of confidence in the tool. Include examples of each type of validity.
- What are the major tests of reliability? Is it necessary to establish more than one measure of reliability for each instrument used in a study? Which do you think is the most essential measure of reliability? Include examples in your answer.
- Is it possible to have a valid instrument that is not reliable? Is the reverse possible? Support your answer with instruments you might use in the clinical setting with your clients.
- What are some ways in which credibility, auditability, and fittingness can be evaluated?
- How do you think the concept of evidence-based practice has changed research utilization models? Is the review of the literature the same when developing a research proposal as it is when implementing the steps of research utilization or an evidence-based practice protocol? Support your position.

KEY POINTS

- Reliability and validity are crucial aspects of conducting and critiquing research.

- Validity refers to whether an instrument measures what it is purported to measure. It is a crucial aspect of evaluating a tool.

- Three types of validity are content validity, criterion-related validity, and construct validity.

- The choice of a validation method is important and is made by the researcher on the basis of the characteristics of the measurement device in question and its utilization.

- Reliability refers to the accuracy-to-inaccuracy ratio in a measurement device.

- The major tests of reliability are as follows: test–retest reliability, parallel or alternate form reliability, split-half reliability, item-to-total correlation, Kuder–Richardson coefficient, Cronbach's alpha, and interrater reliability.

- The selection of a method for establishing reliability depends on the characteristics of the tool, the testing method that is used for collecting data from the standardization sample, and the kinds of data that are obtained.

- Credibility, auditability, and fittingness are criteria for judging the scientific rigour of a qualitative research study.

REFERENCES

Anastasi, A. (1988). *Psychological testing* (6th ed.). New York: Macmillan.

Arminio, J. L., & Hultgren, F. H. (2002). Breaking out from the shadow: The question of criteria in qualitative research. *Journal of College Student Development, 43,* 446–456.

Baker, C. (2007). Globalization and the cultural safety of an immigrant Muslim community. *Journal of Advanced Nursing, 57,* 296–305.

Barnason, S., Zimmerman, L., Atwood, J., Nieveen, J., & Schmaderer, M. (2002). Development of a self-efficacy instrument for coronary artery bypass graft patients. *Journal of Nursing Measurement, 10,* 123–133.

Braden, B., & Bergstrom, N. (1994). Predictive validity of the Braden Scale for pressure sore risk in a nursing home population. *Research in Nursing and Health, 17,* 459–470.

Cameron, J., Chung, A., Coyote, D., Streiner, D., Singh, M., & Stewart, D. (2008). Factor structure and reliability of the Brain Impairment Behavior Scale. *Journal of Neuroscience Nursing, 40*(1), 40–47.

Campbell, D., & Fiske, D. (1959). Convergent and discriminant validation by the matrix. *Psychological Bulletin, 53,* 273–302.

Carruth, A. K. (1996). Development and testing of the caregiver reciprocity scale. *Nursing Research, 45,* 92–97.

Chiovitti, R. F., & Piran, N. (2003). Rigour and grounded theory research. *Journal of Advanced Nursing, 44*(4), 427–435.

Dahinten, S. (2003). Peer sexual harassment in adolescence: The function of gender. *Canadian Journal of Nursing Research, 35,* 56–73.

Dennis, C. L. (2003). The Breastfeeding Self-Efficacy Scale: Psychometric assessment of the short form. *Journal of Obstetric, Gynecologic, & Neonatal Nursing, 32,* 734–744.

Doran, D. M., Harrison, M. B., Laschinger, H. S., Hirdes, J. P., Rukholm, E., Sidani, S., et al. (2006). Nursing-sensitive outcomes data collection in acute care and long-term-care settings. *Nursing Research, 55*(2S), S75–S81.

Emden, C., & Sandelowski, M. (1999). The good, the bad and relative, part two: Goodness and the criterion problem in qualitative research. *International Journal of Professional Nursing Practice, 5*(1), 2–7.

Filion, L., Gélinas, C., Simard, S., Savard, J., & Gagnon, P. (2003). Validation evidence for the French Canadian adaptation of the Multidimensional Fatigue Inventory as a measure of cancer-related fatigue. *Cancer Nursing, 26,* 143–154.

Gillis, A. J. (1997). The Adolescent Lifestyle Questionnaire: Development and psychometric testing. *Canadian Journal of Nursing Research, 29,* 29–46.

Guba, E. G. (1981). Criteria for assessing the trustworthiness of naturalistic enquiries. *Educational Communication and Technology Journal, 29,* 75–91.

Hoskins, C. N. (1988). *The Partner Relationship Inventory.* Palo Alto, CA: Consulting Psychologists Press.

Hoskins, C. N., Haber, J., Budin, W. C., Cartwright-Alcarase, F., Kowalski, M. O., Panke, J., et al. (2001). Breast cancer: Education, counseling and adjustment. A pilot study. *Psychological Reports, 8,* 677–704.

Ibrahim, S. E. R. (2002). Rates of adherence to pharmacological treatment among children and adolescents with attention deficit hyperactivity disorder. *Human Psychopharmacology, 17,* 225–231.

Jack, S. M., DiCenso, A., & Lohfeld, L. (2005). A theory of maternal engagement with public health nurses and family visitors. *Journal of Advanced Nursing, 49,* 182–190.

Lincoln, Y. S. (1995). Emerging criteria for qualitative and interpretive research. *Qualitative Inquiry, 3,* 275–289.

Lincoln, Y., & Guba, E. (1985). *Naturalistic inquiry.* New York: Sage.

McClowry, S. G., Halverson, C. F., & Sanson, A. (2003). A reexamination of the validity and reliability of the School-Age Temperament Inventory. *Nursing Research, 52*, 176–182.

McDowell, I., & Newell, C. (1996). *Measuring health: A guide to rating scales and questionnaires.* New York: Oxford Press.

McGilton, K. S., O'Brien-Pallas, L. L., Darlington, G., Evans, M., Wynn, F., & Pringle, D. M. (2003). Effects of relationship-enhancing program of care on outcomes. *Journal of Nursing Scholarship, 35*, 151–156.

McGilton, K. S., Pringle, D. M., O'Brien-Pallas, L. L., Wynn, F., & Streiner, D. (2005). Development and psychometric testing of the Relational Care Scale. *Journal of Nursing Measurement, 13*, 51–57.

Nunnally, J. C. (1978). *Psychometric theory* (2nd ed.). New York: McGraw-Hill

Nunnally, J. C., & Bernstein, I. H. (1994). *Psychometric theory* (3rd ed.). New York: McGraw-Hill.

Powers, G. C., Zentner, T., Nelson, F., & Bergstrom, N. (2004). Validation of the mobility subscale of the Braden scale for predicting pressure sore risk. *Nursing Research, 53*, 340–346.

Profetto-McGrath, J. (2003). The relationship of critical thinking skills and critical thinking dispositions of baccalaureate nursing students. *Journal of Advanced Nursing, 43*, 569–577.

Resnick, B., Nahm, E. S., Orwig, D., Zimmerman, S. S., & Magaziner, J. (2001). Measurement of activity in older adults: Reliability and validity of the step activity monitor. *Journal of Nursing Measurement, 9*, 275–290.

Santacroce, S. J., Maccarelli, L. M., & Grey, M. (2004). Intervention fidelity. *Nursing Research, 53*, 63–66.

Secco, L. (2002). The Infant Care Questionnaire: Assessment of reliability and validity in a sample of healthy mothers. *Journal of Nursing Measurement, 10*, 97–109.

Sherman, D. W. (1996). Nurses' willingness to care for AIDS patients and spirituality, social support, and death anxiety. *Image, 28*, 205–213.

Smith, D., Edwards, N., Varcoe, C., Martens, P. J., & Davies, B. (2006). Bringing safety and responsiveness into the forefront of care for pregnant and parenting Aboriginal people. *Advances in Nursing Science, 29*(2), E27–E44.

Speziale, H. S., & Carpenter, D. (2007). *Qualitative research in nursing: Advancing the humanistic imperative.* Philadelphia: Lippincott, Williams, & Wilkins.

Tilden, V. P., Nelson, C. A., & May, B. A. (1990). The IPR inventory: Development and psychometric characteristics. *Nursing Research, 39*, 337–343.

Tobin, G. A., & Begley, C. M. (2004). Methodological rigour within a qualitative framework. *Journal of Advanced Nursing, 48*, 388–396.

Waltz, C., Strickland, O., & Lenz, E. (1991). *Measurement in nursing research* (3rd ed.). Philadelphia: F.A. Davis.

Webster, F., Bouck, M. S., Wright, B. L., & Dietrich, P. (2006). Public health nurses' experiences of screening for woman abuse. *Canadian Journal of Nursing Research, 38*, 137–153.

Cherylyn Cameron

CHAPTER 15

Qualitative Data Analysis

LEARNING OUTCOMES

After reading this chapter, the student should be able to do the following:

- Describe the processes of qualitative data analysis.
- Outline the steps common to qualitative data analysis.
- Describe how data are reduced to meaningful units (themes).
- Describe the process of identifying themes and categories and the relationships between them.
- Assess the validity of a data analysis from a study.

KEY TERMS

codes
coding
constant comparative method
data display
data reduction
member checking
thematic analysis
themes

STUDY RESOURCES

evolve Go to Evolve at
http://evolve.elsevier.com/Canada/LoBiondo/Research/
for Weblinks, content updates, and additional
research articles for practice in reviewing
and critiquing.

As discussed in earlier chapters, qualitative analysis is not an analysis of the statistical tests used in the study but an analysis of the qualitative text. The text includes transcripts from interviews, narratives, documents, media such as newspapers and movies, and field notes. Qualitative researchers collect enormous amounts of data, which must be managed carefully: more than 150 pages of transcript can result from 25 interviews. To add to the complexity of qualitative data analysis, many researchers take different approaches to analysis. This chapter expands on the discussion in Chapter 8, in which the analysis of data was introduced in the context of several qualitative research traditions, such as phenomenology, grounded theory, ethnography, and case study.

AUDIOTAPING INTERVIEWS

Interviews are the primary source of data for many qualitative research projects. Although some researchers believe that a tape recorder will inhibit the free flow of discussion, Seidman (1998) and others have found that most participants and interviewers forget about the presence of the tape recorder. Consequently, most researchers audiotape interviews and then transcribe them verbatim into written text. Although not commonly practised, some researchers may consider summarizing or paraphrasing the spoken words (Seidman, 1998). Most researchers wish to use the original words so that their interpretations and personal biases are not juxtaposed with the participant's thoughts. Having the original words allows the reader to check the authenticity of the data.

DATA MANAGEMENT

The open nature of qualitative inquiry typically results in the collection of more data than required. Glesne (2006) referred to the sheer volume of the data collected as "fat data." Consequently, researchers must be methodical in their organization and management of the data. Fortunately, computer software simplifies the storage and retrieval of data. However, researchers are also required to develop a decision or audit trail requiring the tracking of the participants, and the original audiotapes, original and photocopied documents. Moreover, all of the data must be kept secure to maintain confidentiality.

Many computer programs are available to assist researchers with the task of data management, such as ATLAS.ti, Ethnograph, HyperRESEARCH, and QSR NVivo 8. Meadows and Dodendorf (1999) categorized computer programs into the following three types:

1. Code and retrieve programs, which assist in organizing and grouping data

2. Theory builders, which move to a different level of data organization by connecting themes and categories

3. Conceptual network builders, which incorporate graphics with theory-building capabilities

Unlike computer programs used with quantitative data, these programs do not analyze data. Data analysis and interpretation remain largely the task of the researcher. However, using computer programs for orderly organization and grouping of data eases the job of analysis and interpretation for the researcher.

The researcher needs to test software to determine which program will be the most useful. Often, this process is one of trial and error before the most appropriate computer program is found. Although learning new software is very time consuming, the benefits of using computerized software outweigh the time spent researching and learning about it (Speziale & Carpenter, 2007).

OVERVIEW OF DATA ANALYSIS

When does data collection end and data analysis begin? This is a controversial area of qualitative research because not all researchers agree on whether data collection should be completed before analysis begins or whether the two processes ought to take place concurrently. Therefore, the researcher needs to identify the process used.

As mentioned previously, many researchers begin a preliminary analysis as the material accumulates. Typically, the qualitative researcher transcribes all of the interviews, field notes, and observations as they are collected. As each piece of data is transcribed, researchers will begin a preliminary analysis during which they ask themselves what additional data need to be collected. Many researchers feel that the stages of data collection and data analysis should be integrated (Denzin & Lincoln, 2000; Miles & Huberman, 1994; Speziale & Carpenter, 2007), whereas others feel that these stages should be separate (Seidman, 1998).

The overall goal of qualitative data analysis is to make meaning out of massive amounts of text or data, and many methods for analysis are available. Patton (2002) encouraged researchers to do their "very best with . . . full intellectual capacity to fairly represent the data and communicate what the data reveal given the purpose of study" (p. 433). As described earlier, qualitative analysis is not a linear process; rather, it is cyclical, transformative, reciprocal, and iterative. Miles and Huberman (1994, p. 9) identified some common features among different approaches to qualitative data analysis:

- Affixing codes to a set of field notes drawn from observations or interviews

- Noting reflections of other remarks in the margins

- Sorting and shifting though these materials to identify similar phrases, relationships between variables, patterns, themes, distinct differences between subgroups, and common sequences

- Isolating these patterns and processes and commonalities and differences and taking them out to the field in the next wave of data collection

- Gradually elaborating a small set of generalizations that cover the consistencies discerned in the database

- Confronting those generalizations with a formalized body of knowledge in the form of constructs or theories

Guidelines such as those provided in Miles and Huberman's *Qualitative Data Analysis* (1994) described earlier are useful, but they serve only as recommendations. Each qualitative study is unique and is reliant on the creativity, intellect, style, and experience of the researcher.

During the data analysis phase, all researchers fully immerse themselves in the data over a period of weeks to months. This process requires constant reading and rereading of the text until an understanding of what the data conveys is reached (Speziale & Carpenter, 2007. An important part of the data analysis is the interplay between data gathering or questioning and verifying what is heard and understood. Researchers continue to ask whether what they understood before is still relevant after subsequent interviews, observations, and reading of related documents.

Miles and Huberman (1994) referred to three discrete stages of data analysis: data reduction, data display, and conclusion drawing and verification (see Figure 15–1). Many of the common methods used in nursing research fit into this general view of qualitative analysis.

Data Reduction

According to Miles and Huberman (1994), "**data reduction** refers to the process of selecting, focusing, simplifying, abstracting, and transforming the data that appear in written-up field notes or transcriptions" (p. 10). This process is ongoing as data are collected. Initially, the data can be organized into meaningful clusters of data by grouping related or similar data. Often, these clusters or groups of data are labelled as **themes**, or structured meaning units of data that occur frequently in the text. **Thematic analysis** is an important part of organizing data and refers to the process of recognizing and recovering the emergent themes. In the qualitative tradition, as Van Manen (1997) reminded us, "grasping and formulating a thematic understanding is not a rule-bound but a free act of 'seeing' meaning" (p. 79).

Glesne (2006) described several methods to help the researcher discover the meanings embedded

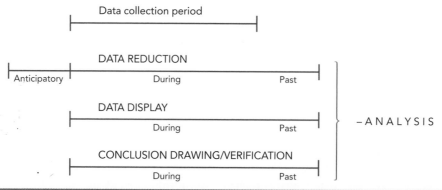

Figure 15–1 Stages of data analysis

From Miles, M. B., & Huberman, A. M. (1994). *Qualitative data analysis*. Thousand Oaks, CA: Sage (Figure 1.3, p. 10). Reprinted by permission of Sage Publications.

in data. The first method is to write memos or keep a reflective journal during the data collection stage, which allows the researcher to record thoughts about the data as these thoughts occur. Analytical files are developed to sort data into general categories, such as interview questions, people, and places, as well as useful quotations from the interviews and relevant quotations from the literature. These files help organize the researcher's thoughts and those of others.

Next, Glesne (2006) recommended the development of rudimentary coding schemes. Coding, as Denzin and Lincoln (2000) described it, "is the heart and soul of whole-text analysis" (p. 780). **Coding** is a progressive marking, sorting, resorting, and defining and redefining of the collected data.

Finally, Glesne (2006) recommended that researchers write themselves monthly field reports as a way of systematically reviewing the progress and determining the next steps. Aside from helping researchers keep track of their progress and communicate progress with other members of the research team, monthly summaries often result in new insights and new ways of approaching the research.

Denzin and Lincoln (2000) provided an overview of the fundamental steps in the coding of data: sampling, identifying themes, building codebooks, and marking texts. Although coding may sound complicated to the novice consumer of research, remember that this process is evolutional: it varies from project to project and from researcher to researcher.

Moreover, remember that meanings are waiting to be discovered, not imposed on the data.

The next step, finding themes, is the most exciting step of the process, which occurs during and after data collection. These themes or basic units of analysis can be entire texts (i.e., interview transcripts, responses to surveys), grammatical segments (words, phrases, sentences, paragraphs), formatting units (rows, pages), or clusters of texts that reflect a single theme. Most researchers try to divide data into units of analysis that do not overlap with others. Theorists approach this step in a variety of ways; for example, grounded theorists recommend that the researcher read the text line by line.

The coding process itself is the analysis (Miles and Huberman, 1994). Glesne (2006) stated that coding is as simple as identifying "what is important and giving it a name (code)" (p. 154). **Codes** are simply tags or labels that are assigned to the themes; often, the code itself is only one to four words long. Major codes may exist along with subcodes. Codes evolve during the analysis; more may be added, and others may be blended together. They mean something to the researcher and are not typically included in the research study. As the coding and themes are fine-tuned and finalized, much of the analysis is completed.

The next step is to build codebooks by organizing codes into lists, composed of either words or numbers that are used by the researcher. Marking the text ensues, in which the codes are assigned to the units of text. During this process, the researcher is immersed in the data, which results in new insights and interpretations.

Some researchers explicitly describe the process of data analysis in their research article. For example, Wuest, Merritt-Gray, Berman, and Ford-Gilboe (2002) described the data analysis of grounded theory with an example of an earlier study by Wuest on women's caring (2001). Wuest read each field note, transcript, or document line by line while asking herself two questions: "What is this a conceptual indicator of?" and "What is going on here?" (Wuest et al., 2002). Codes were assigned to each grouping of data, from sentences, to paragraphs, to whole pages (see Table 15–1 for the code assignments in Wuest's study). The codes (time for self, social interaction, and cultivating the marital relationship) were eventually grouped together into a single category: "replenishing."

In the study by Smith, Edwards, Varcoe, Martens, and Davies (2006) (see Appendix B), data were gathered from several sources, including interviews, supplementary documents, and field notes. The primary investigator used an interpretive descriptive method to analyze the text gathered from stakeholders. Initially, the approach was inductive (see Chapter 6), but it became increasingly deductive (see Chapter 7) as the themes emerged. Smith et al. (2006) reported that they used an iterative cycle of coding, collapsing or combining codes, and reorganizing the coding structure. Thematic patterns were identified as the themes were replicated across different groups and sites.

Cameron (2005) analyzed the transcripts from interviews with 13 participants on their experiences transferring from a college to a university in a collaborative baccalaureate nursing program. She identified an initial set of themes at three points: as they emerged while transcribing the interviews, after relistening to the taped interviews, and following a reading and a rereading of the transcripts. Differences, similarities, contradictions, and gaps in the data were noted as she returned to the original material to confirm the findings. Twenty-nine subthemes emerged from highlighting the students' stories. From these, six major themes surfaced. Table 15–2 shows the coding scheme used to code the transcripts, and Table 15–3 shows how one small section of the text was coded to validate the themes after the data had been collected.

Data Display

The second major step in data analysis is the **data display**. Miles and Huberman (1984) defined data display as "an organized, compressed assembly of information that permits conclusion drawing and action" (p. 11). This display helps us understand what is happening and can be in the form of graphs, flow charts, matrices, or any other visual representation. Like the rest of the analysis, the data display changes as more is known about the phenomenon under study. For example, Smith et al. (2006) (see Appendix B) showed the themes and subthemes resulting from their analysis of the experiences of Aboriginal community-based stakeholders' perspectives on care for pregnant and parenting families in table format. They identified four themes and 14 subthemes (see Table 15–4). Ford-Gilboe, Wuest, and Merritt-Gray (2005) studied how families (i.e., women and their children) promote their

TABLE 15–1 Code Assignments as Described in Wuest et al. (2002)	
Code	Text such as
Time for self	I steal an hour during the day.
Social interaction	I work not only for the money but to get out . . . for the social contacts.
Cultivating the marital relationship	So, after I get the kids to bed, I usually go downstairs and sit with him [partner] for an hour.

From Wuest, J., Merritt-Gray, M., Berman, H., & Ford-Gilboe, M. (2002). Illuminating social determinants of women's health using grounded theory. *Health Care International, 23,* 794–808.

TABLE 15–2 Cameron's (2005) Coding Scheme		
Major Theme	**Subthemes**	**Code**
Academic shock	Workload	AS-Work
	Underprepared	AS-Uprep
	Curriculum	AS-C
	Unfulfilled promises	AS-prom
	Academic shock	AS
Professional transformation	Hospital to community	PT-H to C
	Practice to theory	PT-P to T
	Professionalization	PT-prof
Geographical relocation	Financial	GR-Fin
	Time and commuting	GR-T/C
	University structure	GR-US
	Campus size	GR-Size
	University culture	GR-Cul
	Guinea pigs	GR-GP
Transition stress	Self-doubt	TS-SD
	Going back	TS-GB
	Family and personal responsibility	TS-F
	Rumours	TS-R
	Emotions	TS-E
What social life?	Separation	S-sep
	Loneliness	S-L
	Bonding	S-B
Adaptation	Supports	A-Supp
	Personal attributes	A-P
	Learning the ropes	A-L
	Satisfaction	A-Sat
	Personal change	A-C
	Recommendations – college	A-RC
	Recommendations – university	A-RU

From Cameron, C. (2003). Experiences of transfer students in a collaborative baccalaureate nursing program. *Community College Review, 33*(2), 22–44.

health after leaving male abusive partners. The researchers found that the families limit intrusion by the male partner through a process of strengthening capacity via four subprocesses: providing, regenerating family, renewing self, and rebuilding security. A depiction of the structural components and how the subprocesses relate to the theoretical structure is shown in Figure 15–2.

Although many researchers are fond of figures and charts as part of their data display, profiles or vignettes can also display what is to be learned from the participant's experience. Vignettes of the

participant's experience can summarize what was learned from each participant and can then be shared with each participant for validation (Seidman, 1998). This narrative form transforms the text into a story—a compelling way of sharing meaning.

For example, Cameron (2003) studied the lived experience of transfer students in a collaborative nursing program and, as part of the mixed methodology design, interviewed 13 students. Vignettes were developed for each interview participant, who, in turn, selected a pseudonym that had personal meaning. The vignette was shared

TABLE 15-3 Sample Coding	
Text	**Code**
"The first week of school? - going out of my mind - coming home and crying. It was the expectations, they seem to be going on and on about these expectations that they were expecting of us. I don't think the information that was given to us was, I don't think was clarified properly or they didn't say it in a way to us that made us want to do it. It was . . . I felt very intimidated by the way they were talking to us by the expectations . . . you are going to do this and this and this . . . starting next week. I'm just in there — going out of my mind. . . . I don't know if I am going to be able to do this and it was again the self-doubt. It was I don't think I'm going to be able to handle this. I want to go back to my college. And I remember me and my friends were just outside of our class and we were just like this is unbearable and a couple of my friends wanted to call the college to see if they could get back in and . . . I knew if I could just last this week and last through a month . . . then I will see . . . Because I wasn't going to give up, just then. But it was definitely an eye opening experience. It wasn't at all what expected. The professors were great but they just, it was too much information during that one week of the orientation."	TS-E AS-Work AS-Uprep TS-SD AS-Uprep TS-GB TS-E A-P AS-Uprep AS-Work

From Cameron, C. (2003). Experiences of transfer students in a collaborative baccalaureate nursing program. *Community College Review, 33*(2), 22–44.

TABLE 15-4 Themes and Subthemes in Results from Smith et al. (2006)	
Themes	**Subthemes**
Pregnancy as an opportunity for change	• Wanting children to have the gifts but not the pain of the intergenerational impact of residential schools • Children are highly valued • Parents are highly motivated to heal past hurts and reconnect with self, family, and culture
Safe health care places and relationships	• Nonjudgemental • Respectful • Strengths based • Facilitating healing and trusting relationships
Responsive care	• Holistic • Client directed • Integrating multiple ways of knowing, with greater emphasis on experiential and cultural knowledge
Making intervention safe and responsive	• Reaching out—being visible • Empowerment education • Including fathers and family • Feeding body, mind, and soul

From Smith, D., Edwards, N., Varcoe, C., Martens, P. J., & Davies, B. (2006). Bringing safety and responsiveness into the forefront of care for pregnant and parenting Aboriginal people. *Advances in Nursing Science, 29*(2), E27–E44. Reprinted with permission.

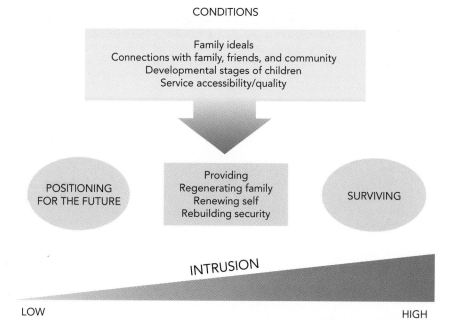

CONDITIONS

Family ideals
Connections with family, friends, and community
Developmental stages of children
Service accessibility/quality

POSITIONING
FOR THE FUTURE

Providing
Regenerating family
Renewing self
Rebuilding security

SURVIVING

INTRUSION

LOW   HIGH

Figure 15–2 Subprocesses in strengthening capacity

From Ford-Gilboe, M., Wuest, J., & Merritt-Gray, M. (2005). Strengthening capacity to limit intrusion: Theorizing family health promotion in the aftermath of woman abuse. *Qualitative Health Research, 15*(4), 483.

with each participant who then had the opportunity to change or modify the description. An example of one vignette follows:

> *Zion, a young minority student, immigrated to Canada as a child. She attended college directly after graduating from high school. She chose the collaborative program because she was aware that the degree would be mandatory for nursing in the future and her mother felt that nursing, as a career choice, was perfect. During the college portion she struggled academically as she was commuting four hours per day. However, through perseverance, she managed to achieve a 'B' average in her second year at college and was admitted to the university portion of the program. Zion rated her transition as fairly difficult. Her primary concern was financial and resulted in the delay of purchase of textbooks and course materials. The ensuing stress led to a breakdown in class. With the intervention of a professor, she stuck it out. Now in the final days of her first year at the university, Zion reflects that she settled in by February and at that point realized that she would not quit and could make it. Driving Zion is her determination and to be a good example for other minority students living below the poverty line. Her motto is "I don't let circumstances determine my outcome". Zion reports that this transition has made her stronger, more self-confident, and that overall she will be a better nurse (Cameron, 2003, p. 120).*

Rich descriptions, such as those found in vignettes or direct quotations bring the data to life and give meaning to people's experiences. Most qualitative research includes selected quotations to illustrate the themes (see Table 15–5) and to provide the reader with the opportunity to understand and validate the themes chosen by the researcher.

TABLE 15–5 Examples of Selected Quotations to Support the Major Themes from Appendix B

Themes	Example of a Quotation
Pregnancy as an opportunity for change	"The real cultural belief is that all children are a gift from God. So no matter what the circumstances . . . if the woman is drinking, if she's doing drugs . . . it doesn't matter [to the importance placed on the child], that child is a gift. And that has an enormous influence on the woman."
Safe places and safe relationships	"It's also the environment, the place; it's warm, friendly and caring and we have time for people. There is a different energy in programs built from an Aboriginal perspective . . . the pace is different . . . the environment is more relaxed, friendly, casual . . . it is a comfortable place to be with couches and the coffee room. There is a mix of staff that is similar to the mix of participants [including some] First Nations staff. We dress differently . . . ."
Responsive care	"Most of it, I truly believe, if I look back over the years . . . it's about 50 to 60% emotional support. I might have an agenda that I'd like to talk about breastfeeding today, but that might be the last thing on their agenda, so if we can't do what's on their mind and their focus, then how can we really reach what we need to do?"
Making intervention strategies safe and responsive	"In the past, the emphasis had always been on perceived rigid rules and regulations coming from the outside. [Though] we wanted to honor our professional code (e.g., nursing standards for practice), we also wanted to honor the cultural codes and protocols of the [local] people. We needed to understand the [local cultural] code, to respect it, to abide by it, and to be guided by it. So that the cultural code was the main code, and the professional code was the add-on piece, rather than the other way around."

Based on Smith, D., Edwards, N., Varcoe, C., Martens, P. J., & Davies, B. (2006). Bringing safety and responsiveness into the forefront of care for pregnant and parenting Aboriginal people. *Advances in Nursing Science, 29*(2), E27–E44.

Conclusion Drawing and Verification

Conclusion drawing begins at the beginning of data collection but is not finalized until the project is completed. Although qualitative research is inductive, most researchers being to draw conclusions as they begin. The challenge for the researcher is to remain open to new ideas, themes, and concepts as they appear.

Conclusion drawing is essentially the description of the relationship between the themes. Grounded theory formalizes this stage through the development of models, leading to theory. Verification occurs as the data are collected; this process can vary from questioning one's own conclusion through the rechecking of the text, to verification by colleagues, to finding new cases and applying the model to them. In grounded theory, researchers use the **constant comparative method**, to compare new data with data previously analyzed.

Miles and Huberman (1994) reminded us that this process of making sense of the data is a skill that we all have. People make sense of the world around them by organizing and interpreting it; this skill is applied to drawing and verifying conclusions. Miles and Huberman listed the following 13 tactics for generating meaning (pp. 245–246):

1. Noting patterns and themes
2. Seeing plausibility
3. Clustering
4. Making metaphors
5. Counting
6. Making contrasts or comparisons
7. Partitioning variables
8. Subsuming particulars into the general
9. Factoring
10. Noting relationships between variables
11. Finding intervening variables
12. Building a logical chain of evidence
13. Making conceptual or theoretical coherence

Refer to Miles and Huberman (1994) for more detail about these tactics.

To verify the emergent themes and subthemes, Smith et al. (2006) consulted with their participants to discuss and critique the findings. Verbatim quotations provided a context for the themes (see Table 15–5). Once a preliminary draft was written, participants were invited to discuss the findings in several three-hour workshops.

Other researchers can use different methods to validate their themes. For example, Bottorff et al. (2004) (see Appendix D) searched the data using NVivo for content related to explanations of dependence, addiction, lack of control over smoking, and experiences associated with cessation. These data were then subjected to a thematic analysis comparing the participants' explanations of addiction. To verify the findings, the research team regularly discussed the analysis and interpretation. Once the initial analysis was complete, secondary analysis took place with a second set of interviews. As a final analysis, further interviews took place with eight selected adolescent to validate the findings.

No matter what method is used, researchers ask themselves, "What have I learned? How do I understand this, make sense of it and see the connections in it?" (Seidman, 1998). The conclusions drawn are simply to "describe, make contributions and contribute to greater understanding" (Glesne, 2006, p. 166). As discussed in Chapter 7, through the processes of reflexivity and bracketing, researchers constantly compare their findings with their own personal beliefs and knowledge to ensure that the analysis reflects the participants' beliefs rather than their own.

SPECIFIC ANALYTIC PROCEDURES

The processes of data analysis vary based on the type of qualitative research. Table 15–6 summarizes the methods of analysis in qualitative methods, including phenomenology, ethnography, grounded theory, and case study. Excerpts from Canadian studies are included to exemplify the methods.

TRUSTWORTHINESS

As described in Chapter 14, rigour in qualitative research is determined by credibility, auditability,

and fittingness as the criteria for evaluation. Trustworthiness is also important when determining the validity of the data interpretation or analysis. To ensure the trustworthiness of their findings, qualitative researchers must ask themselves the following questions (Holloway & Jefferson, 2000):

- *What do you notice?* The researcher has captured some impressions about the data; however, information may be missing.

- *Why do you notice what you notice?* Researchers must consider their own biases and predispositions as they interpret the data to produce trustworthy interpretations.

- *How can you interpret what you notice?* As discussed in Chapter 14, credibility stems from prolonged engagement and persistent observation. To be able to complete a full interpretation, the researcher must spend a sufficient amount of time in the field to build sound relationships with the participants.

- *How can you know that your interpretation is the "right" one?* The quickest way to know whether the interpretation is accurate is through sharing the findings with the participants. This sharing is an integral part of participatory action research, as outlined in Chapter 8, and is referred to in many studies as **member checking**. The researcher is also checking whether the connections between the categories or themes are logical. Inviting other experts to review the data analysis is also an option for many researchers. Some researchers will also analyze their data from several different frameworks (a form of triangulation) to increase the trustworthiness of the data analysis.

Finally, it is important to consider the limitations of the study. Many researchers describe the issues they faced so that the reader will know and understand the research in the proper context (Glesne, 2006).

TABLE 15–6 **Methods of Analysis**

Tradition	Method of Analysis	Example
Phenomenology—includes a variety of traditions	• Immersion in the data: listen to tapes, read and reread transcripts • Identify and extract significant statements • Determine relationships among the extracted statements (themes) • Prepare exhaustive description of the phenomena and the relationship among the themes • Synthesize the themes into a consistent description or statement of the phenomenon under study (essence)	Charlebois & Bouchard (2007): "The Worst Experience": The Experience of Grandparents Who Have a Grandchild with Cancer." Eight grandparents were interviewed. Three central themes emerged: living the worst experience; giving support, a crucial role for grandparents; and feeling supported to carry on. The authors synthesized their findings in this way: "The essence of the phenomenon is described as follows: having a grandchild with cancer is, for all the grandparents in the study, the worst experience they can ever live, a vital duty to support members of the family, a duty that is closely related to the perception they have of their grandparental role, and a need to feel supported by calling upon several strategies to better carry on" (p. 27).
Ethnography	• Immersion in the data • Identify patterns and themes • Complete a cultural inventory • Interpret the findings • Compare the findings with those in the literature	Elliott, Berman, and Kim (2002): "A Critical Ethnography of Korean Canadian Women's Menopause Experience." The authors described their method as follows: "The analysis of the stories began at the onset of data collection. The tapes were listened to numerous times to gain early insight into meaning and understanding of the essence of the whole before determination of themes could occur. This checking of tape to transcription was important when there were language difficulties. A process of 'narrative reduction' was carried out with the verbatim transcripts. Narrative reduction involves retranscribing selected portions to determine narrative forms for detailed analysis. The edited transcripts were coded by content areas and condensed into themes after analysis. Consistent with critical ethnography, analysis of the narratives focused on the stories that the women told about menopause and how culture embedded their experiences" (p. 381).
Grounded theory	• Examine data carefully line by line • Divide data into discrete parts • Compare data for similarities and differences • Compare data with other data continuously in a process—constant comparative method • Cluster codes to form categories • Expand and develop categories or collapse them into one another • Determine relationships between categories	Ford-Gilboe, Wuest, & Merrit-Gray (2005): "Strengthening Capacity to Limit Intrusion: Theorizing Family Health Promotion in the Aftermath of Woman Abuse." The authors described their study as follows: "Initial interviews were coded line by line by all team members using the constant comparative method at a face-to-face meeting. As codes and categories began to solidify, individual coding took place augmented by monthly teleconference discussions and shared memos. Similar codes were grouped together to form categories, which were constantly compared to illuminate their properties (Glaser & Straus, 1967). Hypothesis about the relationships among concepts were generated, tested, and refined (Stern, 1985; Stern & Pyles, 1986)" (p. 481).

TABLE 15–6	Methods of Analysis (cont'd)	
Tradition	**Method of Analysis**	**Example**
Case study	• Identify unit of analysis (person, family, organization) • Code continuously as data are collected • Find commonalities and themes • Analyze field notes • Review description of themes to identify patterns and connections between them	Chircop & Keddy (2003): "Women Living with Environmental Illness." Chircop and Keddy noted: "From the beginning of the data collection the interviews were analyzed case by case, on a continuous basis, according to commonalities or common themes. To arrive at common themes it was necessary to code or identify each interview into units of higher abstraction. The codes of two of the four interviews were peer reviewed for validation purposes. Identified themes were then grounded in a secondary literature review" (p. 374).

Critiquing Qualitative Data Analysis

The general criteria for critiquing qualitative data analysis are proposed in the Critiquing Criteria box; however, remember that many different approaches to data analysis exist. The data analysis is consistent with the research philosophy, the question, and the design. For example, researchers using grounded theory build a case for substantive theory, explaining the phenomenon under study, whereas a phenomenological researcher is interested in expressing the meaning of the phenomenon itself.

Regardless of the study's research method, several commonalities exist among methods used in qualitative data analysis. For example, analysis is conducted alongside the data collection, and in most cases the two processes are interrelated. Researchers become immersed in the data: they listen over and over to the interviews, read and reread the transcripts, and spend substantial time in the field. Although the methods may differ, the text is coded to search for themes and categories through a process of data reduction. The emergent themes are then verified through member checking. As themes emerge, logical connections and relationships between the themes are identified to form a whole picture. The results are displayed in such a manner that the reader can understand and validate the conclusions that the researcher has drawn through the use of diagrams, tables, charts, direct quotations from the participants, and rich descriptions of the findings. In summary, qualitative data analysis takes mounds of disparate data and transforms them into a coherent whole or story to provide meaning about the human experience.

CRITIQUING CRITERIA

1. Is the method of data analysis clearly stated?

2. Is the strategy of data analysis appropriate for the methodology of the study?

3. Are the steps of analysis listed for the reader to follow?

4. Is evidence provided that the researcher's interpretation captures the phenomenon under study?

5. Does the researcher address the credibility, auditability, and fittingness of the data?

Critical Thinking Challenges

- How do researchers determine whether they have spent enough time with the data?
- Is it important for the researcher to personally transcribe the interviews?
- Why do some researchers go back to the literature as themes emerge from the data?
- Often, data analysis takes place as data are collected. How can analysis of the data change the data collection?
- Researchers validate their interpretation of the data through a process of member checking. What happens if the participants indicate that the analysis does not reflect their experience?

KEY POINTS

- Qualitative data are text derived from transcripts from interviews, narratives, documents, media such as newspapers and movies, and field notes.
- Computer software can simplify the storage and retrieval of data.
- Qualitative research data can be managed through the use of computers, but the researcher must interpret the data.
- Data analysis and data collection are parallel processes.
- Qualitative analysis is not a linear process; rather, it is a cyclical and iterative process.
- The three discrete stages of data analysis are data reduction, data display, and conclusion drawing and verification.
- Data are organized into meaningful chunks of data through a clustering of related or similar data and are labelled as themes.
- Coding is the process of progressively marking, sorting, resorting, and defining and redefining the collected data.
- Data display uses graphs, flow charts, matrices, or any other visual representation to assemble data and to allow for conclusion drawing.
- Grounded theorists use the constant comparative method, in which new data are compared with data previously analyzed
- Member checking is the process of checking whether the interpretation is accurate through the sharing of the findings with the participants.

REFERENCES

Bottorff, J. L., Johnson, J. L., Moffat, B., Grewal, J., Ratner, P., & Kalaw, C. (2004). Adolescent constructions of nicotine addiction. *Canadian Journal of Nursing Research, 38*, 22–39.

Cameron, C. (2003). *The lived experience of transfer students in a collaborative baccalaureate nursing program.* Unpublished doctoral dissertation, University of Toronto.

Cameron, C. (2005). Experiences of transfer students in a collaborative baccalaureate nursing program. *Community College Review, 33*(2), 22–44.

Charlebois, S., & Bouchard, L. (2007). "The worst experience": The experience of grandparents who have a grandchild with cancer. *Canadian Oncological Nursing Journal, 17*(1), 26–36.

Chircop, A., & Keddy, B. (2003). Women living with environmental illness. *Health Care for Women International, 24*, 371–383.

Denzin, N., & Lincoln, Y. (2000). *Handbook of qualitative research* (2nd ed.). Thousand Oaks, CA: Sage.

Elliott, E., Berman, H., & Kim, S. (2002) A critical ethnography of Korean Canadian women's menopause experience. *Health Care for Women International, 23*, 377–388.

Ford-Gilboe, M., Wuest, J., & Merrit-Gray, M. (2005). Strengthening capacity to limit intrusion: Theorizing family health promotion in the aftermath of woman abuse. *Qualitative Health Research, 15*, 477–501.

Glaser, B., & Strauss, A. (1967). *The discovery of grounded theory.* Chicago: Aldine.

Glesne, C. (2006). *Becoming qualitative researchers: An introduction* (3rd ed.). Don Mills, ON: Longman.

Holloway, W. & Jeffersen, T. (2000). *Doing qualitative research differently: Free association, narrative and the interview method.* Thousand Oak, CA: Sage.

Meadows, L. M., Dodendorf, D. M. (1999). Data management and interpretation using computers to assist. In B. Crabtree & W. L. Miller (Eds.), *Doing qualitative research* (2nd ed.). Thousand Oaks: CA, Sage.

Miles, B. M., & Huberman, A. M. (1994). *Qualitative data analysis* (2nd ed.). Thousand Oaks, CA: Sage.

Patton, M. (2002). *Qualitative research & evaluation methods* (3rd ed.). Thousand Oaks, CA: Sage.

Seidman, I. (1998). *Interviewing as qualtitative research: A guide for researchers in education and social sciences* (2nd ed.). New York: Teachers College Press.

Smith, D., Edwards, N., Varcoe, C., Martens, P. J., & Davies, B. (2006). Bringing safety and responsiveness into the forefront of care for pregnant and parenting Aboriginal people. *Advances in Nursing Science, 29*(2), E27–E44.

Speziale, H., & Carpenter, D. (2007). *Qualitative research in nursing: Advancing the humanistic imperative* (4th ed.). Philadelphia: Lippincott.

Stern, P. (1985). Using grounded theory method in nursing research. In M. Leininger (Ed.), *Qualitative research methods in nursing* (pp. 149–160). Orlando, FL: Grune & Stratton.

Stern, P., & Pyles, S. (1986). Using grounded theory methodology to study women's culturally based decisions about health. In P. N. Stern (Ed.), *Women, health and culture* (pp. 1–24). Washington, DC: Hemisphere.

Van Manen, M. (1997). *Researching lived experience.* London, ON: Althouse Press.

Wuest, J. (2001). Precarious ordering: Towards a formal theory of women's caring. *Health Care for Women International: Special volume, Using ground theory to study women's health, 22*(1–2), 167–193.

Wuest, J., Merritt-Gray, M., Berman, H., & Ford-Gilboe, M. (2002). Illuminating social determinants of women's health using grounded theory. *Health Care International, 23*, 794–808.

CHAPTER 16

Robin Whittemore
Margaret Grey
Carl Kirton
Mina D. Singh

Quantitative Data Analysis

LEARNING OUTCOMES

After reading this chapter, the student should be able to do the following:

- Differentiate between descriptive and inferential statistics.
- State the purposes of descriptive statistics.
- Identify the levels of measurement in a research study.
- Describe a frequency distribution.
- List measures of central tendency and their use.
- List measures of variability and their use.
- Identify the purpose of inferential statistics.
- Distinguish between a parameter and a statistic.
- Explain the concept of probability as it applies to the analysis of sample data.
- Distinguish between type I and type II errors and their effects on a study's outcome.
- Distinguish between parametric and nonparametric tests.
- List the commonly used statistical tests and their purposes.
- Critically analyze the statistics used in published research studies.

STUDY RESOURCES

evolve Go to Evolve at
http://evolve.elsevier.com/Canada/LoBiondo/Research/
for Weblinks, content updates, and additional research articles for practice in reviewing and critiquing.

KEY TERMS

alpha
analysis of covariance (ANCOVA)
analysis of variance (ANOVA)
chi-square (χ^2)
confidence interval (CI)
correlation
degrees of freedom
descriptive statistics
factor analysis
Fisher's exact probability test
frequency distribution
inferential statistics
interval measurement
kurtosis
level of significance (alpha level)
levels of measurement
Linear Structural Relationships (LISREL)
logistic regression (logit analysis)
mean
measurement
measures of central tendency
measures of variability
median
modality
mode
multiple analysis of variance (MANOVA)
multiple regression
nominal measurement
nonparametric statistics

nonparametric tests of significance
normal curve
null hypothesis
odds ratio
ordinal measurement
p value
parameter
parametric statistics
Pearson correlation coefficient (Pearson *r*, Pearson product moment correlation coefficient)
percentile
population
post hoc analysis
power
probability
range
ratio measurement
sampling error
scatter plots
scientific hypothesis
semiquartile range (semi-interquartile range)
skew
standard deviation (SD)
standard error of the mean
statistic
symmetry
t statistic
type I error
type II error
Z score

The use of statistics pervades the nursing and health care literature. Descriptive and inferential statistics are located in the "Methods" section, the "Results" section, or both sections of a research article. Before you become overwhelmed by the complexity of the information, bear in mind that you do not need to be familiar with or to be able to calculate a large number of complex statistical tests to analyze data. An understanding of which tests are used with which kind of design and which type of data is sufficient. This type of basic understanding will help you to appraise evidence from a research study, which is essential to informing decisions you make in your practice.

As a research consumer, you will not perform the data analysis yourself, but it is important to understand the researcher's challenge in analyzing the data. After carefully collecting data, the researcher is faced with the task of organizing and analyzing the individual pieces of information so that the meaning of study results is clear. The researcher must choose methods of organizing and analyzing the raw data based on the design, the type of data collected, and the hypothesis or question that was tested. Statistical procedures are used to organize and give meaning to the data.

The "Results" section of a research article contains the data generated from the testing of the hypothesis or research questions. These data are the result of analysis using both *descriptive* and *inferential statistics*. An example of what may be found is as follows: "The average length of stay for the control ward participants was 333.5 days (SD = 1068.5), while the average length of stay for the intervention ward participants was 217.5 days (SD = 498.5)" (Forchuk, Martin, Chan, & Jensen, 2005, p. 561) (see Appendix A). The data in Table 1 of the Forchuk et al. article are known as descriptive statistics, which are usually the first set of statistical results in a report or published article.

Statistical details that describe and summarize data are known as **descriptive statistics**. Descriptive statistical techniques reduce data to manageable proportions by summarizing and organizing them. These techniques allow researchers to arrange data visually to give meaning and to help in understanding the sample characteristics and variables before engaging in inferential data analyses. In some studies, descriptive statistics may be the only statistical analysis used. Descriptive statistical techniques include **measures of central tendency**, such as mode, median, and mean; measures of variability, such as range and standard deviation (SD); and some correlation techniques, such as **scatter plots**.

In contrast to descriptive statistics, *inferential statistics* allow researchers to estimate how reliably they can make predictions and generalize findings based on the data. **Inferential statistics** are used by researchers to analyze the data collected and test hypotheses so they can answer the study's research question. Through the use of inferential statistics, researchers can draw conclusions that extend beyond the immediate data of the study. The following is an example of inferential statistics from Forchuk et al. (2005): "The intervention group did not have a significant improvement in global quality of life (control group mean of 4.65, SD = 1.31; intervention mean = 4.78, SD = 1.31, $F(1,22) = 0389$, $P = 0.27$" (p. 562). Samuels-Dennis's (2006) study provides another example: "As predicted, [social assistance] recipients encountered a larger number of stressful life events than employed mothers ($_E = 6.94$, $_{SA} = 8.81$, $t = -2.233$, $p = .028 \ldots$)" (p. 67) (see Appendix C).

The purpose of this chapter is to demonstrate how researchers use descriptive and inferential statistics in nursing research studies so that you, as a research consumer, will be better able to determine the appropriateness of the statistics used and to interpret the strength and quality of the reported findings, their clinical significance, and their applicability to practice. Basic concepts and terminology common in evidence-based practice publications are presented in Chapter 20. The information in this chapter will help you begin to make sense of the statistics used in research papers.

DESCRIPTIVE STATISTICS

Levels of Measurement

Measurement is the assignment of numbers to variables or events according to rules. Every variable in a research study that is assigned a specific number must be similar to every other variable assigned that number. For example, male subjects may be assigned the number 1 and female subjects the number 2. The measurement level is determined by the nature of the object or event being measured. **Levels of measurement** from low to high are nominal, ordinal, interval, and ratio. The levels of measurement are the determining factors of the type of statistics to be used in analyzing data. The higher the level of measurement, the greater the flexibility the researcher has in choosing statistical procedures. Every attempt should be made to use the highest level of measurement possible so that the maximum amount of information will be obtained from the data, as highlighted in Table 16–1. The Critical Thinking Decision Path illustrates the relationship between levels of measurement and appropriate choice of specific descriptive statistics.

Nominal measurement classifies variables or events into categories. The categories are mutually exclusive; the variable or event either has or does not have the characteristic. The numbers assigned to each category are nothing more than labels; such numbers do not indicate more or less of a characteristic. Nominal level measurement can be used to categorize a sample on such information as gender, hair colour, marital status, or religious affiliation.

The study by Samuels-Dennis (2006) of stress and psychological distress in single mothers includes several examples of nominal level measurement, including ethnic or racial background and marital status (see Appendix C). The nominal level of measurement allows the least amount of mathematical manipulation. Most commonly, the frequency of each event is counted, as well as the percentage of the total each category represents.

A variable at the nominal level can also be considered a *dichotomous* or a *categorical* variable. A dichotomous (nominal) variable has only two true values, such as true/false or gender (male/female) (see Chapter 20). Variables that are nominal and categorical still have mutually exclusive categories but have more than two true values, such as marital status (single, married, divorced, separated, or widowed). In both cases, the nominal variables are mutually exclusive. For example, in the Samuels-Dennis (2006) article, the category of ethnic or racial background is both nominal and categorical (see Appendix C). The gender of the client in the Forchuk et al. (2005) article would be considered a dichotomous nominal variable (male/female) (see Appendix A).

Ordinal measurement shows relative rankings of variables or events. The numbers assigned to each category can be compared, and a person in a higher category can be said to have more of an attribute than a person in a lower category. The

TABLE 16–1 Level of Measurement Summary Table			
Measurement	**Description**	**Measures of Central Tendency**	**Measures of Variability**
Nominal	Classification	Mode	Modal percentage, range, frequency distribution
Ordinal	Relative rankings	Mode, median	Modal percentage, range, frequency, percentile, semiquartile range, frequency distribution
Interval	Rank ordering with equal intervals	Mode, median, mean	Modal percentage, range, percentile, semiquartile range, standard deviation
Ratio	Rank ordering with equal intervals and absolute zero	Mode, median, mean	All

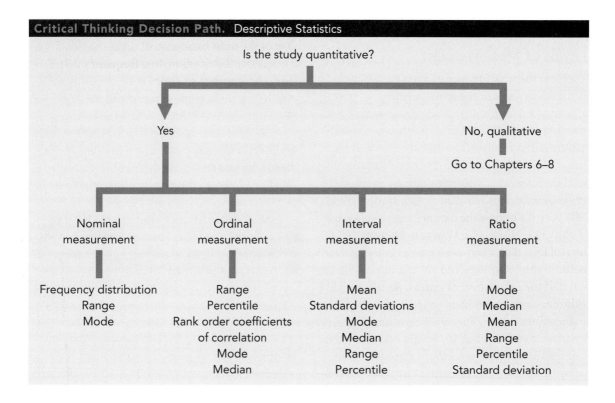

Critical Thinking Decision Path. Descriptive Statistics

Is the study quantitative?

Yes

No, qualitative

Go to Chapters 6–8

Nominal measurement	Ordinal measurement	Interval measurement	Ratio measurement
Frequency distribution	Range	Mean	Mode
Range	Percentile	Standard deviations	Median
Mode	Rank order coefficients of correlation	Mode	Mean
	Mode	Median	Range
	Median	Range	Percentile
		Percentile	Standard deviation

intervals between numbers on the scale are not necessarily equal, and zero is not absolute. For example, ordinal measurement is used to formulate class rankings, in which one student can be ranked higher or lower than another. However, the difference in actual grade point average between students may differ widely. Another example is ranking individuals by their level of wellness and their ability to carry out activities of daily living. Annual income and level of education in the Samuels-Dennis (2006) article are considered ordinal level variables (see Appendix C).

Under the Canadian Heart and Stroke Foundation classification of cardiac failure, individuals can be assigned to one of four classifications. Classification I represents little disease or interference with activities of daily living, whereas classification IV represents severe disease and little ability to carry out the activities of daily living independently, but an individual in class IV cannot be said to be four times sicker than an individual in class I. A similar scale based on an individual's current health status is used to classify an individual's anaesthesia risk.

Ordinal level data are limited in the amount of mathematical manipulation possible. In addition to what is possible with nominal data, medians, percentiles, and rank order coefficients of correlation can be calculated. In most cases, ordinal variables in a scale are treated as interval level measurements when converted to numerical codes. For example, when clients are asked to rate their level of satisfaction with life as "not satisfied," "satisfied," or "very satisfied," their responses are an ordinal measurement. When their ratings are treated numerically and coded as 1, 2, and 3, respectively, their responses are an interval measurement.

Interval measurement ranks events or variables on a scale with equal intervals between the numbers. The zero point remains arbitrary and not absolute. For example, interval measurements are used in measuring temperatures on the Fahrenheit scale. The distances between degrees are equal, but the zero point is arbitrary and does not represent the absence of temperature. Test scores also represent interval data. The differences between test scores represent equal intervals, but a zero does not represent the total absence of knowledge.

In many areas in the social sciences, including nursing, the classification of the level of measurement of intelligence, aptitude, and personality tests is controversial, with some researchers regarding these measurements as ordinal and others as interval. The research consumer needs to be aware of this controversy and to look at each study individually in terms of how the data are analyzed (Knapp, 1990, 1993; Wang, Yu, Wang, & Huang, 1999). Interval level data allow more manipulation of data, including the addition and subtraction of numbers and the calculation of means. Because of this additional manipulation, many argue for the higher classification level. The Spielberger State Anxiety Inventory and the Center for Epidemiologic Studies Depression Scale were used as interval measurements by Davison and associates (2003) to evaluate the effect of an individualized information session on psychological distress in men with prostate cancer and their partners. The Beck Depression Inventory (BDI-II) instrument in the Samuels-Dennis (2006) article is ordinal and was used as an interval level measurement (see Appendix C).

Ratio measurement ranks events or variables on scales with equal intervals and absolute zeros. The number represents the actual amount of the property the object possesses. Ratio measurement is the highest level of measurement but is usually achieved only in the physical sciences. Examples of ratio level data are height, weight, pulse, and blood pressure. All mathematical procedures can be performed on data from ratio scales. Therefore, the use of any statistical procedure is possible as long as it is appropriate to the design of the study.

Helpful Hint

Descriptive statistics assist in summarizing the data. The descriptive statistics calculated must be appropriate to both the purpose of the study and the level of measurement.

FREQUENCY DISTRIBUTION

One of the most basic ways of organizing data is in a frequency distribution. In a **frequency distribution**, the number of times each event occurs is counted, or the data are grouped and the frequency of each group is reported. An instructor reporting the results of an examination could report the number of students receiving each grade or could group the grades and report the number in each group. Table 16–2 shows the results of an examination given to a class of 51 students. The results are reported in several ways. The columns on the left give the raw data tally and the frequency for each grade, whereas the columns on the right give the grouped data tally and grouped frequencies. In another example, a study of stress and psychological distress in single mothers, the results were grouped rather than reported individually for each hospital (Samuels-Dennis, 2006) (see Appendix C).

When data are grouped, the researcher needs to define the size of the group or the interval width so that no score will fall into two groups and each group will be mutually exclusive. The grouping of the data in Table 16–2 prevents overlap; each score falls into only one group. If the grouping had been 70 to 80 and 80 to 90, scores of 80 would have fallen into two categories. The grouping should allow for a precise presentation of the data without serious loss of information. Very large interval widths lead to loss of data information and may obscure patterns in the data. If the test scores in Table 16–2 had been grouped as 40 to 69 and 70 to 99, the pattern of the scores would have been obscured.

Information about frequency distributions may be presented in the form of a table, such as Table 16–2, or in the form of a graph. Figure 16–1 illustrates the most common graph forms: the histogram and the frequency polygon. These two methods are similar in that both plot scores or percentages of occurrence against frequency. The greater the number of points plotted, the smoother the resulting graph. The shape of the resulting graph allows for observations that further describe the data. For example, in their study of parents' knowledge about the use of child safety systems, Snowdon, Polgar,

TABLE 16–2	**Frequency Distribution**				
Individual			Group		
Score	Tally	Frequency	Score	Tally	Frequency
90	|	1	>89	|	1
88	|	1			
86	|	1	80–89	ЖГ ЖГ ЖГ	15
84	ЖГ |	6			
82	||	2	70–79	ЖГ ЖГ ЖГ ЖГ |||	23
80	ЖГ	5			
78	ЖГ	5			
76	|	1	60–69	ЖГ ЖГ	10
74	ЖГ ||	7			
72	ЖГ ||||	9	<59	||	2
70	|	1			
68	|||	3			
66	||	2			
64	||||	4			
62	|	1			
60		0			
58	|	1			
56		0			
54	|	1			
52		0			
50		0			
Total		51			51

Mean, 73.1; standard deviation, +12.1; median, 74; mode, 72; range, 36 (54–90).

Patrick, and Stamler (2006) used histograms to illustrate the rate at which parents transitioned their infant from a rear-facing to a forward-facing seat and the timing of this transition (see Figure 16–2).

MEASURES OF CENTRAL TENDENCY

Measures of central tendency answer questions such as the following: "What does the average nurse think?" "What is the average temperature of clients on a unit?" These measures yield a single number that describes the middle of the group and summarize the members of a sample. In statistics, the three measures of central tendency are the mode, the median, and the mean. Depending on the distribution, these measures may not all give the same answer to the question "What is the average?" Each measure of central tendency has a specific use and is most appropriate to specific kinds of measurement and types of distributions.

Mode.   The **mode** is the most frequent score or result and can be obtained by inspection of the frequency distribution table or graph. Note that a sample distribution can have more than one mode. The number of modes, or peaks, contained in a distribution is called the **modality** of the distribution. The mode is the type of descriptive statistic most appropriately used with nominal data but can be used with all levels of measurement (see Table 16–1). The mode cannot be used for any subsequent calculations and is unstable; in other words, the mode can fluctuate widely from sample to sample from the same population. A change in just one score in Table 16–2 would change the mode from 72.

Median.   The **median** is the middle score—50% of the scores are above it and 50% of the scores are below it. The median is not sensitive to extremes in high and low scores; thus, it is a more accurate

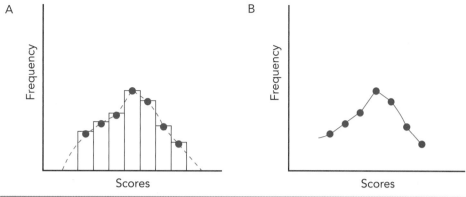

Figure 16–1 Frequency distributions. A, Histogram. B, Frequency polygon.

estimator of central tendency in non-normal distributions. In the series of scores in Table 16–2, the twenty-sixth score will always be the median regardless of how much the high and low scores change. The median is best used when the data are skewed (see "Normal Distribution" in this chapter), and the researcher is interested in the "typical" score. For example, if age is a variable, and a wide range with extreme scores may affect the mean, it would be appropriate to also report the median. The median is easy to find either by inspection or by calculation and can be used with ordinal or higher data, as shown in Table 16–1.

Mean. The **mean** is the arithmetical average of all scores and is used with interval or ratio data (see Table 16–1). Most statistical tests of significance refer to the mean, the most widely used measure of central tendency, which is referred to in general conversations as the *average*. Because the mean is affected by every score, it is affected by extreme scores; however, the larger the sample size, the less effect a single extreme score will have on the mean. For normally distributed populations, the mean is an appropriate measure of central tendency and is generally considered the single best point for summarizing data.

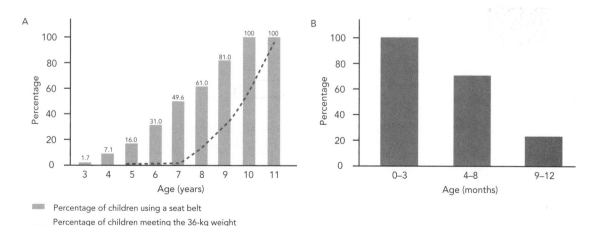

Percentage of children using a seat belt

Percentage of children meeting the 36-kg weight requirement for safely using a seat belt

Figure 16–2 Histograms. A, Premature use of seat belts in children aged 3 to 11 years. B, Use of rear-facing safety seats in infants up to 12 months (*n* = 296).

From Snowdon, A. W., Polgar, J., Patrick, L., & Stamler, L. (2006). Parents' knowledge about use of child safety systems. *Canadian Journal of Nursing Research, 38*(2), 107–108.

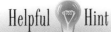

Helpful Hint

Of the three measures of central tendency, the mean is the most stable, the least affected by extremes, and the most useful for other calculations. The mean can be calculated only with interval and ratio data.

Table 16–3 shows how Samuels-Dennis (2006), in her study of stress and psychological distress in single mothers, listed the means and SDs for the study variable, the stress of having started or changed school (see Appendix C). These scores represent the average of each variable and the amount of variation in the scores. For example, the means for the stress of started or changed school were 15, with an SD (variation) of .357, for the employed group and 21, with a SD of .410, for the social assistance group. Summary statistics also may be reported in narrative form, as illustrated by the following excerpt from the study by Secco and Moffatt (2003) of the home environment of Métis, First Nations, and Caucasian adolescent mothers:

> *The final sample . . . consisted of 71 mothers under 20 years of age. The average age was 16.82 years and average educational attainment was 9.55 years . . . . Self-declared ethnicity was recorded as Caucasian 48.7% (n = 38), First Nations 23.1% (n = 18), and Métis 19.2% (n = 15). (pp. 112, 116)*

When comparing the measures of central tendency, the mean is the most stable and the median the most typical of these statistics. If the distribution of a sample is symmetrical and unimodal, the mean, median, and mode will coincide.

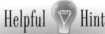

Helpful Hint

Measures of central tendency are descriptive statistics that describe the characteristics of a sample.

NORMAL DISTRIBUTION

The theoretical concept of normal distribution is based on the observation that data from repeated measures of interval or ratio level data will gather at a midpoint in a distribution, approximating the normal curve illustrated in Figure 16–3. In addition, if the means of a large number of samples of the same interval or ratio data are calculated and plotted on a graph, that curve also approximates the normal curve. This tendency of the means to approximate the normal curve is termed the sampling distribution of the means. The mean of the sampling distribution of the means is the mean of the population.

The **normal curve** is unimodal and symmetrical about the mean. The mean, median, and mode are equal. An additional characteristic of the normal curve is that a fixed percentage of the scores falls within a given distance of the mean. As shown in Figure 16–3, about 68% of the scores or means will fall within 1 SD of the mean, 95% within 2 SD of the mean, and 99.7% within 3 SD of the mean.

TABLE 16–3 **Comparison of Stressful Events According to Employment Status**							
Stressful Event	**Employed (n = 48)**			**Social Assistance (n = 48)**			
	%	**x**	**SD**	**%**	**x**	**SD**	**t**
Started/changed school	14.6	.15	.357	20.8	.21	.410	–0.796
Graduated from school	22.9	.23	.425	12.5	.13	.334	1.335
Problems in school	4.2	.04	.202	8.3	.08	.279	–0.838
Failed school	2.1	.02	.144	0	.00	.000	1.000
Got married	2.1	.02	.144	0	.00	.000	1.000
Marital separation	12.5	.13	.334	8.3	.08	.279	0.663
Divorce	0.4	.10	.309	14.6	.15	.357	–0.612

Adapted from Samuels-Dennis, J. (2006). Stress and psychological distress in single mothers. *Canadian Journal of Nursing Research, 38*(1), 59–80.

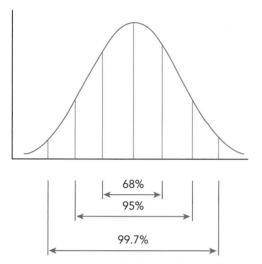

Figure 16–3 The normal distribution and associated standard deviations

Skewness. Not all samples of data approximate the normal curve. Some samples are nonsymmetrical and have the peak off-centre. For example, worldwide individual income has a positive skew, with most individuals in the low-to-moderate range and few in the upper range. The mean in a positive skew is to the right of the median. In contrast, age at death in Canada has a negative skew because most deaths occur at older ages, so the peak of the distribution curve would be to the right of a normal curve. In a negative skew, the mean is to the left of the median. Figure 16–4 illustrates positive and negative skew. In each diagram, the peak is off-centre and one tail is longer.

If the distribution is skewed, the mean will be pulled in the direction of the long tail of the distribution. With a skewed distribution, all three statistics should be reported. For example, national income in Canada is skewed. The mean wage differs from the median wage because the high salaries are so much greater than the low salaries.

Evidence-Based 🔍 Practice Tip

Inspection of descriptive statistics for the sample will indicate whether the sample data are skewed.

INTERPRETING MEASURES OF VARIABILITY

Variability or dispersion is concerned with the spread of data. **Measures of variability** answer questions such as the following: "Is the sample homogeneous or heterogeneous?" "Is the sample similar or different?" If a researcher measures oral temperatures in two samples, one sample drawn from a healthy population and one sample from a hospitalized population, it is possible that the two samples will have the same mean. However, a wider range of temperatures will more likely occur in the hospitalized sample than in the healthy sample. Measures of variability are used to describe these

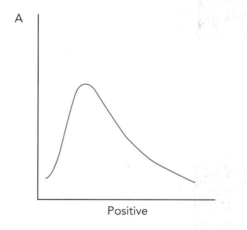

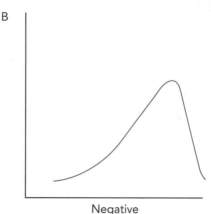

Figure 16–4 Positive and negative skew. A, Positive skew. B, Negative skew.

differences in the dispersion of data. As with measures of central tendency, the various measures of variability are appropriate to specific kinds of measurement and types of distributions.

Helpful 💡 Hint

Remember that descriptive statistics related to variability will enable you to evaluate the homogeneity or heterogeneity of a sample.

Range.   The **range** is the simplest but most unstable measure of variability. Range is the difference between the highest and lowest scores. A change in either of these two scores would change the range. The range should always be reported with other measures of variability. For example, in the Forchuk et al. study (2005), the range of age in the control group was 18 to 83 years, whereas the range of age in the intervention group was 18 to 70 years (see Appendix A). Thus, the range in the control group was 65 years, and in the intervention group, the range was 62 years. Range affects the SD, as discussed below. The range in Table 16–2 is 36, but could easily change with an increase or decrease in the high score of 90 or the low score of 54.

Semiquartile Range.   The **semiquartile range (semi-interquartile range)** indicates the range of the middle 50% of the scores. It is more stable than the range because it is less likely to be changed by a single extreme score. The semiquartile range lies between the upper and lower quartiles, the upper quartile being the point below which 75% of the scores fall and the lower quartile being the point below which 25% of the scores fall. The middle 50% of the scores in Table 16–2 lies between 68 and 78, and the semiquartile range is 10.

Percentile.   A **percentile** represents the percentage of cases a given score exceeds. The median is the 50th percentile, and in Table 16–2, it is a score of 74. A score in the 90th percentile is exceeded by only 10% of the scores. The zero percentile and the 100th percentile are usually dropped.

Standard Deviation.   The **standard deviation (SD)** is the most frequently used measure of variability and is based on the concept of the normal curve (see Figure 16–3). The SD is a measure of average deviation of the scores from the mean and, as such, should always be reported with the mean. The SD takes all scores into account and can be used to interpret individual scores. Because the mean (X) and SD for the examination in Table 16–2 were 73.16 ± 12.1, a student should know that 68% of the grades were between 85.1 and 61. If the student received a grade of 88, he would know that he did better than most of the class, whereas a grade of 58 would indicate that he did not do as well as most of the class. Table 16–3, from the study by Samuels-Dennis (2006), reports the mean and SD of the study variables that contribute to stress and depression. As illustrated in this table, the mean score for the variable "problems in school" for employed women was .04, and the SD was .202. This means that 68% of the women scored between −.162 and .242 on this measure of stress. This table allows the reader to inspect the data and see the variation the data contain (see Appendix C).

The SD is used in the calculation of many inferential statistics. One limitation of the SD is that it is expressed in terms of the units used in the measurement and cannot be used to compare means that have different units. If researchers were interested in the relationship between height measured in centimetres and weight measured in kilograms, it would be necessary to convert the height and weight measurements to standard units or Z scores. The **Z score** is used to compare measurements in standard units. Each of the scores is converted to a Z score, and then the Z scores are used to examine the relative distance of the scores from the mean. A Z score of 1.5 means that the observation is 1.5 SD above the mean, whereas a score of −2 means that the observation is 2 SD below the mean. By using Z scores, a researcher can compare results from scales that use different measurement units, such as height and weight.

Helpful 💡 Hint

Many measures of variability exist. The SD is the most stable and useful because it provides a visual image of how the scores disperse around the mean.

INFERENTIAL STATISTICS

Inferential statistics combine mathematical processes with logic and allow researchers to test hypotheses about a population using data obtained from probability samples. Statistical inference is generally used for two purposes: to estimate the probability that statistics found in the sample accurately reflect the population parameter and to test hypotheses about a population.

In the first purpose, a **parameter** is a characteristic of a *population*, whereas a **statistic** is a characteristic of a *sample*. We use statistics to estimate population parameters. Suppose that we randomly sample 100 people with chronic lung disease and use an interval level scale to study their knowledge of the disease. If the mean score for these subjects is 65, the mean represents the sample statistic. If we were able to study every subject with chronic lung disease, we also could calculate an average knowledge score, and that score would be the parameter for the population. A researcher is rarely able to study an entire population, so inferential statistics provide evidence that allow the researcher to make statements about the larger population from studying the sample.

Both parametric and nonparametric inferential tests can be used in data analyses (see Tables 16–4 and 16–5). Parametric statistical models make assumptions about the distributions of sample values and parameters and thus use means and variances to test significance. Nonparametric tests are used when populations have non-normal distributions or when researchers wish to explore associations among variables. These tests make no assumptions about the distribution of the data.

The example given alludes to two important qualifications of how a study must be conducted so that inferential statistics may be used. First, it was stated that the sample was selected using probability methods (see Chapter 12). Because you are already familiar with the advantages of probability sampling, you know that if we wish to make statements about a population from a sample, that sample must be representative. All procedures for inferential statistics are based on the assumption that the sample was drawn with a known probability. Second, it was stated that the scale had to reach the interval level of measurement. The mathematical operations involved in inferential statistics require this level of measurement. Note that studies that use nonprobability methods of sampling also use inferential statistics. To compensate for the use of nonprobability sampling methods, researchers employ techniques such as sample size estimation using power analysis. The following two Critical Thinking Decision Paths examine inferential statistics and provide matrices that researchers use for statistical decision making.

Evidence-Based 🔍 Practice Tip

Try to determine whether the statistical test chosen was appropriate for the design, the type of data collected, and the level of measurement.

Hypothesis Testing

The second and most commonly used purpose of inferential statistics is hypothesis testing. Statistical hypothesis testing allows researchers to make objective decisions about the outcome of their study and to answer questions such as the following: "How much of this effect is a result of chance?" "How strongly are these two variables associated with each other?" "What is the effect of the intervention?"

The procedures used when making inferences are based on principles of negative inference. In other words, if a researcher studied the effect of a new educational program for clients with chronic

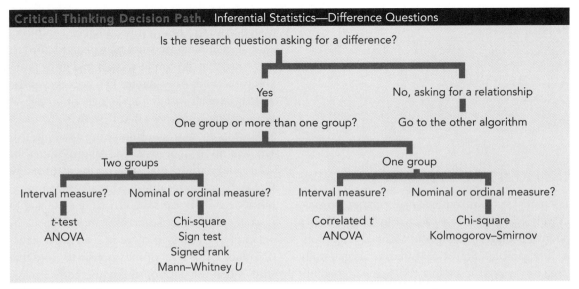

Critical Thinking Decision Path. Inferential Statistics—Difference Questions

ANOVA: analysis of variance.

lung disease, the researcher would actually have two hypotheses: the scientific hypothesis and the null hypothesis. The research or **scientific hypothesis** (H₁) is what the researcher believes the outcome of the study will be. In our example, the scientific hypothesis would be that the educational intervention would have a marked impact on the outcome in the experimental group beyond that in the control group. The **null hypothesis**

(H₀), which is the hypothesis that actually can be tested by statistical methods, would state that no difference exists between the groups. Inferential statistics use the null hypothesis to test the validity of a scientific hypothesis in sample data. The null hypothesis states that no relationship exists between the variables and that any observed relationship or difference is merely a function of chance fluctuations in sampling.

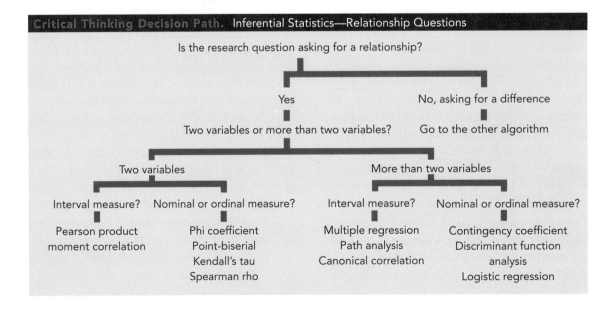

Critical Thinking Decision Path. Inferential Statistics—Relationship Questions

The concept of the null hypothesis is often confusing. An example may help clarify this concept. In the study by Forchuk et al. (2005), the investigators were interested in determining whether a transitional discharge model of care would improve the quality of life of clients undergoing psychiatric treatment (see Appendix A). On the basis of this hypothesis, the authors determined whether the differences found in the dependent variables differed significantly between the intervention group and the control group. The authors would have to use the null hypothesis—that no difference would exist between the intervention and control groups—to test the scientific hypothesis. Forchuk et al. found that men and their partners had significantly lower anxiety and depression after the intervention compared with before the intervention. In other words, the differences between the pretest and post-test scores were large enough that they were unlikely to be caused by chance. Thus, the null hypothesis was rejected.

All statistical hypothesis testing is a process of disproof or rejection. It is impossible to prove that a scientific hypothesis is true, but it is possible to demonstrate that the null hypothesis has a high probability of being incorrect. To reject the null hypothesis, then, is to show support for the scientific hypothesis, which is the desired outcome of most studies reporting inferential statistics.

Helpful Hint

Remember that most samples used in clinical research are samples of convenience, but most researchers use inferential statistics. Although such use violates one of the assumptions of such tests, the tests are robust enough to not seriously affect the results unless the data are skewed in unknown ways.

Probability

The researcher can never *prove* the scientific hypothesis but can show support for it by rejecting the null hypothesis, that is, by showing that the null hypothesis has a high probability of being incorrect. The theory underlying all of the procedures discussed in this chapter is probability theory. Probability is a concept that we talk about all the time, such as the chance of rain, but we have a difficult time defining it. The **probability** of an event is the event's long-run relative frequency in repeated trials under similar conditions. In other words, the statistician does not think of the probability of obtaining a single result from a single study but rather of the chances of obtaining the same result from an idealized study that can be carried out many times under identical conditions. The notion of repeated trials allows researchers to use probability to test hypotheses.

Statistical probability is based on the concept of **sampling error.** The use of inferential statistics is based on random sampling. However, even when samples are randomly selected, the possibility of errors in sampling always exists. Therefore, the characteristics of any given sample may be different from those of the entire population.

Suppose that some researchers have at their disposal a large group of clients with decubitus ulcers and wish to study the average length of time for ulcers to heal with the usual nursing care. If the researchers studied the entire population, they might obtain an average healing time of 50 days, with an SD of 10 days. Now, suppose that the researchers did not have the money necessary to study all of the clients but wished instead to conduct several consecutive studies of these clients. For this study, the researchers first draw a sample of 25 clients, calculate the mean and SD, and replace the subjects in the population before drawing the next sample. If this process is repeated many times in different samples, a different mean for each sample would likely result. For example, the researchers might find that one sample's mean might be 50.5, the next 47.5, and the next 62.5. The tendency for statistics to fluctuate from one sample to another is known as sampling error.

Sampling distributions are theoretical. In practice, researchers do not routinely draw consecutive samples from the same population; usually, they compute statistics and make inferences based on one sample. However, the knowledge of the properties of the sampling distribution—if these repeated samples are hypothetically obtained—permits the researcher to draw a conclusion based on one sample. Such a conclusion is possible because the sampling distribution of the means has certain known properties.

The sampling distribution of the means follows a normal curve, and the mean of the sampling distribution will be the mean of the population. As discussed in the previous section on normal distribution, because the sampling distribution of the means is normal, several other important characteristics are revealed. When scores are normally distributed, 68% of the cases will fall between +1 SD and –1 SD, or the probability is 68 out of 100 that any one randomly drawn sample mean will lie within the range of values between ±1 SD and –1 SD (see Figure 16–3). In the example given, if we drew only one sample, we would have a 68% chance of finding a sample mean that fell between 40 and 60. The SD of a theoretical distribution of sample means is called the **standard error of the mean**. The word *error* is used because the various means that make up the distribution contain an error in their estimates of the population mean. The error is considered to be standard because it implies the magnitude of the average error, just as an SD implies the average variation from one mean. The *smaller* the standard error, the *less* variable are the sample means and the *more accurate* are those means as estimates of the population value.

Although researchers rarely construct sampling distributions, standard error can be estimated because it bears a systematic relationship to the sample SD and the size of the sample. Thus, increasing the size of the sample will increase the accuracy of our estimates of population parameters. It should be intuitive that to increase the size of a sample will decrease the likelihood that one outlying score will dramatically affect the sample mean (see Chapter 12). The other reason that the sampling distribution is so important is that all statistics have sampling distributions. Researchers consult these distributions when making determinations about rejecting the null hypothesis.

Type I and Type II Errors

The researcher's decision to accept or reject the null hypothesis is based on a consideration of the probability that the observed differences are a result of chance alone. Because data on the entire population are not available, the researcher can never flatly assert that the null hypothesis is or is not true. Thus, statistical inference is always based on incomplete information about a population, and errors can occur when making this decision. The two types of errors in statistical inference are type I and type II.

Returning to the example of the study by Samuels-Dennis (2006) of single mothers, one null hypothesis of the study was that no differences in psychological outcomes would exist between employed single mothers and single mothers receiving social assistance. The author reported a significant difference in the number of stressful life events between employed mothers and mothers receiving social assistance. If the differences found were truly a function of chance (because this group of participants was unusual in some way) and if the number of participants was too small, a type I error would occur. A **type I error** is the researcher's incorrect decision to reject the null hypothesis (Kline, 2005). If, however, the researcher had found that the groups did not differ but only a few clients had been studied, a type II error might occur. A **type II error** occurs when the results from the sample data lead to the failure to reject the null hypothesis when it is actually false; this error is also known as beta (β). **Power** is the conditional prior probability of the researcher making a correct decision to reject the null hypothesis when it is actually false (Kline, 2005). A standard value of power of .8 is used to conduct power analyses in studies to determine sample size before the study begins. Power and beta are complementary and sum to 1.00. When power is increased, type II error is decreased and vice versa.

The relationship of the two types of errors is shown in Figure 16–5. When critiquing a study to determine whether a type I error has occurred (rejecting the null hypothesis when it is actually true), the reliability and validity of the instruments used should be considered. For example, if the instruments did not accurately and precisely measure the intervention variables, the conclusion could be that the intervention made a difference when, in reality, it did not. It is critical to consider the reliability and validity of all of the measurement instruments reported (see Chapter 14). In a practice discipline, type I errors usually are considered more serious because if a researcher declares that differences exist where none are present, the potential exists for client care to be affected adversely. Type II errors (accepting the null hypothesis when it is false) may occur if the sample in the study is too small, thereby limiting the opportunity to measure *the treatment effect*, a true difference between two groups. A larger sample size improves the ability to *detect the treatment effect*, that is, the differences between two groups. If no significant difference is found between two groups with a large sample, this finding provides stronger evidence (than with a small sample) not to reject the null hypothesis.

LEVEL OF SIGNIFICANCE

The researcher does not know when an error in statistical decision making has occurred. It is possible to know only that the null hypothesis is indeed true or false if data from the total population are available. However, the researcher can control the risk of making type I errors by setting the level of significance before the study begins (a priori). Slakter, Wu, and Suzuki-Slakter (1991) explained in detail the importance of setting the level of significance before the study is conducted. The **level of significance (alpha level)** is the probability of making a type I error; in other words, the conditional probability of rejecting the null hypothesis when it is actually true. **Alpha** is considered a prior probability because it is set before the data are collected, and it is a conditional probability because the null hypothesis is assumed to be true (Kline, 2005). The minimum level of significance acceptable for nursing research is .05. If the researcher sets alpha, or the level of significance, at .05, the researcher is willing to accept the fact that if the study were done 100 times, the decision to reject the null hypothesis would be wrong five times out of those 100 trials, only if the null hypothesis is true.

If, as is sometimes done, the researcher wants to have a smaller risk of rejecting a true null hypothesis, the level of significance may be set at .01. In this case, the researcher is willing to be wrong only once in 100 trials. The decision as to how strictly the alpha level should be set depends on how important it is not to make an error. For example, if the results of a study are to be used to determine whether a great deal of money should be spent in an area of nursing care, the researcher may decide that the accuracy of the results is so important that an alpha level of .01 is chosen. In most studies, however, alpha is set at .05.

Another concept, called the *p* value, is needed to interpret the alpha value. The **p value** is the conditional probability of obtaining, from the study

Conclusion of test of significance	REALITY	
	Null hypothesis is true	Null hypothesis is not true
Not statistically significant	Correct conclusion	Type II error
Statistically significant	Type I error	Correct conclusion

Figure 16–5 Outcome of statistical decision making

data, a value of the test statistic that is at least as extreme as that calculated from the data given that the null hypothesis is true (Kline, 2005). The *p* value is different from alpha because it is calculated from the sample data and is considered the *exact level of significance* (Gigerenzer, 1993). Thus, if this exact level of significance is less than the conditional prior probability of making a type I error ($p < \alpha$), then the null hypothesis is rejected, and the result is considered statistically significant at that alpha level. For example, if the alpha was set at .05 and the *p* value was found to be .04, then the results are considered statistically significant.

Whatever level of significance is set, the researcher either rejects or accepts the null hypothesis when comparing the statistical results with the preset alpha. For example, in the Samuels-Dennis study (2006), the null hypothesis regarding participants' psychological outcomes was rejected because the variables of the hypothesis were significant at the .05 level or less; in other words, the *p* values were less than alpha (see Appendix C). In the Forchuk et al. (2005) study, however, the researchers failed to reject the null hypothesis and found that the intervention group's quality of life was not significantly improved compared with that of the control group because the *p* values were greater than alpha (see Appendix A).

Perhaps you are thinking that researchers should always use the lowest alpha level possible because it makes sense that they would like to keep the risk of both types of errors at a minimum. Unfortunately, decreasing the risk of making a type I error increases the risk of making a type II error. That is, the stricter the researcher is in preventing the rejection of a true null hypothesis, the more likely is the possibility that a false null hypothesis will be accepted. Therefore, researchers always have to accept more of a risk of one type of error when setting the alpha level.

Another method of determining the level of significance and whether to accept or reject the null hypothesis is called the *critical values method*. In this method, by calculating the estimates of population mean and SD, a range of values is determined from

which one can compare the sample mean findings and decide whether to reject the null hypothesis.

Consider the example of a study in which we want to know the importance of support groups for caregivers of older adults. We ask 100 caregivers to rate the importance of support groups for them using an instrument that ranges from 0 (not important at all) to 100 (very important). If we use Figure 16–3 as the theoretical distribution for our study (a normal distribution with a mean of 50), 68% of the population would score between 40 and 60, and 95% would score between 30 and 70. Thus, our null hypothesis would be that the mean scoring for the population of caregivers would be 50 and the scientific hypothesis would be greater or less than 50. After we complete our measurement with our sample, we find that the sample mean score is 75. This mean is consistent with the scientific hypothesis, and we can be 95% sure that, most of the time, our sample mean would fall under this cutoff, thus giving us confidence in rejecting our null hypothesis. In other words, only five out of 100 times would we obtain this result by chance alone.

Helpful 💡 Hint

Decreasing the alpha level acceptable for a study increases the chance that a type II error will occur. When a researcher is conducting many statistical tests, the probability of some of the tests being significant increases as the number of tests increases. Therefore, when a large number of tests are being conducted, the researcher will often decrease the alpha level to .01.

PRACTICAL AND STATISTICAL SIGNIFICANCE

Statistical significance and practical significance are not the same. When a researcher finds a hypothesis statistically significant, this finding is unlikely to have happened by chance. In other words, if the level of significance has been set at .05, the odds are 19 to 1 that the conclusion the researcher makes on the basis of the statistical test performed on sample data is correct. The researcher would reach the wrong conclusion only five times in 100.

Suppose that a researcher is interested in the effect of loud rock music on the behaviour of laboratory mice. The researcher could design an experiment to study this question and find that loud music makes the mice act strangely. A statistical test suggests that this finding is not the result of chance. However, such a finding may or may not have practical significance, even though the finding has statistical significance. Whereas some would argue that this study might have relevance to understanding the behaviour of teenagers, others would argue that the study has no practical value. Thus, the findings of a study may have statistical significance, but they may have no practical value or significance.

Although researchers should consider the practicality of a problem in the early stages of a research project (see Chapter 3), a distinction between the statistical and practical significance of the findings also should be made when discussing the results of a study. Some people believe that if the findings are not statistically significant, they have no practical value. In the Forchuk et al. (2005) study, the research hypotheses were not statistically supported, yet these nonsupported hypotheses provide as much information about the intervention as do the supported hypotheses. The data allowed the researchers to return to the previous literature in the area and draw from those findings both statistical and practical significance.

Evidence-Based Practice Tip

You will study the results to determine the effectiveness of the new treatment and the size and clinical importance of the effect.

Tests of Statistical Significance

Tests of statistical significance may be parametric or nonparametric. Most studies in nursing research literature use parametric tests that have the following three attributes:

1. The estimation of at least one **population** parameter.
2. Measurement is required at the interval or higher.

3. Assumptions about the variables being studied.

These assumptions usually include that the variable is normally distributed in the overall population.

In contrast to parametric tests, **nonparametric tests of significance** are not based on the estimation of population parameters, so their assumptions about the underlying distribution are less restrictive. Nonparametric tests are usually applied when the variables have been measured on a nominal or ordinal scale.

Some debate surrounds the relative merits of the two types of statistical tests. The moderate position taken by most researchers and statisticians is that **nonparametric statistics**, also called distribution-free tests, are best used when the data cannot be assumed to be at the interval level of measurement or when the sample is small and the normality of the underlying distribution cannot be inferred. If these assumptions can be made, however, most researchers prefer to use **parametric statistics**, which are more powerful and more flexible than nonparametric statistics. Because stringent assumptions for parametric tests makes them more powerful than nonparametric tests researchers are able to formulate simple sample statistics, such as the mean and the SD, which can accurately estimate population parameters with standard sampling distributions to obtain probabilities regarding the null hypotheses.

Researchers use many different statistical tests of significance to test hypotheses; however, the procedure and the rationale for their use are similar from test to test. Once the researcher has chosen a significance level and collected the data, the data are used to compute the appropriate test statistic. Each test has a related theoretical distribution that shows the probable and improbable values for that statistic. On the basis of the statistical result and the values in the distribution, the researcher either accepts or rejects the null hypothesis and then reports both the statistical result and its probability. Thus, a researcher may perform a statistical test called a t test, obtain a value of 8.98, and report that it is statistically significant at the $p < .05$ level.

This means that the researcher had five chances out of 100 to be wrong in concluding that this result could not have been obtained by chance.

The likelihood of finding a statistic that is high enough to be statistically significant is increased as the sample size increases. This likelihood is indicated by the **degrees of freedom**, which are often reported with the statistic and the probability value. Usually abbreviated as *df*, the degree of freedom is the freedom of a score's value to vary depending on the other scores and the sum of these scores; thus, *df* = N–1. For example, imagine you have four numbers represented by letters (a, b, c, and d) that must add up to a total of x; you are free to randomly choose the first three numbers, but the fourth must be chosen to make the total equal to x; thus, your degree of freedom is 3.

To make statistical inferences from data, many types of tests can be conducted. Tables 16–4 and 16–5 show the tests most commonly used for inferential statistics. The test used depends on the level of the measurement of the variables in question and the type of hypothesis being studied. These statistics test two types of hypotheses: that difference exists between groups (see Table 16–4) and that a relationship exists between two or more variables (see Table 16–5). In addition, many types of regression analyses are available to predict the dependent variable. Simple (one independent variable) and multiple regression analyses (several independent variables) are used when the dependent variable is at the interval level or higher. **Logistic regression (logit analysis)** analyzes relationships between multiple independent variables and a dependent variable that is binary, ordinal, or polynomial.

Helpful Hint

Because a researcher has used nonparametric statistics does not mean that the study is not useful. The use of nonparametric statistics is appropriate when measurements are not made at the interval level or the variable under study is not normally distributed.

Evidence-Based Practice Tip

Try to discern whether the test for analyzing the data was chosen because it gave a significant p value. A statistical test should be chosen on the basis of its appropriateness for the type of data collected, not because it gives the answer that the researcher hoped to obtain.

TESTS OF DIFFERENCES

The type of test used for any particular study depends primarily on whether the researcher examines differences in one, two, or three or more groups and whether the data to be analyzed are nominal, ordinal, or interval (see Table 16–4). Suppose that a researcher constructs an experimental study using an after-only design (see Chapter 10). What the researcher hopes to determine is that the two randomly assigned groups are different after the introduction of the experimental treatment. If the measurements taken are at the interval level, the researcher would use the *t* test to analyze the data. If the *t* statistic was found to be high enough to be unlikely to have occurred by chance, the researcher would reject the null hypothesis and conclude that the two groups were indeed more different than would have been expected on the basis of chance alone. In other words, the researcher would conclude that the experimental treatment had the desired effect.

The study discussed earlier by Samuels-Dennis (2006) illustrated the use of the *t* statistic (see Appendix C). In this study, the *t* test was used to determine whether a difference existed between the stress and psychological distress experienced by employed mothers and by mothers receiving social assistance. Samuels-Dennis found that the prevalence of depressive symptoms was significantly higher for the social assistance recipients.

Evidence-Based Practice Tip

Tests of difference are most commonly used in experimental and quasiexperimental designs that provide Level II and Level III evidence.

TABLE 16–4 **Tests of Differences Between Means**				
Level of Measurement	One Group	Two Groups		More than Two Groups
		Related	Independent	
Nonparametric				
Nominal	Chi-square	Chi-square	Chi-square	Chi-square
		Fisher exact probability		
Ordinal	Kolmogorov- Smirnov	Sign test	Chi-square	Chi-square
		Wilcoxon matched pairs		
		Signed rank	Median test	
			Mann-Whitney U	
Parametric				
Interval or ratio	Correlated t	Correlated t	Independent t	ANOVA
	ANOVA (repeated measures)			
			ANOVA	ANCOVA
				MANOVA

ANCOVA: analysis of covariance; ANOVA: analysis of variance; MANOVA: multivariate analysis of variance.

Parametric Tests. The **t statistic** is commonly used in nursing research. This statistic tests whether two group means are different. Thus, the t statistic is used when the researcher has two groups, and the question is whether the mean scores on some measure are more different than would be expected by chance. To use this test, the variables must have been measured at the interval or ratio level, and the two groups must be independent, meaning that nothing in one group helps determine who is in the other group. If the groups are related, as when samples are matched (see Chapter 12), and the researcher also wants to determine differences between the two groups, a paired, or correlated, t test would be used.

The t statistic illustrates one of the major purposes of research in nursing: to demonstrate that differences exist between groups. Groups may be naturally occurring collections, such as age groups, or they may be experimentally created, such as treatment and control groups. Sometimes, a researcher has more than two groups, or measurements are taken more than once. An example of using more than two groups is illustrated in the Wilson (2002) study describing and comparing dependency among dying persons in relation to their care setting. In this study, the researchers used **analysis of variance (ANOVA)**, a test similar to the t test.

Like the t statistic, the ANOVA statistic tests whether group means differ, but instead of testing

TABLE 16–5 **Tests of Association**		
Level of Measurement	Two Variables	More than Two Variables
Nonparametric		
Nominal	Phi coefficient	
	Point-biserial	Contingency coefficient
Ordinal	Kendall's tau	
	Spearman rho	Discriminant function analysis
Parametric		
Interval or ratio	Pearson r	Multiple regression
		Path analysis
		Canonical correlation

each pair of means separately, ANOVA considers the variation between groups and within groups. The ANOVA is usually done with two or more groups by an *F* test rather than multiple pairs of *t* tests. If multiple pairs of *t* tests are done, the type I error rate would increase.

Wilson's (2002) study compared three groups of clients using ANOVA: (a) hospital clients, (b) home care clients who died at home, and (c) home care clients who died in the hospital. The author found that the mean number of days of dependency was highest among those who were transferred to the hospital, *x* = 81.3, and was especially high compared with hospital inpatients (*x* = 13.8). The *F* test was significant at *p* < .01. When more than two groups are compared over time, a variation of the ANOVA is used, the repeated measures ANOVA, because this statistic takes into account the fact that multiple measures at several points in time affect the potential range of scores.

Bierlin, Hadjistavropoulous, Bourgault-Fagnou, and Sagan (2006) conducted a study to assess the needs of older case-coordinated clients receiving community health services by examining changes in cognitive status, physical and mental health status, social support, risk for institutionalization, and service use over a six-month period from initial intake into home care. In this study, repeated measures ANOVA was used to determine whether changes had occurred between baseline and the six-month collection point. Another expansion of the notion of ANOVA is **multiple analysis of variance (MANOVA)**, which is also used to determine differences in group means, but only with more than one dependent variable.

Post hoc Analysis.   When the decision from the ANOVA is to reject the null hypothesis, this indicates that at least one of the means is not the same as the other means. To determine where the difference in means lies, a **post hoc analysis** is conducted. Pairs of means in the main effects and interaction effects are tested to determine whether they are statistically different. Many post hoc analyses are available; the most common include Tukey's

HSD (Honestly Significant Difference), Scheffé, and Bonferroni. This type of analysis is also known as *paired comparisons.*

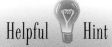

Helpful Hint

A research report may not always refer to the test that was done. The reader can find this information by looking at the tables. For example, a table with *t* statistics will contain a column for "*t*" values, and an ANOVA table will contain "*F*" values.

In other cases, particularly in experimental work, the researcher uses *t* tests or ANOVA to determine whether random assignment to groups was effective in creating groups that are equivalent before introduction of the experimental treatment. In this case, the researcher wants to show that no difference exists among the groups.

In the Samuels-Dennis (2006) study, the author reported that employed mothers and mothers receiving social assistance were comparable at baseline with respect to age ($_E$ = 38.60, SD = 7.203, $_{SA}$ = 40.0, SD = 6.425, *t* = −.990, *p* = .325), but significant differences existed in the number of children currently in their care (x_E = 1.92. SD = .942, $_{SA}$ = 2.42, SD = 1.048, *t* = −2.458, *p* = .016). These results suggested that if differences were found between the two groups, they were likely due to real differences and not to chance. Suppose, however, that these groups had differed on age at baseline. For Samuels-Dennis to conclude that statistically significant differences occurred in stress and psychological distress, she would need to control statistically for educational level by using the technique of **analysis of covariance (ANCOVA)**. ANCOVA also measures differences among group means and uses a statistical technique to equate the groups under study on an important variable.

Nonparametric Tests.   In the example from Samuels-Dennis (2006), the researcher tested whether differences existed in the racial makeup and the educational level of the groups. These two variables are not interval level data, so she could not test this difference with any of the tests discussed thus far.

When data are at the nominal or ordinal level and the researcher wants to determine whether groups are different, the researcher uses another commonly used statistic, the **chi-square** (χ^2). The chi-square is a nonparametric statistic used to determine whether the frequency in each category is different from what would be expected by chance. As with the *t* test and ANOVA, if the calculated chi-square is high enough, the researcher would conclude that the frequencies found would not be expected on the basis of chance alone, and the null hypothesis would be rejected. Although this test is robust and can be used in many different situations, it cannot be used to compare frequencies when samples are small and expected frequencies are less than six in each cell. In these instances, the **Fisher's exact probability test** is used.

When the data are ranks, or are at the ordinal level, researchers have several other nonparametric tests at their disposal: the *Kolmogorov-Smirnov test*, the *sign test*, the *Wilcoxon matched pairs test*, the *signed rank test for related groups*, the *median test*, and the *Mann-Whitney* U *test for independent groups*. Explanation of these tests is beyond the scope of this chapter; readers who desire further information should consult a general statistics book.

Nursing research studies often employ several different statistical tests. The Samuels-Dennis (2006) study illustrated the use of several of these statistical tests. The researcher was interested in comparing the stress and psychological outcomes between two groups of women, and although the clients could not be randomly assigned to the employed or social assistance groups, the researchers needed to determine whether the convenience sampling procedure succeeded in creating equivalent groups. For data measured at the nominal level, such as marital status, the chi-square statistic was used, as mentioned previously. For data measured at the interval level, such as the BDI-II scale, the *t* test was used. Finally, to test the differences between the two groups, the chi-square method was used for nominal variables, such as racial makeup.

TESTS OF RELATIONSHIPS

Researchers often are interested in exploring the *relationship* between two or more variables. Such studies use statistics that determine the **correlation**, or the degree of association, between two or more variables. Tests of the relationships between variables are sometimes considered to be descriptive statistics when they are used to describe the magnitude and direction of a relationship of two variables in a sample and the researcher does not wish to make statements about the larger population. Such statistics also can be inferential when they are used to test hypotheses about the correlations that exist in the target population.

Null hypothesis tests of the relationships between variables assume that no relationship exists between the variables. Thus, when a researcher rejects this type of null hypothesis, the conclusion is that the variables are, in fact, related. Suppose that a researcher is interested in the relationship between the age of clients and the length of time it takes them to recover from surgery. As with other statistics discussed, the researcher would design a study to collect the appropriate data and then analyze the data using measures of association. In the example, age and length of time until recovery can be considered interval level measurements. The researcher would use a test called the **Pearson correlation coefficient**, **Pearson *r***, or **Pearson product moment correlation coefficient**. Once the Pearson *r* is calculated, the researcher consults the distribution for this test to determine whether the value obtained is likely to have occurred by chance. Again, the research reports both the value of the correlation and its probability of occurring by chance.

Correlation coefficients can range in value from −1.0 to +1.0 and also can be zero. A zero coefficient means that no relationship exists between the variables. *A perfect positive correlation* is indicated by a +1.0 coefficient and a *perfect negative correlation* by a −1.0 coefficient. We can illustrate the meaning of these coefficients by using the example from the previous paragraph. If no relationship exists between the age of the client and the time required for the client to recover from surgery, the researcher would find a correlation of zero. However, a correlation of +1.0 would mean the older the client, the longer the recovery time. A negative coefficient would imply that the younger the client, the longer the recovery time. Figure 16–6 illustrates a perfect positive correlation, a perfect negative correlation, and no correlation. A correlation value of 0 to .2 is considered weak to none, a value of .2 to .4 is weak, a value of .4 to .6 is moderate, a value of 6 to .8 is strong, and a value of .8 to 1.0 is very strong (Bluman, 2006).

Of course, relationships are rarely perfect. The magnitude of the relationship is indicated by how close the correlation comes to the absolute value of 1. Thus, a correlation of −.76 is just as strong as a correlation of +.76, but the direction of the relationship is opposite. In addition, a correlation of .76 is stronger than a correlation of .32. When a researcher tests hypotheses about the relationships between two variables, the test considers whether the magnitude of the correlation is large enough not to have occurred by chance. This is the meaning of the probability value or the p value reported with correlation coefficients. As with other statistical tests of significance, the larger the sample, the greater the likelihood of finding a significant correlation. Therefore, researchers also report the degrees of freedom associated with the test performed.

An example of a descriptive, correlational study is provided by Decaire, Bédard, Riendeau, and Forrest (2006) who examined incidents in a psychiatric setting and the relationships with staff and client characteristics. The researchers found that a significant negative correlation existed between nonviolent experience and departmental experience ($r(10) = -.73, p = .017$). Staff members with higher levels of departmental experience had a lower frequency of nonviolent incidents. They also found that a significant positive correlation existed between the age of the staff member and the frequency of violent incidents ($r(10) = .74, p = .014$). Nominal and ordinal data also can be tested for relationships by nonparametric statistics. When two variables being tested have only two levels (e.g., male/female; yes/no), the phi coefficient can be used to express relationships. When the researcher is interested in the relationship between a nominal variable and an interval variable, the point-biserial correlation is used. Spearman's rho is used to determine the degree of association between two sets of ranks, as is *Kendall's tau*. All of these correlation coefficients may range in value from −1.0 to +1.0. These tests are shown in Table 16–5.

Nursing problems are rarely so simple that they can be explained by only two variables. When researchers are interested in studying complex relationships among more than two variables, they use techniques other than those discussed thus far. When researchers are interested in understanding more about a problem than just the relationship between two variables, they often use a technique called **multiple regression**, which measures the relationship between one interval level dependent

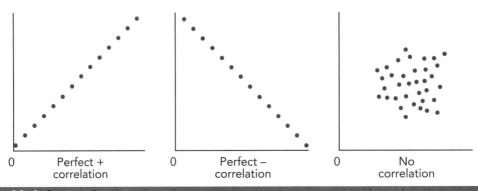

| 0   Perfect + correlation | 0   Perfect − correlation | 0   No correlation |

Figure 16–6 Scatter plots

variable and several independent variables. Multiple regression is the expansion of correlation to include more than two variables and is used when the researcher wants to determine what variables contribute to the explanation of the dependent variable and to what degree.

For example, a researcher may be interested in determining what factors help women decide to breastfeed their infants. A number of variables, such as the mother's age, previous experience with breastfeeding, number of other children, and knowledge of the advantages of breastfeeding, might be measured and then analyzed to see whether they, separately and together, predict the length of breastfeeding. Such a study would require the use of multiple regression. The results of such a study might help nurses know that a younger mother with only one other child might be more likely to benefit from a teaching program about breastfeeding than an older mother with several other children.

The reader of research reports often will see multiple regression techniques described as *forward solution*, *backward solution*, or *stepwise solution*. These techniques are used in multiple regression to find the smallest group of variables that will account for the greatest proportion of variance in the dependent variable. In the forward solution, the independent variable with the highest correlation with the dependent variables is entered first, and the next variable is the one that will increase the explained variance the most. In the backward solution, all variables are entered into the solution, and each variable is deleted to see whether the explained variance drops significantly. The stepwise solution is a combination of the two approaches. In general, all of the approaches give similar, although not identical, results.

Suppose that the individual who was researching breastfeeding was interested in not just breastfeeding but also maternal satisfaction. *Canonical correlation* is used with more than one dependent variable. If the data are nominal or ordinal, the contingency coefficient or discriminant function analyses are used. (These last tests are beyond the scope of this text; further information can be found in statistical texts.)

Samuels-Dennis (2006) was interested in understanding to what extent employment status and stressful events predict depression among single mothers. A regression analysis was conducted, and the results indicated that age, number of children, employment, and stressful events explained 40.6% of the variance in depressive symptoms, with employment status being the primary contributor ($\beta = .591$, $p = .000$). These data allowed her to build on the past research that she reviewed and to suggest both future descriptive and intervention research, thus moving the data toward evidence-based practice.

Evidence-Based Practice Tip

Tests of relationship are usually associated with nonexperimental designs that provide Level IV evidence. Establishment of a strong, statistically significant relationship between variables often lends support for replicating the study to increase the consistency of the findings and provide a foundation for developing an intervention study.

THE USE OF CONFIDENCE INTERVALS

A **confidence interval (CI)** is a range of values, based on a random sample, which often accompanies measures of central tendency and measures of association and provides the nurse with a measure of precision or uncertainty about the sample findings. In other words, the CI gives an estimated range of values, which is likely to include an unknown population parameter calculated from a given set of sample data.

Typically, investigators record their CI results as a 95% degree of certainty; sometimes, the degree of certainty is recorded as 99%. Today, professional journals often require investigators to include CIs as one of the statistical methods used to interpret study findings. Even when CIs are not reported, they can be easily calculated from study data. The method for performing these calculations is widely available in statistical texts.

Lenhardt, Seybold, Kimberger, Stoiser, and Sessler (2002) attempted to answer the following clinical question: "Does local warming of the insertion site result in successful cannulation?" These investigators tested the use of a warming device and measured the first-attempt cannulation success rates in those who had active warming (device on) compared with those who had passive warming (device off) (see Table 16–6). The CI helps us place the study results in context for all clients similar to those in the study (generalization).

As a result of the calculated CI for the Lenhardt et al. (2002) study, it can be stated that in neurosurgical clients (the study population), 95 out of 100 times when a Thermamed hand warmer is used, the nurse will have a successful insertion on the first attempt anywhere from 10% to 62%. Knowing these ranges helps nurses to make important decisions about implementing change in practice or applying an intervention to a client (clinical significance of the study results).

The practitioner might think differently about changing or adopting a new intervention if the CI is large, for example, 2 to 170. The wide interval means that the relative benefit (in the case of a good outcome) or reduction in risk (in the case of a bad outcome) is anywhere from 2% to 170%. With such large numbers, the clinical significance is widely variable and, depending on the experiment, may or may not be worth the effort, expense, or uncertainty. From a statistical standpoint, such a large CI indicates that the study was not sufficiently powered; in other words, the study did not enroll enough study clients to provide meaningful results (see Chapter 12). As the number of clients enrolled in a study increases, the CI narrows.

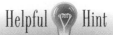

Helpful Hint

When evaluating whether you should spend time reviewing an article, examine the article's tables. The information you need to answer your clinical question should be contained in one or more of the tables.

Harm Studies

The odds ratio in logistic regression can be used in exploring clinical questions of harm, when investigators want to determine whether an individual has been harmed by being exposed to a particular event. In this type of study, investigators select the outcome they are interested in (e.g., pressure ulcers) and try to determine whether any one factor explains those who have and do not have the outcome of interest. The measure of association that best describes the analyzed data is the **odds ratio**, which communicates the probability of an event. An odds ratio is calculated by dividing the odds in the treated or exposed group by the odds in the control group. Investigators present an odds ratio of factors in study tables; thus, calculation of the odds ratio is rarely necessary. The interpretation of the odds ratio is straightforward and presented in Table 16–7. Note that the null value for the odds ratio is equal to 1.

The use of the odds ratio to describe the probability of an event is illustrated by a study in which investigators sought to determine risk factors for the death of full-term, postneonatal, healthy infants born to young mothers (Phipps, Blume, & DeMonner, 2002). The authors used a large data set ($N = 1,830,350$) of mothers 12 to 29 years of age who had delivered healthy babies. The investigators wanted to determine whether the death of

TABLE 16–6	**Active Warming Versus Passive Warming Before Insertion of Peripheral Venous Cannulas in Neurosurgical Clients**			
Outcome	Active Warming	Passive Warming	RBI (95% CI)	NNT (CI)
Successful insertions on first attempt	94%	72%	30% (10 to 62)	5 (3 to 13)

Data from Lenhardt, R., Seybold, T., Kimberger, O., Stoiser, R., & Sessler, D. (2002). Local warming and insertion of peripheral venous cannulas: Single blinded, prospective randomised controlled trial and single blinded crossover trial. *British Journal of Medicine, 325,* 409–412.
CI: confidence interval; NNT: number needed to treat; RBI: relative benefit increase.

TABLE 16–7 **Interpretation of Odds Ratios**		
	Type of Outcome	
Odds ratio	Adverse outcome, e.g., myocardial infarction	Beneficial outcome, e.g., adherence
Less than 1, e.g., 0.375	Intervention better	Intervention worse
Equal to 1	Intervention no better/worse	Intervention no better/worse
More than 1, e.g., 4.0	Intervention worse	Intervention better

an infant was more likely to occur within the first year after birth to young mothers compared with infants born to older mothers. The result of the study's main outcome stratified by age is described in Table 16–8. For both unadjusted and adjusted odds, as the mother's age declines, the probability of death of an infant in the postneonatal period increases (the odds ratio gets larger). Healthy, full-term infants born to mothers younger than 15 years of age are three to four times more likely to die within their first year compared with infants born to mothers 23 to 29 years of age. The study was not designed to determine which factors are associated with death. However, the authors indicated that unmeasured social factors could have a potential association; further studies are needed to test the validity of this association. With this evidence, a nurse could justify the need for increased home care visits to younger mothers in the immediate postpartum period. Another nurse can use this evidence to start a nurse-managed support group for babies born to younger mothers.

Harm data, with their measure of probabilities, help nurses identify factors that may or may not contribute to an adverse or beneficial outcome. This information is useful for the nursing plan of care, program planning, and client and family education.

Meta-Analysis

Meta-analysis is not a type of study design but a research method that statistically combines the results of multiple studies (usually randomized controlled trials) to answer focused clinical questions through an objective appraisal of carefully synthesized research evidence (see Chapter 11). People sometimes use the terms *meta-analysis* and *systematic review* interchangeably; however, a meta-analysis is a quantitative approach to a systematic review.

Systematic review is the process whereby the investigators find all relevant studies, published and unpublished, on the topic or question. At least two members of the review team independently assess the quality of each study, include or exclude studies based on pre-established criteria, statistically combine the results of individual studies, and present a balanced and impartial summary of the findings that represents a "state of the science" conclusion about the evidence supporting the benefits and risks of a given health care practice (Stevens, 2001). Each meta-analysis is a complex project and, as such, is conducted by a multidisciplinary team of clinicians, health scientists, clinical epidemiologists, meta-analytic statisticians, evidence-based practice librarians, and informatics specialists.

In the evidence-based hierarchy, the findings of a meta-analysis are considered to provide the strongest evidence available to the clinician because they summarize large amounts of information

TABLE 16–8 **Odds Ratios for Postneonatal Mortality Associated with Maternal Age Groups**		
Maternal Age (y)	**Crude OR**	**Adjusted OR***
≤15	4.1 (3.4, 4.8)	3.0 (2.5, 3.6)
16–17	3.1 (2.8, 3.5)	2.4 (2.1, 2.7)
18–19	2.5 (2.3, 2.8)	2.0 (1.8, 2.3)
20–22	1.8 (1.6, 2.0)	1.5 (1.4, 1.7)
23–29	1.0	1.0

From Phipps, M., Blume, J., & DeMonner, S. (2002). Young maternal age associated with increased risk of postneonatal death. *Obstetrics and Gynecology, 100,* 481–486.
Data are given as OR (95% confidence interval).
*Adjusted for maternal race/ethnicity, adequacy of prenatal care utilization, and marital status.
OR: odds ratio.

derived from multiple experimental studies investigating the effect of the same intervention. A methodologically sound meta-analysis is more likely than an individual study to identify the true effect of an intervention because the meta-analysis limits bias.

In a **systematic review**, the meta-analysis quantitatively combines the data from the selected experimental studies by using their measures of association (see Table 16–5). An odds ratio is the statistic of choice for use in a meta-analysis. The same interpretation of odds ratio described in Table 16–7 applies to the odds ratios seen in a meta-analysis.

The usual manner of displaying data from a meta-analysis is by a pictorial representation known as a blobbogram, accompanied by a summary measure of effect size in odds ratio. In the meta-analysis depicted in Figure 16–7, the investigators were interested in comparing the efficacy of a beta-agonist given by a metered-dose inhaler with a chamber versus a nebulizer on hospital admission in children under 5 years of age (Castro-Rodriquez and Rodrigo, 2004). The investigators searched the literature for randomized controlled trials with children under 5 years of age with acute asthma who were treated in the emergency department and were randomized to receive either a metered-dose inhaler with a chamber or a nebulizer. The investigators found six trials that met this criterion (see Figure 16–7). The study groups are represented by a fraction; for example, in the trial published by Closa, 4 of 17 children in the metered-dose inhaler with a chamber group were admitted to the hospital and 4 of 17 children in the nebulizer group were admitted to the hospital. In the centre of the figure, each trial in the analysis is represented by a horizontal line. The findings from each study are represented as a blob or square (the measured effect) on the vertical line. The size of the blob or square (sometimes just a small vertical line) reflects the amount of information in that study. The width of the horizontal line represents the 95% CI. A vertical line is the line of no effect (odds ratio = 1). When the CI of the result (horizontal line) crosses the line of no effect (vertical line), then the differences in the effect of the treatment are not statistically significant. If the CI does not cross the vertical line, then the study results are statistically significant.

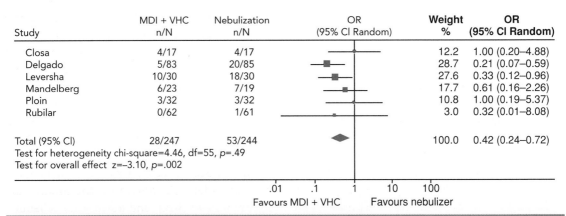

Study	MDI + VHC n/N	Nebulization n/N	OR (95% CI Random)	Weight %	OR (95% CI Random)
Closa	4/17	4/17		12.2	1.00 (0.20–4.88)
Delgado	5/83	20/85		28.7	0.21 (0.07–0.59)
Leversha	10/30	18/30		27.6	0.33 (0.12–0.96)
Mandelberg	6/23	7/19		17.7	0.61 (0.16–2.26)
Ploin	3/32	3/32		10.8	1.00 (0.19–5.37)
Rubilar	0/62	1/61		3.0	0.32 (0.01–8.08)
Total (95% CI)	28/247	53/244		100.0	0.42 (0.24–0.72)

Test for heterogeneity chi-square=4.46, df=55, p=.49
Test for overall effect z=–3.10, p=.002

.01   .1   1   10   100
Favours MDI + VHC   Favours nebulizer

Figure 16–7 Systematic review with meta-analysis data showing the efficacy of a beta-agonist given by metered-dose inhaler with a valved holding chamber (MDI + VHC) versus a nebulizer in children under 5 years of age with acute exacerbation of wheezing or asthma in the emergency department on hospitalization.

From Castro-Rodriquez, J., & Rodrigo, G. (2004). Beta-agonists through metered-dose inhaler with valved holding chamber versus nebulizer for acute exacerbation of wheezing or asthma in children under 5 years of age: A systematic review with meta-analysis. *Journal of Pediatrics, 145*(2), 172–177. CI: confidence interval; MDH: metered-dose inhaler; OR: odds ratio; VHC: valved holding chamber.

In the blobbograms in Figure 16–7, only two of the six studies do not cross the line of no effect: study 2 published by Delgado and study 3 published by Leversha. Because the analysis line does not cross the line of no effect, these studies have statistically significant findings. In columns 4 and 5 of the figure, the investigators have also provided the numerical equivalent of each blobbogram. Other important information and additional statistical analysis may accompany the blobbogram, such as a test to determine the degree to which the results of each of the individual trials are mathematically compatible (heterogeneity). (The reader is referred to a book of advanced research methods for discussion.)

In Figure 16–7, the summary odds ratio for all of the studies combined is represented by a diamond. In this case, after statistically pooling the results of each of the controlled trials, these studies, statistically combined, favour the metered-dose inhaler with a chamber for preventing hospitalization of children under 5 years of age, and this option is statistically significant. If this meta-analysis were methodogically sound, it would support the clinical practice of providing children under 5 years of age with asthma exacerbation with a metered-dose inhaler with a chamber to prevent hospitalization.

ADVANCED STATISTICS

Sometimes, researchers are interested in even more complex problems. For example, Fisher, Wells, and Harrison (2004) conducted a cross-sectional study to identify predictors of pressure ulcers in adults in acute care hospitals. The authors had a sample size of nearly 2000 clients, approximately 12% of whom had a pressure ulcer. The results of the logistic regression revealed that the variables of age, male gender, and nutrition were significant predictors of pressure ulcers. For example, the odds of having a pressure ulcer when nutrition was a deficit was twice as high for males as for females (odds ratio = 2.29, $p = .03$). On the basis of a proposed model, the relationships between the independent and dependent variables were tested using logistic regression analysis. Logistic regression is a form of advanced statistics used when a researcher wishes to confirm the relationship of a set of categorical data (data that have a discrete value).

This notion of testing specific relationships in a specific order can be extended further to test hypothesized variables that are made up of several measures. A technique called structural equation modelling tests path models made up of variables that are not actually measured. For example, a researcher might study the concept of self-esteem and use three different measures to determine subjects' levels of self-esteem. The researcher would test how carefully these three measures gauge self-esteem by testing a measurement model using a software package such as LISREL, AMOS, EQS, or Mplus. For example, Cummings, Estabrooks, Midodzi, Wallin, and Hayduk (2007) tested theories about a theoretical model of organizational influences on research utilization by nurses, and the **Linear Structural Relationships (LISREL)** software gave the researchers the opportunity to study complex interactions among variables simultaneously.

Another advanced technique often used in nursing research is factor analysis. Factor analysis helps us understand concepts more fully and contributes to our ability to measure concepts reliably and validly (see Chapter 14). **Factor analysis** takes a large number of variables and groups them into a smaller number of factors to reduce a set of data so that it may be easily described and used. Factor analysis is also used for instrument development and theory development.

In instrument development, factor analysis is used to group individual items on a scale into meaningful factors or subscales. Secco (2002), for example, was interested in assessing perceptions of competence in the maternal role function of infant care providers. She developed the Infant Care Questionnaire (ICQ) and tested it for reliability and validity in a sample of healthy, low-risk, primiparous and multiparous mothers of term infants. Factor analysis was used to determine whether the scale measured the concepts that it was intended to measure. Many other statistical techniques are available to nurse researchers.

THE USE OF STATISTICS

Statistics are used in nursing research to describe the samples of research studies and to test for hypothesized differences or associations in the sample. Knowing the characteristics of the sample of a research study allows for determining the population for whom the results will be generalized. For example, if a study sample was primarily Caucasian with a mean age of 42 years (SD 2.5), the findings may not be applicable to elderly Punjabi men and women. The cultural, demographic, or clinical factors of an elderly population of a different ethnic group may contribute to different results. Thus, understanding the descriptive statistics of a study assists in determining the applicability of findings to different practice settings.

Statistics are also used to test hypotheses proposed by the researchers. Inferential statistics used to analyze data (i.e., t test, F test, r coefficient) and the associated significance level (p value) indicate the likelihood that the association or difference found in any study is due to chance or to a true difference between groups. The closer the p value is to zero, the less likely the association or difference of a study is due to chance. Thus, inferential statistics provide an objective way to determine whether the results of the study are likely to be a true representation of reality (Brown, 1999; Munro, 2001).

Evidence-Based Practice Tip

A basic understanding of statistics will improve your ability to assess the effect of the independent variable on the dependent variable and related client outcomes for your client population and practice setting.

Critiquing Guide *Descriptive and Inferential Statistics*

Many students who have not had a course in statistics think they cannot critique the statistics of research. However, students should be able to critically analyze the use of statistics even if they do not understand the derivation of the numbers presented. What is most important in critiquing this aspect of a research study is that the procedures for summarizing and analyzing the data make sense in light of the purpose of the study (see the Critiquing Criteria box).

Before deciding whether the statistics employed make sense, return to the beginning of the study and determine the purpose. Although all studies use descriptive statistics to summarize the data obtained, many studies use inferential statistics to test specific hypotheses. In an exploratory study, it is possible that only descriptive statistics will be presented because their purpose is to describe the characteristics of a population.

Just as the hypotheses or research questions should flow from the purpose of a study, so should the hypotheses or research questions suggest the type of analysis that will follow. The hypotheses or the research questions should indicate the major variables that are expected to be presented in summary form. Each of the variables in the hypotheses or research questions should be followed in the "Results" section with appropriate descriptive information.

After studying the hypotheses or research questions, the reader should proceed to the "Methods" section. Using the operational definition provided, identifying the levels of measurement employed to measure each of the variables listed in the hypotheses or research questions. From this information, the reader should be able to determine the measures of central tendency and variability that should be employed to summarize the data. For example, you would not expect to see a mean used as a summary statistic for the nominal variable of gender. In all likelihood, gender would be reported as a frequency distribution. The means and SD should be provided for measurements performed at the interval level. The sample size is another aspect of the "Methods"

CRITIQUING CRITERIA

*Descriptive and
Inferential Statistics*

1. Were appropriate descriptive statistics used?

2. What level of measurement is used to measure each of the major variables?

3. Is the sample size large enough to prevent one extreme score from affecting the summary statistics used?

4. What descriptive statistics are reported?

5. Were these descriptive statistics appropriate to the level of measurement for each variable?

6. Are appropriate summary statistics provided for each major variable?

7. Does the hypothesis indicate that the researcher is interested in testing for differences between groups or in testing for relationships? What is the level of significance?

8. Does the level of measurement permit the use of parametric statistics?

9. Is the size of the sample large enough to permit the use of parametric statistics?

10. Has the researcher provided enough information to decide whether the appropriate statistics were used?

11. Are the statistics used appropriate to the problem, the hypothesis, the method, the sample, and the level of measurement?

12. Are the results for each of the hypotheses presented clearly and appropriately?

13. If tables and graphs are used, do they agree with the text and extend it, or do they merely repeat it?

14. Are the results understandable?

15. Is a distinction made between practical significance and statistical significance? How is it made?

section that is helpful when evaluating the researcher's use of descriptive statistics. The larger the sample, the less chance that one outlying score will affect the summary statistics.

If tables or graphs are used, they should agree with the information presented in the text. The tables and charts should be clearly and completely labelled. If the researcher presents grouped frequency data, the groups should be logical and mutually exclusive. The size of the interval in grouped data should not obscure the pattern of the data, nor should it create an artificial pattern. Each table and chart should be referred to in the text, but each should add to the text, not merely repeat it. Each table or graph should have an obvious connection to the study being reported.

In reading a table such as Table 16–3, the reader should first look at the heading. The title should give an indication of the information in the table. Next, the reader should review the column headings. Do these headings follow from the title? Is each heading clear, and are any nonstandard abbreviations explained? Are the statistics contained in the table appropriate to the level of measurement used? In

Table 16–3, the column headings follow from the title. Each study variable is listed, along with its mean and SD. Mean and SD are appropriate statistics because these data were regarded as interval data.

After evaluating the descriptive statistics, inferential statistics can then be evaluated. The first place to begin critiquing the inferential statistical analysis of a research report is with the hypothesis or research question. If the hypothesis or research question indicates that a relationship will be found, you should expect to find indices of correlation. If the study is experimental or quasiexperimental, the hypothesis would indicate that the author is looking for differences between the groups studied, and you would expect to find statistical tests of differences between means that test the effect of the intervention.

As you read the "Methods" section of the article, again consider the level of measurement the author has used to measure the important variables. If the level of measurement is interval or ratio, the statistics most likely will be parametric statistics. But if the variables are measured at the nominal or ordinal level, the statistics used should be nonparametric. Also, consider the size of the sample and remember that samples need to be large enough to permit the assumption of normality. If the sample is quite small, for example, 5 to 10 subjects, the researcher may have violated the assumptions necessary for inferential statistics to be used (see Chapter 12). Thus, the important question is whether the researcher has provided enough justification to use the statistics presented.

Finally, consider the results as they are presented. Enough data should be presented for each hypothesis or research question to determine whether the researcher actually examined each one. The tables should accurately reflect the procedure performed and be in harmony with the text. For example, the text should not indicate that a test reached statistical significance, whereas the tables indicate that the probability value of the test was above .05. If the researcher has used analyses that are not discussed in this text, you may want to refer to a statistics text to decide whether the analysis was appropriate to the hypothesis or research question and the level of measurement.

The reader should critique two other aspects of the data analysis. The study should not read as if it were a statistical textbook. The results should be presented clearly enough that the average reader can determine what was done and what the results were. In addition, the author should attempt to make a distinction between the practical and the statistical significance of the evidence related to the findings. Some results may be statistically significant, but their practical importance may be doubtful in terms of applicability to a client population or clinical setting. In this case, the author should note the deficiency. Alternatively, you may find yourself reading a research report that is elegantly presented, but you come away with a "so what?" feeling. Such a feeling may indicate that the practical significance of the study and its findings have not been adequately explained in the report. From an evidence-based practice perspective, a significant hypothesis or research question should contribute to improving client care and clinical outcomes.

Note that the critical analysis of a research article's statistical analysis is not conducted in a vacuum. The adequacy of the analysis can only be judged in relation to the other important aspects of the article: the problem, the hypotheses, the research question, the design, the data collection methods, and the sample. Without consideration of these aspects of the

research process, the statistics themselves have very little meaning. Statistics can be misleading; thus, the researcher must use the appropriate statistic for the problem. For example, a researcher may sometimes use a nonparametric statistic when it appears that a parametric statistic is appropriate. Because parametric statistics are more powerful than nonparametric statistics, the result of the parametric analysis may not have been what the researcher expected. However, the nonparametric result might be in the expected direction, so the researcher reports only that result.

EXAMPLE OF THE USE AND CRITIQUE OF STATISTICS

The purpose of the study by Forchuk et al. (2005) was to determine the cost and effectiveness of a transitional discharge model of care with clients who have a chronic mental illness (see Appendix A). The statement of purpose implies that the investigators were interested in looking at differences between groups, thereby suggesting an experimental design that provides Level II evidence. Therefore, the reader should expect that the analysis will consist of statistical tests that examine differences between means, such as t tests or ANOVA.

In the Forchuk et al. (2005) study, sample characteristics were adequately described. In this difficult to reach follow-up sample, attrition was high (i.e., 141 out of 390 initially recruited), and the final sample size was 249. If the participants who did not complete the study differed from those who completed the study, the findings would be difficult to interpret (i.e., those who completed the program had fewer problems). Dependent variables consisted of quality of life, health care utilization, and levels of functioning and were measured over time at discharge and 1 month and 12 months after discharge. The investigators were interested in looking at differences between the intervention program group and the standard care control group that received the transitional discharge intervention. Various statistical tests were used to examine differences depending on the level of measurement. Dependent variables calculated at the interval level were compared using repeated measures ANOVA.

These tests are appropriate to the study design and the hypotheses because the researchers were interested in differences between the two groups. The results for each of the hypotheses were presented and suggested differences in some of the outcomes between the two groups. The tables agreed with the text, and the results were understandable to the reader. The discussion pointed out limitations to the study. Clear implications for practice were found, and they supported the practical significance of the study. The statistical level of significance was set at .05 and was consistent throughout the article. Therefore, the researchers' statistics were appropriate to the study's purpose, design, method, sample, and levels of measurement.

Critical Thinking Challenges

- Discuss the ways a researcher might use a computer to analyze data and present the descriptive statistical results of a study.
- What is the relationship between the level of measurement a researcher uses and the choice of a statistical procedure? How is this level of measurement associated with the level of evidence in the study design?
- What type of visual representation can be used to demonstrate the use of correlations? Use examples from clinical practice to illustrate the difference between positive and negative correlations.
- A classmate from research class tells you that it is ridiculous for the instructor to ask students to critique the descriptive statistics used in a study when none of the students has taken a statistics course. Would you agree or disagree with her claim? Defend your position.
- What assumptions are violated when a clinical research study uses a convenience sample and applies inferential statistics?
- What are the advantages and disadvantages of decreasing the alpha level for a study? What is the relationship between setting an alpha level and type I and type II errors?
- Discuss the parameters for using nonparametric statistics in a study and its impact on the usefulness of applying the evidence provided by the findings in practice.
- A research study's findings are not considered significant at the .05 level; are they deemed to provide evidence that is applicable to practice? Justify your answer.

KEY POINTS

- Descriptive statistics are a means of describing and organizing data gathered in research.
- The four levels of measurement are nominal, ordinal, interval, and ratio. Each is associated with appropriate descriptive techniques.
- Measures of central tendency describe the average member of a sample. The mode is the most frequent score, the median is the middle score, and the mean is the arithmetical average of the scores. The mean is the most stable and useful of the measures of central tendency and, with the SD, forms the basis for many inferential statistics.
- The frequency distribution presents data in tabular or graphic form and allows for the calculation or observations of characteristics of the distribution of the data, including skewness, **symmetry**, modality, and **kurtosis**.
- In nonsymmetrical distributions, the degree and direction of the pull of the peak off-centre are described in terms of **skew**.
- The ranges reflect differences between high and low scores.
- The SD is the most stable and most useful measure of variability. It is derived from the concept of the normal curve. In the normal curve, sample scores and the means of large numbers of samples gather around the midpoint in the distribution, with a fixed percentage of the scores falling within given distances of the mean. This tendency of means to approximate the normal curve is called the sampling distribution of the means. A Z score is the SD converted to standard units.
- Because the sampling distribution of the means follows a normal curve, researchers are able to estimate the probability that a certain sample will have the same properties as the total population of interest. Sampling distributions provide the basis for all inferential statistics.
- Inferential statistics allow researchers to estimate population parameters and to test hypotheses about populations from sample data. The use of these statistics allows researchers to make objective decisions about the outcome of the study. Such decisions are based on the rejection or acceptance of the null hypothesis, which states that no relationship exists between the variables.
- If the null hypothesis is accepted, this result indicates that the findings are likely to have occurred by chance. If the null hypothesis is rejected, the researcher accepts the scientific hypothesis that a relationship exists between the variables that is unlikely to have been found by chance.

- Statistical hypothesis testing is subject to two types of errors: type I and type II.

- A type I error is the researchers' incorrect decision to reject the null hypothesis

- A type II error occurs when the results from the sample data lead to the failure to reject the null hypothesis when it is actually false; this error is also known as beta (β).

- The researcher controls the risk of making a type I error by setting the alpha level, or level of significance. Unfortunately, reducing the risk of a type I error by reducing the level of significance increases the risk of making a type II error.

- The results of statistical tests are reported to be significant or nonsignificant. For statistically significant results, the probability of occurring is less than .05 or .01, depending on the level of significance set by the researcher.

- Commonly used parametric and nonparametric statistical tests include tests for differences between means, such as the *t* test and ANOVA, and tests for differences in proportions, such as the chi-square test.

- Tests that examine data for the presence of relationships include the Pearson *r*, the sign test, the Wilcoxon matched pairs, the signed rank test, and multiple regression.

- Advanced statistical procedures include *path analysis*, LISREL, and factor analysis.

- The most important aspect of critiquing statistical analyses is the relationship of the statistics employed to the problem, design, and method used in the study. Clues to the appropriate statistical test to be used by the researcher should stem from the researcher's hypotheses. The reader also should determine whether all of the hypotheses have been presented in the article.

- A basic understanding of statistics will improve your ability to think about the level of evidence provided by the study design and findings and their relevance to client outcomes for your client population and practice setting.

REFERENCES

Bierlin, C., Hadjistavropoulous, H., Bourgault-Fagnou, M., & Sagan, M. (2006). A six-month profile of community case coordinated older adults. *Canadian Journal of Nursing Research, 38*, 32–50.

Bluman, A. J. (2006). *A brief version elementary statistics: A step by step approach.* New York: McGraw-Hill.

Brown, S. J. (1999). *Knowledge for health care practice: A guide to using research evidence.* Philadelphia: WB Saunders.

Castro-Rodriquez, J., & Rodrigo, G. (2004). Beta-agonists through metered-dose inhaler with valved holding chamber versus nebulizer for acute exacerbation of wheezing or asthma in children under 5 years of age: A systematic review with meta-analysis. *Journal of Pediatrics, 145*, 172–177.

Cummings, G. G., Estabrooks, C. A., Midodzi, W. K., Wallin, L., & Hayduk, L. (2007). Influence of organizational characteristics and context on research utilization. *Nursing Research, 56*(4), S24–S39.

Davison, B.J., Goldenberg, S. L., Gleave, M. E., & Degner, L. F. (2003). Provision of individualized information to men and their partners to facilitate treatment decision making in prostate cancer. *Oncology Nursing Forum, 30*, 107–114.

Decaire, M. W., Bédard, M., Riendeau, J., & Forrest, R. (2006). Incidents in a psychiatric forensic setting: Association with patient and staff characteristics. *Canadian Journal of Nursing Research, 38*, 68–80.

Fisher, A. R., Wells, G., & Harrison, M. B. (2004). Factors associated with pressure ulcers in adults in acute care hospitals. *Advances in Skin & Wound Care, 17*, 80–90.

Forchuk, C., Martin, M. L., Chan, Y. L., & Jensen, E. (2005). Therapeutic relationships: From psychiatric hospital to community. *Journal of Psychiatric and Mental Health Nursing, 12*, 556–564.

Gigerenzer, G. (1993). The superego, the ego, and the id in statistical reasoning. In G. Keren & C. Lewis (Eds.), *A handbook for data analysis in the behavioural sciences: Vol. 1. Methodological issues* (pp. 311–339). Hillsdale, NJ: Erlbaum.

Kline, R. B. (2005). *Beyond significance testing: Reforming data analysis methods in behavioral research.* Washington, DC: American Psychological Association.

Knapp, T. R. (1990). Treating ordinal scales as interval scales: An attempt to resolve the controversy. *Nursing Research, 39*, 121–123.

Knapp, T. R. (1993). Treating ordinal scales as ordinal scales. *Nursing Research, 42*, 184–186.

Lenhardt, R., Seybold, T., Kimberger, O., Stoiser, R., & Sessler, D. (2002). Local warming and insertion of peripheral venous cannulas: Single blinded prospective randomised controlled trial and single blinded randomized crossover trial. *British Journal of Medicine, 325*, 409–412.

Munro, B. H. (2001). *Statistical methods for health care research* (4th ed.). Philadelphia: Lippincott.

Phipps, M., Blume, J., & DeMonner, S. (2002). Young maternal age associated with increased risk of post-neonatal death. *Obstetrics and Gynecology, 100,* 481–486.

Samuels-Dennis, J. (2006). Stress and psychological distress in single mothers. *Canadian Journal of Nursing Research, 38,* 59–80.

Secco, L. (2002). The Infant Care Questionnaire: Assessment of reliability and validity in a sample of healthy mothers. *Journal of Nursing Measurement, 10,* 97–110.

Secco, M. L., & Moffatt, M. E. K. (2003). The home environment of Métis, First Nations, and Caucasian adolescent mothers: An examination of quality and influences. *Canadian Journal of Nursing Research, 35*(2), 106–125.

Slakter, M. J., Wu, Y. W. B., & Suzuki-Slakter, N. S. (1991). Statistical nonsense at the .00000 level. *Nursing Research, 40,* 248–249.

Snowdon, A. W., Polgar, J., Patrick, L., & Stamler, L. (2006). Parents' knowledge about use of child safety systems. *Canadian Journal of Nursing Research, 38,* 98–114.

Stevens, K. (2001). Systematic reviews: The heart of evidence-based practice. *AACN Clinical Issues: Advanced Practice in Acute and Critical Care, 12,* 529–538.

Wang, S., Yu, M., Wang, C., & Huang C. (1999). Bridging the gap between the pros and the cons in treating ordinal scales as interval scales from an analysis point of view. *Nursing Research, 48,* 226–229.

Wilson, D. M. (2002). The duration and degree of end-of-life dependency of home care clients and hospital in-patients. *Applied Nursing Research, 15,* 81–86.

Geri LoBiondo-Wood

Mina D. Singh

CHAPTER 17

Presenting the Findings

LEARNING OUTCOMES

After reading this chapter, the student should be able to do the following:

- Discuss the difference between a study's "Results" section and the "Discussion" section.
- Identify the format of the "Results" section.
- Determine whether both statistically supported and statistically unsupported findings are discussed.
- Determine whether the results are objectively reported.
- Describe how tables and figures are used in a research report.
- List the criteria of a meaningful table.
- Identify the format and components of the "Discussion of the Results" section.
- Determine the purpose of the "Discussion" section.
- Discuss the importance of including the generalizations and limitations of a study in the report.
- Determine the purpose of including recommendations in the study report.
- Discuss how the strength, quality, and consistency of evidence provided by the findings are related to a study's limitations, generalizability, and applicability to practice.

KEY TERMS

confidence interval   374

findings   369

generalizability   375

limitations   371

recommendation   376

good tables   372

STUDY RESOURCES

evolve Go to Evolve at
http://evolve.elsevier.com/Canada/LoBiondo/Research/
for Weblinks, content updates, and additional research
articles for practice in reviewing and critiquing.

The ultimate goals of nursing research are to develop nursing knowledge and to promote evidence-based nursing practice, thereby supporting the scientific basis of nursing. From the viewpoint of the research consumer, the analysis of the results, interpretations, and the generalizations that a researcher generates from a study becomes a highly important piece of the research report. After the analysis of the data, the researcher puts the final pieces of the jigsaw puzzle together to view the total picture with a critical eye. This process is analogous to evaluation, the last step in the nursing process. In the final sections of the report, after the statistical procedures have been applied, the researcher relates the statistical or numerical findings to the theoretical framework, literature, methods, hypotheses, and problem statements.

The final sections of published research reports are generally titled "Results" and "Discussion," but other topics, such as limitations of findings, implications for future research and nursing practice, recommendations, and conclusions, may be separately addressed or subsumed within these sections. The format of the "Results" and "Discussion" is contingent upon the stylistic considerations of the author and the journal. The function of these final sections is to relate all aspects of the research process, as well as to discuss, interpret, and identify the limitations and generalizations relevant to the investigation, thereby furthering research-based practice.

The process that both the investigator and the research consumer use to assess the results of a study is depicted in the Critical Thinking Decision Path. The goal of this chapter is to introduce the purpose and content of the final sections of a research investigation, in which the data are presented, interpreted, discussed, and generalized. An understanding of what an investigator presents in these sections will help the research consumer critically analyze an investigator's findings.

FINDINGS

The **findings** of a study are the results, conclusions, interpretations, recommendations, generalizations, and implications for future research and nursing practice, which are separated into two major areas: the results and the discussion of the results. The "Results" section focuses on the results or statistical findings of a study, and the "Discussion" section focuses on the remaining topics. For both sections, as well as all other sections of a report, the same rule applies: the content must be presented clearly, concisely, and logically.

Evidence-Based Practice Tip

Evidence-based practice is an active process that requires you to consider how, and if, research findings are applicable to your client population and practice setting.

Results

The "Results" section of a research report is the data-bound section where the researcher presents the quantitative data or numbers generated by the descriptive and inferential statistical tests. The results of the data analysis set the stage for the interpretations or "Discussion" section that follows the results. The "Results" section should then reflect the question or hypothesis tested. The information from each hypothesis or research question should be sequentially presented. The tests used to analyze the data should be identified. If the author does not explicitly state the exact test that was used, then the values obtained should be noted. The researcher typically provides the numerical values of the statistics and states the specific test value and probability level achieved (see Chapter 16). Examples of statistical tests and the corresponding statistical values can be found in Table 17–1.

Novices should not be intimidated by the numbers and symbols. Although these numbers are important, they are only one piece of the whole; the research process is much more important. Whether research consumers superficially understand statistics or have an indepth knowledge of statistics, they can expect to find the study results clearly stated. Thus, the presence or absence of any statistically significant results should be noted. For the conceptual meanings of the numbers found in studies, refer to the discussion in Chapter 16.

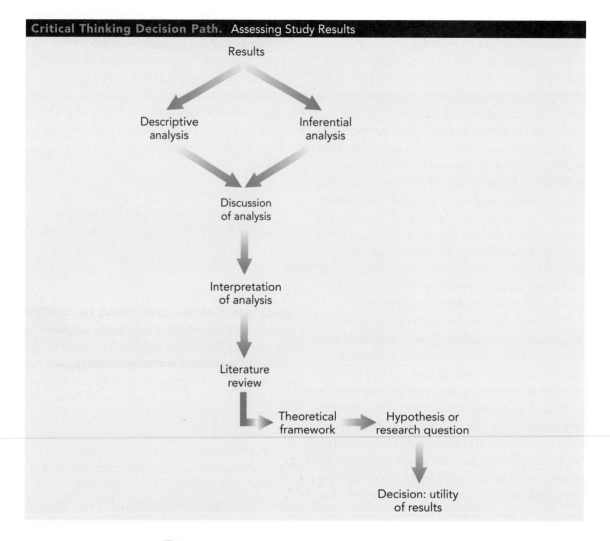

Critical Thinking Decision Path. Assessing Study Results

Results

Descriptive analysis

Inferential analysis

Discussion of analysis

Interpretation of analysis

Literature review

Theoretical framework

Hypothesis or research question

Decision: utility of results

Helpful Hint

In the "Results" section of a research report, the descriptive statistics are generally presented first, followed by the results of each hypothesis or research question tested.

The researcher is bound to present the data for all of the hypotheses posed or research questions asked (e.g., whether the hypotheses were accepted, rejected, supported, or not supported). If the data supported the hypotheses, it might be assumed

TABLE 17–1   Examples of Reported Statistical Results

Statistical Test	Examples of Reported Results
Mean	$M = 118.28$
Standard deviation	$SD = 62.5$
Pearson correlation	$r = .39, p < .01$
Analysis of variance	$F = 3.59, df = 2, 48, p < .05$
t test	$t = 2.65, p < .01$
Chi-square	$\chi^2 = 2.52, df = 1, p < .05$

that the hypotheses were proven, but this is not necessarily true. It only means that the hypotheses were supported, and the results suggest that the relationships or differences tested, which were derived from the theoretical framework, were probably logical in that study's sample.

Novice research consumers might also think that if a researcher's results are not supported statistically or are only partially supported, the study is irrelevant or possibly should not have been published. This is also not true. If the data are not supported, the research consumer should not expect the researcher to bury the work in a file. Reviewing and understanding unsupported studies is as important for a research consumer as it is for the researcher. Information obtained from unsupported studies can often be as useful as data obtained from supported studies.

Unsupported studies can be used to suggest **limitations** of particular aspects of a study's design and procedures. Data from unsupported studies may suggest that current modes of practice or current theory in an area may not be supported by research and therefore must be re-examined and researched further. Data help generate new knowledge, as well as prevent knowledge stagnation.

Generally, the results are interpreted in a separate section of the report. At times, the research critiquer may find that the "Results" section contains the results and the researcher's interpretations, which are more commonly found in the "Discussion" section. Integrating the results with the discussion in a report is the decision of the author or the journal editor. Both sections may be integrated when a study contains several segments that may be viewed as separate subproblems of a major overall problem.

When presenting the results, the investigator should demonstrate objectivity. The following quotation illustrates the appropriate way to express results:

The frequency of incidents varied according to diagnosis (χ^2 (5) = 14.69, p = .012). Patients with a diagnosis of schizophrenia or psychotic disorder were responsible for the greatest number of incidents (observed = 29,

expected = 17.7). Those with a diagnosis of substance abuse disorder or with a deferred diagnosis were the perpetrators of fewer incidents than expected (observed = 1, expected = 5.4 and 4.8, respectively). (Decaire, Bédard, Riendean, & Forrest, 2006, p. 73)

Investigators would be accused of lacking objectivity if they stated the results in the following manner:

The results were not surprising as we found a significant relationship between lower physical and social functioning and higher fatigue, as we expected.

Opinions or reactionary statements to the data in the "Results" section are therefore avoided. Box 17–1 provides examples of objectively stated results.

BOX 17–1 Example of Objective Statements in the Results Section

- ". . . Drug use in the CCS [Canadian Campus Survey] is generally lower than that among 13th-graders" (Adlaf, Gliksman, Demers, & Newton-Taylor, 2003, p. 37).

- "The intervention group did not have a significant improvement in global quality of life (control group mean of 4.65, SD = 1.31; intervention mean = 4.78, SD = 1.31, $F(1,22) = 0.38$, $P = 0.27$" (Forchuk, Martin, Chan, & Jensen, 2005, p. 562) (see Appendix A).

- "The majority of students in the sample (93%) reported experiencing at least one form of sexual harassment during the preceding two months, with higher rates reported by girls (95%) than boys (89%): χ^2 (df = 1, N = 565) = 6.63, p < .05)" (Dahinten, 2003, p. 63).

- "There were two antecedent and sustaining categories that represented the values and actions necessary for caring to occur. These categories were respecting the patient and not taking the patient's behaviour personally" (Chiovitti, 2008, p. 209).

- "Dyspnea frequency and severity in LTC [Long Term Care] were related to oxygen therapy (r = .18 and r = .21, respectively [p<.05])" (Doran et al., 2006, p. S79).

The critiquer of a study should consider the following points when reading a "Results" section:

- The investigators responded objectively to the results in the discussion of the results.

- In the discussion of the results, the investigators interpreted the results, with a careful reflection on all aspects of the study that preceded the results.

- The data presented are summarized. Many data are generated, but only the critical summary numbers for each test are presented. Examples of summarized data are the means and standard deviations of age, education, and income. Including all data is too cumbersome. The results can be viewed as a summation section.

- The condensation of data is done both in the written text and through the use of tables and figures. Tables and figures facilitate the presentation of large amounts of data.

- Results for the descriptive and inferential statistics for each hypothesis or research question are presented. No data should be omitted even if insignificant.

In the study in Appendix C, Samuels-Dennis (2006) developed tables to present the results visually. Table 17–2 provides demographic descriptive results about the study's subjects; Table 17–3 provides the results for testing comparisons of stressful events according to employment status. Tables allow researchers to provide a more visually thorough explanation and discussion of the results. If tables and figures are used, they must be concise. Although the text is the major mode of communicating the results, the tables and figures serve a supplementary but independent role. The role of tables and figures is to report results with details that the investigator does not enter into the text. This does not mean that the content of tables and figures should not be mentioned in the text. The amount of detail that the author uses in the text to describe the specific tabled data varies with the needs of the researcher.

A good table meets the following criteria:

- It supplements and economizes the text.

- It has precise titles and headings.

- It does not repeat the text.

An example of a table that meets these criteria can be found in Table 2 in the study by Smith, Edwards, Varcoe, Martens, and Davies (2006) (see Appendix B, Table B-2), which shows the study's themes and subthemes. Visualizing the findings of a study is easier if the reader has a table that clearly summarizes the results, as this table does. Providing a description of each theme in the text of the article would have taken a lot of space, and the results would have been difficult to visualize. The table developed by the researchers allows the reader not only to visualize the concepts quickly but also to assess the results (see Table 17–4).

TABLE 17–2 Sociodemographic Characteristics of Single Mothers, by Employment Status				
	Employment (n = 48)		Social Assistance (n = 48)	
Race	n	%	n	%
Caucasian	14	29.2	21	43.8
Afro-Canadian	27	56.3	11	22.9
Native	1	2.1	1	2.1
South Asian	1	2.1	9	18.8
Asian	4	8.3	1	2.1
Latino	1	2.1	3	6.3
Arabic	0	0.0	1	2.1
Other	0	0.0	1	2.1

Adapted from Samuels-Dennis, J. (2006). Relationship among employment status, stressful life events, and depression in single mothers. *Canadian Journal of Nursing Research, 38*(1), 68.

TABLE 17-3 Comparison of Stressful Events According to Employment Status							
	Employed (n = 48)			Social Assistance (n = 48)			
Stressful Event	%	x	SD	%	x	SD	t
Started or changed school	14.6	.15	.357	20.8	.21	.410	−0.796
Graduated from school	22.9	.23	.425	12.5	.13	.334	1.335
Problems in school	4.2	.04	.202	8.3	.08	.279	−0.838
Failed school	2.1	.02	.144	0	.00	.000	1.000
Got married	2.1	.02	.144	0	.00	.000	1.000

Adapted from Samuels-Dennis, J. (2006). Relationship among employment status, stressful life events, and depression in single mothers. *Canadian Journal of Nursing Research, 38*(1), 69.

Helpful Hint

A well-written "Results" section is systematic, logical, concise, and drawn from all of the analyzed data. All that is written in the "Results" section should be geared to letting the data reflect the testing of the problems and hypotheses. The length of this section depends on the scope and breadth of the analysis.

Evidence-Based Practice Tip

As you reflect on the results of a study, think about how the results fit with previous research on the topic and the strength and quality of available evidence on which to base clinical practice decisions.

Discussion of the Results

In the final section of the report, the investigator interprets and discusses the results of the study. In the discussion section, a skilled researcher makes the data come alive. The researcher interprets and gives meaning to the numbers in quantitative studies or the concepts in qualitative studies. The reviewer may ask where the investigator extracted the meaning that is applied in this section. If the researcher does the job properly, the discussion will return to the beginning of the study, where a problem statement was identified and independent and dependent variables were related on the basis of a theoretical framework (see Chapter 2) and literature

TABLE 17-4 Themes and Subthemes in Results	
Themes	Subthemes
Pregnancy as an opportunity for change	• Wanting children to have the gifts but not the pain of the intergenerational impact of residential schools • Children are highly valued • Parents are highly motivated to heal past hurts and reconnect with self, family, and culture
Safe health care practices and relationships	• Nonjudgemental • Respectful • Strengths based • Facilitating healing and trusting relationships • Holistic
Responsive care	• Client directed • Integrating multiple ways of knowing, with greater emphasis on experiential and cultural knowledge • Reaching out—being visible
Making intervention safe and responsive	• Empowerment education • Including fathers and family • Feeding body, mind, and soul

From Smith, D., Edwards, N., Varcoe, C., Martens, P. J., & Davies, B. (2006). Bringing safety and responsiveness into the forefront of care for pregnant and parenting Aboriginal people. *Advances in Nursing Science, 29*(2), E34.

review (see Chapter 5). In this section, the researcher discusses the following:

- The supported and the nonsupported data
- The limitations or weaknesses of a study in light of the design and the sample or data collection procedures
- How the theoretical framework was supported
- Additional or previously unrealized relationships suggested by the data

Even if the data are supported, the reviewer should not believe the conclusions to be the final word. Statistical significance is not the end point of a researcher's thinking, and low p values may not be indicative of research breakthroughs. To the critiquer, this means that statistical significance in a research study does not always mean that the results of a study are clinically significant. As the body of nursing research grows, so does the profession's ability to critically analyze beyond the test of significance and assess a research study's applicability to practice. Chapter 20 reviews methods used to analyze the usefulness of research findings. Within the nursing literature, discussion of clinical significance and evidence-based practice has also emerged (Goode, 2000; Ingersoll, 2000; Melnyk & Fineout-Overholt, 2002).

As indicated throughout this text, many important pieces in the research puzzle must fit together for a study to be evaluated as a well-done project. Therefore, researchers and reviewers should accept statistical significance with prudence. Statistically significant findings are not the sole means of establishing the study's merit. Remember that accepting statistical significance only means acceptance that the sample mean is the same as the population mean, which may not be true (see Chapter 16).

Another way to assess whether the findings from one study can be generalized is to calculate a confidence interval. A **confidence interval** quantifies the uncertainty of a statistic or the probable value range within which a population parameter, for example, the mean, is expected to lie. The width of the confidence interval gives the researcher some idea about

the uncertainty surrounding the unknown parameter. A very wide interval may indicate that more data should be collected before anything very definite can be said about the parameter. Confidence intervals are more informative than the simple results of hypothesis tests (where we decide "reject H_0" or "fail to reject H_0") because they provide a range of plausible values for the unknown parameter.

To illustrate, the study by Adlaf et al. (2003) used confidence intervals around rates to present population patterns of illicit drug use among Canadian university undergraduates relative to nonuniversity samples (see Table 17–5). The researchers explained that, to evaluate sample differences, they assessed whether estimates of the comparisons samples were bounded by the Canadian Campus Survey confidence intervals.

The process used to calculate a confidence interval is beyond the scope of this text, but references are provided for further explanation (Bluman, 2006; Gardner and Altman, 1986; Wright, 1997). Other aspects of the study, such as theory, sample, instrumentation, and methods, should also be considered.

When the results are not statistically supported, the researcher returns to the theoretical framework and analyzes the earlier thinking process. The results of nonsupported hypotheses do not require the investigator to go on a fault-finding tour of each piece of the project. Such a course can become an overdone process. All research has weaknesses. This analysis is an attempt to identify the weaknesses and to suggest the possible or actual problems in the study. At times, the theoretical thinking is correct, but the researcher finds problems or limitations that could be attributed to the tools (see Chapter 14), the sampling methods (see Chapter 12), the design (see Chapters 10 and 11), or the analysis (see Chapters 15 and 16). Therefore, when the results are not supported, the investigator attempts a fact-finding tour rather than a fault-finding tour. The purpose of the discussion, then, is not to show humility or one's technical competence but rather to enable the reviewer to judge the validity of the

TABLE 17–5   Percentage Reporting Past-Year Drug Use: Canadian Campus Survey Versus Other Populations

Drug	CCS 1998	US MTF (College) 1998 (n = 1440)	US CAS (College) 1999 (n = 13,986)	Ontario 13th-Graders 1997 (n = 917)	Ontario 13th-Graders 1999 (n = 447)	Ontario 18–29-year-olds 1998 (n = 332)
Cannabis	28.7 (25.6–31.8)	35.9	27.4	31.9 (29.7–34.1)	43.3 (29.6–58.1)	25.6 (20.4–31.7)
Cocaine	1.6 (1.3–2.0)	4.6	3.6	2.1 (0.6–3.6)	6.4 (1.8–19.9)	2.7 (1.3–5.8)
Crack	—*	1.0	0.9	0.8 (0.1–1.3)	1.1 (0.3–4.1)	NA
LSD	1.8 (1.2–2.5)	4.4	3.7	7.1 (3.3–10.9)	6.9 (2.0–21.2)	NA
MDMA	2.4 (1.4–3.3)	3.9	4.7	3.9	7.8	NA

From Adlaf, E., Gliksman, L., Demers, L., Demers, A., & Newton-Taylor, B. (2003). Illicit drug use among Canadian university undergraduates. *Canadian Journal of Nursing Research, 35*(1), 36.
*Data suppressed owing to unreliability; entries in parentheses are 95% confidence intervals; *n*'s vary due to missing values.
CAS: Campus Alcohol Survey; CCS: Canadian Campus Survey; LSD: lysergic acid diethylamide; MDMA: methylenedioxymethamphetamine; MTF: Monitoring the Future Survey; NA: not available.

interpretations drawn from the data and the general worth of the study.

In the "Discussion" section, the researcher ties together all the loose ends of the study and returns to the beginning to assess whether the findings support, extend, or counter the theoretical framework of the study. From this point, reviewers of research can begin to think about clinical relevance, the need for replication, or the germination of an idea for further research study. Finally, the reviewer of a research article should find the results section either in separate sections or subsumed within the "Discussion" section, and the results section should include generalizability and recommendations for future research, as well as a summary or a conclusion.

Generalizations (**generalizability**) are inferences that the data are representative of similar phenomena in a population beyond the study's sample. Reviewers of research are cautioned not to generalize beyond the population on which a study is based. Rarely, if ever, can one study be a recommendation for action. Beware of research studies that may overgeneralize. An example of making a sweeping generalization is concluding that all clients waiting for cardiac bypass can benefit from preoperative teaching and support when the study sample consisted of Caucasian male adults, 50 to 70 years of age. Attention must be paid to the limitations section of an article to note what the researchers have considered to affect the generalizability of their study findings. Generalizations that draw conclusions and make inferences within a particular situation and at a particular time are appropriate.

An example of an appropriate generalization is drawn from the study conducted by Secco et al. (2007), who assessed the factors affecting the postpartum depressive symptoms of adolescent mothers. When discussing the sample in light of the results, the researchers appropriately noted the following:

Convenience sampling, recruitment from only two high-risk settings, and attrition of participants are limitations that diminish generalizability of study findings to other settings and adolescent mothers. Self-selection bias is a factor that operates when adolescents who chose to participate differ in some manner from the population of adolescent mothers. Consequently, generalizability of study findings outside the current sample to other communities, ethnic groups, and SES characteristics is limited. (p. 52)

This type of statement is important for reviewers of research. It helps guide thinking in terms of a study's clinical relevance and suggests areas for further research (see Chapter 20).

In a qualitative study, the limitations may be stated differently, as Chiovitti (2008) wrote:

> *One of the purposes of this qualitative study was to specify, not generalize, the conditions and actions of caring. Consequently, as conditions change, it is expected that the theoretical formulation presented will also change to meet new conditions, different settings and samples. Therefore, what cannot be found in the actual data, at the time of the study, is one of the limitations. (p. 208)*

Chiovitti (2008) noted the issues of a qualitative study to prevent a sweeping transferability of findings, leading to misinterpretations of the results. An example of how the limitations in a qualitative study can affect transferability is provided by Edwards and Donner (2007). These authors conducted a descriptive, interpretive study to explore and describe the work of critical care nurses in sharing and discussing their knowledge about clients with other members of the health care team. The overall theme of "filling out the picture" for others by passing along knowledge about the client's status, client responses over time, interventions that had been beneficial, and the client as a person. The authors noted that the limitations of a small size, the use of one facility, and a stable period in the intensive care unit (ICU) will affect the transferability of their findings to other ICUs and different nursing units. Edwards and Donner concluded that more research needs to be done in this area.

One study does not provide all of the answers, nor should it. The final steps of evaluation are critical links to the refinement of practice and the generation of future research. Evaluation of research, like evaluation of the nursing process, is not the last link in the chain but a connection between findings that may serve to improve nursing theory and nursing practice.

Helpful Hint

It has been said that a good study is one that raises more questions than it answers. So, the research consumer should not view an investigator's review of limitations, generalizations, and implications of the findings for practice as a lack of research skills but as the beginning of the next step in the research process.

The final area that the investigator integrates into the "Discussion" section is the recommendations. The **recommendations** are the investigator's suggestions for the study's application to practice, theory, and further research. These suggestions require the investigator to reflect on the question, "What contribution to nursing does this study make?" (Box 17–2 provides examples of recommendations for future research and implications for nursing practice.) This evaluation places the study in the realm of what is known and what needs to be known before being used. Nursing has grown tremendously over the last century through the efforts of many nursing researchers and scholars. This thought is critical and has been reaffirmed by many nurse researchers in the past decade, such as Gortner (2000) and Hinshaw (2000).

BOX 17-2 Examples of Research Recommendations and Practice Implications

RESEARCH RECOMMENDATIONS

- "To test total effects of the predictors, rather than direct effects only, we believe that analysis strategies such as structural equation modelling may be more appropriate" (Tourangeau, Giovannetti, Tu, & Wood, 2002, p. 85).

- "To assess the impact and response of providing emotional support and education to patients on the waiting list for elective CA [coronary angiography], a prospective interventional cohort study could be designed to allocate patients awaiting elective CA to 2 groups: one group receiving weekly tracking telephone calls with an educational component and the other group not receiving treatment" (de Jong-Watt & Arthur, 2004, p. 247).

- "Future research is needed to determine appropriate interventions to promote prenatal expectations of infant care emotionality among adolescent mothers" (Secco et al., 2007, p. 52).

PRACTICE IMPLICATIONS

- "This study produced two important findings about nurse staffing. First, nurse staffing was related to client safety outcomes for a sample of medical and surgical nursing clients. The lower the proportion of professional nursing staff employed on the unit, the higher the medication errors and wound infections.

As well, the less experienced the nursing staff, the higher the number of wound infections on a unit" (McGillis-Hall, Doran, & Pink, 2004, p. 44).

- "Nurses and other care providers therefore need to understand the cultural manifestations and context of postpartum depression . . . . Opportunities for social support (e.g., networking initiatives, immigrant women centres) can be especially advantageous to women as they address a range of needs, including isolation, instrumental and emotional support, and access to information about community resources" (Sword, Watt, & Krueger, 2006, p. 724).

- "The higher rates of harassment among Grade 9 students, coupled with other empirical evidence showing that sexual harassment begins in the lower grades, suggest that prevention efforts should be instituted well before children reach high school" (Dahinten, 2003, p. 69).

- "These results need to be considered in developing health care interventions to enhance well-being and decrease distress for caregivers. These interventions may include educating caregivers on how to provide emotional support or manage behavioural problems, and linking caregivers to community resources to increase mastery and improve their emotional health (Singh & Cameron, 2005, p. 24).

Critiquing the Results and Discussion

The results and the discussion of the results are the researcher's opportunity to examine the logic of the hypothesis posed, the theoretical framework, the methods, and the analysis (see the Critiquing Criteria box). This final section requires as much logic, conciseness, and specificity as employed in the preceding steps of the research process. The research consumer should be able to identify statements on the type of analysis that was used and whether the data statistically supported the hypothesis. These statements should be straightforward and not reflect bias (see Tables 17–3 and 17–4 and Box 18-1, page 387). Auxiliary data or serendipitous findings also may be presented. If such auxiliary findings are presented, they should be stated as dispassionately as

were the hypothesis data. The statistical test used also should be noted, as well as the numerical value of the data (see Tables 17–1, 17–3, and 17–4). The presentation of the tests, the numerical values found, and the statements of support or nonsupport should be clear, concise, and systematically reported. For illustrative purposes that facilitate readability, the researchers should present extensive findings in tables rather than in the text.

The "Discussion" section should interpret the data, gaps, limitations, and conclusions of the study, as well as provide recommendations for further research. Drawing these aspects into the study should give the research consumer an understanding of the relationship between the findings and the theoretical framework. Statements reflecting the underlying theory are necessary, whether or not the hypotheses were supported.

If the findings were not supported, the consumer should—as the researcher did—attempt to identify, without fault finding, possible methodological problems. Finally, a concise presentation of the study's generalizability and the implications of the findings for practice and research should be evident. The last presentation can help the research consumer begin to rethink clinical practice, provoke discussion in clinical settings (see Chapter 20), and find similar studies that may support or refute the phenomena being studied to more fully understand the problem.

CRITIQUING CRITERIA

1. Are the results of each hypothesis presented?

2. Is the information regarding the results concisely and sequentially presented?

3. Are the tests that were used to analyze the data presented?

4. Are the results presented objectively?

5. If tables or figures are used, do they meet the following standards?
    a. They supplement and economize the text.
    b. They have precise titles and headings.
    c. They do not repeat the text.

6. Are the results interpreted in light of the hypotheses and theoretical framework and all of the other steps that preceded the results?

7. If the data are supported, does the investigator provide a discussion of how the theoretical framework was supported?

8. If the data are not supported, does the investigator attempt to identify the study's weaknesses and strengths, as well as suggest possible solutions for the research area?

9. Does the researcher discuss the study's clinical relevance?

10. Are any generalizations made, and, if so, are they within the scope of the findings or beyond the findings?

11. Are any recommendations for future research stated or implied?

12. What is the study's strength of evidence?

Critical Thinking Challenges

- Defend or refute the following statement: "All results should be reported and interpreted whether or not they support the hypothesis (hypotheses)."

- What type of knowledge does the researcher draw on to interpret the results of a study? Is the same type of knowledge used when the results of a study are not statistically significant?

- Do you agree or disagree with the statement that a good study raises more questions than it answers? Support your view with examples.

- How is it possible for research consumers to critique the findings and recommendations of a reported study? How could you use the Internet for critiquing the findings of a study?

- Now that nursing students and nurses have access to reports of clinical problems (i.e., critiques of multiple studies available on a clinical topic) or critiques of individual studies of a clinical topic published in *Evidence-Based Nursing*, as well as published meta-analyses on clinical topics, why is it necessary for them to read and critique research studies on their own? Justify your response.

KEY POINTS

- The analysis of the findings is the final step of a research investigation. In this section, the research consumer will find the results presented in a straightforward manner.

- All results should be reported whether or not they support the hypothesis. Tables and figures may be used to illustrate and condense data for presentation.

- Once the results are reported, the researcher interprets the results. In this presentation, usually titled "Discussion," the consumer should be able to identify the key topics being discussed. The key topics, which include an interpretation of the results, are the limitations, generalizations, implications, and recommendations for future research.

- The researcher draws together the theoretical framework and makes interpretations based on the findings and theory in the section on the interpretation of the results. Both statistically supported and unsupported results should be interpreted. If the results are not supported, the researcher should discuss the results reflecting on the theory, as well as possible problems with the methods, procedures, design, and analysis.

- The researcher should present the limitations or weaknesses of the study. This presentation is important because it affects the study's generalizability. The generalizations or inferences about similar findings in other samples also are presented in light of the findings.

- The research consumer should be alert for sweeping claims or overgeneralizations that a researcher may state. An overextension of the data can alert the consumer to possible researcher bias.

- The recommendations provide the consumer with suggestions regarding the study's application to practice, theory, and future research. These recommendations furnish the critiquer with a final perspective of the utility of the investigation's findings in practice.

REFERENCES

Adlaf, E. M., Gliksman, L., Demers, A., & Newton-Taylor, B. (2003). Illicit drug use among Canadian university students. *Canadian Journal of Nursing Research, 35,* 24–43.

Bluman, A. J. (2006). *Elementary statistics: A brief version.* New York: McGraw-Hill.

Chiovitti, R. F. (2008). Nurses' meaning of caring with patients in acute psychiatric hospital settings: A grounded theory study. *International Journal of Nursing Studies, 45*(2), 203–223.

Dahinten, V. S. (2003). Peer sexual harassment in adolescence: The function of gender. *Canadian Journal of Nursing Research, 35,* 56–73.

Decaire, M. W., Bédard, M., Riendean, J., & Forrest, R. (2006). Incidents in a psychiatric forensic setting: Association with patient and staff characteristics. *Canadian Journal of Nursing Research, 38,* 68–80.

de Jong-Watt, W. J., & Arthur, H. M. (2004). Anxiety and health-related quality of life in patients awaiting elective coronary angiography. *Heart & Lung, 33,* 237–248.

Doran, D. M., Harrison, M. B., Laschinger, H. S., Hirdes, J. P., Rukholm, E., Sidani, S., et al. (2006). Nursing-sensitive outcomes data collection in acute care and long-term-care settings. *Nursing Research, 55*(2S), S75–S81.

Edwards, M., & Donner, G. (2007). The efforts of critical care nurses to pass along knowledge about patients. *Canadian Journal of Nursing Research, 39,* 138–154.

Forchuk, C., Martin, M.-L., Chan, Y.-C., & Jensen, E. (2005). Therapeutic relationships: From psychiatric hospital to community. *Journal of Mental Health Nursing, 12,* 556–564.

Gardner, M. J., & Altman, D. G. (1986). Confidence intervals rather than p values: Estimation rather than hypothesis testing. *British Medical Journal: Clinical Research, 292,* 746–750.

Goode, C. J. (2000). What constitutes the "evidence" in evidence-based practice. *Applied Nursing Research, 13,* 222–225.

Gortner, S. (2000). Knowledge development in nursing: Our historical roots and future opportunities. *Nursing Outlook, 48,* 60–67.

Hinshaw, A. S. (2000). Nursing knowledge for the 21st century: Opportunities and challenges. *Journal of Nursing Scholarship, 32,* 117–123.

Ingersoll, G. L. (2000). Evidence-based nursing: What it is and what it isn't. *Nursing Outlook, 48,* 151.

McGillis-Hall, L., Doran, D., & Pink, G. H. (2004). Nurse staffing models, nursing hours, and patient safety outcomes. *Journal of Nursing Administration, 34,* 41–45.

Melnyk, B. M., & Fineout-Overholt, E. (2002). Key steps in evidence based practice: Asking compelling questions and searching for the best evidence. *Pediatric Nursing, 28,* 262–263, 266.

Samuels-Dennis, J. (2006). Relationship among employment status, stressful life events, and depression in single mothers. *Canadian Journal of Nursing Research, 38,* 59–80.

Secco, M. L., Profit, S., Kennedy, E., Walsh, A., Letourneau, N., & Stewart, M. (2007). *Journal of Obstetric, Gynecologic, & Neonatal Nursing, 36,* 47–54.

Singh, M., & Cameron, J. (2005). Psychosocial aspects of caregiving to stroke patients. *AXON, 27*(1), 18–24.

Smith, D., Edwards, N., Varcoe, C., Martens, P. J., & Davies, B. (2006). Bringing safety and responsiveness into the forefront of care for pregnant and parenting Aboriginal people. *Advances in Nursing Science, 29*(2), E27–E44.

Sword, W., Watt, S., & Krueger, P. (2006). Postpartum health, service needs, and access to care experiences of immigrant and Canadian-born women. *Journal of Obstetric, Gynecologic, & Neonatal Nursing, 35,* 717–727.

Tourangeau A. E., Giovannetti P., Tu J. V., & Wood M. (2002) Nursing-related determinants of 30-day mortality for hospitalized patients. *Canadian Journal of Nursing Research, 33*(4), 71–88.

Wright, D. B. (1997). *Understanding statistics: An introduction for the social sciences.* London: Sage.

PART FIVE

Critiquing Research

Evolution in a Program of Research Focusing on Family Violence, Caregiving, and Women's Health

Programs of research evolve in unpredictable ways depending on the findings of previous studies, opportunities for collaboration, and successes and failures in applications for funding. My current program of research began with my first research study, my master of nursing thesis, a grounded theory study of family caregiving for children with chronic middle ear disease. I had a generous mentor in my supervisor, Phyllis Noerager Stern, who was an expert in grounded theory. This first research experience was exciting and interesting because the research approach allowed me to learn about family issues from the perspective of the families themselves, and developing a beginning theory was useful for both nurses and families.

As a new faculty member who was expected to develop a program of research and to obtain funding locally, I built on my thesis research by conducting a similar study with Aboriginal families. This research was followed by a small study of family caregiving for relatives with Alzheimer's disease. Throughout this research, I became very conscious that family caregivers were largely women who carried the brunt of caring, sometimes at great personal cost, including disruption to family relationships. I entered the summer doctoral program at Wayne State University with this in mind.

At this same time, my colleague Marilyn Merritt-Gray and I began a grounded theory study of women leaving abusive partners. Our goal was to fill the gap in our theoretical knowledge about the process of leaving. As a community mental health nurse, Marilyn felt the need for a framework to guide her practice and help women understand where they were, where they were headed, and how to get there.

Our initial findings, funded by a local grant, allowed us to obtain a larger local grant to develop the *theory of reclaiming self*. We became affiliated with the Muriel McQueen Fergusson Centre for Family Violence Research and began to collaborate with professionals and survivors of abusive relationships, who were concerned that, despite their best efforts, the incidence of intimate partner violence (IPV) in their rural area remained high. Together, we engaged in a participatory action study to determine the sociocultural influences on the meanings of and responses to woman abuse. This participatory study helped enhance the visibility of domestic violence and resulted in community actions to help women and change common understandings or attitudes that allowed abuse to continue.

This work took place over several years, when I was also spending summers in doctoral work at Wayne State University. There I met Jacquelyn Campbell, an international expert in domestic violence, who introduced me to a wide range of feminist thought and emphasized IPV as a nursing and health issue. In my doctoral research, I combined feminist theory and grounded theory and studied women's caring across the lifespan, developing the theory of *precarious ordering*. An important finding in this study was that women who were caring for family members who in the past had abused them, or with whom they had very strained relationships, had more difficulty gaining control of their health and had poorer health outcomes. My two areas of interest, IPV and women's caring, had begun to intersect!

Following graduation, I grappled with the challenge of getting national funding. Combining my interest in IPV and my colleague Marilyn Ford-Gilboe's interest in single motherhood led to a program of research focusing on single-parent families after leaving abusive relationships. This work has been well funded by the Medical Research Council, the National Health Research and Development Program, and, currently, the Canadian Institutes of Health Research (CIHR). Our first study built on the leaving study and focused on health promotion in single-parent families after leaving, using a feminist grounded theory perspective. We developed the theory of *strengthening capacity to limit intrusion* and noted that women in the study had many health issues related to IPV that had persisted for as long as 20 years after leaving the abusive partner. Yet little was known about the long-term health consequences of IPV.

This finding led to the development of a CIHR "New Emerging Team" focusing on the long-term health effects of IPV. The team recruited 309 women who had been out of abusive relationships no longer than three years to participate in structured interviews and health assessments annually for five years. Our goal is to apply structural equation modelling to discover the relationships between social, personal, and economic resources; abuse history; health outcomes; and health services use. The Women's Health Effects Study (WHES), a longitudinal design, is being supported by CIHR operating grants. The findings of the WHES, combined with the intrusion theory we developed, are currently being used to develop a health advocacy intervention to help women manage their symptoms and reduce intrusion in their lives, which we hope to test in a pilot study.

Similarly, my caregiving research has evolved from a qualitative to a quantitative focus. With further CIHR funding, Marilyn Hodgins and I assembled a caregiving team to develop an instrument measuring selected concepts in the grounded theory of precarious ordering, with the goal of testing the relationships among past relationships, obligation, health, and health promotion in women caregivers of adult family members. We surveyed over 250 caregiving women and found that past relationships and obligation accounted for significant variance in health outcomes. With funding from the Alzheimer Society, we are beginning a second study that replicates the first study but will include repeated data collection to capture changes in health and health promotion over time.

The final portion of my program of research also stems from the study of women who left abusive partners. Although the theory of reclaiming self was useful for these women, it did not help us understand the experiences of some women who remain with their partners and whose relationships become nonviolent. With funding from the Social Sciences and Humanities Research Council (SSHRC), our research team conducted a grounded theory study of how women achieve nonviolence, and we developed a theory, *shifting the pattern of abusive control*. Although violence cessation was important to women staying, equally important for some women was men reinvesting in the relationship. We realized that to fully understand how relationships shift when they become nonviolent, we needed to understand men's perspective on how their relationships changed when they ceased to be abusive toward their partners. This study was also funded by SSHRC and is ongoing.

What is most interesting to me is how my program of research has evolved methodologically and substantively in response to each study's findings and the collaborative opportunities that have arisen. I have an affinity for grounded theory research and likely approach most research with the mindset of a grounded theorist. But each study raises essential questions that cannot always be answered by the method the researcher likes best. Research partnerships with experts in diverse approaches are essential to build teams with the methodological versatility needed to move from inductive to deductive to intervention research. These partnerships are needed to provide the necessary knowledge for nursing practice to respond to the enormous challenges of the effects of family violence on individuals, families, and communities.

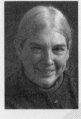

Judith Wuest
RN, BScN, MN, PhD
Canadian Institutes of
  Health Research
  Investigator
Professor, Faculty of
  Nursing
University of New Brunswick
Fredericton, New Brunswick

Helen J. Streubert Speziale
Cherylyn Cameron

CHAPTER 18

Critiquing Qualitative Research

LEARNING OUTCOMES

After reading this chapter, the student should be able to do the following:

- Identify the influence of stylistic considerations on the presentation of a qualitative research report.
- Identify the criteria for critiquing a qualitative research report.
- Evaluate the strengths and weaknesses of a qualitative research report.
- Describe the applicability of the findings of a qualitative research report.
- Construct a critique of a qualitative research report.

KEY TERMS

auditability 421
credibility 421
fittingness 421
saturation 421
theoretical sampling 420
transferability
trustworthiness 386

STUDY RESOURCES

evolve Go to Evolve at
http://evolve.elsevier.com/Canada/LoBiondo/Research/
for Weblinks, content updates, and additional
research articles for practice in reviewing
and critiquing.

Nursing research is accelerating at an unprecedented rate. The contributions nurse scientists are making to health care are evident in the fields of nursing, medicine, and health care, as well as in business journals. Nurse researchers are partnering at an ever-increasing rate with other health care professionals to develop, implement, and evaluate a variety of evidence-based interventions to improve client outcomes. The methods used to develop evidence-based practice include quantitative, qualitative, and mixed research approaches. Added to the increase in the number of research studies and publications is the growing number of nursing research projects that are accepted and funded by private and public organizations. This willingness of private and public entities to invest in nursing research attests to the quality of work being conducted by nursing researchers. Although quantitative, qualitative, and mixed research methods are all important to the ongoing development of sound evidence-based practice for nurses, this chapter focuses on the criteria used to determine the quality of a qualitative research report. To illustrate the critiquing process, two published research reports, as well as critiquing criteria, are presented. The criteria are then used to demonstrate the process of critiquing a qualitative research report.

STYLISTIC CONSIDERATIONS

Qualitative research differs from quantitative research in some very fundamental ways. Qualitative researchers seek to discover and understand concepts, phenomena, or cultures. Creswell (2003) stated that "qualitative research is exploratory and researchers use it to explore a topic when the variables and theory base are unknown" (pp. 74–75). In a qualitative study, you should not expect to find hypotheses; theoretical frameworks; dependent and independent variables; large, random samples; complex statistical procedures; scaled instruments; or definitive conclusions about how to use the findings. Because the purpose of qualitative research is to describe or explain concepts, phenomena, or cultures, the report is generally written in a way that allows the researcher to convey the full meaning and richness of the phenomena or cultures being studied. Narrative comments, including subjective remarks, are necessary to convey this depth and richness.

The goal of the qualitative research report is to describe in as much detail as possible the "insider's" or emic view of the phenomenon being studied. The emic view is the view of the person experiencing the phenomenon that reflects his or her culture, values, beliefs, and experiences. The qualitative researcher hopes to produce in the report an understanding of what it is like to experience a particular phenomenon or to be part of a specific culture.

One of the most effective ways to help the reader understand the emic view is to use quotations reflecting the phenomenon as experienced. For this reason, the qualitative research report has a more conversational tone than a quantitative report. In addition, data are frequently reported using concepts or phrases, which the researcher calls themes (see Chapter 8) as a way of describing large quantities of data in a condensed format.

To clearly demonstrate the application of a theme and how it helps the reader understand the emic view, consider an example from a report by Bottorff et al. (2004), who explored adolescents' understanding of nicotine addiction (see Appendix D). Six themes were identified as the adolescent constructions of nicotine addictions, one of which was described as "nicotine addiction as repeated use." The following quotation was used to demonstrate this theme:

> *When you're a smoker you get used to smoking at different points in the day. Like, it's weird to think, but certain times, like before I go to bed, I have to have a cigarette. As soon as I wake up and have my coffee I have a cigarette . . . . There's certain times where . . . when I'm driving I have to have a cigarette . . . I smoke a lot more when I'm driving just because it's what I do, like, I drive and I smoke. It's natural to me now. [17-year-old, daily smoker]. (Bottorff et al., 2004, p. 28)*

When writing a research report, the qualitative researcher's role is to illustrate the richness of the data and convey to readers the relationship between the themes identified and the quotations shared. This process is essential to documenting the rigour of the research, which is called **trustworthiness** in a qualitative research study. However, the richness of the participant's story or experience gathered in a qualitative research study cannot be shared in its entirety in a journal publication.

Page limitations imposed by journals frequently limit research reports to 15 pages, although some journals, such as *Qualitative Health Research*, by virtue of their readership, are committed to publishing lengthier reports. Note, however, that the criteria for publication of research reports are not based on a specific type of research method (i.e., quantitative or qualitative). The primary goal of journal editors is to provide their readers with high-quality, informative, timely, and interesting articles. To meet this goal, editors prefer to publish manuscripts that have scientific merit, present new knowledge, and engage their readership. The challenge for the qualitative researcher is to meet these editorial requirements within the page limit imposed by the journal of interest.

Although guidelines for the authors of qualitative and quantitative research reports are generally listed in each journal or are available from the journal editor, nursing journals do not generally offer their reviewers specific guidelines for evaluating these reports. The editors do, however, make every attempt to ensure the reviewers are knowledgeable in the method and subject matter of the study. But this determination is often made based on the reviewer's self-identified area of interest. Research reports are often evaluated based on the ideas or philosophical viewpoint of the reviewer, who may have strong feelings about particular types of qualitative or quantitative research methods. Therefore, authors usually clearly state the qualitative approach used and, if appropriate, its philosophical base.

Fundamentally, the principles for evaluating different qualitative research approaches are very similar. Research consumers are concerned with the plausibility and trustworthiness of the researcher's account of the research and its relevance to current or future theory and practice, or both (Horsburgh, 2003). Box 18–1 provides general guidelines for evaluating qualitative research, and Box 18–2 provides guidelines for evaluating grounded theory. For information on specific guidelines for evaluation of phenomenology, ethnography, grounded theory, and historical and action research, see Speziale and Carpenter (2007). For additional information on the specifics of qualitative research design, see Chapters 7 and 8.

APPLICATION OF QUALITATIVE RESEARCH FINDINGS IN PRACTICE

As already stated, one of the purposes of qualitative research is to describe, understand, or explain phenomena. Phenomena are events perceived by our senses, such as pain and losing a loved one. In addition to seeking to understand phenomena, qualitative research can give voice to those who have been disenfranchised and have no history (Barbour & Barbour, 2003; Schepner-Hughes, 1992). Unlike quantitative research, prediction and control of phenomena are not the aim of the qualitative inquiry. Therefore, qualitative results are applied differently than more traditional quantitative research findings. As Barbour and Barbour (2003) stated:

> *rather than seeking to import and impose templates and methods devised for another purpose, qualitative researchers and reviewers should look . . . for inspiration from their own modes of working and collaborating and seek to incorporate these, forging new and creative solutions to perennial problems, rather than hoping that these will simply disappear in the face of application of pre-existing sets of procedures. (p. 185)*

The application of qualitative findings will necessarily be context bound; in other words, findings may be applicable only in certain circumstances (Russell & Gregory, 2003). As Lincoln and Guba stated in 1985, "the trouble with generalizations is

BOX 18–1 Critiquing Guidelines for Qualitative Research

STATEMENT OF THE PHENOMENON OF INTEREST

1. Is the phenomenon of interest clearly identified?
2. What is the justification for using a qualitative method?
3. What are the philosophical underpinnings of the research method?

PURPOSE

1. What is the purpose of the study?
2. What is the projected significance of the work to nursing?

METHOD

1. Is the method used to collect data compatible with the purpose of the research?
2. Is the method adequate to address the phenomenon of interest?
3. If a particular approach is used to guide the inquiry, does the researcher complete the study according to the processes described?

SAMPLING

1. What type of sampling is used? Is it appropriate given the particular method?
2. Are the informants who were chosen appropriate to inform the research?

DATA COLLECTION

1. Is the data collection focused on human experience?
2. Does the researcher describe the data collection strategies (i.e., interview, observation, field notes)?
3. What are the procedures for collecting data?
4. Is the protection of human participants addressed?
5. Is saturation of the data described?

DATA ANALYSIS

1. What strategies are used to analyze the data?
2. Has the researcher remained true to the data?
3. Does the reader follow the steps described for data analysis?
4. Does the researcher address the credibility, auditability, and fittingness of the data? (See Chapter 14 for a complete discussion.)

Credibility

a. Do the participants recognize the experience as their own?
b. Has adequate time been allowed to fully understand the phenomenon?

Auditability

a. Can the reader follow the researcher's thinking?
b. Does the researcher document the research process?

Fittingness

a. Are the findings applicable outside of the study situation?
b. Are the results meaningful to individuals not involved in the research?
c. Is the strategy used for analysis compatible with the purpose of the study?

FINDINGS

1. Are the findings presented within a context?
2. Is the reader able to apprehend the essence of the experience from the report of the findings?
3. Are the researcher's conceptualizations true to the data?
4. Does the researcher place the report in the context of what is already known about the phenomenon? Was the existing literature on the topic related to the findings?

CONCLUSION, IMPLICATIONS, AND RECOMMENDATIONS

1. Do the conclusions, implications, and recommendations give the reader a context in which to use the findings?
2. Do the conclusions reflect the study findings?
3. What are the recommendations for future study? Do they reflect the findings?
4. How has the researcher made explicit the significance of the study to nursing theory, research, or practice?

that they don't apply to particulars" (p. 110). Thus, if a qualitative researcher studies the pain experience of individuals undergoing bone marrow biopsy, for example, the application of these findings will be confined to individuals who are similar to those in the study.

BOX 18–2   Critiquing Guidelines for Research Using the Grounded Theory Method

STATEMENT OF THE PHENOMENON OF INTEREST

1. What is the phenomenon of interest, and is it clearly stated for the reader?

2. What is the justification for using a grounded theory method?

PURPOSE

1. What is the explicit purpose for conducting the research?

2. What is the projected significance of the work to nursing?

METHOD

1. Is the method used to collect data compatible with the purpose of the research?

2. Is the method adequate to address the research topic?

3. What approach is used to guide the inquiry? Does the researcher complete the study according to the processes described?

SAMPLING

1. What type of sampling procedure is used? Is it appropriate for the method?

2. What major categories emerged?

3. What events, incidents, or actions pointed to these major categories?

4. What categories led to theoretical sampling?

5. After the theoretical sampling was completed, how representative did the categories prove to be?

DATA GENERATION

1. What were the data collection strategies? Were they appropriate for a grounded theory study?

2. How did theoretical formulations guide data collection?

3. How were human subjects protected?

DATA ANALYSIS

1. What strategies were used to analyze the data?

2. How does the researcher address the credibility, auditability, and fittingness of the data?

3. Does the researcher clearly describe how and why the core category was selected?

EMPIRICAL GROUNDING OF THE STUDY FINDINGS

1. Are the concepts grounded in the data?

2. How are the concepts systematically related?

3. Are conceptual linkages described, and are the categories well developed? Do they have conceptual density?

4. Are the theoretical findings significant? If yes, to what extent?

5. Was data collection comprehensive and analytical? Were interpretations conceptual and broad?

6. How does the researcher relate the study findings to existing literature?

CONCLUSIONS, IMPLICATIONS, AND RECOMMENDATIONS

1. How do the conclusions, implications, and recommendations give readers a context in which to use the findings?

2. Do the conclusions reflect the study findings?

3. What are the recommendations for future research? Are they appropriate?

4. Is the significance of the study to nursing practice made explicit?

Adapted with permission from Streubert, H. J. (1998). Evaluating the qualitative research report. In G. LoBiondo-Wood & J. Haber (Eds.), *Nursing research: Methods, critical appraisal, and utilization* (4th ed., pp. 445–465). St. Louis, MO: Mosby; and Strauss, A., & Corbin, J. (1990). *Basics of qualitative research: Grounded theory procedures and techniques.* Newbury Park, CA: Sage. Adapted with permission.

In another example, a study of depression in children with chronic disease should not be viewed as having direct application to adults suffering from chronic disease. The findings must either be used within a specific context or additional studies must be conducted to validate the applicability of the findings across contexts. Hence, nurses who wish to use the findings of qualitative research in their practices must first validate them, either through their own observations or through interaction with groups similar to the original study participants, to determine whether the findings accurately reflect wider experiences. In spite of the limitations associated with qualitative research findings, Glesne (2006) stated that qualitative research findings can be used to create solutions to practical problems. Qualitative research also has the ability to contribute to the evidence-based practice literature (Cesario, Morin, & Santa-Donato, 2002; Gibson & Martin, 2003).

Evidence-Based Practice Tip

Nurses using qualitative research findings should ask whether the evidence provided in the study enhances their understanding of particular client care situations.

Qualitative outcome analysis (QOA) can assist researchers to employ the findings of a qualitative study to develop interventions and then to test those selected. Morse, Penrod, and Hupcey (2000) offered "(QOA) [as a] systematic means to confirm the applicability of clinical strategies developed from a single qualitative project, to extend the repertoire of clinical interventions, and evaluate clinical outcomes" (p. 125). QOA allows the researcher or clinician to implement interventions based on the client's expressed experience of a particular clinical phenomenon. Application of knowledge discovered during qualitative data collection adds to our understanding of clinical phenomena by selecting interventions that are based on the client's experience. QOA is considered a form of evaluation research and, as such, has the potential to add to evidence-based practice literature either at Level V or at Level VI, depending on how the study was designed.

Another use of qualitative research findings is to initiate examination of important concepts in nursing practice, education, or administration. Caring, for example, is considered a significant concept in nursing; therefore, studying its multiple dimensions is important. Using a qualitative approach, Wilkin and Slevin (2004) explored the meaning of caring for intensive care nurses. The researchers posited that although caring has been studied extensively, little research has been conducted in the highly technological area of critical care. The authors identified that caring in an intensive care setting was a "process of competent physical and technical action imbued with affective skills" and confirmed that "to care is human and the capacity to care is affirmed and actualised in caring for the critically ill patient and their relatives" (p. 50). Wilkin and Slevin's study adds to the existing body of knowledge on caring and extends the current state of nursing science by examining a specific area of nursing practice and the experience of caring by critical care nurses.

Evidence-Based Practice Tip

Qualitative research studies can be used to guide practice when they are applied within a context. The nurse should ask the following question: "Does this study provide me with a direction for caring for a particular client group?"

Finally, qualitative research can be used to discover information about phenomena of interest that can lead to instrument development. Usually, qualitative methods are used to direct the development of structured research instruments as part of a larger empirical research project. Instrument development from qualitative research studies is useful to practising nurses because it is grounded in the reality of human experience with a particular phenomenon. For example, after an initial qualitative exploration of the phenomenon, the researcher may develop a survey to collect data related to specific variables.

Critiquing of a Qualitative Research Study

CRITIQUE #1

The study "Promoting Participation: Evaluation of a Health Promotion Program for Low Income Seniors" by Rosanne Buijs, Janet Ross-Kerr, Sandra O'Brien Cousins, and Douglas Wilson, published in the *Journal of Community Health Nursing* (2003), is critiqued. The article is presented in its entirety and is followed by the critique on pages 401–403. (From *Journal of Community Health Nursing, 20*, 93–107. Reprinted with permission.)

Promoting Participation: Evaluation of a Health Promotion Program for Low Income Seniors

Rosanne Buijs, RN, MSc
Centre for Health Promotion Studies
University of Alberta
Edmonton, Alberta

Janet Ross-Kerr, RN, PhD
Faculty of Nursing
University of Alberta
Edmonton, Alberta

Sandra O'Brien Cousins, EdD
Faculty of Physical Education and Recreation
University of Alberta
Edmonton, Alberta

Douglas Wilson, MD
Department of Public Health Sciences
University of Alberta
Edmonton, Alberta

This article describes a qualitative evaluation of the Seniors Active Living in Vulnerable Elders (ALIVE) program, a 10-month health promotion program for low income seniors. Program interventions delivered in seniors' apartment buildings included exercise classes, health information sessions (i.e., health corners), and newsletters. The evaluation examined program participation, program impacts, and how the program worked. The most frequent reason for joining the program was recognizing the benefits of exercise, and the most frequent reason for not attending the program was having other priorities. The main participant impact was "feeling better." Specific impacts were also noted in physical, mental, and social domains. Fun, program delivery adaptations, autonomy, social interactions, and staff–participant relationships were discovered to be important program processes. These processes all contributed to participants' "comfort" in the program. How and why the program worked is examined in relation to Pender's (1996) revised health promotion model and implications for nursing are indicated.

Seniors are an important target population for health promotion programs. The increasing numbers and age of this population have become a major demographic trend in western industrialized nations (Bernard, 2000). The impact of this trend on health care systems is expected to be considerable because increased health care utilization and expenditure occur during the senior years (Heidrich, 1998). Although health promotion and education programs have been used to assist young and middle-aged populations to maintain or improve their health status, such programs have not been employed extensively in older populations. However, health promotion programs have the potential to ameliorate or postpone health declines associated with aging, which in turn can increase quality of life and decrease health care costs (Schuster, 1995).

The Seniors Active Living in Vulnerable Elders (ALIVE) program was developed by a team of multidisciplinary researchers from the disciplines of nursing, physical education, pharmacy, nutrition, and sociology as part of a three-phase research study. The goal of the three-phase study was to promote independent living and to enhance quality of life for low-income seniors. The first phase examined the health status, attitudes, and health practices of the target population. Findings from the first phase showed that key background variables of age, cognitive status, physical status, and exercise habits were likely to be determinants of independent living. All of the variables except physical status contributed to increased social activity and group participation, which in turn influenced quality of life. Based on these findings, a health promotion program was developed, and the second phase was a pilot study of this program that included 35 participants from three low income seniors' apartment buildings. The third phase was a randomized controlled trial of the phase two health promotion program, now named the Seniors ALIVE program. Fourteen apartment buildings were involved in the third phase: 7 buildings receiving the intervention (the Seniors ALIVE program) and 7 buildings comprising the control group (with no intervention). The three-phase study was overseen by a program coordinator who was a master's prepared nurse and a qualified fitness instructor. Two evaluations of the Seniors ALIVE program were conducted, one quantitative and one qualitative. The purpose of this article is threefold:

1. To describe the qualitative evaluation of the Seniors ALIVE program in the seven intervention apartment buildings.

2. To discuss the findings in relation to Pender's (1996) revised health promotion model.

3. To suggest some implications for nursing including how nurses can encourage participation of seniors in health promotion programs.

These are important nursing interventions because participation in such programs can improve health and quality of life.

The Seniors ALIVE program was delivered for 10 months in seven seniors' apartment buildings in a large western Canadian city. All residents of these buildings have low incomes and are able to manage activities of daily living independently. The program consisted of three interventions: exercise classes providing a place to learn and practice active living, health corners providing a place to discuss health concerns, and newsletters providing health information. These interventions were expected to increase seniors' independence by improving their physical health (i.e., flexibility) and their quality of life by increasing their independence and functional health. The majority of program staff were university students in nursing, physical education, pharmacy, and nutrition who were recruited by their respective instructors. When insufficient numbers of students were available for the program, staff was hired from the community.

The 1-hr exercise classes were based on the Fit for Your Life strength training program (Fiatarone, 1996). The program coordinator, who was a qualified Fit for Your Life instructor, trained and supervised the staff who delivered the exercise classes. The biweekly classes included a warm-up, slow motion and progressively loaded resistance training for all major muscle groups, brief cardiovascular exercise, and a cool down. One- to 3-lb hand-held weights and resistance bands were used for the strength training. Each participant was encouraged to work at individually appropriate intensity and resistance loads.

At the health corners, seniors could have individual health consultations with nursing students who were supervised by the program coordinator. Health corners were held on a drop-in basis for 2-hr periods weekly or biweekly, with the average visit lasting 5 to 10 min. The health corners were usually held in a common room in the apartment building where furniture was arranged to provide a "waiting area" and a "consultation area." The consultation area consisted of a table and two chairs set apart from the waiting area for privacy. In addition to the health consultation, the nurse offered to monitor blood pressure and pulse rate. For about 10% of the health corners, pharmacy students were available for medication consultations and nutrition students for diet consultations.

Newsletters served as an important form of communication between staff and seniors. Seven four-page newsletters issued during the 10-month period were prepared by the program coordinator using a large-size font with a reading level between Grade 6 and 7. The newsletter contained information about the program such as the time and location of the exercise classes and the health corners and also articles on health related topics, such as exercise, sleep, bladder health, and healthy low cost recipes. Positive feedback about the seniors' progress in the program was included to encourage continued participation. Newsletters were placed under the apartment doors of registered program participants approximately once a month.

LITERATURE REVIEW AND STUDY PURPOSE

Evaluating the outcome of health promotion programs for seniors has been challenging. For example, when Heidrich (1998) reviewed 42 studies from 1980 to 1998 to examine the health behaviors of community-dwelling seniors who practiced two or more concurrent health behaviors, the benefits experienced by seniors could not easily be related to improved health outcomes. There are several reasons why it is difficult to measure health outcomes in seniors. First, an aging body makes the efficacy of physical health interventions more difficult to demonstrate. Second, there is a shorter life expectancy during which to measure changes (Arnold, Kane, & Kane, 1986). Third, seniors' undesirable health habits may be more difficult to change than those of younger adults because they have existed for a longer time. Finally, seniors are more likely than younger adults to have other circumstances unrelated to the health condition of interest that may confound, dilute, or block the effects of an intervention, making evaluation difficult (Rakowski, 1986).

Previous seniors' health promotion program evaluations have focused on the outcomes with respect to physical health (Heidrich, 1998). A more comprehensive, informative approach to evaluating these programs should also include an examination of functional health and the impact of program processes on health. Functional health, based on the ability to perform the tasks of daily living, is well documented in the literature as an important health outcome for seniors (Haber, 1999; Heidrich, 1998; Penning & Chappell, 1993), because it contributes to their independence (Gatz, 1995; Haber, 1999) and quality of life (Williams, 1994). Quality of life is a multidimensional concept referring to overall life satisfaction and includes both behavioral competence and psychological well-being.

Under ideal circumstances, interventions used in health promotion programs are expected to produce an outcome of improved health for participants. However, a number of intermediary steps, processes, or mechanisms occur between interventions and outcomes. The metaphor of a "black box" has been used to describe these intermediary steps because they are not well understood (Pearson et al., 2001; Swanson & Chapman, 1994). Figure 18C1–1 illustrates the relation of program interventions, the black box, and outcomes of the Seniors ALIVE program. The three program interventions, exercise classes, health corners, and newsletters are expected to produce the outcomes of increased independence and quality of life. The black box represents the unknown, intermediary steps in this chain of events.

Looking inside this black box will provide information about the inner functioning of a program and contribute to understanding how and why the program works. The possible benefits of learning more about the black box include being able to design interventions, utilize resources, and measure outcomes more effectively (Pearson et al., 2001).

Variables from Pender's (1996) revised health promotion model were used to assist in the interpretation of data from the Seniors ALIVE qualitative evaluation. This model explains the motivation for health promoting behavior by integrating a number of constructs from social cognitive and expectancy-value theory. Behavior specific thoughts and feelings important in the performance of health promoting behavior are classified into two groups: prior related behavior and personal factors. Prior related behavior consists of the following variables: perceived benefits of action, perceived barriers to action, perceived self-efficacy (i.e., an individual's

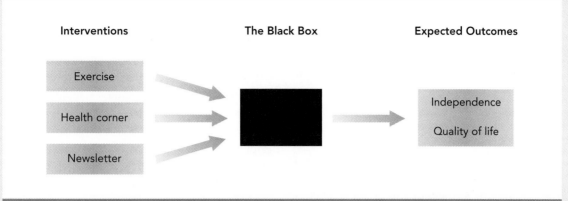

Figure 18C1–1 The Seniors ALIVE program and the black box

judgement about whether or not he or she can do the behavior), and activity-related affect (i.e., an individual's subjective feeling states before, during, and after performing a behavior such as delight or disgust). Personal factors include interpersonal influences (including social support) and situational influences (i.e., an individual's perceptions of feeling compatible, related, and safe). Motivation for action is further influenced by the immediate factors of commitment to a plan of action and competing demands or preferences.

The purpose of this study was to determine the impact of the Seniors ALIVE program on the participants and to understand how and why these impacts occurred by examining the intermediary steps between the interventions and the outcomes (the black box). The qualitative evaluation described in this article was conducted at the end of the 10-month trial of the Seniors ALIVE program and was guided by the following research questions:

1. What factors influenced seniors' participation in the program?

2. How did the program impact seniors who attended?

3. How did the program work (i.e., the black box)?

METHOD

Evidence from the literature suggests that not only are qualitative methods appropriate to answer questions seeking to understand phenomena about which little is known (Hammell, Carpenter, & Dyck, 2000; Morse & Field, 1995), but they can yield insights about which aspects of a program contribute to successful outcomes (Broughton, 1991). They are also ideal for looking at program outcomes such as quality of life (Patton, 2002). Qualitative methods were therefore most appropriate for this evaluation because the purposes of the study were to investigate program processes that were not well understood (the black box) and to assess program outcomes including quality of life.

Participant Selection

First, recruitment for the Seniors ALIVE program will be described because this provided the sampling frame for the qualitative evaluation. Letters advertising the Seniors ALIVE program were placed under each senior's door and the program coordinator attended regularly scheduled tenant meetings to speak about the program and answer questions. Any senior living in the buildings where the program was offered could attend the program, but only those who registered were considered participants for data collection purposes. This procedure was an ethical consideration to ensure voluntary, informed consent. At the completion of the Seniors ALIVE program, there were 90 seniors participating whose mean age was 76 years (range = 57–94 years). Twenty seniors withdrew before completion of the program; some reasons were declining health and relocation. Although the male:female ratio in the apartment buildings was approximately 25% men and 75% women, only 8% of program participants were men and 92% were women.

At the completion of the Seniors ALIVE program, the 90 participants were asked if they would be willing to be contacted by the researcher doing the qualitative evaluation. All those who agreed (44 out of 90) received a letter explaining the qualitative evaluation, and within a few days were contacted by telephone to ask if they wished to participate. Twenty-six individuals (3 men and 23 women) agreed to participate but 3 of them were reclassified as partial program withdrawers because they had withdrawn from the exercise classes (although they continued to attend the health corners). The final sample of program participants was 23 (2 men and 21 women) with an average age of 76 years and a range of 61 to 90 years.

Seniors who were full participants in the 10-month program were the principal informant group. However, to provide a variety of perspectives, three other small groups were included in the study. Recruitment procedures for these groups were as follows:

1. Program Withdrawers: Letters were sent to the 20 individuals who had withdrawn from the program inviting them to contact the researcher if they wished to participate. Three contacts were made, and 1 individual agreed to be interviewed. The three individuals identified in the participant group who had withdrawn from the exercise classes were included in the withdrawers group for analysis, making a final sample of four program withdrawers (1 man and 3 women) with an average age of 77 years and a range of 74 to 84 years.

2. Program Staff: The 10 program staff working at the end of the program were contacted by phone and invited to attend a focus group. If they did not attend the focus group, they were then asked to participate in individual interviews. Six staff participated; 3 in a focus group and 3 in individual interviews.

3. Family Members of Program Participants: Four family members were recruited from seven names supplied by program participants (one family member could not be contacted, and two declined to participate).

This study was approved by the University of Alberta Health Research Ethics Board. A small thank-you gift, valued under $5.00, was provided as an incentive for all respondents because the success of recruitment was initially uncertain.

Sample Size

A convenience sample was used rather than a probability sample, as is used in quantitative research (Sandelowski, 1995). In this evaluation, all of those recruited by procedures approved by an ethics board were included, and no one in the sampling frame was purposively excluded. In addition, the final sample of seniors and staff represented a broad variety of perspectives including all seven of the program sites and all three of the interventions. Although determining an adequate sample size in qualitative research does not use rigid rules, a general principle is that a sample should be small enough to permit deep analysis and large enough to result in new understanding (Sandelowski, 1995). Because a deep analysis and new understanding were achieved in this evaluation it can be assumed that there was an adequate sample size. In addition, program participants were interviewed to the point of data saturation, meaning that no new findings emerged during the last interviews.

Data Collection and Analysis

Individual semistructured interviews were conducted with 34 participants; 3 program staff participated in a focus group interview. All of the interviews were audio-taped.

Content analysis was used to analyze the data. This method involves reducing a volume of qualitative material and identifying core consistencies and meanings (Patton, 2002). The following steps were used:

1. The interviews were transcribed (9 by a typist and 26 by Rosanne Buijs, who was the qualitative researcher).

2. Each interview was divided into separate units of meaning called "data bits" (Dey, 1993).

3. The data bits were then coded and classified using these main categories: exercise, health corner, newsletter, staff, participant characteristics, and social interactions.

4. Data from each of the four informant groups (program participants, family members of program participants, program withdrawers, and program staff) were analyzed separately.

5. The analysis of each informant group was then compared with that of the other groups.

The strength of this evaluation includes the large number of interviews with program participants and the use of four different informant groups. Also check-coding, described by Miles and Huberman (1994) as a good reliability check, was used on three occasions to verify the coding. Check-coding involved recoding a previously coded interview and then comparing results of the two codings. In addition, four participants and two staff members were contacted for follow up feedback on the analysis. These member checks confirmed the analysis.

One limitation of this qualitative evaluation was the use of an incentive that could have led to biased data, because participants may have wanted to please the interviewer. The number of participants in the staff focus group (i.e., three) was smaller than the ideal number of six to nine (Krueger, 1994). Because this was a convenience sample, findings cannot be generalized to other populations.

RESULTS

The results are reported in two parts. First, the results concerning participation factors and program impacts are briefly outlined. A more detailed discussion is available (Buijs, 2001). Second, the results that contribute directly to an understanding of the black box are reported.

Participation and Impact

The most frequent factors influencing participation reported by participants were perceived benefits, encouragement by others, a positive social program atmosphere, and having fun. Barriers to participation, reported by participants, were other priorities, deteriorating health, and forgetting to come. Some participants stopped attending when there were program changes, such as new times, days, and instructors. These changes occurred because schedules of the program staff, who were also university students, changed with each new university term. Not getting along with particular program participants was given as a reason why other residents in the building did not join. Eighty-five percent of participants demonstrated self-efficacy, because they were confident that they would be able to do the exercises before they attended the first class. The same percentage of program participants reported that they were physically active in their younger years.

Program impacts noted by respondents spanned physical, mental, and social domains (see Figure 18C1–2), including both positive and negative impacts. The most frequently reported impact was "feeling better," expressed by participants as "It [the program] sort of perked my whole self up," or "You feel more alive" and having more "energy." Specific physical impacts described were being more flexible, having increased strength, noting some weight loss, and experiencing less pain. On the other hand, three people who did not continue exercise classes noted more aches after exercising.

Staff members gave examples of mental impacts. One senior who "never came out of his apartment . . . was at each and every health corner" and another senior's "concentration skills were better" after 1 month of participation. Staff said participants "left with smiles on their faces . . . like they felt better about themselves." However,

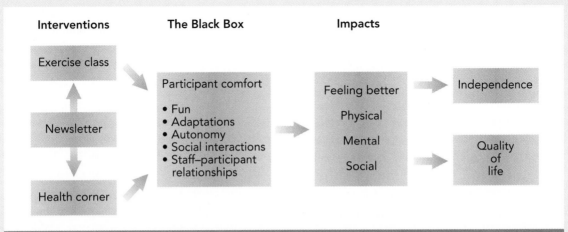

Interventions   **The Black Box**   **Impacts**

Exercise class

Participant comfort

- Fun
- Adaptations
- Autonomy
- Social interactions
- Staff–participant relationships

Feeling better

Physical

Mental

Social

Independence

Quality of life

Newsletter

Health corner

Figure 18C1–2 How the Seniors ALIVE program worked

termination of the experimental program was upsetting for some participants. One staff explained "they thought I would always come there . . . they never could really understand."

There were also positive and negative social interactions. For example the program "just seemed to bring people out of their shell." The health corners were "a very social time." On the other hand, there was one example of two participants whose relationship deteriorated because of an interaction that happened during the program. Staff noted "little cliques" and commented that sometimes "familiarity breeds contempt."

The Black Box

An overwhelming majority of participants and staff expressed enthusiastic support for this program. Participants ranked the three program components in the following order of preference: exercise classes, the health corners, and the newsletters. Five key program processes that linked program interventions and impacts were having fun, adapting program delivery, providing opportunities for autonomy, encouraging social interaction, and developing meaningful staff–participant relationships. Together these processes contributed to participant "comfort" in the program. Figure 18C1–2 illustrates the relation of the five key processes of the black box to the interventions and program impacts.

Fun.   Both staff and participants talked about enjoyment and fun in the program. One staff member said, "I'd say why did you come and they'd say, 'cause we heard it was fun.'" Participants said "this program . . . was a fun time" and "there was a lot of enjoyment with [the program]."

Program Delivery Adaptations.   The ability of the program staff to be adaptable was an important element of the program. For example, one of the staff members recounted the time one of the participants died between one class and the next. She said, "we didn't [do all the exercises] because there was talk because someone died." The encouragement of individual exercise adaptations also demonstrated this theme of adaptability in program delivery. One participant remarked that "I couldn't hold [the weights] this way . . . so [the exercise leader] would let me reverse my hand to do it this way." In the health corners, this adaptation was seen by the willingness of the nurses to occasionally go to the seniors' apartments for a "home visit" when the seniors could not come to the nurse.

Autonomy.   Autonomy, the freedom to act and to make independent choices, was encouraged in the Seniors ALIVE Program. Seniors were not pressured to join or stay in the program. Informed consents were signed by all seniors participating in the program. Seniors exercised autonomy when they chose which classes to attend and when they chose the amount and type of participation in each class.

Social Interactions.   The importance of the social aspects of the program was described by staff, participants, and family members. The program was compared to an "ice- breaker for [participants] to get to know each other," leading to increases in the amount and depth of social interactions. Seniors developed friendships during the program. For example, one staff member said, "people would come by themselves at first . . . then I'd see the same two ladies . . . come together and it seemed like they became friends." Over time several staff noticed that the seniors became more open with them and shared more of their problems. Attending the Seniors ALIVE Program was a social event that participants eagerly anticipated. A participant noted, "we always sort of looked forward to [the program] . . . . We'd have our chit chat . . . you got to know the other ones on a first name basis." One family member reported that her relative told her, "I was bored . . . [but with the program] I don't feel bored."

Staff–Participant Relationships.   Staff interacted with the participants in a caring and empathetic way by adjusting the program to fit participant needs in various ways. For example, one of the exercise leaders would arrive 1/2 hr early for class so she would have a chance to interact with the seniors before her class. Another staff member conveyed information to a participant outside of regular program hours. Staff made occasional "home visits" in special circumstances.

Program staff listened to the seniors and noted this was an important part of their job. As one staff remarked, "You can never be too busy . . . because what they [seniors] have to say is important." One participant said that the health corner nurse was such a good listener she felt she could have told the nurse her "whole life's history."

Participants were very positive about program staff. Some of the participants mentioned a particular staff member by name despite the fact that most seniors had difficulty remembering specific details of the program. For example, one senior, who had forgotten receiving the newsletters, remembered the name of the health corner nurse and there was a softness that came into her voice as she spoke her name.

Mutual gift giving at the termination of the program demonstrated that these bonds were mutual and reciprocal. One staff member described herself as being both a "teacher" and a "student" of the seniors. Staff relationships with seniors were described as being like that of a "granddaughter."

Comfort.   Both staff and one program participant's family member talked about the program being "comfortable" for the seniors. For example, one exercise instructor said, "If they felt comfortable, they came." A family member noted that "[the participants] felt safe there and asking questions was comfortable for them." Although seniors did not directly talk about comfort themselves, it was assumed that they experienced a significant level of comfort because of the pleasure and fun they experienced during the Seniors ALIVE program.

DISCUSSION

Program Impacts

This study provided evidence that the goals of the Seniors ALIVE program to promote independence and quality of life were achieved (see Figure 18C1–2). Independence was influenced in two ways: First, the program supported seniors' independence by encouraging them to choose the extent of their own participation (i.e., working at their own pace); second, some specific program impacts (i.e., becoming more physically flexible) directly contributed to participants' ability to perform activities of daily living (such as vacuuming). The majority of program impacts resulted in participants generally "feeling better" and hence contributed to improving their quality of life (i.e., overall life satisfaction).

Application to Pender's Revised Health Promotion Model

Overall, the findings support the variables of Pender's Revised Health Promotion Model. For example, 85% of program participants had the prior related behavior of being physically active in their younger years. Perceived benefits were the most frequent reason given for participation. Reasons given for missing classes or withdrawing could all be classified as perceived barriers. Perceived self-efficacy or the estimated confidence in their ability to perform a health behavior was evident because 85% of participants had no concerns about their ability to do the exercises before they attended the first class. Activity-related affect included having fun and the positive or negative feelings associated with other participants and staff of the program.

Social contact with other participants and staff contributed to social support, which is one of the determinants of health (Federal, Provincial and Territorial Advisory Committee on Population Health, 1994) and also plays an important role in the development and maintenance of active living (Frankish, Milligan, & Reid, 1998). In addition, this social contact contributed to Pender's (1996) variable of interpersonal influences. Because the program was offered in their apartment buildings, at least some participants came to the program already knowing other participants. Although the majority of these interpersonal relationships were positive, some were negative. Liking or not liking other participants or staff were both given as reasons for attending or not attending the program. Awareness of these existing relationships was an important factor in understanding the best way to facilitate program delivery in each building. For example, where the relationships are positive, staff encouragement of participant–participant interactions would be appropriate and likely enhance social support. On the other hand, when the relationships were negative such encouragement would not be appropriate and arranging seating to accommodate personal likes and dislikes would be particularly important.

The social contact in the program gave participants opportunities to deepen existing relationships and establish new relationships with other participants. One long-term impact of the program was the change in the participants' social relationships, which continued even after the completion of the program. It is important to consider this program impact when evaluating programs offered in places where seniors live in a common location.

Strong and meaningful relationships developed between staff and participants. These relationships were enhanced by the readiness and ability of staff to listen to the seniors, to encourage autonomy and to adapt program delivery. The literature supports providing as many opportunities for autonomy as possible, because personal control is one of the indicators of successful aging and helps to maintain quality of life as individuals age (Baltes, 1994). A personal sense of control is also highly correlated with good mental health (Zautra, Reich, & Newsom, 1995).

The increasing openness of seniors with staff over time suggests that staff–participant relationships became stronger and more meaningful as the program progressed. If this is true, it follows that the full implementation of a program will not be realized until these relationships are fully developed. As Downie, Tannahill, and Tannahill (1997) pointed out, a health promotion program cannot be expected to be fully effective if it is not fully implemented. Hence, program evaluations should carefully describe the length and quality of staff–participant relationships because this will affect the validity of the evaluation.

Environments in which individuals feel compatible, connected, and safe are one of the situational influences thought to influence health promoting behavior in Pender's (1996) Revised Health Promotion Model. *Comfort* was the term used by staff and family members to describe this optimal environment in the Seniors ALIVE program. Program staff were an essential ingredient of the "comfortable" environment. Staff used their judgment and skill to balance the needs of the program with the needs of individual participants. The more effectively staff can balance these needs, the more likely seniors will feel "comfortable" in the program.

Nursing Implications

The Seniors ALIVE program was developed, implemented, and evaluated by a multidisciplinary team of health professionals including leadership contributions by nurses. In addition to implementing a beneficial health promotion program that extended beyond the discipline of nursing, the multidisciplinary approach benefitted faculty and program staff who learned to appreciate the expertise of the other disciplines through their shared experience. Nurses should be encouraged to seek opportunities for multidisciplinary collaboration because it has the potential to be beneficial for nurses, their colleagues, and seniors.

The findings of this study indicate that participants experienced many benefits from program involvement, including an increase in independence and quality of life. An important nursing intervention was to motivate and encourage seniors to attend the programs so that they could experience the benefits. Pender's (1996) model can be used as a framework to encourage participation in health promotion activities. For example, in the Seniors ALIVE program, the initial advertising letter, the regular newsletters, and the information presented by the program coordinator at resident meetings were designed to maximize the perception of the benefits of participation. In addition, the program addressed several participation barriers previously identified in the literature (Connell, Davies, Rosenberg, & Fisher, 1988) by being offered in the day time, at no cost, in a familiar location requiring no transportation. Staff encouraged hesitant seniors to observe an exercise class before they participated, thus providing an opportunity to estimate their ability to do the exercises (self-efficacy) in relation to an actual class. The fun, program flexibility, encouragement of positive social interactions, and development of positive staff–participant relationships all had positive impacts on activity-related affect. Together these elements contributed to a comfortable environment that was a positive situational influence.

Seniors' communal residences are ideal locations for community nurses to implement health promotion programs. Transportation is a participation barrier for some seniors. The provision of a program in the seniors' residence eliminated this barrier. In addition, using their residence as the location for the program provided opportunities to build social relationships in the buildings, which in most cases were beneficial.

The use of more than one intervention in the program was beneficial because each one addressed different needs. At times, seniors stopped attending the exercise classes when their health declined, but they were still able to attend the health corners. The newsletter disseminated health information and also supported the other two interventions by encouraging continued participation. Providing several linked interventions has the potential to meet the needs of more seniors and hence to increase the numbers participating in health promoting activities.

Having staff who are capable of delivering adaptable programs is an especially important consideration when working with seniors. Because aging occurs at different rates it is very unlikely that "one program will fit all." The ability to adapt a program means that the individual needs of more seniors can be met. Carefully choosing and providing adequate training for program staff will ensure optimal program delivery.

This program focused on one target population. Are the program processes found to be important in this program of similar importance for other age groups? Another area for future research is an exploration of gender differences in program participation in that very few men participated in this program. Because staff were so important in program delivery, the question of how a health promotion program led by peers would perform, is also of interest.

REFERENCES

Arnold, S., Kane, R. L., & Kane, R. A. (1986). Health promotion and the elderly: Evaluating the research. In K. Dychtwald (Ed.), *Wellness and health promotion for the elderly* (pp. 326–344). Rockville, MD: Aspen.

Baltes, M. (1994). Aging well and institutional living: A paradox? In R. Abeles, H. Gift, & M. Ory (Eds.), *Aging and quality of life* (pp. 185–201). New York: Springer.

Bernard, M. (2000). *Promoting health in old age.* Buckingham, England: Open University Press.

Broughton, W. (1991). Qualitative methods in program evaluation. *American Journal of Health Promotion, 5*, 461–465.

Buijs, R. (2001). *A qualitative evaluation of the Seniors ALIVE Program.* Unpublished master's thesis, University of Alberta, Edmonton, Canada.

Connell, C., Davies, R., Rosenberg, A., & Fisher, E. (1988). Retiree's perceived incentives and barriers to participation in health promotion activities. *Health Education Research, 3*, 325–330.

Dey, I. (1993). *Qualitative data analysis.* London: Routledge.

Downie, R. S., Tannahill, C., & Tannahill, A. (1997). *Health promotion: Models and values.* Oxford, England: Oxford University Press.

Federal, Provincial and Tenitorial Advisory Committee on Population Health. (1994). *Strategies for population health.* Ottawa, Canada: Health Canada.

Fiatarone, M. (1996). *Fit for your life exercise program.* Boston: Hebrew Rehabilitation Center.

Frankish, C. J., Milligan, C. D., & Reid, C. (1998). A review of relationships between active living and determinants of health. *Social Science and Medicine, 47*, 287–301.

Gatz, M. (1995). Questions that aging puts to preventionists. In L. Bond, S. Cutler, & A. Grams (Eds.), *Promoting successful and productive aging* (pp. 36–50). Thousand Oaks, CA: Sage.

Haber, D. (1999). *Health promotion and aging.* New York: Springer.

Hammell, K., Carpenter, C., & Dyck., I. (Eds.). (2000). *Using qualitative research: A practical introduction for occupational and physical therapists.* New York: Churchill Livingstone.

Heidrich, S. M. (1998). Health promotion in old age. *Annual Review of Nursing Research, 16*, 173–195.

Krueger, R. (1994). *Focus groups: A practical guide for applied research.* Thousand Oaks, CA: Sage.

Miles, M., & Huberman, A. (1994). *Qualitative data analysis.* Thousand Oaks, CA: Sage.

Morse, J., & Field, P. (1995). *Qualitative research methods for health professionals.* Thousand Oaks, CA: Sage.

Patton, M. Q. (2002). *Qualitative research and evaluation methods.* Thousand Oaks, CA: Sage.

Pearson, T., Lewis, S., Wall, S., Jenkins, P., Nafziger, A., & Weinehall, L. (2001). Dissecting the "black box" of community intervention: Background and rationale. *Scandinavian Journal of Public Health, 29*(56), 5–12

Pender, N. J. (1996). *Health promotion in nursing practice.* Stanford, CT: Appleton & Lange.

Penning, M., & Chappell, N. (1993). Age-related differences. In T. Stephens & D. Fowler Graham (Eds.), *Canada's health promotion survey 1990: Technical report* (pp. 247–255). Ottawa, Canada: Minister of Supply & Services Canada.

Rakowski, W. (1986). Research issues in health promotion: Programs for the elderly. In K. Dychtwald (Ed.), *Wellness and health promotion for the elderly* (pp. 313–326). Rockville, MD: Aspen.

Sandelowski, M. (1995). Focus on qualitative methods: Sample size in qualitative research. *Research in Nursing & Health, 18*, 179–183.

Schuster, C. (1995). Have we forgotten the older adults? An argument in support of more health promotion programs for and research directed toward people 65 years and older. *Journal of Health Education, 26*, 338–344.

Swanson, J., & Chapman. L. (1994). Inside the black box: Theoretical and methodological issues in conducting evaluation research: Using a qualitative approach. In J. M. Morse (Ed.), *Critical issues in qualitative research methods* (pp. 66–93). Thousand Oaks, CA: Sage.

Williams, T. F. (1994). Rehabilitation in old age. In R. Abeles, H. Gift, & M. Ory (Eds.), *Aging and quality of life* (pp. 121–132). New York: Springer.

Zautra, A., Reich, J., & Newsom, J. (1995). Autonomy and sense of control among older adults: An examination of their effects on mental health. In L. Bond, S. Cutler, & A. Grams (Eds.), *Promoting successful and productive aging* (pp. 153–170). Thousand Oaks, CA: Sage.

INTRODUCTION TO CRITIQUE #1

The article "Promoting Participation: Evaluation of a Health Promotion Program for Low Income Seniors" (Buijs, Ross-Kerr, Cousins, & Wilson, 2003), an example of program evaluation, uses qualitative methodology. Although this study does not align itself with a specific qualitative research tradition, it is useful as a model to explore the methodology associated with qualitative research. The article is critiqued to determine the quality, rigour, and usefulness of the research as a model. The criteria for critique #1 are identified in Box 18–1.

Statement of the Phenomenon of Interest

The purpose of the article was to evaluate the health promotion program Seniors Active Living in Vulnerable Elders (ALIVE), which was clearly articulated in the title, abstract, and study purpose. Developed by a multidisciplinary team, the project was a three-phase study to promote independent living and to improve the quality of life for seniors. The target population was seniors with a low income. The rationale behind the selection of low-income seniors was not included.

The first phase collected data on the health status, attitudes, and health practices of low-income seniors. Based on the findings, a health promotion program was developed and delivered in a pilot study with 35 participants in the second phase. The third phase included a randomized controlled trial of the health promotion program with two evaluations, one qualitative and one quantitative.

The authors indicated that their work is important because programs such as ALIVE can improve health, and evaluation of such programs is necessary to measure the actual program impact.

Purpose

The purpose of the study was to determine the impact of the Seniors ALIVE program and to understand the how and the why of the research process. The intermediary steps between interventions and outcomes, the how and the why, are referred to in the black box (see Figure 18C1–1). The authors described the purpose of the article in addition to the research questions. Although both are clearly stated, the reader may be confused because the purpose and research questions do not correlate. For example, one of the purposes was to discuss Pender's health promotion model in relation to the findings; however, this purpose was not part of the original research questions. Moreover, the original purpose did not include the recommendation of strategies for encouraging participation in health promotion programs. However, the reporting of strategies that emerge from the research is typical of qualitative research, which chronicles unintended outcomes.

Method

In the methods section, the authors stated that qualitative methods are ideal to assess program outcomes, particularly when the research processes are not well understood. Although many researchers align themselves with a specific epistemological perspective, these researchers did not. The lack of an epistemological perspective is acceptable because, as Patton (2002) stated, "the methods of qualitative inquiry now stand on their own as a reasonable way to find out what is happening in programs and other human settings" (p. 137). Patton (2002) also supported the notion that qualitative methods can answer questions related to program evaluation and development.

Both quantitative and qualitative methods were used to evaluate the ALIVE program; however, the authors did not refer to the quantitative methods. Although the purpose of this article was to report the qualitative findings, the reader would have benefited from a brief overview of both the quantitative and the qualitative aspects of the research to achieve a more holistic understanding of the study.

Sampling

Convenience sampling was used because participants volunteered to be studied. To provide several perspectives, four groups were included in the study. The primary informant group was the program participants. Ninety seniors completed the ALIVE program, with 23 agreeing to participate in the evaluation component. To gather data from seniors who were potentially dissatisfied with the program, all people who had withdrawn were invited to participate; of those, four people agreed. Inclusion of the withdrawn participants is important because their perspectives may have been very different from those who completed the program. Program staff and family members were also interviewed. Three of the staff members participated in a focus group rather than individual interviews. Informed consents were obtained. Interviews were conducted until the data were saturated (i.e., no new data emerged).

The researchers indicated that the number of participants allowed for a broad base of perspectives, yet the numbers were small enough for deep analysis. For a qualitative study, 34 participants is at the larger end of the continuum. Concern about large sample sizes (generally over 50) in qualitative research is related to the expectation that in-depth, detailed analysis will be difficult (Sandelowski, 1995). However, in this study, the size of the sample should not be considered too large since the phenomenon studied is very specific, allowing for thorough analysis.

Data Collection

Data were collected primarily through semi-structured interviews, which were audiotaped. Little information was shared regarding who interviewed the participants, how many interviews were conducted, and the length of each interview. Moreover, the authors did not include samples of the questions. Readers would appreciate a more comprehensive description of the data collection; however, the authors may have had to cull details in this area

to produce a manuscript within the page allowance established by the journal publisher.

Data Analysis

The authors were careful to provide a detailed, step-by-step explanation of the data analysis, which provided a clear description of the process. They identified the method of content analysis, which was used to reduce the large volume of data from the sample to identify the core meanings. Variables, such as social support and commitment, from Pender's revised health promotion model were used to interpret the data. The analysis supported the study design and the research questions. The limitations of the analysis were described, and the reader was discouraged from generalizing the findings to other populations, as is appropriate to qualitative research. However, the authors discussed the strengths of using different informant groups and their validation lent reliability to the data. Additionally, seeking convergence from different perspectives (informant groups) is a form of triangulation that can lend credibility to a study (Carnevale, 2002). To increase reliability, coding was verified, and six participants confirmed the analysis. Member checking to verify the results is an important step in establishing the study's credibility.

Findings

The authors were clear and comprehensive in reporting the findings separately in response to the research questions. To provide authenticity to the findings, a series of quotations were provided from the participants, allowing the voices of the seniors to be heard. The discussion of the findings was limited because a more detailed report is available in the first author's thesis (Buijs, 2001). The most frequent factors affecting participation were listed in the findings, and barriers were identified. The impacts of the program were also listed in Figure 18C1–2. Based on the findings, modifications to the original model (see Figure 18C1–1) were suggested by the literature review; consequently, the authors redrew the relationships between the interventions, the process (the black box), and the impact as protrayed in Figure 18C1–2. The findings were related to the literature review and what is known about health promotion programs.

Conclusions, Implications, and Recommendations

The authors discussed the program's impact and application to Pender's Health Promotion Model and concluded that the essential ingredient of the Seniors ALIVE program is comfort—the optimal environment for participation and health promotion. The authors concluded that the participants experienced many benefits, such as independence and improved quality of life, and that Pender's model could be used as a framework to encourage independence. Although specific recommendations were made, the concept of comfort was not discussed explicitly in the section on nursing implications. Some suggestions for future research were offered; however, limitations were not discussed, making it difficult to determine the generalizability of the findings.

Overall, the study was well written and is easily accessible to readers. The findings are significant to nurses involved in community-based health promotion programs and to health practitioners interested in improving the quality of life for seniors. The study is also a good example of research conducted by a multidisciplinary team, in this case, with representation from nursing, physical education, and public health services.

CRITIQUE #2 The study "Women's Health in Northern British Columbia: The Role of Geography and Gender" by Beverly D. Leipert and Linda Reutter, published in the *Canadian Journal of Rural Medicine* (2005), is critiqued. The article is presented in its entirety and is followed by the critique on pages 419–422. (From *Canadian Journal of Rural Medicine*, *10*(4), 241–253. © 2005 Society of Rural Physicians of Canada.)

WOMEN'S HEALTH IN NORTHERN BRITISH COLUMBIA: THE ROLE OF GEOGRAPHY AND GENDER

Beverly D. Leipert, PhD, RN
Chair, Rural Women's Health Research
Associate Professor, Faculty of Health Sciences and Faculty of
   Medicine and Dentistry
University of Western Ontario
London, Ontario

Linda Reutter, PhD, RN
Professor, Faculty of Nursing
University of Alberta
Edmonton, Alberta

INTRODUCTION

Various factors and conditions, labelled determinants of health, and the complex interactions among these determinants are now known to have a profound effect on health.[1] Determinants of health include income and social status, social support networks, education, employment and working conditions, social environments, physical environments, biology and genetic endowment, personal health practices and coping skills, healthy child development, health services, gender, and culture.[1] In this paper we discuss how geographic location affects women's health in a northern Canadian setting, with emphasis on the determinants of physical and social environments and gender.

The physical environment includes factors in the natural environment such as air and water quality, geography and distance, as well as factors in the human-made environment such as community and road design, and housing and workplace safety.[1] Reports about the effects of the physical environment on health in northern Canada[2,3] tend to focus on the natural environment with minimal attention to the human-made environment. There is limited knowledge on how the natural and human-made environments influence the health of women.

Social environments include societal norms and values, social stability, diversity, safety, good working relationships and cohesive communities.[1] Social factors such as low availability of emotional support, low social participation, and social exclusion limit life prospects, supportive networks, life chances and self-esteem; these factors prove damaging at all societal levels, from the individual through to the community.[1,4] Little is known about the nature of social environments in northern settings and the effects of these environments on women's health.

Gender is a social construct based more in human culture than in biological difference.[1] Gender affects health through the "array of socially determined roles, personality traits, attitudes, behaviours, values, relative power and influence that society ascribes to the two sexes on a differential basis" (p. 17).[1] Although minimal research has focused on the health of women in isolated settings, research that exists indicates that these settings create challenges for women's health. Health services provided by family physicians, public health nurses, and specialist services such as obstetricians either do not exist, are intermittent, or are limited in range and quality.[3,5,6] Issues of confidentiality and anonymity exist when women seek care in small communities, and lack of transportation to care elsewhere exacerbates access problems. The values and priorities of male physicians, the dominant care providers in small communities, often influence the practices of female physicians, nurses and other health care providers, thus compromising women's access to the type of care and provider they desire.[6] Because traditional roles of wife and mother are favoured in small communities, education and career opportunities for women are limited.[7–10] In addition, small communities have limited employment opportunities and access to high paying positions in the resource-based industries are largely denied women.[11] Although northern women may obtain employment, employment is often not permanent, respected, adequately remunerated, or is not work in which they can take pride.[12] These challenges not only limit women's health, they also compromise women's life chances.

Research indicates that understanding the contexts of women's lives is crucial to the advancement of women's health.[13–15] While studies employing quantitative research methods identify some aspects of northern women's health, in-depth qualitative understanding of the effects that a northern place has on women's health is needed. The study on which this paper is based used a qualitative research design to examine how women perceive and maintain their health within northern British Columbia (BC), Canada. This study seeks to enrich understanding of the northern social environment so that social support, which is key to northern women's health,[13] can be advanced. This paper describes one aspect of the study, namely factors in the northern context that influence women's health. Findings of the study that describe how women address factors to maintain their health in northern BC are reported elsewhere.[13]

METHODS

This study was conducted in northern BC, where most communities depend upon a single resource-based industry such as forestry, mining or fishing. The largest city in northern BC, Prince George, has a population of 80 000; however, most communities are much smaller—some contain fewer than 15 residents—and are typically remote from each other and from larger centres. Many people in northern BC live on isolated farms and ranches.

The study was conducted using a feminist grounded theory method. Feminist grounded theory seeks to generate a theory that explains how a central problem for women is resolved or processed.[16,17] The feminist grounded theory research process attends to tenets of feminist research such as respect for participants, avoidance of oppression and usefulness of findings. In addition, feminist inquiry considers not only women's individual voices and experiences, but also larger sociopolitical, economic, and cultural structures that influence women's lives.[18]

Ethical approval for the study was obtained from the University of Alberta and the University of Northern British Columbia. Women were recruited from 2 health regions in northern BC. Inclusion criteria were: able to read and write English, over 20 years of age, and have lived in northern settings for a minimum of 2 years. To reach women in remote areas, recruitment strategies included radio and television interviews about the research, publishing recruitment information in community newspapers and posting study information in feed and tack stores, grocery stores, and clothing shops in small communities. Recruitment information included the purpose of the study (identifying how living in the north influences women's health), the inclusion criteria and the study procedures. Recruitment efforts were very successful; over 100 women from throughout the 2 northern health regions telephoned, emailed or applied in person for the research.

In compliance with the feminist grounded theory method,[16,17] the final sample of 25 women was selected using purposeful and theoretical sampling. Initially, women were selected to represent diverse geographical locations (cities, towns, villages, ranches, farms), ages and cultural backgrounds. In theoretical sampling, study participants are selected throughout the course of the research for their ability to enrich and enlarge upon themes and codes emerging from the ongoing analysis. Theoretical sampling also ensures that participants will provide contradictory as well as confirmatory evidence.[19] The recommended sample size for a grounded theory study is approximately 30 to 50 interview instances.[20] In this study, 75 interview instances were included (25 women, each interviewed 3 times).

First and second interviews were 1.5–2 hours in length and were tape recorded. Third interviews, which were about a half hour, were not tape recorded, but comments were noted and incorporated in the analysis. First interviews occurred in the women's homes and work places. Due to weather, distance and time constraints, three-quarters of the second interviews and all third interviews were conducted by telephone.

In first and second interviews, women were asked open-ended questions about how they maintained their health, how the northern context influenced their health, and how northern BC could be healthier for women. After each interview, each participant was provided with a summary of the analysis of her interview and invited to comment in a subsequent interview on the accuracy and completeness of the analysis and on emerging categories and relationships. These comments were incorporated into the data and analysis of the study. Third interviews provided each participant with an opportunity for final commentary on the emerging theory.

In addition to interviews, observations about geographical terrain, distance, road conditions and isolation were collected during travels to farms, ranches and small northern communities. Written documents such as maps, tourist guides, locally produced histories, newspapers and northern poetry enriched understanding of northern history, culture, and social and physical environments.

Data were analyzed using the constant comparative method of grounded theory.[16,19] Data analysis in grounded theory research occurs concurrently with data collection.[16,19] Each interview tape was transcribed verbatim and then reviewed while listening to the tape to determine accuracy and to facilitate analytical thinking. With the assistance of the NVivo computer program, transcripts were then reviewed line by line and coded for categories. NVivo is designed for qualitative researchers who need to combine subtle coding with qualitative linking, shaping, searching and modelling. It is ideal for those working with complex data and for deep levels of analysis. Emerging categories were constantly compared to determine their nature and significance and their relationships to each other.[19] Second and third interview questions clarified, elaborated and verified emerging categories, subcategories and relationships. Consistent with the grounded theory method, data from the literature relevant to emerging categories and relationships also informed the analysis. Data collection and analysis ceased when no new information or insight was forthcoming about the categories and their relationships, and when the theory seemed to be elaborated in complexity and clear in its articulation of the central problem and the process used to address it.[19]

RESULTS

The findings of this research revealed that northern women develop a process of resilience to address the central problem of vulnerability to health risks.[13] This vulnerability was influenced by the northern context and women's marginalization within that context. In this paper, we discuss findings regarding the northern context and effects of this context on women's health.

The Sample

The final sample consisted of 25 women of diverse backgrounds (Table 18C2–1). The majority of women were 20–60 years of age, had post high school education, were married or living common-law, employed full-time or part-time, in good health and of relatively adequate financial status. They

TABLE 18C2–1	Sociodemographic Information on the 25 Study Participants
Variable	No. of Participants
Age	
20–30	2
31–40	5
41–50	6
51–60	7
61–70	2
71–80	2
81–90	1
Education	
<Grade 9	2
Grade 9–13	8
Trade/Technical diploma	8
University undergraduate degree	6
University graduate degree	1
Marital status	
Married or common-law	14
Divorced / Separated	5
Widowed	2
Never married	4
Employment	
Currently employed	
Full-time	10
Part-time	7
Not employed outside the home	3
Retired	5
Rating of health	
Good	16
Fair	8
Poor	1
Annual household income, $	
<10 000	2
11 000–20 000	6
21 000–30 000	1
31 000–40 000	5
41 000–50 000	2
51 000–60 000	4
61 000–70 000	1
71 000–80 000	2
>80 000	2

represented various geographical locations including cities, towns, villages, a community with under 20 residents, ranches and farms. Culturally, one woman was Métis, one woman was First Nations, 2 were of Asian background, 3 were of European background, and the remaining 18 participants claimed Canadian Caucasian heritage. Each woman selected a pseudonym and these pseudonyms are used throughout this article when referring to study participants.

The Northern Context

The importance of the northern context to women's health can be attributed to the north's historical location, and its physical, sociocultural and political environments.

Historical Location

Because of the severe climate, social isolation and relative absence of material resources, indigenous peoples and early settlers needed to be self-reliant, hard working, and able to live off the land.[21] These attributes survive in the north today. Casey, a ranch woman in the study, noted that women are still expected to carry on the tradition of living off the land by having large gardens and canning and preserving food. Other historical elements include a heritage of control of the north by outsiders, impoverishment of indigenous populations, emphasis on rapid, profit-oriented resource development and exploitation, and limited ability of local northern residents to control their destinies.[21] Fluctuations in the economy, globalization of markets and the political view of northern settings as primarily locations for resource extraction have created and perpetuate northern communities of insecurity and transience.

Because of resource-based employment opportunities, northern regions have been comprised largely of relatively younger populations who come north in search of work. When resource-based economies fluctuate and jobs are lost, young people move elsewhere in search of employment.

Consequences of this demographic shift include inconsistency and decline in the quantity, quality and nature of goods and services in northern communities, and instability, insecurity and the under-resourcing of northern communities.

The Physical Environment

Climate, distance and geography, pollution, and dependence upon resource-based employment were noted by women in the study as problematic. Long periods of cold weather exacerbate physical problems such as arthritis and make getting around difficult, especially for elderly women and women with physical disabilities. Christine, a woman who had lived 23 years in the north, noted that winter weather results in being "housebound . . . more depression and anxiety." Several women noted that the long, cold, dark winter season also contributes to the depressive condition termed seasonal affective disorder. Leah, a young northern woman, stated, "Winter is so damn depressing here. Seasonal affective disorder syndrome—half the town has it." Gill[8] noted that, especially in February, the incidence of mental disorders (known as 'cabin fever' or 'housewife psychosis') among northern women reaches its peak. Travelling in the north is time consuming, expensive and hazardous. Long distances, poor road conditions and large logging trucks make travel dangerous, especially in winter. Barbara summed up many northern women's perspectives when she stated: "I'm really stranded here for 6 months of the year. It's my own fear of driving on winter roads."

For some women, though, the physical environment provided accessible and affordable opportunities for outdoor recreation, such as skating, hiking and swimming. These activities were valued if women had good physical and mental health, and the time and finances to participate. Women who enjoyed solitary activities could better cope with the isolation engendered by northern distance and winter weather.

Women in this study were concerned about pollution in northern environments caused by resource-based industries such as pulp mills. Jocelyn lived near a pulp mill town and perceived that "a mill town is not the healthiest place to live," and Mary observed that "living here in Prince George is the only time I've had asthma . . . . I really feel that it has to do with the pollution due to the pulp mills." Still, women may be reluctant to complain too loudly about the pollution because it is the resource-based industries that provide jobs and income for their families.

Although the north provides resource-based employment, the precarious nature of the employment due to decline in resources and international influences can result in unstable communities, decline in the diversity and quality of good and services, and threats to community security and sustainability. Casey, a ranch woman, noted that, as a result of a mine closure, "the population has gone down . . . . The elementary school may close. The fall fair's no longer held." Diminishing employment within the north and consequent seeking of jobs outside of the north weaken the community because fewer people are available to sustain it. This affects women's quality of life, as women often assume—or are designated—the responsibility to deal with contexts of diminishing goods and services.

The Sociocultural Environment

Overfamiliarity, outsider status and lack of resources were the primary negative sociocultural factors noted by women in the study.

In spite of—or perhaps because of—the vast distances between people and communities, over-familiarity can lead to lack of anonymity and compromised confidentiality. Over-familiarity occurs when people in small isolated communities become visible and identifiable, with the result that unduly intimate and personal liberties may be taken and presumptions made.[22] Park explained how being known can interfere with women's abilities to access services:

> *If somebody's car was parked at the women's centre . . . people kind of assume that she's gone there to get help . . . . When you're going to see a counsellor, you may be seeing*

her in other social functions as well . . . so women probably feel their confidentiality is at stake . . . . In bigger cities, nobody knows where you're going for help.

Being an outsider in a community can also be a problem for women in small northern communities. An outsider is someone who is different from the dominant community culture and characteristics, and is unconnected to family or other personal ties in the community.[23] Outsiders tend to experience less inclusion and more exclusion. Conversely, an insider is someone who has been a long time resident of a community and who is intimate with the community's norms and assumptions.[24] Insiders are included and valued.

Outsider status is created in several ways in northern communities. Outsider women who are new to the community or who have identities, associations and experiences that are seen to be somehow different may be deemed outsiders. Christine, a woman who moved to the north from elsewhere, explained how being new and unfamiliar may act to create outsider status:

. . . when you first move up here . . . you don't have the network of people that you may have had . . . . You have to develop that and it takes time. Small communities may be very friendly once you get into them, but they can be very cold as well . . . . Possibly they want you to prove yourself.

Women who return to a community after leaving may also find that they have become outsiders because they now subscribe to different norms and values. Outsider women experience more limited employment opportunities, social isolation and marginalization than women who are perceived as insiders.

Insider status can be achieved in several ways. Casey, originally an 'outsider' woman, suggested that marrying an 'insider' man can facilitate inclusion:

My father-in-law was very highly regarded in the community. I took my husband's surname when we married . . . that was

definitely an in. And I think it expedited my acceptance into the community.

Rose, a woman who moved to the north and has lived there for many years, pointed out that becoming an insider requires an initial acceptance of community norms and political awareness:

You have to prove yourself as being acceptable. You have to meet the principles of the community. You have to not be intrusive, you have to take people as they are, and know where the hierarchy is in a bigger community, the political base of the community. You have to be willing to respect their attitude, even if you don't agree with it. There's got to be that acceptance period. Once you're accepted, you're family.

For some women, achieving insider status is problematic. Mary, an Aboriginal human services worker, described several instances where her children or clients "had to try to defend themselves against people who are not of the same race as them." Ruhi, a young South Asian woman who had recently immigrated to Canada, noted that new immigrants may be pressured by their cultural community to minimize their culture and conform to the Canadian way of life. Women who do not subscribe to insider behaviours such as becoming married and having children are likely to have more problems achieving insider status in the north. Elizabeth, Casey, Leah and Marie, women who were single or child free, noted how the "couples and child oriented" nature of their communities affected their mental health. Elizabeth stated: "As a single person, you never quite fit in." Casey noted that since she and her husband now have their niece living with them and so 'have a child,' she feels more included in community events than when she did not have a child.

The northern sociocultural environment was less problematic for women who had adequate finances, time, good health and interests that coincided with those in the north. Women with adequate finances could purchase resources within and outside the north, women with adequate time could travel to resources, women with good health did not need resources that could not be accessed in the north, and women who enjoyed the north or who did not realize the potential of resources such as enhanced cultural amenities did not expect or miss these in the north.

The Political Environment

The political environment in the north can be characterized by 2 elements: undervaluing of the north and undervaluing of women. Undervaluing had profound effects on northern women's health.

Undervaluing of the north is reflected in misunderstanding, exploitation, lack of commitment and lack of political power and support. Misunderstanding results from minimal contact between southern and northern residents. Southerners rarely travel north, thus "they think we're still mukluks and sleighs, and sled dogs. They figure Prince George is a little one-horse town where the horse died" (Signe).

Undervaluing of the north is also evident in the exploitation of northern natural resources and the inequities that exist between northern and southern locations. As Christine noted: "We northerners don't get our share of resources. We provide all sorts of stuff for the province but we don't get back in return." Several women identified a lack of commitment to the north by human services professionals as an important manifestation of undervaluing. Health care professionals come to the north for various reasons: because jobs are available, to obtain professional experience, and for more generously remunerated employment.[25,26] However, they may have little intention of staying in the north. Unhappy and uncommitted care providers compromise women's health. As women in the study explained: "Some of the people hate it here. And when you don't like where you are, you don't do a good job" (Christine). Jocelyn noted: "I have never gone to the same doctor twice . . . . it seems that every time I see a doctor, I have to start over." Thus, northern women and northern communities often benefit very little

or not at all from the rich experience gained by workers in their communities. This type of situation, where the north is undervalued by workers, compromises consistency of care and the building and sustaining of northern communities.

Lack of political power was also recognized as evidence of the undervaluing of the north. Sparse populations result in fewer elected positions and thus, less representation in government, as reflected in Elizabeth's comment:

> *The political attitude—it's that we don't exist. There's not enough of us in the north to vote to make a difference, so we're totally ignored.*

Lack of political power was seen as leading to under-resourcing of northern communities, and this under-resourcing could lead to dissatisfaction and depopulation of the north. For example, Marie had decided to leave the north for more resources elsewhere so that she could obtain "the quality of life I want to lead."

Undervaluing of women in the north is most clearly seen in the undervaluing of women's roles and perspectives. Women described this undervaluing as reflecting a "redneck" attitude, one that favours men's values, interests and behaviours, and traditional oppressive roles for women. Leah, a young single woman, stated: "It's a really redneck mentality here. The man's the breadwinner. I don't see a lot of choices for women here." Rhoda stated:

> *The woman's place is in the house chewing the leather [laughs]. . . . It's about that sign I saw (when I was travelling): "Lexington, Kentucky: Where Men Are Men and Women Are Glad of It." That's the kind of attitude around here. . . . that's partly why there's violence and drinking and it's like an old time western movie.*

However, even traditional roles such as mothering were sometimes not respected. Eileen, a single mother who had grown up in the north, moved away for several years, and then returned, observed:

I noticed a lack of respect for me as a mother and as a thinking person, particularly by men in the community. There's this idea that men and women are on different sides. . . . There isn't easy mixing between the sexes here. Everything is more gender labelled.

Undervaluing of women may also result from the nature of employment in northern communities. Resource-based industries tend to be male-oriented and prefer male employees; few of the pulp mills, for example, employ female foresters. Eileen noted:

The resource-based work place isn't integrated in terms of gender. . . . The pulp mills are male work places, and the offices are run by women.

In addition, small northern communities do not have many opportunities for well paying, satisfying work for women. Jobs for women tend to be in low status, traditional and low paying sectors. Gender segregation at work can accentuate and sustain gender segregation and the undervaluing of women at home and in society at large.

Undervaluing of women was clearly exemplified in the attitudes of some physicians. Women felt undervalued when physicians did not respect them, or denigrated them, and when they excluded women as equal partners in their care. The following comments provide a beginning appreciation of physician attitudes and behaviours that women in the study experienced:

When I asked for a second opinion, my doctor was quite rude. He wanted to know who I thought I was that I should ask for a second opinion. . . quite arrogant, and he told my husband and me to prepare ourselves for the fact that it was cancer. (Vicki)

My doctor said that it was absolutely none of his concern about doing follow-ups for patients, and didn't I know that he was a very busy person, and didn't I know that it was my responsibility if I wanted a follow up with a specialist, and he had no more time to spend on my file. (Vicki)

Asking for a second opinion and for specialist consultation indicates women's commitment to self-care and empowerment. Such requests require courage and initiative in the north because these requests often involve substantial travel and expense, and the assertiveness to endure responses of unsupportive physicians. Although female physicians were often perceived as more caring and respectful of women, female physicians are rare in the north and their practices fill up quickly. To deal with physician shortages and attitudes, geographical challenges and women's desires for respectful holistic care, women often turned to public health nurses and other care providers. Alice noted: "You can go to the health unit. The public health nurses really open their doors."

"Listening," "respect," "preventive medicine" and "helping me—and I underline *helping* me—do what I could to be responsible and knowledgeable regarding my body, health, mind and emotions" were rarely experienced but highly valued approaches in physician care that women in this study talked about.

The political undervaluing of the north and of women was less problematic for women who were less dependent on the north, less committed to the north, or who were able to leave the north for respites and resources. These women were able to avoid or negate some of the undervaluing and provide themselves with hope and sustaining experiences. However, women needed time, finances, knowledge and awareness in order to avoid or address the undervaluing they perceived in the north.

Marginalization of Northern Women

Marginalization as experienced by women in the study related to experiencing inequitable access to resources necessary to achieve and maintain health when compared with non-northern women and men within the northern context. Marginalization that northern women experience can be characterized by 4 aspects: isolation, limited options, limited power and being silenced.

Isolation

Women in the north are isolated first and foremost by the physical environment, especially in winter. However, isolation is also created by social and political environments. Women in the study believed that northern social and political environments isolated women from each other. Although northern beliefs in traditional gender roles may favour women-only groups for traditional activities such as child care, women-only associations for other reasons, such as for self help or to advocate for women, may be seen as problematic, perhaps because these associations are perceived as 'subversive' or threatening to the status quo. Park, a director of a women's centre, explained:

> People have the perception that they [staff in women's resource centres in small northern communities] are a bunch of men-hating, lesbian women and that the Centre is there to rip the family apart.

Park noted that lesbian relationships can expose women to safety issues and "affect their mental, emotional, and physical health" because these women may feel they must keep their relationships "in the closet" due to lack of acceptance of diversity in small northern communities.

Social and political environments can also isolate women in the north by creating unstable and chronic underfunding of women's centres in small communities. Underfunding limits the social and other resources that these centres can provide for women. In the few communities where women's centres exist, they provide vital—and often the only—services that facilitate women's health, particularly from a holistic health promotion perspective. Park noted that men sometimes access centre services as well. Limits to and losses of these centres contribute significantly to the isolation of northern

women and restrict the ability to make change at personal and community levels.

In addition to isolating women from women, the social and political environments also isolate women from men. Marie observed: "We have loggers, miners, ranchers and there's this macho sense, there's this real male camaraderie, and it excludes women." Women attributed the social diversion of the sexes to the dominance of the male culture in the north. Exclusion of women and segregation of the sexes can sustain and foster isolation and oppression of women.[27]

The north can also create isolate through the fostering of a social status as 'outsider,' as someone who lives in the community but is not truly part of the community. Outsider women experience greater social isolation and marginalization than insider women. For example, in small communities, outsider women may be isolated from the few employment opportunities that exist. Leah, a woman who grew up in the north, noted that for women new to her community

> It is so hard for them because they didn't grow up here and people know that. You have to be friends with someone to 'get in,' you can't just be a new person [to be included or hired].

Limited Options

The limited quantity, quality and diversity of goods, services and education available in the north also reflect and impact upon the status of northern women. Goods that are limited include diverse and affordable food, especially fresh fruit and vegetables, and clothing and goods for women and children. Because women in the north often do most of the shopping for their families, limitations in these goods is especially problematic for women. One participant stated: "You're either buying the really low, low quality stuff or you're paying top dollar." It is perhaps reflective of the undervaluing of women that small communities have a greater selection of goods related to the northern male lifestyle, for example, hunting weapons, outdoor recreational vehicles, and farming, ranching and forestry related supplies.

Daycare services, supports for parenting and relationships, and artistic and cultural opportunities were some of the services and experiences that women found restricted. For example, Park noted that the women's centre had only "one full-time counsellor—it's not for the full year and it's a contract position." This was inadequate because over 100 women come yearly for one-on-one counselling to the centre. Eileen noted that "there were no services that were oriented to treating the whole family" when her marriage broke down. Limitations in services constrained women's abilities to obtain resources that could support them in employment, personal situations and family relationships. Limited cultural experiences in music and the arts made living in the north harder because the relief from the harshness of the north and the enhanced quality of life that these experiences could provide were not available.

Women found particularly problematic the limitations in traditional and alternative health services and in health promotion and disease prevention services. Limited numbers of nurses, physicians, hospitals, mental health and other services exist in the north. The north has difficulty recruiting and retaining health professionals, and recent health care reforms and personnel shortages have resulted in the elimination or downsizing of health care sites. Women's options were thus compromised and they often had to put up with inadequate care:

> *There's more depression up here in women than in men. And yet, from what I can see, physicians' solution is drugs . . . not counselling. Without counselling, I would never have come out of my depression. I would never have learned to turn it around. (Christine)*

> *It's the amount of time that doctors spend with you—10 minutes at the most and . . . I always feel that I'm being pushed out the door. (Rhoda)*

> *The first thing my doctor says to me is "The government pays me to see eight patients a day and you're the twelfth." I didn't feel like I was going to get any kind of quality check-up or interview and he was very quick and brusque with me. (Barbara)*

Although women in urban areas may experience similar limitations, in rural and remote areas women are more compromised because they have fewer or no other options; they may not be able to access a second opinion or change care providers because they don't exist in their communities or close by. Medical specialists, such as psychiatrists, from southern urban areas occasionally fly to northern communities to provide care for a few days. Sometimes clinics are held in remote northern communities. Women felt that this was inconsistent and second-rate care and, for the most part, ineffective.

Quality of care was also compromised by the knowledge and attitudes of physicians. Women felt that their health issues were often dismissed or downplayed by physicians, as displayed in attitudes that

> *. . . women bring on a lot of their own illness, that whatever a woman has that she's responsible for it directly. If a man has it—he's the bread winner so he deserves to have [care]. (Barbara)*

Disrespect of the contexts of women's lives and of their needs was evident, as Elizabeth, a single woman, vividly articulates:

> *That man was brutal, but he was the only gynecologist. . . . I just thought "this man shouldn't even be a doctor." He was rough, and he says to me, "Well, if you're going to have kids, you better have them now." And I said, "Well, I'm not into being a single parent." [He says] "Well, what's the matter? Good looking girl like you, you should be able to find a man." I would have asked to go somewhere else but there was nowhere else to go.*

When the nature of women's lives and their perspectives are not taken into account, or when care is difficult to access, women may choose to forego care, or they may receive care that does not fit with their values or lifestyle and that is not timely or appropriate. As a result, women may live with disease and illness longer, experience increased complications of treatment due to advanced illness and endure compromised recovery.

To avoid or minimize the impact of inadequate and inappropriate health care, women wanted to prevent health problems and promote their health. Services that women favoured included massage, midwifery, naturopathic services, health education, and social and counselling services. However, these services either do not exist in most northern communities, are provided in inadequate ways, or are not included in the national health insurance plan. Women thought that physicians were often ill-informed about, or did not appreciate, the value of health promotion and illness prevention services, and that physicians needed "a more open mind" regarding alternative health care. Christine summarized the values of several women in the study when she stated that she appreciated that her physician "told me about people to see about different holistic medicines." Physician discomfort with women's requests for alternative health care services and limited availability of other health care professionals, such as public health nurses who could advise women, resulted in under use or ineffective use of health promotion and illness prevention services. Consequently, northern women often live with pain, discomfort and illness that could be prevented, and that is not treated in a timely, valued and effective manner.

In addition to limitations in goods and services, women also noted limitations in education. Women valued education because, especially in the under-resourced north, "women have to have the information to be responsible for themselves" (Elizabeth), and because education would enhance women's self-esteem and sense of agency, especially for women in low socioeconomic situations. Mary, an Aboriginal woman who works with low-income Aboriginal women, explained:

> *A lot of [my clients] want to just be able to take a course, just to feel good that they can do something. . . . you know, 'cause if they can do one course, maybe they can do this [other activity to improve their lives] and, you know, [it] branches off from there.*

Women felt that improving women's education would also strengthen families. Lilac stated: "A woman needs an education. You educate a boy, you educate a man. You educate a girl, you educate a family."

In spite of the benefits of education, educational resources are limited in the north. Libraries, health education personnel and community colleges are not readily accessible due to distance and weather. Computers and the creation of the University of Northern British Columbia in the north in 1994 have increased the ability of northern women to acquire information and education. However, women must still have the money, time and self-confidence to access these resources. Often they must also relocate to Prince George to access on-campus university classes and other educational resources. Study participants believed that women in the north live in a patriarchal culture that does not privilege the advancement of women. Thus, girls and women may not be encouraged or supported to access educational resources or achieve academic success.

The politics of funding for education seems to be an ongoing problem in the north. Although more affordable technology such as satellite dishes, computers and the Internet are facilitating distance learning, this technology is only available to women who have the funds and technology such as electricity and telephone services to access these education resources.

Limited Power

Aspects of limited power were evident in women's descriptions of their agency and activities and in observational data. Several women suggested that women's voices and perspectives are not valued because northern communities are segregated by gender, with women occupying the less powerful role:

> *There's this idea that men and women are on different sides. I think it's partly pure sexism. That women don't have anything interesting to say. (Eileen)*

> *I hate to say this in this day and age, but women don't feel that they have a lot of power in a lot of rural communities . . . it's like stepping back in time 40 years. (Rosie)*

Within the north, women's lives are often linked to economic dependence on men who are employed in the resource industries. This limits women's power. Marie noted that women's dependence on resource-based economies may compel them to tolerate gender inequities to sustain employment for their husbands. "If you're blatant about it [feminism] and open about it, it's not really good, because you might be ostracized or not accepted." In a small community with few jobs, non-acceptance could cost one one's livelihood.

Women's economic dependence is further perpetuated by the assumption that housewives and mothers do not need to be responsible for their own economic well-being and that women's primary responsibility is to home and family, as Eileen's comments reveal:

> *If you're going to be a 'real' woman—quotes around that, right—and be married and have a family or be a mother, you don't do that kind of thing [have a well paying job].*

In addition, few well paying and satisfying jobs exist for women in the north, and the limited access to education compromises women's acquisition of well paying and satisfying employment that might be available.

Religious beliefs that foster traditional attitudes can further compromise northern women's power. Leah observed:

> *A large religious population here probably contributes to the lack of opportunity for women with beliefs such as "men are the bread winners, women belong at home raising the children."*

Marie believed that while the church fosters a sense of community, it may also result in rigidity of values, whereby people become "so dogmatic . . . they don't want to actively listen and even consider the possibility that there could be other answers."

Limited power that results from religious and male values was most often noted by older and single women and by women who had university education and life experiences outside the north. It may well be that women who are aware of other ways of being and who have independent life experiences may be better able to locate northern women's power—or lack thereof—in the structures of northern communities.

Being Silenced

Women in the study noted the importance of having a voice. The overwhelming response to recruitment initiatives indicates that northern women have a great desire for a voice in health-related matters, and suggests that northern women often do not have the opportunity for such participation.

The silencing of northern women's experience and their desire for voice were revealed in several of the women's comments about the research:

> *How wonderful it is that someone's finally sitting down and reaching out to women and finding out what people are thinking. This is so needful. I talked last time about women not having a voice—well, this is giving women a voice. (Jocelyn)*

> *I admire you so much for having done this [research]. Our . . . voices wouldn't be heard if it wasn't for you drawing them out and possibly putting them where they will be heard. (Amelia)*

> *I think what you're doing is really valuable. This [research] needs to be done because men have been in control for so long and women have just had to go along with it. They've had no say. They've had no say at all. (Signe)*

Other indicators of northern women being silenced include the limited number of women in public positions of authority and decision-making. For example, during this study the Prince George city council of 10 elected members included only 2 women. Prince George has had only one female mayor in its almost century-long existence. Representation of northern women in elected provincial and federal government positions is also very much in the minority. Women's lack of representation in public venues reflects social, political and gender roles and power structures inherent in northern resource-based communities.[28]

The importance of women having a voice was also evident in women's stated preference for face-to-face interviews, rather than written surveys or telephone interviews. Although women would be listened to in telephone interviews, it seems that the women felt that they would not 'really be heard.' Face-to-face interviews in women's communities and across their kitchen tables were important in conveying respect, facilitating communication and understanding, and decreasing the silence that many northern women experiences. Casey, a ranch woman, explained:

> . . . a lot of times up here we get a lot of phone research . . . and the people at the end of the line don't care. It's all written out for them. . . . It's just cold. . . . Whereas a face-to-face encounter—there's a body there, there's warmth, there's humanity. There's a connection.

Fred, a woman who has lived in the north all her life, valued face-to-face research because it afforded her the opportunity to evaluate the respect for her, and to voice concerns and be heard:

> . . . seeing the person is seeing their face . . . a lot of communication is body language, that they aren't a threatening person . . . not laughing at you. . . . A voice on the phone— it's really impersonal. What you're doing is listening and you did a good job of it.

DISCUSSION

This study revealed how the historical, physical, sociocultural and political contexts of the north influence northern women's health by contributing to their marginalization. More specifically, the marginalization experienced by women in northern BC was characterized by isolation, limited options of good, services and education, limited power and being silenced.

While there is considerable research focusing on marginalization related to race, ethnicity and socioeconomic exclusion, less attention has been directed to marginalization resulting from geographical location and gender. Geographers and social and political scientists have discussed marginalization in the north in terms of the terrain, distance and sociopolitical and economic factors, such as the lack of political power and economic dependence on a single resource.[8,12,21,29,30] This study reveals important new information about the relationship of geography and gender and implications for women's health. For example, this study found that the depth and scope of factors in the northern context such as extensive distances and isolation, prolonged severe climates, power and sociocultural aspects of relationships, and fewer health and human service resources make northern women's needs more acute, their solution options more limited, and their plight more problematic. Moreover, a 'pile-up' or accumulation of contextual factors such as isolation and severe climate and limited personal and social resources increase northern women's marginalization and health challenges.

Hall, Stevens and Meleis[27] note that one's identity, associations, experiences and environments can all form the basis of an individual's or a group's marginalization. Various attitudes and behaviours such as discrimination, scapegoating, stigmatizing and segregation may also serve to marginalize and exclude women.[4,27] This study confirms, clarifies and extends information about factors of marginalization and exclusion that affect women's health in northern settings. For example, this study revealed that women without male partners may be stigmatized and excluded in northern settings and that this may be seen as legitimate because of patriarchal male-dominated values and behaviours that are promoted within socioeconomic contexts in northern communities.

A strength of this study is that it provides beginning information about diverse women's lives in northern settings. The study included northern women who were elderly, young and middle-aged; disabled and able-bodied; poor, middle-class and wealthy; Caucasian and from minority cultures; and women from remote, rural and urban locations. Thus, this research extends understanding about how geography intersects with other determinants of health in remote northern settings. Nevertheless, the small study sample limits the depth and scope of understanding about the health and lives of northern women. Research is especially needed regarding the health and marginalization of northern women who are physically disabled, elderly, low income, lesbian, single/widowed/divorced, and about those who live in particularly remote settings. Given the size and nature of the sample, the findings regarding health provider attitudes and behaviours may not be reflective of health providers as a whole; therefore, additional research that explores human service provider attitudes and behaviours from the perspective of consumers and providers would be beneficial. Participatory action research and research that uses interviews, focus groups and other methods that privilege women's voices and experiences would enrich understanding and would foster respect, inclusion and empowerment as northern women 'come to voice' in research.

CONCLUSIONS

This study has relevance for rural and northern health care practice and northern women's health. To strengthen northern women's access to quality health care, equitable inclusion and empowerment, increased efforts must be made to recruit and retain human service professionals in the north, especial-

ly female public health nurses, nurse practitioners and physicians who will provide respectful and appropriate care and who are comfortable with the professional and personal aspects of living and working in small northern communities.[25,31,32] Northern health practitioners must be able to work in environments that are culturally diverse, where lack of anonymity, scarcity of resources and isolation characterize life, and where they may be regarded as outsiders.[6,32–34] In addition, health care practitioners must include women as equal partners in health care and realize that women are experts of their own lives.

Human service providers in northern settings must include in their practices advocacy for healthy public policy, community development and coalition building approaches. These activities, if conducted for and with women,[6,14,35] help to give power and recognition to northern women, make the most of limited resources and draw enriched resources to northern communities.

In 2002, a national report on health care in Canada[3] highlighted the need to improve health and access to health care for people in rural and remote communities. When national reports include initiatives and suggestions proposed by women in geographically isolated settings, such as the women in this study, health care practice and women's health in rural and remote settings will significantly improve.

Acknowledgement: This research was supported by an Isaac Walton Killam Memorial Scholarship from the University of Alberta.

Competing interests: None declared.

REFERENCES

1. Health Canada. (1996). *Towards a common understanding: Clarifying the core concepts of population health.* Ottawa, ON: Health Canada.

2. Health Canada; Ministry of Health and Ministry Responsible for Seniors. (1995). *Report of the northern and rural health task force.* Victoria, BC: Health Canada.

3. Romanow, R. J. (2002). *Building on values: The future of health care in Canada.* Saskatoon, SK: Commission on the Future of Health Care in Canada. Retrieved August 18, 2005, from http://www.hc-sc.gc.ca/english/pdf/romanow/pdfs/HCC_Final_Report.pdf

4. Guildford, J. (2000). *Making the case for social and economic inclusion.* Halifax, NS: Health Canada.

5. Health Canada. (2002). *Rural health in rural hands.* Retrieved August 18, 2005, from http://www.phac-aspc.gc.ca/rh-sr/rural_hands-mains_rurales_e.html

6. Leipert, B. (1999). Women's health and the practice of public health nurses in northern British Columbia. *Public Health Nursing, 16,* 280–289.

7. Leipert, B. (Ed.). (1998). *Northern voices: Health, community, and economic perspectives in northern British Columbia.* Prince George, BC: University of Northern British Columbia.

8. Gill, A. (1984). Women in northern resource towns. In *Social science in the north: Communicating northern values* (Occasional Publication No. 9). Ottawa, ON: Association of Canadian Universities for Northern Studies.

9. Luxton, M. (1980). *More than a labor of love: Three generations of women's work in the home.* Toronto, ON: The Women's Press.

10. Young, J. (1997). *Farm women's perceptions of health and work.* Unpublished master's thesis, University of Alberta, Edmonton, Alberta, Canada.

11. Wall, M. (1993). Women and development in northwestern Ontario. In C. Southcott (Ed.), *Provincial hinterland: Social inequity in northwestern Ontario.* Halifax, NS: Fernwood Publishing.

12. Heald, S. (1991). Projects and subjects: Women, the north, and job creation. In T. Dunk (Ed.), *Social relations in resource hinterlands.* Thunder Bay, ON: Lakehead University.

13. Leipert, B., & Reutter, L. (2005). Developing resilience: How women maintain their health in northern geographically isolated settings. *Qualitative Health Research, 15*(1), 49–65.

14. Leipert, B., & Reutter, L. (1998). Women's health and community health nursing practice in geographically isolated settings: A Canadian perspective. *Health Care for Women International, 19,* 575–588.

15. Walters, V., Lenton, R., & Mckeary, M. (1995). *Women's health in the context of women's lives.* Ottawa, ON: Minister of Supply and Services Canada.

16. Glaser, B. (1992). *Basics of grounded theory analysis: Emergence vs. forcing.* Mill Valley, CA: Sociology Press.

17. Keddy, B., Sims, S., & Stern, P. (1996). Grounded theory as feminist research methodology. *Journal of Advanced Nursing, 23,* 448–453.

18. MacDonald, M. (2001). Finding a critical perspective in grounded theory. In R. Schreiber & P. Stern (Eds.), *Using grounded theory in nursing.* New York: Springer.

19. Glaser, B. (1978). *Theoretical sensitivity.* Mill Valley, CA: Sociology Press.

20. Morse, J. (1994). Designing funded qualitative research. In N. Denzin & Y. Lincoln (Eds.), *Handbook of qualitative research.* Thousand Oaks, CA: Sage.

21. Coates, K., & Morrison, W. (1992). *The forgotten north: A history of Canada's provincial norths.* Toronto, ON: James Lorimer & Company.

22. McNeely, A., & Shreffler, M. (1998). Familiarity. In H. Lee (Ed.), *Conceptual basis for rural nursing.* New York: Springer.

23. Bailey, M. (1998). Outsider. In H. Lee (Ed.), *Conceptual basis for rural nursing.* New York: Springer Publishing Company.

24. Myers, D. (1998). Insider. In H. Lee (Ed.), *Conceptual basis for rural nursing.* New York: Springer.

25. Belzer, E. (1999). *What health professionals need to know: How to survive and thrive in rural and underserved practices.* Kansas City, MO: National Rural Health Association.

26. Delaney, R., & Brownlee, K. (1996). Ethical dilemma in northern social work practice. In R. Delaney, K. Brownlee, M. & Zapf (Eds.), *Issues in northern social work practice.* Thunder Bay, ON: Lakehead University.

27. Hall, J., Stevens, P., & Meleis, A. (1994). Marginalization: A guiding concept for valuing diversity in nursing knowledge development. *ANS Advanced in Nursing Science, 16*(4), 23–41.

28. Delaney, R., Brownlee, K., & Zapf, M. (Eds.). (1996). *Issues in northern social work practice.* Thunder Bay, ON: Lakehead University.

29. McCann, L., & Gunn, A. (1998). *Heartland and hinterland: A regional geography of Canada* (3rd ed.). Scarborough, ON: Prentice Hall.

30. Weller, G. (1993). Hinterland politics: The case of northwestern Ontario. In C. Southcott (Ed.), *Provincial hinterland: Social inequity in northwestern Ontario.* Halifax, NS: Fernwood.

31. Bushy, A. (2000). *Orientation to nursing in the rural community.* London: Sage.

32. Bushy, A., & Leipert, B. (2005). Factors that influence students in choosing rural nursing practice: A pilot study. *Rural and Remote Health, 5,* 387. Retrieved August 18, 2005, from http://rrh.deakin.edu.au/articles/subviewnew.asp?ArticleID=387

33. Canitz, B. (1990). *Everything for everyone and no one for you: Understanding nursing turnover in northern Canada.* Toronto, ON: University of Toronto.

34. Dunkin, J. (1998). Applying interventions in rural areas. In C. Helvie (Ed.), *Advanced practice nursing in the community.* London: Sage.

35. Denton, M., Hadjukowski-Ahmed, M., Connor, M., & Zeytinoglu, U. (1999). *Women's voices in health promotion.* Toronto, ON: Canadian Scholars' Press.

INTRODUCTION TO CRITIQUE #2

The research report "Women's Health in Northern British Columbia: The Role of Geography and Gender" (Leipert & Reutter, 2005) is critically examined for its rigour as a grounded theory study, its contribution to nursing, and its usefulness in practice. The criteria identified in Box 18–2 which are specific to grounded theory research, are used to guide the critique.

Statement of the Phenomenon of Interest

Leipert and Reutter (2005) clearly stated the phenomenon of interest. They indicated that although interest in women's health is becoming more pervasive, research does not adequately address the importance of geography and gender, even though these factors are considered important determinants of health. Leipert and Reutter chose to explore the experiences of gender and geography by studying women in northern British Columbia.

The authors described the determinants of health, emphasizing the components of the physical environment factors. The authors also indicated that prior reports have focused on the natural environment and the effects on health but ignored the impact of the man-made environment on women's health. A description of the minimal research on the challenges affecting the health status of women who live in isolated settings followed. Finally, the authors presented their argument as to why in-depth research on understanding the impact of geography is needed to understand the context of the lives and health of women in northern British Columbia.

Evidence-Based Practice Tip

Qualitative studies are particularly helpful in answering research questions about a concept or phenomenon that is not well understood or adequately covered in the literature.

Purpose

The purpose of qualitative research studies is often consistent with the identified statement of the problem. In this case, Leipert and Reutter (2005) stated that the purpose of their study was "to enrich understanding of the northern social environment so that social support, which is key to northern women's health, can be advanced" (p. 242).

The authors explained that the significance of the study, which is found in the "Conclusions" section of the report, is to inform health care practitioners about the professional and personal aspects of living and working in small northern communities. Understanding the sociocultural contexts of small northern communities will assist health practitioners in providing culturally relevant care and advocating for healthy public policy and community development.

Method

The method used in this study is clearly identified as feminist grounded theory (Leipert & Reutter, 2005). The authors stated that this method was used to generate a theory that will explain a central problem for women, provide respect for participants, avoid oppression, and consider, in addition to the women's experience, the larger sociopolitical, economic, and cultures processes. According to Speziale and Carpenter (2007), "grounded theory is a qualitative research approach used to explore the social processes that present within human interaction" (p. 133). The grounded theory method was appropriate for this study and yielded the expected results.

Missing from the declaration of the method, however, is the tradition on which the study was based. The references in the data analysis section are primarily from Glaser, one of the leading grounded theorists, along with Strauss and Corbin. It is important to understand which tradition of grounded theory informed this study because they differ. For example, the work of Glaser (1978, 1992,

1998, 2001) has been described as inductive, as opposed to the work of Strauss and Corbin (1990, 1998), which has been described as inductive-deductive (Maijala, Paavilainen, & Astedt-Kurki, 2003). For the reader to determine whether the research approach was executed fully and properly, it is necessary to return to the original work of Glaser (1978) because little is offered in Leipert and Reutter's (2005) article regarding the specifics of the method they used. So, for the novice reader, a primary source on grounded theory is necessary to fully understand the authors' research process.

Sampling

Leipert and Reutter (2005) stated that purposive sampling was used for data collection, which is appropriate for a grounded theory study. Purposive or purposeful sampling provides the qualitative researcher with the opportunity to recruit participants who are knowledgeable about the phenomenon under study. Participants are recruited for the purpose of providing rich descriptions based on their personal experiences. In this case, Leipert and Reutter (2005) recruited women who represented diverse backgrounds based on geographical location, ages, and cultural backgrounds.

The researchers also stated that theoretical sampling was used following the initial purposive sampling. In **theoretical sampling**, which is used primarily in grounded theory, individuals are interviewed in an effort to further develop specific aspects of the emerging theory. In this case, Leipert and Reutter (2005) stated that the "study participants were selected throughout the course of the research for their ability to enrich and enlarge upon themes and codes emerging from the ongoing analysis [which] also ensures that participants will provide contradictory as well as confirmatory evidence" (p. 243).

However, the authors did not discuss how representative the categories proved to be after using this sampling procedure. For the reader to fully appreciate the use of theoretical sampling, the researchers could have explained what led to theoretical sampling and how it affected theory development. Again, the limited explanation of the use of theoretical sampling may be a result of the page limitation imposed by the journal.

The authors carefully described how they recruited participants through a number of strategies, including radio and television advertisements, newspaper advertisements, and information posted in the stores of small communities. Their efforts were rewarded, with over 100 women responding to the search. Twenty-five women were purposively selected from this pool and interviewed three times. The authors indicated that the recommended sample size for grounded theory is 30 to 50 interview instances, and their study included a total of 75 interview instances. Data collection stopped when no further information was forthcoming or the data was saturated. **Saturation** is a term used in qualitative research to signify the repeating nature of information and the end of data collection.

Leipert and Reutter (2005) reported that before the data collection process, permission to conduct the study was obtained from the institutional review boards of both the universities of Alberta and Northern British Columbia. The researchers did not state why two reviews were necessary. In spite of the ethical approval, the authors did not indicate how the participants were protected, how confidentiality was maintained, or how consent was obtained. Although these steps and precautions are assumed in most studies, researchers should explicitly state how they addressed these ethical concerns, either in the methods or sampling section.

Data Generation

During the first two interviews of the study, the women responded to open-ended questions about "how they maintained their health, how the northern context influenced their health, and how northern BC could be healthier for women" (Leipert & Reutter, 2005, p. 243). Open-ended questions allow participants to fully describe their experiences (Speziale & Carpenter, 2007). The first two interviews lasted between 1.5 and 2 hours and were audiotaped and transcribed. The first interview occurred in the women's workplace or home. Subsequent interviews were primarily conducted on the telephone. The questions and means of recording the interviews were appropriate. The third interview was shorter and not tape-recorded, and the researchers noted the participants' comments in writing. Not taping and transcribing the third interview could have threatened the confirmability of the data.

The authors did not describe the time interval between interviews. One way to ensure the credibility of findings is to have a period of prolonged engagement with the subject matter. Because the reader does not have this information, it is difficult to conclude whether the authors met this criterion for credibility.

In compliance with the feminist method, the researchers provided the participants with summaries of each interview and asked them in the third interview to comment on the emerging theory. By allowing the participants to confirm that this theory was true to their experiences, the researchers met this criterion for credibility.

Although interviews were the primary tool for data generation in this study, the researchers' observations about the geographical environment were noted, and written documents, such as tourist guides, publications with local history, and newspapers, were collected to assist the researchers in understanding northern culture, history, and social–political context.

Data Analysis

Data generation and analysis are iterative processes in grounded theory. Data collection is followed by data analysis, which is followed by more data collection. The analysis leads the researcher to ask other questions of the data to build a strong theory. Leipert and Reutter (2005) reported that they used the constant comparative method. True to this strategy, the researchers reported that data collection and analysis were completed simultaneously. They further described how theoretical coding,

using NVivo software, was used to guide theory development. The researchers narrated the development of their ideas by describing the concepts that supported their conceptual categories. This process was further substantiated through the use of quotations from the participants.

Generally speaking, the measures of rigour in qualitative research are its **credibility**, **auditability**, and **fittingness** or **transferability**. In this study, the researchers reported that the first check, credibility, was obtained by the amount of time spent with the informants and by doing informant or member checks. Member checking is a process of returning to the informants and asking them whether the data reported represent their experience of the phenomenon under study.

Auditability (also called the audit trail) is the second check for rigour. The question to ask is as follows: "Did the researcher present enough information for me to see how the raw data lead to the interpretation?" Leipert and Reutter did not describe the development of an audit trail thus calling into question the rigour of the study.

The third check, the fittingness or transferability of the data, is based on asking the following question: "Is there enough detail here for me to evaluate the relevance and importance of these data for my own practice or for use in research or theory development?" The details provided should allow the research consumer to determine whether the results of the study in question can be applied to another setting or context. Overall, the study meets most of the criteria for confirmability.

Finally, when judging the quality of data analysis, the reader must ask the following: "Has the researcher shared enough with me so that I can judge the results?" In this article, the authors provided readers with a rich contextual narrative. The text is compelling, and the concepts are easily understood. In addition to sharing the core variable and the subprocesses, Leipert and Reutter described the northern context, including the historical location and the physical, sociocultural, and political environments. Once the context is understood, the authors concluded that northern women are marginalized, which is caused by their isolation, limited options, limited power, and lack of voice.

Empirical Groundings of the Study Findings

When evaluating the findings, the reader must ask a number of questions related to the theoretical concepts identified. In Leipert and Reutter's study, the subjective comments of the participants are interwoven with the authors' narratives. It is clear from the participants' quotes that the authors' theoretical concepts are grounded in the interview data. So although the concepts are validated, Leipert and Reutter do not provide a clear description of their theory explaining the linkages between the concepts. In many grounded theory studies, the theoretical model is displayed in a schematic drawing of the model. In this study, however, the authors have not clarified how each of the identified four aspects leading to the marginalization of women specifically affects women's health. This paper studies the social processes within human interactions essential to ground theory; however, the research study is more explorative because it is limited to description rather than the generation of theory to explain how geographic location affects women's health in a northern Canadian setting.

Conclusions, Implications, and Recommendations

The depth of the discussion and conclusion that appear in the article are appropriate. The authors presented the implications of their theoretical formulations, as well as the overall conclusions of their findings. They also placed the findings in context by sharing their recommendations and comparing what they found with the findings of authors who have studied similar topics. A number of future research questions were offered, and the significance of the work was made clear in the opening paragraph of the "Conclusions" section.

Overall, the research is well reported and offers the reader an insight into the role of gender and geography in women's health in northern British Columbia. The article's rich commentary helps the reader understand the experiences of these women. However, rather than building theory, these research results contribute to a descriptive understanding of the environment's impact on women's health. Although this contribution is an important research direction, the reader is left without a clear understanding of why grounded theory was used because the theory was not clearly explained and no plan was elaborated to further refine and test the theory. Based on the conclusions, the researchers could have achieved the same outcome by using phenomenology as the method because the purpose of phenomenology is to understand human experience. Perhaps the theory development was addressed in other publications as the authors indicated that they reported how women addressed factors to maintain their health elsewhere.

In summary, the findings of the study are useful and can lead to further study. The authors indicated some future direction for research. However, the conclusions of the study leave the reader without a clear understanding of the purpose of developing a substantive theory given that no plan was elaborated either to use the theory or further develop it.

Evidence-Based Practice Tip

Qualitative research may generate basic knowledge, hypotheses, and theories to be used in the design of other types of qualitative or quantitative studies. However, qualitative research is not necessarily a preliminary step to another type of research. It is a complete and valuable end in itself.

Critical Thinking Challenges

- Discuss the similarities and differences between the stylistic considerations of reporting a qualitative study versus a quantitative study in a professional journal.
- Are critiques of qualitative studies by consumers of research, in the role of either a student or a practising nurse, valid? Which type of qualitative study is the most difficult for consumers of research to critique? Discuss what assumptions led you to this determination.
- Discuss how one would go about incorporating qualitative research in evidence-based practice. Give an example.

REFERENCES

Barbour, R. S., & Barbour, M. (2003). Evaluating and synthesizing qualitative research: The need to develop a distinctive approach. *Journal of Evaluation in Clinical Practice, 9,* 179–186.

Bottorff, J. L., Johnson, J. L., Moffat, B., Grewal, J., Ratner, P., & Kalaw, C. (2004). Adolescent constructions of nicotine addiction. *Canadian Journal of Nursing Research, 38,* 22–39.

Buijs, R. (2001). *A qualitative evaluation of the Seniors ALIVE Program.* Unpublished master's thesis, University of Alberta, Edmonton, Canada.

Buijs, R., Ross-Kerr, J., Cousins, S., & Wilson, D. (2003). Promoting participation: Evaluation of a health promotion program for low income seniors. *Journal of Community Health Nursing, 20,* 93–107.

Carnevale, F. (2002). Authentic qualitative research and the quest for methodological rigour. *Canadian Journal of Nursing Research, 34,* 121–128.

Cesario, S., Morin, K., & Santa-Donato, A. (2002). Evaluating the level of evidence of qualitative research. *Journal of Obstetric, Gynecological and Neonatal Nursing, 31,* 708–714.

Creswell, J. W. (2003). *Research design: Qualitative, quantitative, and mixed methods approaches* (2nd ed.). Thousand Oaks, CA: Sage.

Gibson, B. E., & Martin, D. K. (2003). Qualitative research and evidence-based physiotherapy practice. *Physiotherapy, 89,* 350–358.

Glaser, B. G. (1978). *Theoretical sensitivity: Advances in methodology of grounded theory.* Mill Valley, CA: Sociology Press.

Glaser, B. G. (1992). *Basics of grounded theory analysis. Emergence vs. forcing.* Mill Valley, CA: Sociology Press.

Glaser, B. G. (1998). *Doing grounded theory: Issues and discussions* (2nd ed.). Mill Valley, CA: Sociology Press.

Glaser, B. G. (2001). *The grounded theory perspective: Conceptualizing contrasted with description.* Mill Valley, CA: Sociology Press.

Glesne, C. (2006). *Becoming qualitative researchers: An introduction* (3rd ed.). New York: Longman.

Horsburgh, D. (2003). Evaluation of qualitative research. *Journal of Clinical Nursing, 12,* 307–312.

Leipert, B. D., & Reutter, L. (2005). Women's health in northern British Columbia: The role of geography and gender. *Canadian Journal of Rural Medicine, 10,* 241–253.

Lincoln, Y. S., & Guba, E. (1985). *Naturalistic inquiry.* Beverly Hills, CA: Sage.

Maijala, H., Paavilainen, E., & Astedt-Kurki, P. (2003). The use of grounded theory to study interaction. *Nursing Research, 11,* 40–58.

Morse, J. M., Penrod, J., & Hupcey, J. E. (2000). Qualitative outcome analysis: Evaluating nursing interventions for complex clinical phenomena. *Journal of Nursing Scholarship, 32,* 125–130.

Patton, M. (2002). *Qualitative research and evaluation methods* (3rd ed.). Thousand Oaks, CA: Sage.

Russell, C. K., & Gregory, D. M. (2003). Evaluation of qualitative research studies. *Evidence-Based Nursing, 6,* 36–40.

Sandelowski, M. (1995). Sample size in qualitative research. *Research in Nursing and Health, 18,* 179–183.

Schepner-Hughes, N. (1992). *Death without weeping: The violence of everyday life in Brazil.* Berkeley, CA: University of California Press.

Speziale, H. J. S., & Carpenter, D. R. (2007). *Qualitative research in nursing: Advancing the humanistic imperative* (3rd ed.). Philadelphia: Lippincott.

Strauss, A., & Corbin, J. (1990). *Basics of qualitative research: Grounded theory procedures and techniques.* Newbury Park, CA: Sage.

Strauss, A., & Corbin, J. (1998). *Basics of qualitative research. Techniques and procedures for developing grounded theory.* Thousand Oaks, CA: Sage.

Streubert, H. J. (1998). Evaluating the qualitative research report. In G. LoBiondo-Wood & J. Haber (Eds.), *Nursing research: Methods, critical appraisal and utilization* (4th ed., pp. 445–465). St. Louis, MO: Mosby.

Wilkin, K., & Slevin, E. (2004). The meaning of caring to nurses: An investigation into the nature of caring work in an intensive care unit. *Journal of Clinical Nursing, 13,* 50–59.

Judith A. Heermann

Betty J. Craft

Mina D. Singh

CHAPTER 19

Critiquing Quantitative Research

LEARNING OUTCOMES

After reading this chapter, the student should be able to do the following:

- Identify the purpose of the critiquing process for a quantitative research report.
- Describe the criteria of each step of the critiquing process for a quantitative research report.
- Evaluate the strengths and weaknesses of a quantitative research report.
- Discuss the implications of the findings of a quantitative research report for nursing practice.
- Construct a critique of a quantitative research report.

KEY TERMS

research base
scientific merit

STUDY RESOURCES

evolve

http://evolve.elsevier.com/Canada/LoBiondo/Research/
for Weblinks, content updates, and additional
research articles for practice in reviewing
and critiquing.

As reinforced throughout each chapter of this book, it is important not only to conduct and read research but also to use research for evidence-based practice. As nurse researchers increase the depth (quality) and breadth (quantity) of research methods from descriptive research designs to randomized clinical trials, the data to support clinical interventions and quality outcomes are becoming more readily available. Each published study, regardless of its design, reflects a *level of evidence*, but the critique of each study goes well beyond the level of evidence produced by the design. When critiquing a research study, examine each component to determine the merit of the report. Key to the critique is the strength of evidence that each study produces individually and collectively.

This chapter presents critiques of two studies that test research questions with different quantitative designs. The critiquing criteria designed to assist research consumers in judging the relative value of a research report are found at the end of previous chapters. These critiquing criteria have been summarized to create an abbreviated set of questions that will be used as a framework for the two sample research critiques (see Table 19–1). These critiques exemplify the process of evaluating reported research for potential application to practice, thus extending the **research base** for nursing. For clarification, readers are encouraged to refer to the earlier chapters for detailed presentations of the critiquing criteria and explanations of the research process. The criteria and examples in this chapter apply to quantitative studies using experimental, quasiexperimental, and nonexperimental research designs that provided Level II, III, and IV evidence.

TABLE 19–1 **Major Content Sections of a Research Report and Related Critiquing Guidelines**	
Section	**Questions to Guide Evaluation**
Problem statement and purpose (see Chapter 4)	1. What is the problem or purpose of the research study? 2. Does the problem or purpose statement express a relationship between two or more variables (e.g., between an independent and a dependent variable)? If so, what is the relationship? Is it testable? 3. Does the problem statement or purpose specify the nature of the population being studied? What is it? 4. What significance of the problem—if any—has the investigator identified?
Review of the literature and theoretical framework (see Chapters 2 and 5)	1. What concepts are included in the review? Of particular importance, note those concepts that are the independent and dependent variables and how they are conceptually defined. 2. Does the literature review make the relationships among the variables explicit or place the variables within a theoretical or conceptual framework? What are the relationships? 3. What gaps or conflicts in knowledge of the problem are identified? How is this study intended to fill those gaps or resolve those conflicts? 4. Are the references cited by the author mostly primary or secondary sources? Give an example of each. 5. What are the operational definitions of the independent and dependent variables? Do they reflect the conceptual definitions?
Hypotheses or research questions (see Chapter 4)	1. What hypotheses or research questions are stated in the study? Are they appropriately stated? 2. If research questions are stated, are they used in addition to hypotheses or to guide an exploratory study? 3. What are the independent and dependent variables in the statement of each hypothesis or research question? 4. If hypotheses are stated, is the form of the statement statistical (null) or research? 5. What is the direction of the relationship in each hypothesis, if indicated? 6. Are the hypotheses testable?

TABLE 19–1 Major Content Sections of a Research Report and Related Critiquing Guidelines—cont'd

Section	Questions to Guide Evaluation
Sample (see Chapter 12)	1. How was the sample selected? 2. What type of sampling method is used in the study? Is it appropriate to the design? 3. Does the sample reflect the population as identified in the problem or purpose statement? 4. Is the sample size appropriate? How is it substantiated? 5. To what population may the findings be generalized? What are the limitations in generalizability?
Research design (see Chapters 10 to 11)	1. What type of design is used in the study? 2. What is the rationale for the design classification? 3. Does the design seem to flow from the proposed research problem, theoretical framework, literature review, and hypothesis?
Internal validity (see Chapter 9)	1. Discuss each threat to the internal validity of the study. 2. Does the design have controls at an acceptable level for the threats to internal validity?
External validity (see Chapter 9)	1. What are the limits to generalizability in terms of external validity?
Research approach (see Chapters 7 and 11)	1. Does the research approach fit with the purpose of the study? 2. If used, is a mixed method approach appropriate for the study?
Methods (see Chapter 13)	1. What data collection methods are used in the study? 2. Are the data collection procedures similar for all subjects?
Legal–ethical issues (see Chapter 6)	1. Have the rights of subjects been protected? How? 2. What indications are given that informed consent of the subjects was ensured?

Instruments (see Chapter 13)	1. Physiological measurement
	  a. Is a rationale given for why a particular instrument or method was selected? If so, what is it?
	  b. What provision is made for maintaining the accuracy of the instrument and its use, if any?
	2. Observational methods
	  a. Who did the observing?
	  b. How were the observers trained to minimize bias?
	  c. Did the observers have an observational guide?
	  d. Were the observers required to make inferences about what they saw?
	  e. Is there any reason to believe that the presence of the observers affected the behaviour of the subjects?
	3. Interviews
	  a. Who were the interviewers? How were they trained to minimize bias?
	  b. Is there evidence of any interviewer bias? If so, what is it?
	4. Questionnaires
	  a. What is the type or format of the questionnaires (e.g., Likert, open-ended)? Are they consistent with the conceptual definitions?
	5. Available data and records
	  a. Are the records that were used appropriate to the problem studied?
	  b. Were the data used to describe the sample or for hypothesis testing?

Reliability and validity (see Chapter 14)	1. What type of reliability is reported for each instrument? 2. What level of reliability is reported? Is it acceptable? 3. What type of validity is reported for each instrument? 4. Does the validity of each instrument seem adequate? Why?

TABLE 19–1	**Major Content Sections of a Research Report and Related Critiquing Guidelines—cont'd**
Section	**Questions to Guide Evaluation**

Analysis of data (see Chapters 15 and 16)	1. What level of measurement is used to measure each of the major variables?
	 2. What descriptive or inferential statistics are reported?
	 3. Were these descriptive or inferential statistics appropriate to the level of measurement for each variable?
	 4. Are the inferential statistics used appropriate to the intent of the hypotheses?
	 5. Does the author report the level of significance set for the study? If so, what is it?
	 6. If tables or figures are used, do they meet the following standards?
	    a. They supplement and economize the text.
	    b. They have precise titles and headings.
	    c. They do not repeat the text.

Conclusions, implications, and recommendations (see Chapter 19)	1. If hypothesis testing was done, were the hypotheses supported or not supported? 2. Are the results interpreted in the context of the problem or purpose, hypothesis, and theoretical framework or literature reviewed? 3. What does the investigator identify as possible limitations or problems in the study related to the design, methods, and sample? 4. What relevance for nursing practice does the investigator identify, if any? 5. What generalizations are made? 6. Are the generalizations within the scope of the findings or beyond the scope of the findings? 7. What recommendations for future research are stated or implied?
Application and utilization for nursing practice (see Chapter 20)	1. Does the study appear to be valid? In other words, do its strengths outweigh its weaknesses? 2. Do other studies have similar findings? 3. What risks or benefits are involved for clients if the research findings are used in practice? 4. Is direct application of the research findings feasible in terms of time, effort, money, and legal–ethical risks? 5. How and under what circumstances are the findings applicable to nursing practice? 6. Should these results be applied to nursing practice? 7. Would it be possible to replicate this study in another clinical practice setting?

STYLISTIC CONSIDERATIONS

As an evaluator, you should be aware of several aspects of the world of publishing before you begin to critique research studies. First, different journals have different publication goals and target specific professional markets. For example, the *Canadian Journal of Nursing Research* publishes articles on the conduct or results of research in nursing. Although the *Canadian Oncology Nursing Journal* also publishes research articles, because its emphasis is broader, readers of this journal will also encounter clinical and theoretical articles relating to knowledge, experience, trends, and policies in oncological nursing. Consequently, the style and content of the manuscript will vary according to the type of journal to which it is being submitted.

Second, the author of a research article prepares the manuscript using both personal judgement and specific guidelines. *Personal judgement* refers to the researcher's expertise that is developed in the course of designing, executing, and analyzing the study. As a result of this expertise, the researcher is in a position to judge which content is most important to communicate to the profession. The decision is a function of the following:

- The research design: experimental or nonexperimental
- The focus of the study: basic or clinical
- The audience to whom the results will be most appropriately communicated

The guidelines are provided by each journal for preparing research manuscripts for publication and usually the following major headings are essential sections of a research manuscript or research report:

- Introduction
- Methodology
- Results
- Discussion

Depending on the stylistic considerations related to the author's preferences and the journal's requirements, the content included in each of the above mentioned sections is specific to those sections of the research report.

Stylistic variations (as factors influencing the presentation of the research study) are very distinct features of a research report and can deter from the focus of evaluating the reported research for **scientific merit**. Constructive evaluation is based on objective appraisal of the study's strengths and limitations. This step precedes consideration of the relative worth of the findings for clinical application to nursing practice. Judgements of the scientific merit of a research study are the hallmark of promoting a sound evidence base for quality nursing practice.

CRITIQUE #1 — The study "Using the Theory of Planned Behaviour to Predict Exercise Intention in Obese Adults" by François Boudreau and Gaston Godin, published in the *Canadian Journal of Nursing Research* (2007), is critiqued. The article is presented in its entirety and is followed by the critique on pages 437–438. (From *Canadian Journal of Nursing Research*, 39(2), 112–125. © McGill University School of Nursing. Reprinted with permission.)

USING THE THEORY OF PLANNED BEHAVIOUR TO PREDICT EXERCISE INTENTION IN OBESE ADULTS

François Boudreau, MSc, PhD (c)
Nursing Sciences Department
Université du Québec à Trois-Rivières, Trois-Rivières, Québec

Gaston Godin, PhD
Faculty of Nursing
Université Laval, Sainte-Foy, Québec

The purpose of this cross-sectional study was to use Ajzen's Theory of Planned Behaviour (TPB) as a theoretical framework for understanding the intention to be physically active among a group of obese individuals. Individuals (n = 96) classified as obese (BMI ≥ 30 kg/m²) completed a self-administered questionnaire assessing intention to be physically active and its theoretically related variables. The TPB explained 66% of the variance in physical activity intentions. Significant independent predictors of intention were perceived behavioural control (β = .40) and attitude (β = .36). The consideration of past behaviour (β = .32) explained an additional 7% of the variance. These findings support the idea that, in designing interventions for obese individuals, nurses should focus on developing skills to overcome barriers to physical activity and on developing a positive attitude towards this behaviour.

Keywords: Obesity, physical activity, intention, Theory of Planned Behaviour

Today, regular physical activity must be considered a critical part of the treatment for obesity. In primary care settings, nurses are in a position to assess and manage obesity in patients (Banning, 2005). However, one study found that only 32% of nurses believed they were effective in counselling to promote a change in lifestyle in order to reduce obesity (Steptoe, Doherty, Kendrick, Rink, & Hilton, 1999). According to Hardeman, Griffin, Johnston, Kinmonth, and Wareham (2000), health education interventions addressing the problem of obesity would be more effective if explicitly based on methods of behaviour modification that have shown to be effective in other contexts. For instance, in order to develop theory-based health education interventions to promote leisure-time physical activity in obese individuals, nurses should first identify the key correlates of the behaviour under study in the target population. This would enable nurses to identify the content of the intervention messages, select appropriate methods, and develop material specifically adapted to the characteristics of the target population. Such interventions would have greater likelihood of success.

It is reported in the literature that the Theory of Planned Behaviour (TPB) (Ajzen, 1991) "may have a valuable contribution to make to developing effective interventions aimed at behaviour change, especially among individuals where motivation to act cannot be taken for granted" (Hardeman et al., 2002, p. 151). According to the TPB, the proximal determinant of behaviour is the intention to adopt or not to adopt that behaviour, while the proximate determinants of the intention to adopt a behaviour are the individual's attitude, subjective norm, and perceived behavioural control with respect to adopting the behaviour. Attitude represents one's evaluation of the perceived benefits and drawbacks of adopting a given behaviour (e.g., "My doing physical activities in my free time during the next month would be good/bad"). Subjective norm reflects the perceived expectations of specific individuals or groups regarding one's adoption of a given behaviour (e.g., "In your opinion, are the people who are most important to you in favour or not in favour of your regular participation in one or more physical activities in your free time during the next month?"). Lastly, perceived behavioural control is determined by the individual's perception of the presence or absence of resources and opportunities as well as perceived obstacles and impediments regarding adoption of the target behaviour (e.g., "To me, participating in one or more physical activities in my free time during the next year appears difficult/easy"). Perceived behavioural control can also influence behaviour directly, when it closely approximates actual control.

In short, the TPB could prove useful for identifying the determinants of regular leisure-time physical activity among obese individuals. Identification of these determinants would, in turn, be useful in nursing practice for developing health education interventions aimed at promoting physical activity in these individuals. To the best of our knowledge, the TPB has not been applied in the study of exercise among obese individuals. Thus, the aim of this study was to use the TPB to examine intention to engage in regular physical activity among a group of obese individuals. The main research question was: *Can attitude, subjective norm, and perceived behavioural control explain physical activity intentions?* To address this question, the following hypotheses were formulated: 1. *A significant portion of variance will be explained by a combination of attitude, subjective norm, and perceived behavioural control. 2. The relative importance of attitude, subjective norm, and perceived behavioral control will vary.*

METHOD

Participants and Procedure

This study consisted of the secondary analysis of data from a cross-sectional survey on cardiovascular risk factors among a sample of the population served by a Local Community Health Service Centre in the province of Quebec, Canada. The goal of the survey was to determine the overall prevalence and distribution of cardiovascular risk factors. Briefly, a sample of 900 randomly selected individuals between the ages of 35 and 64 was identified. These individuals were mailed a package containing a self-administered questionnaire, a return envelope, and a covering letter—signed by the principal investigator and the health coordinator of the Local Community Health Service Centre—describing the purpose of the survey and soliciting the individual's cooperation. The recipients were advised that their responses would be confidential and that no name would appear on the questionnaire. All of the study procedures were approved by an ethics review board. Two follow-up reminders were sent, one after the first week and one after the fourth week. Overall, 558 completed questionnaires were returned, for a participation rate of 63%. Among the 558 respondents, 96 were classified as obese according to their BMI (≥ 30 kg/m^2).

Measures

The psychosocial variables assessed were intention, attitude, subjective norm, and perceived behavioural control. The chosen time frame of 1 year for measuring the psychosocial variables was the same as that used in a province-wide survey conducted by a Quebec government agency (Daveluy, Pica, Audet,

Courtemanche, & Lapointe, 2000). That survey was adapted to make the results comparable to those of the present population survey. In order to standardize the definition of physical activity for all participants, the following two statements were included at the top of each page of the questionnaire: "Physical activity includes all activities, such as sports, outdoor activities, physical fitness, and brisk walking," and "Participation in physical activity is considered regular when done for 20 to 30 minutes per session at least three times a week." Although the determinants of physical activity could vary according to the three components of physical activity (frequency, intensity, and duration) (Courneya & McAuley, 1994), the wording of the questions in this study was oriented towards frequency, as this dimension reflects the behavioural aspect.

Intention. Two items were used to assess intention. The first asked, "Do you intend to participate regularly in one or more physical activities for 20 to 30 minutes per session in your free time during the next year?" The response was recorded on a five-point scale (1 = definitely not, 5 = definitely). The second stated, "I intend to participate regularly in one or more physical activities for 20 to 30 minutes per session in my free time during the next year" (1 = strongly disagree, 5 = strongly agree). The two items correlated at .75 ($p < .01$) and the mean of the sum was taken as the intention score. Test-retest reliability for this question has been verified several times, with the values varying between .65 (Godin, Valos, Shephard, & Desharnais, 1987) and .77 (Valois, Godin, & Bertrand, 1992).

Attitude. Attitude towards adoption of the behaviour was measured on six five-point items on a semantic differential scale. Each of the six scales appeared following the statement "I think that participating regularly in one or more physical activities in my free time during the next year would be. . . ." The bipolar adjectives used were *unpleasant/pleasant, boring/interesting, useless/useful, tiresome/stimulating, disadvantageous/advantageous,* and *unreasonable/reasonable.* The score for attitude

was expressed as the average of the sum of the six pairs of adjectives. Internal consistency was verified using Cronbach's alpha coefficient; an appropriate value of .82 was found. Test-retest reliability for this measure has been reported as .81 (Valois et al., 1992).

Subjective Norm. The participants were asked the following question: "In your opinion, are the people who are most important to you in favour or not in favour of your participating regularly in one or more physical activities in your free time during the next year?" This item was measured on a five-point scale (1 = strongly not in favour, 5 = strongly in favour). Test-retest reliability for a measure similar to that used in this study produced a value of .66 (Courneya & McAuley, 1995).

Perceived Behavioural Control. Three items adapted from Nguyen, Potvin, and Otis (1997) were used to assess perceived behavioural control in the following format: "To me, participating in one or more physical activities in my free time during the next year appears. . ." *very difficult/very easy, complicated/straightforward, unachievable/achievable;* five-point scales were used. The mean of the three scales was taken as a composite score for PBC. Cronbach's alpha coefficient indicated an appropriate value of .92. Test-retest reliability of such a measure of perceived behavioural control is reported as .63 (Valois et al., 1992).

Past Behaviour. The role of past behaviour in the TPB as discussed by Conner and Armitage (1998) was retained on the basis of a meta-analytic review indicating that it may play an important role in predicting intention to be physically active (Hagger, Chatzisarantis, & Biddle, 2002). Past behaviour was assessed using a simple self-report question: "How often have you participated in one or more physical activities for 20 to 30 minutes per session during your free time in the last 3 months?" (1 = never, 2 = less than once a month, 3 = two or three times a month, 4 = once a week, 5 = twice a week, 6 = three times a week, 7 = four times a week).

This method of assessing behaviour is based on previous validated studies (Gionet & Godin, 1989; Godin, Jobin, & Bouillon, 1986). Test-retest reliability for this scale was .64 (Godin et al., 1986). In the previous studies, concurrent validity was established against measures of maximum oxygen intake (VO2 max), body fat, and muscular endurance.

Age, gender, and BMI were also assessed. Based on respondents' self-reported weight (kg) and height (m),[2] BMI was calculated as weight (kg)/height (m).[2] The weight classification recommended by the WHO Expert Consultation on Obesity was used: thus, BMI between 25.0 kg/m^2 and 29.9 kg/m^2 denoted "overweight" and BMI of 30.0 kg/m^2 or greater represented "obesity" (World Health Organization, 2000).

Statistical Analysis

The data were analyzed using the SPSS statistical package (Version 10.0). The hypotheses concerning TPB were tested according to Ajzen's (1991) recommendations. First, Pearson product-moment correlations were calculated to examine the interrelationships between the TPB variables and additional variables. Then, a hierarchical regression analysis was conducted to predict intention to be physically active based on the TPB variables and additional variables.

RESULTS

A total of 96 individuals were classified as obese based on their BMI (≥ 30). Four questionnaires were excluded because of missing data on the TPB variables. Thus, data analysis was based on the responses of 92 participants (49% female). The average age of the participants was 47.7 years ($SD = 7$); 29% of participants had completed post-secondary education, 58% had completed high school, and 13% had not completed high school. The measure of past behaviour indicated that 47.8% of respondents had not participated in any leisure-time physical activity during the previous 3 months, whereas 21.8% had been physically active three or more times per week.

Intercorrelations, mean scores, and standard deviations of the variables are presented in Table 19C1–1. The correlation matrix of the variables revealed positive correlations between intention and attitude ($r = .65, p < .01$), perceived behavioural control ($r = .72, p < .01$), and past behaviour ($r = .62, p < .01$). Subjective norm was weakly positively correlated with intention ($r = .25, p < .05$). No correlation was observed between intention and age ($r = .11, p > .05$), gender ($r = -.18, p > .05$), or BMI ($r = .14, p > .05$).

The results of the hierarchical regression analysis are presented in Table 19C1–2. In the first step,

TABLE 19C1–1	**Intercorrelations, Mean Scores, and Standard Deviations of the Theoretical Model and Additional Variables**									
	1	2	3	4	5	6	7	8	M	SD
1. Intention[a]	–	.65**	.25*	.72**	.62**	.11	-.18	.14	3.94	0.86
2. Attitude[a]		–	.33**	.44**	.31**	.04	-.11	.12	4.19	0.58
3. Subjective norm[a]			–	.19	.02	.01	.11	.02	4.25	0.82
4. Perceived behavioural control[a]				–	.46**	.06	-.16	.17	3.58	0.87
5. Past behaviour[b]					–	.18	-.14	.12	3.22	2.22
6. Age						–	-.24*	.07	47.74	6.97
7. Gender[c]							–	-.20	.51	0.50
8. BMI								–	33.89	4.33

[a]Mean score varying from 1 to 5.
[b]Mean score varying from 0 to 16 times per month.
[c]0 = female; 1 = male.
*$p < .05$; **$p < .01$.

TABLE 19C1–2	**Hierarchical Regression Analysis of Intention from Theoretical Model and Additional Variable**					
Predictor	R	R^2	ΔR^2	F for change	β^1	β^2
Step 1	.81	.66	.66	56.01*		
Attitude					.42*	.36*
Subjective norm					.01	.04
Perceived behavioural control					.53*	.40*
Step 2	.86	.73	.07	25.55*		
Past behaviour						.32*

$R^2 = .73$; $p < .0001$.
β^1: standardized regression coefficients for first step.
β^2: final standardized regression coefficient.

attitude and perceived behavioural control accounted for 66% of the variance in intention ($F(3,88) = 56.01$, $p < .0001$). In the second step, the addition of past behaviour added 7% of the explained variance in intention ($F(1,87) = 25.55$, $p < .0001$). In order of relative importance, the standardized regression coefficients indicated that perceived behavioural control ($\beta = .40$, $p < .0001$), attitude ($\beta = .36$, $p < .0001$), and past behaviour ($\beta = .32$, $p < .0001$) were the most important variables in predicting intention to be physically active.

DISCUSSION

The goal of this study was to verify the utility of the Theory of Planned Behaviour to predict the intention of obese people to participate in free-time physical activity on a regular basis. The results indicate that intention is associated firstly with perceived behavioural control and secondly with having a favourable attitude towards this behaviour. A third determinant, past behaviour (which is not part of the TPB), also helped to explain intention. Thus, the results of this study suggest that TPB is an appropriate theoretical framework for understanding the determinants of motivation to be physically active with respect to obese individuals. Also, though secondary to the main goal of the study, self-reports of recent physical activity indicate that nearly half of the respondents had a sedentary lifestyle. Only one person out of five reported participating in physical exercise on a regular basis.

Regarding the first hypothesis, a significant portion of the variance in intention ($R^2 = 66\%$) was explained by the TPB variables. This was higher than the average reported by Godin and Kok (1996) for prediction of exercise among different segments of the population; indeed, a value of 42% was derived from 21 applications regarding prediction of exercise intention. However, the regression values from individual studies varied from 13% to 66%. For instance, Biddle, Goudas, and Page (1994) (R^2 of .62), Ajzen and Driver (1992) (R^2 of .66), and Kimiecik (1994) (R^2 of .66) report values in the same range as that found in the present study. Therefore, the present observed value in terms of explained variance is not unusual.

Concerning the second hypothesis, it was observed that attitude ($\beta = .36$) and perceived behaviour ($\beta = .40$) had similar standardized regression coefficients. These results are consistent with those observed by Godin and Kok (1996) and Hagger et al. (2002) for application of the TPB in the context of physical activity. Subjective norm was not a significant determinant of intention to engage in leisure-time physical activity on a regular basis. Therefore, perceived social norm can be considered of little importance to obese individuals regarding intention to exercise. This observation is congruent with several reviews of the scientific literature showing a weak correlation between subjective norm and intention to adopt various behaviours (Armitage & Conner, 2001; Godin & Kok, 1996), including participation in physical activity (Hausenblas, Carron, & Mack, 1997).

Perceived behavioural control can be viewed as the combined influence of two components: self-efficacy (ease or difficulty of adopting a behaviour), and controllability (the extent to which engagement is up to the person) (see Ajzen, 2002, for a review). Therefore, the perception of ease or difficulty of adopting a behaviour depends on the individual's evaluation of (1) available opportunities, and (2) the presence or absence of the necessary time, money, or ability. For the obese person, there is true difficulty in moving, because of body weight. Thus, nurses working with obese clients should have them begin slowly, with light exercise, and to slowly add frequency, intensity, and duration as the person's physical abilities improve.

The intention of obese individuals to engage in regular physical activity was also explained by attitude. This suggests that respondents who expressed an intention to be physically active perceived more advantages than disadvantages to engaging in regular physical exercise. This finding is congruent with that of Sarkin, Johnson, Prochaska, and Prochaska (2001), who also found that for individuals with excess weight (BMI ≥ 25 kg/m^2), intention to engage in moderate physical activity was associated with the perceived advantages of exercising. Thus, in designing health education interventions, nurses should provide exercise-related information stressing the benefits of participating in some form of physical activity (Jones, Sinclair, & Courneya, 2003).

The additional contribution of past behaviour was in the same range as the values reported by Conner and Armitage (1998) following their TPB meta-analysis. These authors found that, after taking into account the TPB determinants, past behaviour explained a further 7.2%, on average, of the variance in intention. The role of past behaviour as a predictor of exercise intention has also been documented for various population subgroups (Blanchard, Courneya, Rodgers, Daub, & Knapik, 2002; Godin, Vezina, & Leclerc, 1989). The results of the present study with a group of obese individuals are in line with these observations. Although past exercise behaviour does not provide any

insights into intervention strategies, as discussed by Ajzen (1991), it does suggest that it is important for nurses to find ways of increasing obese individuals' number of active days so that these persons may strengthen their intention to adopt an active lifestyle. Indeed, in the present study the respondents who were physically active during the previous few months exhibited the strongest intention to exercise during the next year.

Limitations

This study has a number of limitations. Firstly, the classification of obese was based on self-reported height and weight. This may have underestimated the actual number of obese people. Indeed, it has been documented that height and weight are often overestimated and underestimated by respondents (Newell, Girgis, Sanson-Fisher, & Savolainen, 1999; Niedhammer, Bugel, Bonenfant, Goldberg, & Leclerc, 2000). Secondly, the assessment of physical activity was based on self-reported leisure-time physical activity. Even though the questionnaire that was used has been validated in several studies (e.g., Godin et al, 1986), an objective measure may be more appropriate for use with obese individuals (Westerterp, 1999). Thirdly, according to the TPB (Ajzen, 1991) the main constructs of attitude, subjective norm, and perceived behavioural control are determined by underlying beliefs (i.e., behavioural, normative, and control). Ultimately, these are the beliefs that guide the development of educational interventions. However, they were not elicited in this study, thus limiting the identification of the content of an intervention. Future studies should provide this important information. A final limitation was the cross-sectional design of the study and reliance on intention measure as the dependent variable. The scientific literature recognizes, however, that intention is a reliable predictor of future exercise behaviour. In fact, based on several applications of Ajzen's theory in the field of exercise behaviour, the explained variance of exercise by intention only was 27% (Godin & Kok, 1996). Consequently, an intention measure is an acceptable proxy for exercise behaviour.

Implications for Nursing Practice

Overall, the results of this study suggest that, in designing effective health education interventions to promote regular leisure-time physical activity in obese individuals, nurses should favour the development of a sense of control over behaviour. In other words, nurses should help obese individuals to develop the skills needed to overcome barriers. Nurses should also support the development of a positive attitude towards exercise. In this regard, a health education intervention that highlights positive outcomes and minimizes negative outcomes could be an appropriate approach. Also, from a public health perspective, nurses should endeavour not to place the overall responsibility exclusively on the obese person but to take his or her environment and social context into account.

Finally, in order to motivate obese individuals to initiate regular leisure-time physical activity, nurses should use innovative strategies for delivering health education messages. Telecommunication and computer technologies can be an ideal medium for promoting leisure-time physical activity (Marcus, Nigg, Riebe, & Forsyth, 2000). In this regard, a promising and relatively new approach in health education is computerized tailoring. According to Kreuter and Skinner (2000), tailoring can be defined as "any combination of information or change strategies intended to reach one specific person, based on characteristics that are unique to that person, related to outcome of interest, and have been derived from an individual assessment" (p. 1). It is interesting to note that this definition is congruent with the nursing process—that is, individualization of interventions based on the client's needs (Bakken, 2001). The results of a recent systematic review confirm the conclusions drawn in earlier reviews and position papers: tailoring is a promising means of promoting a health diet and possibly physical activity as well (Kroeze, Werkman, & Brug, 2006).

REFERENCES

Ajzen, I. (1991). The Theory of Planned Behavior. *Organizational Behaviour and Human Decision Processes, 50,* 179–211.

Ajzen, I. (2002). Perceived behavioral control, self-efficacy, locus of control, and the Theory of Planned Behavior. *Journal of Applied Social Psychology, 32,* 665–683.

Ajzen, I., & Driver, B. L. (1992). Application of the Theory of Planned Behavior to leisure choice. *Journal of Leisure Research, 24,* 207–224.

Armitage, C. J., & Conner, M. (2001). Efficacy of the Theory of Planned Behavior: A meta-analytic review. *British Journal of Social Psychology, 40,* 471–499.

Bakken, S. (2001). Interactive health communication technology: Where do clinical nursing interventions fit into the picture? *Applied Nursing Research, 14,* 173–175.

Banning, M. (2005). The management of obesity: The role of the specialist nurse. *British Journal of Nursing, 14,* 139–144.

Biddle, S., Goudas, M., & Page, A. (1994). Social-psychological predictors of self-reported actual and intended physical activity in a university workforce sample. *British Journal of Sports Medicine, 28,* 160–163.

Blanchard, C. M., Courneya, K. S., Rodgers, W. M., Daub, B., & Knapik, G. (2002). Determinants of exercise intention and behavior during and after phase 2 cardiac rehabilitation: An application of the Theory of Planned Behavior. *Rehabilitation Psychology, 47,* 308–323.

Conner, M., & Armitage, C.J. (1998). Extending the Theory of Planned Behavior: A review and avenues for further research. *Journal of Applied Social Psychology, 28,* 1429–1464.

Courneya, K. S., & McAuley, E. (1994). Are there different determinants of the frequency, intensity, and duration of physical activity? *Behavioral Medicine, 20,* 84–90.

Courneya, K. S., & McAuley, E. (1995). Reliability and discriminant validity of subjective norm, social support, and cohesion in an exercise setting. *Journal of Sport and Exercise Psychology, 17,* 325–337.

Daveluy, C., Pica, L., Audet, N., Courtemanche, F., & Lapointe, F. (2000). *Enquête sociale et de santé 1998.* Quebec: Institut de la statistique du Quebec.

Gionet, N. J., & Godin, G. (1989). Self-reported exercise behavior of employees: A validity study. *Journal of Occupational Medicine, 31,* 969–973.

Godin, G., Jobin, J., & Bouillon, J. (1986). Assessment of leisure time exercise behavior by self-report: A concurrent validity study. *Canadian Journal of Public Health, 77,* 359–362.

Godin, G., & Kok, G. (1996). The Theory of Planned Behavior: A review of its applications to health-related behaviors. *American Journal of Health Promotion, 11,* 87–98.

Godin, G., Valois, P., Shephard, R. J., & Desharnais, R. (1987). Prediction of leisure-time exercise behavior: A path analysis (LISRELV) model. *Journal of Behavioral Medicine, 10,* 145–58.

Godin, G., Vezina, L., & Leclerc, O. (1989). Factors influencing intentions of pregnant women to exercise after giving birth. *Public Health Reports, 104,* 188–195.

Hagger, M. S., Chatzisarantis, N. L. D., & Biddle, S. J. H. (2002). A meta-analytic review of the theories of reasoned action and planned behavior in physical activity: Predictive validity and the contribution of additional variables. *Journal of Sport and Exercise Psychology, 24,* 3–32.

Hardeman, W., Griffin, S., Johnston, M., Kinmonth, A. L., & Wareham, N. J. (2000). Interventions to prevent weight gain: A systematic review of psychological models and behaviour change methods. *International Journal of Obesity and Related Metabolic Disorders, 24,* 131–143.

Hardeman, W., Johnston, M., Johnston, D. W., Bonetti, D., Wareham, N. J., & Kinmonth, A. L. (2002). Application of the Theory of Planned Behaviour in behaviour change interventions: A systematic review. *Psychology and Health, 17,* 123–158.

Hausenblas, H. A., Carron, A. V., & Mack, D. E. (1997). Application of the theories of reasoned action and planned behavior to exercise behavior: A meta-analysis. *Journal of Sport and Exercise Psychology, 19,* 36–51.

Jones, L. W., Sinclair, R. C., & Courneya, K. S. (2003). The effects of source credibility and message framing on exercise intentions, behaviors, and attitudes: An integration of the elaboration likelihood model and prospect theory. *Journal of Applied Social Psychology, 33,* 179–196.

Kimiecik, J. (1994). Predicting vigorous physical activity of corporate employees: Comparing the theories of reasoned action and planned behavior. *Journal of Sport and Exercise Psychology, 14,* 192–206.

Kreuter, M. W., & Skinner, C. S. (2000). Tailoring: What's in a name? *Health Education Research, 15,* 1–4.

Kroeze, W., Werkman, A., & Brug, J. (2006). A systematic review of randomized trials on the effectiveness of computer-tailored education on physical activity and dietary behaviors. *Annals of Behavioral Medicine, 31,* 205–223.

Marcus, B. H., Nigg, C. R., Riebe, D., & Forsyth, L. H. (2000). Interactive communication strategies: Implications for population-based physical-activity promotion. *American Journal of Preventive Medicine, 19,* 121–126.

Newell, S. A., Girgis, A., Sanson-Fisher, R. W., & Savolainen, N. J. (1999). The accuracy of self-reported health behaviors and risk factors relating to cancer and cardiovascular disease in the general population. *American Journal of Preventive Medicine, 17,* 211–229.

Nguyen, M. N., Potvin, L., & Otis, J. (1997). Regular exercise in 30- to 60-year-old men: Combining the stages-of-change model and the Theory of Planned Behavior to identify determinants for targeting heart health interventions. *Journal of Community Health, 22,* 233–246.

Niedhammer, I., Bugel, I., Bonenfant, S., Goldberg, M., & Leclerc, A. (2000). Validity of self-reported weight and height in the French GAZEL cohort. *International Journal of Obesity and Related Metabolic Disorders, 24,* 1111–1118.

Sarkin, J. A., Johnson, S. S., Prochaska, J. O., & Prochaska, J. M. (2001). Applying the transtheoretical model to regular moderate exercise in an overweight population: Validation of stages of change measure. *Preventive Medicine, 33,* 462–469.

Steptoe, A., Doherty, S., Kendrick, T., Rink, E., & Hilton, S. (1999). Attitudes to cardiovascular health promotion among GPs and practice nurses. *Family Practice, 16,* 158–163.

Valois, P., Godin, G., & Bertrand, R. (1992). The reliability of constructs derived from attitude-behavior theories: An application of generalizability theory in the health sector. *Quality and Quantity, 26,* 291–305.

Westerterp, K. R. (1999). Assessment of physical activity level in relation to obesity: Current evidence and research issues. *Medicine and Science in Sports and Exercise, 31*(Suppl. 11), S522–525.

World Health Organization. (2000). *Obesity: Preventing and managing the global epidemic* (WHO Technical Report Series #894). Geneva: Author.

AUTHORS' NOTE

Comments or queries may be directed to François Boudreau, Nursing Sciences Department, Université du Québec à Trois-Rivières, P.O. Box 500, Trois-Rivières, Quebec G9A 5H7 Canada. Telephone: 819-376-5011, ext. 3465. Fax: 819-376-5048. E-mail: Francois.Boudreau@uqtr.ca.

INTRODUCTION TO CRITIQUE #1

The article "Using the Theory of Planned Behaviour to Predict Exercise Intention in Obese Adults" (Boudreau & Godin, 2007) is examined in terms of its quality and the potential usefulness of the findings for application to nursing practice.

Title

The title of the article captures the essence of the study succinctly.

Abstract

The abstract meets the requirements of a good abstract; it contains the purpose, the sample size, the method, the findings, and a short concluding statement.

Problem and Purpose

The authors stated that the overall objective of the study was "to use the TPB [theory of planned behaviour] to examine intention to engage in regular physical activity among a group of obese individuals" (Boudreau & Godin, 2007, p. 114). The significance of the problem was briefly stated as follows: "the TPB could prove useful for identifying the determinants of regular leisure-time physical activity among obese individuals . . . and has not been applied in the study of exercise among obese individuals" (Boudreau & Godin, 2007, p. 114). This problem statement is very brief and should present a more persuasive argument.

Review of Literature and Definitions

Although the literature review is very short, it establishes for the reader the importance of having nurses successfully assist clients in managing their obesity through behaviour modification. For example, the authors state that "health education interventions addressing the problem of obesity would be more effective if explicitly based on methods of behaviour modification that have shown to be effective in other contexts" (p. 113). Note, however, that only three studies were cited. The authors could have offered more explanation of the problem of obesity, which would have established greater significance to their present study; however, because the objective of the study was to apply the TPB to a new group of clients, the focus, instead was on the model.

The studies cited were within 10 years of the article's publication date, which means that the literature review was up-to-date. The authors used a number of primary sources (e.g., Ajzen, 1991) but also relied on some secondary sources regarding behaviour modification (e.g., Hardeman et al., 1999). The literature review provides an adequate basis for the present study as the review identified the need to use the TPB to develop theory-based health education interventions.

Development of a Conceptual Framework

The definitive conceptual framework of the study, the TPB, was explained. The authors defined the three proximate determinants of attitude, subjective norm, and perceived behavioural control toward intention. However, the underlying beliefs of the TPB—behavioural, normative, and control—were not explored in this study. A visual model of the TPB would have helped the reader understand which parts of the model were studied and which parts were omitted. Thus, the major variables for the study would be "intention," "attitude," "subjective norm," and "behavioural."

Hypotheses and Research Question

The authors explicitly stated the research question as follows (p. 114): "Can attitude, subjective norm, and perceived behavioural control explain physical activity intentions?" The two hypotheses were expressed as follows (p. 114): "A significant portion of variance will be explained by a combination of attitude, subjective norm, and perceived behavioural control" and "The relative importance of attitude, subjective norm, and perceived behavioural control will vary."

Sample

The sample consisted of 900 randomly selected individuals between the ages of 35 and 64 years. Of these, 558 individuals responded, yielding a response rate of 63%, which is remarkably high. It appears that the only inclusion criterion was a body mass index (BMI) greater than or equal to 30 kg/m². Power analysis was not done prior to the data collection or post hoc to determine the power of the test in having a sample size of 96. This omission is probably due to the limitations of using secondary data from a previous study. Because the data had already been collected, the sample size could not be increased and, thus, the power of the test could also not be increased.

Research Design

The authors stated that their study "consisted of the secondary analysis of data from a cross-sectional survey on cardiovascular risk factors among a sample of the population served by a Local Community Health Service Centre" in Quebec (p. 114). Details on the previous cross-sectional design were omitted. Later in the article, the authors stated that "the chosen time frame of 1 year for measuring the psychosocial variables was the same as that used in a province-wide survey . . ." (p. 115). This statement may lead the reader to think that the study used a longitudinal design, but data from these individuals were collected only once, although it probably took one year to obtain responses from all 96 individuals.

The independent or explanatory variables of this study are attitude, subjective norm, and perceived behavioural control. The dependent or outcome variable is intention.

Internal Validity

Although threats to internal validity are germane to experimental research, researchers need to pay attention to factors in a nonexperimental design that may potentially compromise a study. Possible threats to internal validity include history and mortality.

History is important to acknowledge in this age of widespread media campaigns directed at obesity. In this study, mortality could have been identified in terms of attrition rates, but was not appropriate here because the data were secondary and thus had already been collected.

Potential bias is associated with self-reports, which was acknowledged in the study under "Limitations."

External Validity

Generalizability is limited to the sample because the individuals were from a specific geographical area in Canada; thus, generalizing to other populations would be limited.

Legal–Ethical Issues

Ethical approval was received from an ethics review board. Because a health coordinator signed the cover letter, it can be inferred that approval for the study was obtained from the Local Community Health Service Centre. In many cases, smaller health agencies do not have an ethics review board and thus rely on the ethics approval process from a university or hospital.

The authors stated that the recipients' responses would be confidential and that no names appeared on the questionnaires.

Instruments

From the conceptual framework, the reader anticipates that the authors collected information on demographics, attitude, subjective norms, perceived behavioural control, and intention. The demographic information collected was age, gender, height, and weight, which were used to determine the BMI in keeping with the conceptual framework. Although the authors stated that "a province-wide survey conducted by a Quebec government agency . . . was adapted to make the results comparable to those of the present population" (p. 115), it is not clear what they meant—whether the items were changed or the two clarification statements on physical activity were added. It appears that from this survey, respondents were asked questions addressing intention, attitude, subjective norm, perceived behavioural control, and past behaviour. A detailed explanation of the content of the items of each survey was provided for the reader to understand their fit in the study. The scoring of the subscales was explained to help the reader understand the results.

Reliability and Validity

The reliability results of these separate constructs, attitude, subjective norm, and perceived behavioural control, were assessed or quoted from the literature, but no information was provided on the validity of the survey. Reliability is a necessary but not sufficient condition for validity (see Chapter 14). Validity is needed to determine whether the instrument measures what it is intended to measure. The reliability coefficients of these subscales ranged from adequate (.63) to high (.92). The internal consistency reliability was not stated for the subjective norm and the past behaviour subscales.

Analysis and Findings of the Data

The variables mentioned in the article are either on a nominal or interval scale of measurement. Gender and type of education are measured on a nominal scale, whereas age, BMI, attitude, subjective norm, perceived behavioural control, and past behaviour constitute interval levels of measurement.

Descriptive statistics were reported as means and standard deviations in both Table 19C1–1 and the text, where a small amount of repetition of the results highlighted the findings. Correlation analyses and level of significance (.05) were appropriately conducted for obtaining information on whether the association between the variables to proceed to regression analysis. The results to support the first hypothesis are listed in Table 19C1–1, and in the text, "attitude and perceived behavioural control accounted for 66% of the variance in

intention" (p. 117), and when "past behaviour" was added to the regression equation, another 7% was explained. The results to support the second hypothesis are in Table 19C1–2 and are discussed in the text as follows: "In order of relative importance, the standardized regression coefficients indicated that perceived behavioural control . . . attitude . . . and past behaviour . . . were the most important variables in predicting intention to be physically active" (p. 119).

Discussion

The findings were explained within the context of previous research and the TPB with the conclusion that "TPB is an appropriate theoretical framework for understanding the determinants of motivation to be physically active with respect to obese individuals" (p. 119).

Conclusions, Implications, and Recommendations

The first research hypothesis, that a significant portion of variance will be explained by a combination of attitude, subjective norm, and perceived behavioural control, is not fully supported in this study. The authors found that the subjective norm did not contribute to the variance and thus was not a predictor of the participants' intention. Past behaviour was added as a predictor variable and contributed to explaining intention.

The second research hypothesis, that the relative importance of attitude, subjective norm, and perceived behavioural control will vary, was again partially supported as the subjective norm was found not to be important in this group of individuals.

Interpretations of self-report biases, or not examining the underlying assumptions of the TPB toward the development of educational interventions, are consistent with the study's limitations. The ways in which this evidence can be integrated into developing nursing education interventions were clearly articulated.

CRITIQUE #2 The study "Self-Efficacy of Staff Nurses for Health Promotion Counselling of Patients at Risk for Stroke" by Cheryl Mayer, Mary-Anne Andrusyszyn, and Carroll Iwasiw, published in *AXON* (2005), is critiqued. The article is presented in its entirety and is followed by the critique on pages 452–454. (From *AXON* 26(4), 14–21. Reprinted with permission from *Canadian Journal of Neuroscience Nursing*.)

Codman Award Paper: Self-Efficacy of Staff Nurses for Health Promotion Counselling of Patients at Risk for Stroke

Cheryl Mayer, RN, MScN

Mary-Anne Andrusyszyn, RN, EdD

Carroll Iwasiw, RN, EdD

ABSTRACT

The effect of nurses' confidence to counsel patients at risk of stroke in selected health promotion areas: smoking cessation, exercise and nutrition was examined. Bandura's (1986) self-efficacy and Knowles' adult learning theories provided the theoretical underpinnings for the study. This was a quasi-experimental design in which neuroscience nurses (N=23) from a quaternary hospital completed questionnaires prior to, immediately after, and 2 months post completion of a self-directed learning manual (SDL). The researcher-designed manual was designed to enhance learning about the risk factors for stroke and the importance of stroke prevention. Along with reflective activities and pre-post test, strategies for counseling high-risk, stroke-prone individuals in areas of smoking cessation, exercise, and nutrition were also integrated.

The Health Promotion Counseling Self-Efficacy Scale (Tresolini, Saluja, and Stritter, 1995), consisting of 10 self-efficacy subscales relating to self-confidence in knowledge and ability to counsel in health promotion areas, was used to capture the nurses' self-report of self-efficacy. Using a 5-point Likert Scale,

nurses also rated their amount of agreement or disagreement about health promotion counseling in practice. Overall, self-efficacy levels for both knowledge and counseling increased significantly (p<.01) from pre- to immediately post completion of the manual, and decreased slightly at two-month follow-up. This pattern was evident in all health promotion areas measured except for knowledge in exercise (p=.015). Nurses' attitudes about aspects of health promotion practices correlated significantly (p<.05) at two-month follow-up with all health promotion areas. Results of this study support the usefulness of a self-directed learning manual as a teaching strategy for health promotion counseling of individuals at risk of stroke.

Keywords: professional education, self-directed learning, self-efficacy, stroke prevention

As the third leading cause of death and disability in Canada, stroke is one of the most devastating events experienced by humans (Bahle, 1998). Many stroke victims would rather die than live with disability and without dignity and quality in their lives. Increasing numbers of elderly persons, coupled with a doubling of stroke risk every decade after age 55, mandate attention to stroke risk reduction (Bahle). It is important to recognize that the consequences of stroke extend beyond individuals and families to Canadian society. The direct and indirect costs of stroke are estimated to be $2.7 billion annually (Canadian Stroke Systems Coalition, 2001).

Recognition of a transient ischemic attack (TIA) provides an opportunity to prevent a subsequent stroke (Gorelick, 1995, 2002). One of every three Canadians possesses at least one risk factor for heart disease and stroke, and the identification and management of modifiable risk factors in high-risk patients is one of the most important and effective strategies for reducing the incidence of this disease (Ingall, 2000). One strategy is to promote and facilitate the adoption of healthy lifestyle practices in these individuals.

The need to prepare health care professionals who are skilled in health promotion practices has become increasingly important (Laschinger, McWilliam, & Weston, 1999). Primary care nurses are crucial to identifying factors that place individuals at risk for suffering a stroke, and then counselling them about the signs and symptoms of impending stroke and the importance of gaining control over the risk factors (Schretzman, 2001).

To maintain competencies and enhance self-efficacy in this area, nurses need sources of information that are accessible, cost-effective, and supported by the workplace (Nolan, 1998; Purdy, 1997). However, traditional didactic methods of teaching, which have predominated in nurse education, have not generally fostered self-directed learning and reflection. Nor have they been practical in the current nursing work environment. Thus, a strategy that encourages self-directed learning and reflection, and can be completed at a time, place, and pace that fit the learner's schedule can be an alternative to traditional education (Knowles, 1990).

Self-directed learning can be achieved by reading professional journals, using the internet, attending professional workshops and seminars (DiMauro, 2000), and working through educational modules at an individually determined pace, without the aid of an instructor (Holtzman, 1999). It is reasonable to suggest that a self-directed learning manual may be an effective educational strategy to promote the self-efficacy of nurses for counselling patients at risk of stroke. The purpose of this study, therefore, was to examine the effect of a self-directed learning manual on neuroscience nurses' self-efficacy for counselling patients identified as being at risk for stroke.

THEORETICAL FRAMEWORK

Knowles's (1990) adult learning theory and Bandura's (1986) self-efficacy theory provided the theoretical frameworks for this study. Adult learning theory, or andragogy, posits that adults move from dependency to self-directness, reflect upon their past experiences as sources for learning, are ready to learn when placed in new roles or situations, and want to apply any new knowledge gained using a problem-solving approach (Knowles, 1990). Adults are ready to learn once they identify a need to know something to complete a task. Successful task completion requires enhanced self-esteem and a belief in one's self. Internal priorities such as increased job satisfaction can enhance self-esteem or build a sense of accomplishment or self-efficacy through goal achievement. Knowles (1990) suggested that programs should be developed using these principles and that educators should establish an atmosphere for learning that is cooperative in nature. Further, he proposed that educators should: encourage learners to assess their own learning needs, base learning objectives on these assessments, plan varying activities to achieve the objectives, and allow learners to evaluate if the learning was successful. Thus, educators become facilitators as they support a shift from a didactic or teacher-driven model to a self-directed learning approach.

According to Bandura (1986), self-efficacy is an individual's perception of confidence in one's own ability to perform a specific task or behaviour, and is acquired through an individual's exploration and processing of four sources of efficacy: performance accomplishments or mastery experiences, vicarious experiences or symbolic role-modeling, verbal persuasion, and emotional and physiological arousal. Performance accomplishments or mastery experiences provide immediate evidence of whether or not one can succeed at a particular behaviour; it is the strongest predictor of self-efficacy. Past successful experiences tend to raise self-efficacy and unsuccessful experiences tend to lower it. Once experience and success have created a strong sense of efficacy in an individual, failure is unlikely to affect it. Vicarious experiences gained by observing another person's successes and failures, especially one who is perceived to be similar, such as a peer, tend to raise self-efficacy to execute the particular behaviour. Understanding how one's emotional state or physiological factors (stress, fatigue, arousal, aches, pains, or fear) can subconsciously debilitate performance, and receiving positive feedback from a credible individual (verbal persuasion) can raise an individual's self-efficacy to execute a behaviour successfully.

The information individuals use to gauge their sense of efficacy must be processed and interpreted (Bandura, 1986). This cognitive processing plays a powerful role in the final judgments of efficacy. Self-efficacy judgments determine how much effort individuals will expend on a task and how long they will persevere at completing it. For individuals to execute a task successfully, they must believe they can perform the behaviour that leads to the desired outcome. Before they can believe they can perform the behaviour, however, they must acquire the necessary knowledge to execute it. Strategies must be put in place that will facilitate the development of this knowledge and perceptions of self-efficacy.

Educational strategies that incorporate the sources of efficacy information, such as: combining explanations with modeling, providing information on specific strategies, setting specific short-term and long-term goals, and giving explicit feedback to individuals about their performance can enhance self-efficacy development (Laschinger & Tresolini, 1999). In the current study, a self-directed learning manual, developed according to principles of Adult Learning Theory (Knowles, 1990) provided the sources of efficacy information (Bandura, 1986).

LITERATURE REVIEW

Research and theoretical literature about nurses' self-directed learning, nurses' self-efficacy for health promotion, self-efficacy in other contexts, and stroke prevention and the nurse's role, were reviewed. Most relevant literature was from the 1990s, possibly reflective of a time in health care when resources were limited and nontraditional approaches for staff education were developed.

Nurses' Self-Directed Learning

The most common definition of self-directed learning is that of Knowles (1975): a process in which individuals take the initiative with or without the help of others in diagnosing their learning needs, formulating learning goals, identifying human and material resources for learning, choosing and implementing appropriate learning strategies, and evaluating learning outcomes. From this, self-directed learners have been characterized as possessing maturity; able to identify learning needs, objectives, resources, and strategies; capable of pursuing learning strategies and evaluating learning outcomes (Iwasiw, 1987). Nurses who are unable to direct their own learning will not have the skills necessary to meet changes in health care (O'Shea, 2003).

Self-directed learning is a collaborative process between learners and teachers (Hewitt-Taylor, 2001), and to be self-directed in continuing education, learners must be able to seek, analyze and utilize information effectively (Lunyk-Child, et al., 2001). Didactic teaching methods may not be an efficient strategy for self-directed learners (Nolan & Nolan, 1997a).

In two studies, registered nurses were reported to spend 152 hours (Dixon, 1991) and 217 hours (Emblen & Gray, 1990) in continuing professional learning activities in one year. As well, nurses scored significantly higher on a scale measuring readiness for self-directed learning than students in law and adult education (Oddi, 1988). These results suggest that nurses tend to be self-directed and motivated to seek additional education.

In addition to self-directed learning, a self-paced strategy may be effective for nursing staff development (O'Very, 1999). Self-paced learning is a method that takes the training to the individual and presents information in a brief, compartmentalized form that allows learners to complete according to their own schedule. It incorporates the adult learning principles of autonomy and self-direction, and provides a convenient way for health care providers to continue learning (Holtzman, 1999; Jenkins, Carlson, & Herrick, 1998; Sparling, 2001). Although initial design and implementation can be time-consuming, these manuals can be cost-effective. Lipe et al. (1994) demonstrated a restoration of 4.5 full-time equivalents per year from the classroom back to the patient care area, when nurses completed learning activities on their own time or during slow times on their units. Additionally, they cited an increase in compliance with mandatory inservice programs from 40% to 95%.

In a study addressing the learning needs of nurses upgrading their education from diploma to degree status, Morris (1999) compared the effectiveness of self-study and didactic sessions. Students in the didactic group (n=6) show a slightly higher improvement in knowledge than self-study students (n=5). In response to open-ended questions, the self-study group reported they like the opportunity for self-pacing.

Continuing education for credentialing of nurses working in a maternal/newborn unit in the military was provided efficiently and effectively through self-study modules that spanned a year. By 2001, the program had been established for 10 years and involved 460 hospitals and more than 9,000 nurses. The programs were theory-based, cost-effective, and portable. Practice hours were not lost because of staff leaving the work area for educational sessions, and staff appreciated the relatively low cost and the ability to complete the manual at a time and place of their choosing. Close to 90% of students achieved a mark of 90% on regular testing. However, accommodating different educational backgrounds of participating nurses and maintaining motivation for test completion were challenges (Rivero, 2001).

Nurses' Self-Efficacy for Health Promotion

Health promotion is a concept long emphasized in nursing education and self-efficacy for health promotion counselling has been studied. Laschinger and Tresolini (1999) compared the self-efficacy of third year baccalaureate nursing students (n=41) with fourth year medical students (n=60) for their knowledge and ability to engage in health promotion counselling. The Health Promotion Counselling Self-Efficacy Scale (HPCSES) developed by Tresolini, Saluja, and Stritter (1995) was used. Nursing students were significantly more efficacious than medical students on both overall knowledge and ability to counsel patients about health promotion.

Using a modified version of the HPCSES (Tresolini, et al., 1995) Laschinger et al., (1999) examined self-efficacy to counsel among nursing and medical students attending a Canadian University in a two-group, pre-post design. Nursing students' (n=11) self-efficacy scores for counselling were significantly higher than medical students' (n=31) scores, with the difference sustained at three-month follow-up (t40=2.30, p=0.05). Although the sample size was small, the study provided useful information about the importance of incorporating a health promotion focus in the professional curriculum.

Other Self-Efficacy Studies

Self-efficacy theory has been used as a framework to evaluate continuing education in nursing. Davis and Hodnett (2002) assessed labor and delivery nurses' self-efficacy and views for labor support, and described nurses' perception of factors assisting and preventing the provision of labor support. Continuing education for advanced practice in pharmacology has been evaluated using self-efficacy theory (Murdock & Neafsey, 1995; Neafsey & Shellman, 2002; Neafsey, 1998). Neafsey concluded that measurement of self-efficacy was a useful adjunct in post-instruction evaluation and may be a cost-effective alternative to longitudinal impact evaluation.

In the clinical setting, Ockene et al., (2000, 2002) concluded, from studies addressing relapse and maintenance issues for smoking cessation, that predictors of relapse included low self-efficacy, and that brief interventions during medical visits were cost-effective and increased self-efficacy. Other self-efficacy studies include activity levels following cardiac surgery (Gortner & Jenkins, 1990), family caregivers' adaptation to the stresses of the role (DiBartolo, 2002), quality of life post-stroke (Robinson-Smith, 2002), adherence to treatment regimens and preventative behaviours in patients with auto immune deficiency disorder (Demmer, 2003; Murphy, Lu, Martin, Hoffman, & Marelich, 2002; Simoni, Frick, Lockhart, & Liebovitz, 2002), and the effectiveness of health promotion counselling for overweight adolescent nursing students in Taiwan (Chen, et al., 2001).

Stroke Prevention and Role of the Nurse

Hakim, Silver, & Hodgson (1998) proposed that best-practice stroke care in Canada must include prevention. Sacco (2001) published an account of controlled trials that demonstrated stroke risk can be reduced by blood pressure control, lipid lowering agents, surgery for carotid stenosis, warfarin for atrial fibrillation, and anti-platelet agents. This account also listed what is currently known about modifiable risk factors, i.e., hypertension, atrial fibrillation, other cardiac diseases, hyperlipidemia, diabetes, cigarette smoking, physical inactivity, carotid stenosis, and TIA.

Recognition of TIA and the identification and management of modifiable risk factors are the most important and effective strategies for reducing the incidence of this disease (Ingall, 2000). Based on literature examining the success of nurse-led clinics in cardiac disease, Schretzman (2001) concluded that there is at present a window of opportunity to develop the role of the nurse in the secondary prevention of stroke. How to facilitate the development and assess the effectiveness of this role has not been researched.

Summary

Studies of nursing students' self-efficacy for health promotion have been conducted. However, staff nurses' self-efficacy for counselling and means to enhance their self-efficacy for health promotion, have not been investigated. Although studies are limited in number, theory-based, self-directed learning manuals meant to be completed at a time, place, and pace of the learner's choosing are effective in professional education. They are portable, cost-effective, and widely accepted by nurses.

Self-efficacy is a reliable predictor of behaviour change in a variety of contexts. In stroke prevention, high-risk individuals can be targeted for specific health promotion programs. However, nurses' confidence to undertake this counselling is not known. It is reasonable, therefore, to determine the self-efficacy of neuroscience nurses to deliver risk factor counselling to patients at risk of stroke and to assess the influence of a self-directed learning manual on their self-efficacy.

HYPOTHESES AND RESEARCH QUESTION

The purpose of this study was to evaluate the self-efficacy of staff nurses to deliver risk factor modification counselling, after completion of a self-directed learning manual, to patients on a general neuroscience unit who have been identified as being at risk for stroke.

Hypotheses

Upon completion of a self-directed learning manual, immediate post self-efficacy scores (time two) will be significantly higher than pre self-efficacy scores (time one/baseline) in neuroscience nurses delivering health promotion counselling.

There will be no difference in the self-efficacy scores two months after completing the manual (time three) when compared to immediate post self-efficacy scores (time two). There will be a positive correlation between self-efficacy scores and attitudes about risk factor counselling.

Research Question

What is the relationship between neuroscience nurses' post-test self-efficacy scores and selected demographic variables?

METHODS

Design

A quasi-experimental, pre-post test, one-group design, was used to assess the self-efficacy of registered nurses (RNs) employed as staff nurses on a neuroscience unit in a quaternary care hospital to engage in counselling with patients at risk for stroke. Nurses completed a researcher-designed, self-directed learning manual focused on three areas of risk reduction: smoking, nutrition, and exercise. The subjects were their own controls.

The manual, based on the principles of adult learning theory, incorporated the sources of efficacy information and contained pre- and post-tests for assessing learning needs. Included were activities to enhance learning, promote critical thinking and reflection, encourage users to value and share experiential learning, and guide users to evaluate the success of counselling. Literature from medical and nursing journals about stroke prevention, risk factor identification and management was evidence-based and current. The warning signs and symptoms of TIA, risk factors for developing vascular disease, and strategies to promote smoking cessation, exercise, and proper nutrition were addressed. Expert faculty critiqued the manual at each stage of development for its consistency with the foundational theories and readability. Experts in stroke care reviewed the manual for content relevance. The manual was to be completed at a time, place and pace of each nurse's choosing.

Sample

Convenience sampling was used to recruit nurses from the neuroscience unit at one quaternary hospital with an all-RN staff. Envelopes (N=76) containing a letter of information detailing the study expectations, demographic questionnaire, baseline self-efficacy questionnaire, and consent form were placed in all nurses' mailboxes. With an alpha level of 0.05 (two-tailed), power of 80%, and a standard deviation for the difference score of 0.5, a sample size of 22 was required to detect a 10% change (absolute change of 0.3) in the pre-post self-efficacy score. The original sample consisted of 27 participants with a final data-producing sample of 23 (30.3%) nurses.

Instrumentation

The Health Promotion Counselling Self-Efficacy Scale (HPCSE) developed by Tresolini, Saluja, and Stritter (1995), that consists of 10 self-efficacy subscales: five relating to self-confidence in knowledge of three areas of health promotion and five relating to confidence in ability to convey this knowledge to patients in a clinical setting, was used in this study. Alpha reliability coefficients for knowledge and counselling subscales for each health domain across three data collection time points ranged from [0.71 to 0.94 (Laschinger, et al., 1999)]. Scale items referred to behaviours related to maintaining health in three areas: smoking, nutrition, and exercise. Counselling self-efficacy scores for each health promotion areas were created by summing and averaging items measuring confidence in nurses' ability to counsel clients. Knowledge self-efficacy scores for each health promotion areas were computed in the same manner. Averaged subscale scores were computed. Response scales ranged from one to four with high scores indicating high self-efficacy. At baseline, Cronbach's alpha reliability coefficient on all scales was acceptable at .81.

Five items designed to assess the contribution of sources or enhancers of efficacy information to nurses' confidence were measured on a four-point Likert-type scale. A high score indicated a strong perceived contribution of a particular learning experience or source of efficacy information to nurses' confidence in health promotion counselling. Attitudes of health promotion behaviour were assessed by asking the extent of agreement of disagreement to four questions about the importance of health promotion, using a five-point Likert scale (Laschinger, et al., 1999).

Data Collection Procedures

Approval from the Institutional Ethics Review Board, permission from the nursing manager of the clinical neuroscience unit and the hospital's professional practice leader of nursing were obtained. A questionnaire package was placed in nurses' individual mailboxes. Signed consent forms and the demographic and baseline self-efficacy questionnaires were returned to the administrative assistant (AA) of the stroke clinic who assigned a code to each participant. The AA delivered the manuals and the post-manual (time two) questionnaire to participants, who were asked to complete the learning manual and return the time two questionnaire within six weeks. At six weeks, the AA sent a reminder letter and a new questionnaire to those who had not returned a completed questionnaire. Two months after receiving the completed time two questionnaire, the AA mailed the time three questionnaires and subsequent reminder as needed.

Data Analysis

The Statistical Package for Social Sciences Program (SPSS) (Version 10 SPSS Inc., 1999) was used for analysis. Four of the 27 (15%) did not complete the time two or time three questionnaires even after being sent a reminder letter.

Frequency counts were compiled and estimated proportions were reported for all categorical demographic data such as age, sex, years in nursing practice, whether the participants were involved in continuing education, and roles outside the workplace. The summated scores of each scale were grouped according to concepts. Subscale means and standard deviations for each of three time points were computed; the assumption was made that data from the summated rating scales could justifiably be treated as interval rather than ordinal data (Nullay, 1978).

Hypotheses one and two: Single factor, repeated-measures analyses of variance (ANOVA) were conducted, using an alpha level of .01, to determine if there was a significant effect for the influence of the self-directed learning manual on the self-efficacy of nurses to counsel individuals at risk of stroke. Where a significant effect existed, Tukey's post hoc procedures were employed.

Hypothesis three and research question: Pearson Product-Moment Correlations were computed to determine if significant relationships existed between nurses' attitudes about health promotion and self-efficacy scores at each time point. Relationships between demographic variables (age, sex, years of practice as an RN, educational preparation, years in neuroscience nursing, enrolment in an educational program, and other roles and responsibilities) and post-test self-efficacy scores were determined in the same way.

RESULTS

Sample Description

In the data-producing sample of 23 participants (30% response rate), all but two were female. Most participants had college preparation (n = 18) with three participants having a baccalaureate degree. Two received their nursing education in a hospital-based program. Their ages ranged from 22 to 60 years (M = 37.11, SD = 10.94) with the number of years in nursing practice ranging from one to 30 (M = 12.17, SD = 10.02). Thirteen participants (57%) were involved in additional educational activities. Of the 13 who indicated they were involved in additional roles, 61.5% (n = 8) were involved in childcare, 7.7% (n = 1) in eldercare and 30.8% (n = 4) in roles 'other' than the above. These 'other' roles were not described.

Hypotheses Testing

Means and standard deviation scores for knowledge and counselling self-efficacy at time one, time two, and time three are presented in Table 19C2–1. Overall, scores for both knowledge and counselling self-efficacy increased from time one to time two and decreased slightly at time three.

TABLE 19C2–1 Knowledge and Counselling Self-Efficacy Scores* Across Time (N=23)		
	Time 1	Time 2	Time 3
Self-Efficacy	Mean (SD)	Mean (SD)	Mean (SD)
Knowledge			
Smoking	2.46 (.67)	3.67 (.67)	3.52 (.56)
Exercise	2.78 (.54)	3.66 (1.74)	3.47 (.56)
Nutrition	2.61 (.65)	3.24 (.70)	3.48 (.65)
Counselling			
Smoking	2.38 (.64)	3.45 (1.01)	3.44 (.56)
Exercise	2.62 (.62)	3.50 (1.53)	3.41 (.64)
Nutrition	2.50 (.68)	3.14 (.77)	3.37 (.77)

*Scale range 1-4

As predicted in hypotheses one and two, neuroscience nurses' self-efficacy for counselling was significantly higher at time two and unchanged at time three. The hypotheses were supported.

Smoking Cessation Knowledge and Counselling Self-Efficacy. The repeated measures ANOVA revealed a significant effect for nurses' smoking cessation knowledge [$F(1.47, 32.23) = 9.22, p < .01$] and counselling self-efficacy [$F(2, 44) = 18.44, p < .01$] over time. Tukey's post-hoc procedure (HSD = 0.89; a = .05 and HSD = 0.49; a = .05 respectively) revealed that time two and three scores were significantly higher than time one scores. The effect size (h2) for within-subjects was calculated. Approximately 18% of the variance of scores for knowledge self-efficacy and 31% of the variance of scores for counselling self-efficacy were explained by time. The h2 values (0.18 and 0.31) are the equivalent of an f (effect size) value of .47 and .67 respectively and represent a large effect size (Cohen, 1988).

Exercise Knowledge and Counselling Self-Efficacy. For exercise knowledge self-efficacy, the repeated measures ANOVA revealed an effect approaching significance [$F(1.25, 27.50) = 4.61, p = .015$]. Tukey's post-hoc procedure (HSD = 0.96; a = .05) revealed this difference to be between time one and time two (0.88). There was no significant difference between time two and three scores. The effect size for within-subjects (h2=0.11) is equivalent to an f value of .35 [moderate to large effect (Cohen, 1988)].

The analysis revealed a significant effect [$F(1.39, 30.65) = 7.17, p < .01$] for exercise counselling self-efficacy. Tukey's post-hoc procedure (HSD = 0.76; a = .05) revealed that time two and three scores were significantly higher than time one scores, with no significant difference between time two and three scores. The effect size for within subjects (h2 = 0.14) was calculated. Approximately 14% of the variance of scores for exercise counselling self-efficacy can be explained by time. The h2 value of .14 is the equivalent of an f (effect size) value of .40 or borderline large effect size (Cohen, 1988).

Nutrition Knowledge and Counselling Self-Efficacy. The repeated measures ANOVA revealed a significant effect for nurses' nutrition knowledge [$F(2, 44) = 27.80, p < .01$)] and counselling self-efficacy [$F(2, 44) = 23.56, p < .01$] over time. Tukey's post-hoc procedure (HSD = 0.29; a = .05 and HSD = 0.32; a = .05 respectively) revealed that time two and three scores were significantly higher than time one scores. There was no significant difference between time two and three scores. The effect size (h2) for within subjects was calculated. Approximately 24% of the variance of scores for nutrition knowledge self-efficacy and 20% of the variance of scores for nutrition counselling self-efficacy were explained by time. The h2 values (0.24 and 0.20) are the equivalent of an f (effect size) value of .32 (medium effect size) and .50 (large effect size) respectively (Cohen, 1988).

As predicted in hypothesis three, there was a positive correlation between self-efficacy scores and attitudes about risk factor counselling. Pearson Product-Moment Correlations are presented in Table 19C2–2. All time three correlations were significant.

The research question asked if there was a relationship between neuroscience nurses' post-test self-efficacy scores and selected demographic variables. Pearson Product-Moment Correlations between post-test self-efficacy scores and selected demographic values (age, gender, education, years in nursing practice and additional responsibilities) did not reveal any significant relationships.

SUMMARY OF RESULTS

With the exception of exercise knowledge self-efficacy scores at time two, significant differences were found in the nurses' knowledge and counselling self-efficacy scores over time. There were significant increases between time one and two scores and no significant differences between time two and three scores. Despite the relatively small sample size, the effect size magnitude was mainly moderate to large. The relationship between nurses' attitudes and self-efficacy scores correlated positively and significantly at time three. There were no significant relationships between post self-efficacy scores and the selected demographic variables.

DISCUSSION

Although the advantages of using a self-directed learning manual as an educational strategy to enhance professional education have been studied (Holtzman, 1999; O'Very, 1999; Rivera, 2001), this is the first known study to examine the self-efficacy of neuroscience nurses to execute a behaviour after completing such a manual. Except for exercise knowledge self-efficacy, the nurses' knowledge and risk factor counselling self-efficacy following completion of a self-directed learning manual was increased. This study supports the use of a self-directed manual to increase knowledge and counselling self-efficacy, and validates aspects of Bandura's self-efficacy theory.

Generally, nurses' confidence in their knowledge was higher than their confidence about counselling. These findings are consistent with those of Laschinger and Tresolini (1999) and Laschinger et al., (1999), and can be partially explained by Bandura's (1986) notion of self-efficacy magnitude. Specifically, individuals may have high self-efficacy for less difficult aspects of a set of behaviours.

While there was no significant improvement in exercise knowledge self-efficacy, exercise counselling self-efficacy scores were significantly increased. A possible explanation is that nurses initially were confident about exercise knowledge and the manual did not contribute any additional knowledge. Since prior knowledge was not measured, the manual may not have contained the appropriate learning materials

TABLE 19C2–2	**Pearson Product-Moment Correlations Between Health Promotion Attitudes and Self-Efficacy Scores at Three Time Points (N=23)**		
	Correlations		
	Attitudes about health promotion		
Self-Efficacy	Time 1	Time 2	Time 3
Smoking Cessation			
Knowledge	.15	.21	.62*
Counselling	.17	.01	.58*
Exercise			
Knowledge	.03	.32	.68*
Counselling	.17	−.17	.60*
Nutrition			
Knowledge	.32	.26	.61*
Counselling	.30	.20	.59*

*p=.05

or sources to facilitate an improvement in the nurses' overall knowledge. It may be difficult to increase exercise knowledge through readings alone. Open-ended questions or an analysis regressing the nurses' health promotion subscales on items intended to assess the sources of efficacy information provided by the self-directed learning manual might have been helpful. Interestingly, there is a noticeable difference in the standard deviations at time two for both exercise knowledge and exercise counselling self-efficacy (1.74 and 1.53 respectively). This deviation may partially explain why there was no significant finding for exercise knowledge self-efficacy.

Nurses' self-efficacy levels decreased slightly but not significantly from post-completion of the manual to two-month follow-up. The pattern was consistent across the three health promotion areas and provides support for the utility of the manual. Measurement of self-efficacy has been found to be a useful adjunct in post-instruction evaluation of continuing education (Neafsey, 2002) and may be a cost-effective alternative to longitudinal impact evaluation. These findings may be explained by the theory. Bandura (1986) stated that once experience and success have created a strong sense of efficacy in an individual, there is reason to believe that the specific behaviour will hold up over time.

There was a positive correlation between self-efficacy scores and attitudes about health promotion (hypothesis three) at time three. Bandura (1986) stated that self-efficacy beliefs serve as motivators for engaging in and persisting with specific behaviours. Health promotion is a process. It might be that nurses had time to use knowledge, implement counselling, and receive feedback. Performance attainment may have led to more positive attitudes. From a methodological perspective, it is not known how attentive to detail the nurses were when reading and answering the questions. Many were sent reminder letters and some may have hurriedly completed the questionnaires. When using a questionnaire, it can only be assumed the responses are an accurate indication of behaviours.

No notable differences were found between the nurses' post-test self-efficacy scores and selected demographic variables. This may have been because the sample size was too small for correlations to emerge.

In summary, after completion of a researcher developed, self-directed learning manual, the nurses' self-efficacy to counsel patients at risk for stroke and attitudes about health promotion increased significantly, and the increase was maintained. The results of this study suggest that learning experiences that incorporate focused sources of efficacy information can have an impact on health promotion counselling self-efficacy. The consistency of the results provides encouraging support for the use of Bandura's theory (1986) as a framework to guide strategies to develop health promotion skills of health professionals (Laschinger & Tresolini, 1999).

LIMITATIONS

The results of this study, although encouraging, must be viewed with caution. The sample consisted of neuroscience nurses in a single quaternary hospital who may not be comparable to nurses in general units or hospitals where exposures to stroke care experiences may vary. Future studies could be expanded to include nurses in other hospitals and other neuroscience units. Even though self-directed learning manuals are useful, it is important to remember that they may not be congruent with all learning styles or previous educational experiences. As well, the manual was not developed in accordance with all tenets of self-directed learning. For some nurses, having to complete the manual within six weeks may not have provided a comfortable pace. The study was based on self-reported confidence levels, performance was not observed or evaluated. Seventy per cent of nurses on the unit did not participate. These nurses may have perceived they had sufficient knowledge in this area or were overworked and did not have extra time in which to participate in a research study. In this study, the nurses' prior knowledge of the subject material or prior health promotion knowledge were not measured. As a self-directed, volunteer sample, the nurses who did respond may be a special group who are self-directed and value continuing education and research. This may limit the generalizability of the results and the potential usefulness of the self-directed learning manual as an educational strategy to a varied population.

There was only one follow-up two months after completion of the module. Even though self-efficacy to deliver health promotion counselling was improved and held up over time, it is not known if this would be sustained over a longer period. However, since the study was based on the assumptions of self-efficacy theory, these limitations may be offset (Laschinger & Tresolini, 1999). Despite these limitations, the results provide previously unavailable data on the self-efficacy of neuroscience nurses to counsel individuals at risk of stroke and provide a basis for future research.

CONCLUSIONS

Despite limitations in the study design, neuroscience nurses' self-efficacy in knowledge and counselling in selected health promotion areas increased significantly after completion of a self-directed learning manual. As self-efficacy scores improved, so did attitudes about health promotion in daily practice. Overall, the self-directed learning manual appeared to provide nurses with the appropriate learning experiences, and encouraged them to observe counselling and take opportunities to practise counselling. In conclusion, the results support Knowles's (1990) adult learning theory, Bandura's (1986) self-efficacy theory, and the potential future use of these theories as frameworks to guide educational strategies for continuing education for professional nurses.

ABOUT THE AUTHORS

Cheryl Mayer, RN, MScN, is the advanced practice nurse for the secondary prevention clinic for stroke at London Health Sciences Centre and Mary-Anne Andrusyszyn, RN, EdD and Carroll Iwasiw, RN, EdD, are associate professors in the School of Nursing at the University of Western Ontario, London, ON. They are co-founding editors of the International Journal of Nursing Education Scholarship. If you have any questions or comments about the paper, please contact Cheryl Mayer, Urgent TIA Clinic/Stroke Prevention Program, LHSC/University Campus, London, Ontario N6A 5A5, (519) 663-3674 (office), Cheryl.Mayer@lhsc.on.ca

REFERENCES

Bahle, J. (1998). Stroke prevention screening program. *Journal of Vascular Nursing, 16*(2), 35–37.

Bandura, A. (1986). *Social foundations of thought and action: A social cognitive theory.* Englewood Cliffs, NJ: Prentice Hall.

Canadian Stroke Systems Coalition. (2001). Creating a Canadian stroke system. *Canadian Medical Association Journal, 164,* 1853–1855.

Chen, M., Huang, L., Wang, E. K., Cheng, N., Hsu, C., Hung, L., & Shiao, Y. (2001). The effect of health promotion counselling for overweight adolescent nursing students in Taiwan. *Public Health Nursing, 18,* 350–356.

Cohen, J. (1992). A power primer. *Psychological Bulletin, 112*(1), 155–159.

Cohen, J. (1998). *Statistical power analysis for the behavioral sciences* (2nd ed.). Hillsdale, NJ: Erlbaum Associates.

Davis, B. L., & Hodnett, E. (2002). Labor support nurses' self-efficacy and views about factors influencing implementation. *Journal of Obstetrical, Gynecological, and Neonatal Nursing, 21,* 48–56.

Demmer, C. (2003). HIV prevention in the era of new treatments. *Health Promotion Practitioner, 4,* 449–456.

DiBartolo, M. C. (2002). On her terms. *Journal of Gerontological Nursing, 28*(10), 55–56.

DiMauro, N. M. (2000). Continuing professional development. *The Journal of Continuing Education in Nursing 31*(2), 59–62.

Dixon, E. A. (1991). Brief: Nurse readiness and time spent in self-directed learning. *The Journal of Continuing Education in Nursing, 22,* 215–218.

Emblen, J. D., & Gray, G. T. (1990). Comparison of nurses' self-directed learning activities. *The Journal of Continuing Education in Nursing, 21,* 56–61.

Gorelick, P. B. (1995). Stroke prevention. *Archives of Neurology, 52,* 347–355.

Gorelick, P. B. (2002). New horizons for stroke prevention. *Lancet, 1*(3), 149–156.

Gortner, S., & Jenkins, L. (1990). Self-efficacy and activity level following cardiac surgery. *Journal of Advanced Nursing, 15,* 1132–1138.

Hakim, A. M., Silver, F., & Hodgson, C. (1998). Is Canada falling behind international standards for stroke care? *Canadian Medical Association Journal, 159,* 671–673.

Hewitt-Taylor, J. (2001). Self-directed learning: Views of teachers and students. *Journal of Advanced Nursing, 36,* 496–504.

Holtzman, G. (1999). The development of a self directed module for orientation of nursing students to multiple inpatient clinical areas. *Journal of Nursing Education, 38*, 380–382.

Ingall, T. J. (2000). Preventing ischemic stroke: Current approaches to primary and secondary prevention. *Postgraduate Medicine, 107*(6), 34–36, 39–42, 47–50.

Iwasiw, C. (1987). The role of the teacher in self-directed learning. *Nurse Education Today, 7*, 49–55.

Jenkins, T. B., Carlson, J. H., & Herrick, C. A. (1998). Developing self-directed learning modules. *Journal of Nursing Staff Development, 14,* 17–22.

Knowles, M. S. (1975). *Self-directed learning: A guide for learners and teachers.* Englewood Cliffs, NJ: Cambridge Adult Education, Prentice Hall Regents.

Knowles, M. S. (1990). *The adult learner: A neglected species* (4th ed.). Houston: Gulf Publishing.

Laschinger, H., & Tresolini, C. (1999). An exploratory study of nursing and medical students' health promotion counselling self-efficacy. *Nurse Education Today, 19*, 408–418.

Laschinger, H., McWilliam, C., & Weston, W. (1999). Nursing and medical students' health promotion counselling self-efficacy. *Journal of Nursing Education, 38*(8), 347–356.

Laschinger, H. K. (1996). Undergraduate nursing students' health promotion counselling self-efficacy. *Journal of Advanced Nursing, 24,* 36–41.

Lipe, D. M., Reeds, L. B., Prokop, J. A., Phelps, B. L., Menousek, L. F., & Bryant, M. M. (1994). Mandatory inservice programs using self-learning modules. *Journal of Nursing Staff Development, 10,* 167–172.

Lunyk-Child, O. L., Crooks, D., Ellis, P. J., Ofosu, C., O'Mara, L., & Rideout, E. (2001). Self-directed learning, faculty and student perceptions. *Journal of Nursing Education, 40,* 116–123.

Morris, J. (1999). Evaluation of open-learning material designed for part of the diploma level research module for pre-post registration nurses. *Nurse Education Today, 19,* 601–609.

Murdock, J. E., & Neafsey, P. J. (1995). Self-efficacy measurements: An approach for predicting practice outcomes in continuing education? *The Journal of Continuing Education in Nursing, 26*(4), 158–165.

Murphy, D. A., Lu, M. C., Martin, D., Hoffman, D., & Marelich, W. D. (2002). Results of a pilot intervention trial to improve antiretroviral adherence among HIV positive patients. *Journal of Association of Nurses in AIDS Care, 13*(6), 57–59.

Neafsey, P. J. (1998). Immediate and enduring changes in knowledge and self-efficacy in APNs following computer-assisted home study of The Pharmacology of Alcohol. *The Journal of Continuing Education in Nursing, 29,* 173–181.

Neafsey, P. J., & Shellman, J. (2002). Knowledge and self-efficacy of community health nurses concerning interactions of prescription medicines with over-the-counter agents and alcohol. *Journal of Gerontology Nursing, 18*(9), 30–39.

Nullay, J. (1978). *Psychometric theory* (2nd ed.). New York: McGraw-Hill.

Nolan, J., & Nolan, M. (1997a). Self-directed and student-centred learning in nurse education: 1. *British Journal of Nursing, 6,* 103–107.

Nolan, P. (1998). Competencies drive decision-making. *Nursing Management, 29*(3), 27–29.

O'Shea, E. (2003). Self-directed learning in nurse education: A review of the literature. *Journal of Advanced Nursing, 43,* 62–70.

O'Very, D. (1999). Self-paced: The right pace for staff development. *The Journal of Continuing Education in Nursing, 30,* 182–187.

Ockene, J. K., Emmons, K. M., Mermetstein, R. J., Perkins, K. A., Bonollo, D. S., Voorhees, C. C., & Hollis, J. F. (2000). Relapse and maintenance issues for smoking cessation. *Health Psychology, 19*(1 Suppl.), 17–31.

Ockene, J., Ma, Y., Zapka, J., Pbert, L., Valentine-Goins, K., & Stoddard, A. (2002). Spontaneous cessation of smoking and alcohol use among low-income pregnant women. *American Journal of Preventative Medicine, 23,* 150–159.

Oddi, L. F. (1988). Comparison of self-directed learning scores among graduate students in nursing, adult education, and law. *The Journal of Continuing Education in Nursing, 17,* 178–181.

Purdy, M. (1997). Humanist ideology and nurse education: Limitations of humanist educational theory in nurse education. *Nurse Education Today, 17,* 196–202.

Rivero, C. (2001). A model for self-directed learning in a military facility. *Military Medicine, 166,* 711–713.

Robinson-Smith, G. (2002). Prayer after stroke: Its relationship to quality of life. *Journal of Holistic Nursing, 20,* 352–356.

Sacco, R. L. (2001). Newer risk factors for stroke. *Neurology, 57*(5, Suppl. 2), S31–S34.

Schretzman, D. (2001). Acute ischemic stroke. *Dimensions of Critical Care Nursing, 20*(2), 14–21.

Simoni, J. M., Frick, P. A., Lockhart, D., & Liebovitz, D. (2002). Mediators of social support and antiretroviral adherence among an indigent population in New York City. *AIDS Patient Care, 16,* 431–439.

Sparling, L. A. (2001). Enhancing the learning in self-directed learning modules. *Journal for Nurses in Staff Development, 17*(4), 199–205.

Tresolini, C. P., Saluja, G., & Stritter, F. (1995, April). *Assessing medical students' self-efficacy in health promotion counselling: A pilot study.* Presented at the annual meeting of the American Educational Researchers Association, San Francisco, CA.

INTRODUCTION TO CRITIQUE #2

The article "Self-Efficacy of Staff Nurses for Health Promotion Counselling of Patients at Risk for Stroke" (Mayer, Andrusyszyn, & Iwasiw, 2005) is examined in terms of its quality and the potential usefulness of the findings for application to nursing practice.

Title

The title matches the major purpose of this study.

Abstract

The abstract meets the requirement of thoroughness; it contains the purpose, the sample size, the research design, a very brief description of the instrument, the findings, and the results.

Problem and Purpose

The authors stated that the purpose of the study was to "evaluate the self-efficacy of staff nurses to deliver risk factor modification counselling, after completion of a self-directed learning manual, to patients on a general neuroscience unit who have been identified as being at risk for stroke" (Mayer et al., 2005, p. 17).

The identification of the research problem is very well organized, with an easy flow of the linkages. Mayer et al. (2005) outlined the significance of the study by stating the risk and impact of having a stroke and the direct and indirect costs of stroke. Next, the authors stated that preparation of health professionals in health promotion practices is increasingly important to reduce the risk of a stroke. The concepts of competencies, self-efficacy, and self-directed learning are highlighted as components of this preparation. The rationale for the study was explicitly stated as follows:

> The need to prepare health care professionals who are skilled in health promotion practices has become increasingly important. . . . Primary care nurses are crucial to identifying factors that place individuals at risk for suffering a stroke, and then counselling them about the signs and symptoms of impending stroke and the importance of gaining control over the risk factors. (p. 15)

Review of Literature and Definitions

The literature review was well organized. In a systematic matter, it tied together the core elements of the risk of stroke, self-directed learning and self-efficacy, and stroke prevention and the role of the nurse. The use of subheadings increased the readability of the literature review. Mostly primary sources (e.g., Bandura, 1986; Knowles, 1990) were used, with the additional of a few secondary sources (e.g., Nullay, 1978; Purday, 1997). Most sources were within 10 years of publication, and those over 10 years old are landmark studies. Although the research on the study's topic is considerable, as articulated in the literature review, the authors identified a gap in the literature by commenting that "staff nurses' self-efficacy for counselling and means to enhance self-efficacy for health promotion have not been investigated [and] nurses' confidence to undertake counselling is not known" (p. 17).

Theoretical Framework

The theoretical framework consisted of Knowles's (1990) adult learning theory and Bandura's (1986) self-efficacy theory. The linkages of these theories to support the study are clearly articulated.

Hypotheses and Research Question

Mayer et al. (2005) explicitly stated the research hypotheses as follows (p. 17):

1. "Upon completion of a self-directed learning manual, immediate post self-efficacy scores (time two) will be significantly higher than pre self-efficacy scores (time one/baseline) in neuroscience nurses delivering health promotion counselling."

2. There will be no difference in the self-efficacy scores two months after completing the manual (time three) when compared to immediate post self-efficacy scores (time two)."

3. "There will be a positive correlation between self-efficacy scores and attitudes about risk factor counselling."

The authors offered only one research question. It flows from the research problem, the literature review, and the theoretical framework and was stated as follows: "What is the relationship between neuroscience nurses' post-test self-efficacy score and selected demographic variables?" (p. 17).

Sample

The study had no exclusion criteria and only one inclusion criterion in that the sample of nurses had to work in the neuroscience unit. A nonprobability convenience sample was used from a single hospital with staff composed of registered nurses, limiting generalizability to the sample itself.

A letter of information was sent to 76 nurses, with 27 responding, for a response rate of 30%, which is considered good. Power analysis revealed that 22 participants were required to detect a 10% change in scores. Thus, the final sample size of 23 was adequate.

Research Design

The authors explicitly stated that the study was a quasiexperimental, pretest–post-test, one-group design. Participants acted as their own controls. The intervention was the researcher-designed, self-directed learning manual to be completed at a time, place, and pace suitable for each nurse. A repeated measures component was also included, in which data were collected at baseline (premanual), time two (postcompletion of the manual), and time three (two months after completion of the manual). This design is consistent with the purpose of the research.

The major dependent variable of this study was self-efficacy, which was subdivided into two variables, knowledge and counselling ability. All dependent variables are all interval-level variables. The only independent variable was the manual. Demographic variables, such as age, sex, years of experience as a registered nurse, educational preparation, years in neuroscience nursing, enrolment in an educational program, and other roles and responsibilities, were used to determine relationships with the post-test scores.

Internal Validity

The authors made no mention of possible threats to internal validity that would inordinately decrease confidence in the results.

External Validity

Generalizability is limited to the sample because of the effect of nonprobability convenience sampling. Another issue is the self-selection method used. The authors acknowledged that this volunteer sample "may be a special group who are self-directed and value education and research" (p. 20), thus limiting the generalizability of the results.

Legal–Ethical Issues

Approval for the study was obtained from the Institutional Ethics Review Board, and the relevant permissions from hospital leaders were obtained. The informed consent form was signed, and participants were anonymous to the researchers owing to the coding by the administrative assistant.

Instruments

The major measurement instrument used was the Health Promotion Counselling Self-Efficacy Scale (HPCSE), which consisted of 10 self-efficacy subscales. The scoring system was briefly explained for the reader; the response scores ranged from 1 to 4, with higher scores indicating greater self-efficacy. The scoring system was also explained so that the meaning of the summated values would be understood.

A demographic survey appears to have been developed requesting information on age, sex, years of experience as a registered nurse, educational preparation, years in neuroscience nursing, enrolment in an educational program, and other roles and responsibilities.

Reliability and Validity

Past reliability information was given for the HPCSE; in other words, the internal consistency and test–retest coefficients ranged from .71 to .94, which is acceptable to good. Cronbach's alpha was .81, which is good. The authors did not provide information on the validity of the HPCSE.

Results

A description of the participants' results is detailed in the text (p. 18); use of a table format makes it easier for the reader to examine the results. Evidence to support hypotheses one and two are detailed in Table 19C2–1 and in the text as follows: "neuroscience nurses' self-efficacy for counselling was significantly higher at time two and unchanged at time three" (p. 19). The results to support hypothesis three are in Table 19C2–2 and expressed in the text as follows: "there was a positive correlation between self-efficacy scores and attitudes about risk factor counselling [health promotion]" (p. 19). With regard to the research question, no significant demographic variables correlated with the post-test self-efficacy scores.

The researchers also examined other relationships, such as nurses' smoking cessation knowledge and counselling self-efficacy over time. These results were found to be significant. Because the analysis of variance compared the three time period means in the same procedure for both knowledge and counselling, the post hoc procedure was conducted to determine which pair of means was significant, and the researchers found that the time two and three scores were significantly higher than time one scores for both smoking cessation knowledge and counselling self-efficacy.

Similarly, comparisons were made for exercise knowledge self-efficacy, exercise counselling self-efficacy, nutrition knowledge, and nutrition counselling self-efficacy. When a difference is found, the strength of that difference is measured by the effect size. In these results, the effect sizes ranged from .32 to .50, which the authors qualified as varying degrees of medium to large.

Overall, the findings related to each hypothesis are clearly stated, and the authors made good use of tables for illustrating these detailed results for the reader.

Discussion

The findings of this study are appropriately related to previous studies on self-directed learning and self-efficacy.

Limitations and Conclusion

The authors discussed the data collection in a single hospital as a limitation and recommended future studies to expand the sampling. Limitations around learning styles and their effect on self-directed learning were raised. Self-reporting was discussed because it may have affected the results regarding self-efficacy. The issue of sustainability after two months must be investigated.

The conclusion appropriately summarized the findings in relation to educational strategies for continuing education.

Critical Thinking Challenges

- Discuss the ways in which the stylistic considerations of a journal affect the researcher's ability to present the research findings of a quantitative study.
- Are critiques of quantitative studies valid when conducted by a student or a practising nurse? What level of quantitative study is best for consumers of research to critique? What assumptions did you use to make this determination?
- What is essential for the consumer of research to use when critiquing a quantitative research study? Discuss the ways you might use Internet resources now or in the future when critiquing studies.

REFERENCES

Ajzen, I. (1991). The Theory of Planned Behavior. *Organizational Behaviour and Human Decision Processes, 50*, 179–211.

Boudreau, F., & Godin, G. (2007). Using the Theory of Planned Behaviour to predict exercise intention in obese adults. *Canadian Journal of Nursing Research, 39*, 112–125.

Hardeman, W., Griffin, S., Johnston, M., Kinmonth, A. L., & Wareham, N. J. (2000). Interventions to prevent weight gain: A systematic review of psychological models and behavior change methods. *International Journal of Obesity and Related Metabolic Disorders, 24*, 131–143.

Mayer, C., Andrusyszyn, M.-A., & Iwasiw, C. (2005). Self-efficacy of staff nurses for health promotion counselling of patients at risk for stroke. *AXON, 26*(4), 14–21.

PART SIX

Application of Research: Evidence-Based Practice

RESEARCH VIGNETTE
Barbara Davies

CHAPTER 20
Use of Research in Practice

Nursing Best Practice

*Give to the world the best you have
and the best will come back to you.*
                    —Author unknown

As a graduating student in nursing at the University of Toronto in 1974, I was asked to supply a quotation about my philosophy of life to accompany my yearbook photograph. I still recall being perplexed about what to state and spending considerable time searching sources. Eventually, I selected the above quotation about doing your "best." Little did I know that more than 30 years later, I would be the co-director of the Nursing Best Practice Research Unit at the University of Ottawa, a dynamic collaboration with the politically active Registered Nurses' Association of Ontario.

It is fascinating to contemplate the forces that influenced my career development and, in particular, the development of my research program on evidence-based practice. Clearly, one of the influential people in my early career was Donna Diers, the Dean of Nursing at Yale University. I was employed as a clinical instructor at Yale and recall Donna passionately pleading about the need for nursing research to provide the data to demonstrate the "power" of nursing care to improve health. She strongly encouraged teaching staff at Yale to conduct nursing research that "would make a difference in practice."

My Ph.D. supervisor, Ellen Hodnett, who holds the Heather M. Reisman Chair in Perinatal Nursing Research at the University of Toronto, also influenced my knowledge and skills related to best practice. Ellen is one of the early leaders of the Cochrane Collaboration, an international research initiative to answer substantive clinical questions by conducting systematic reviews of published and unpublished research. Cochrane Reviews strive to determine the most effective health care interventions. Ellen was the lead author of a review about the provision of labour support to women at childbirth.

Continuous labour support provides the benefits of reduced use of analgesia or anaesthesia, reduced number of births by Caesarean section, and reduced reports by women of negative labour experiences. Simultaneously, another Cochrane Review about fetal health surveillance concluded that intermittent fetal auscultation was preferable to electronic fetal monitoring for low-risk women owing to reduced rates of Caesarean section with auscultation. Although the provision of labour support and the use of intermittent fetal auscultation were recommended by the Society of Obstetricians and Gynaecologists of Canada and the World Health Organization, several observational studies found that the majority of low-risk women giving birth in Canada were not receiving either of these beneficial interventions. Thus, the challenge of my doctoral work was to create a knowledge transfer intervention to improve practice to be consistent with recommendations from the Cochrane Collaboration and clinical practice guidelines.

The creation of this type of knowledge transfer intervention was a stimulating process. A multifaceted intervention, including an educational workshop for nurses, was developed. The workshop included tools for applying research results to practice. Assessment forms, protocols based on the research results, and case study exercises were included.

The intervention received positive evaluations from the participating nurses, and the majority of staff nurses (>80%) attended the workshop. I am proud to report that this labour support workshop, which was first offered in 1995 as part of my Ph.D. research, is still being offered regularly in 2008 by our regional Perinatal Partnership Program in Eastern and Southeastern Ontario. (A note of caution for others who are considering the development of similar knowledge transfer interventions to improve practice: Many nurses have extensive experience, and it is important to recognize their knowledge and expertise. Using a respectful, collaborative approach works well. Ask nurses what they think is needed to improve practice to be consistent with research results and you will likely hear some excellent ideas.)

Shortly after completing my Ph.D. in 2000, I received a Career Scientist award from the Ministry of Health and Long-Term Care in Ontario for a five-year program of research on maternal–infant knowledge transfer. It was exciting to be selected for provincial recognition in a tough competition but rather daunting to meet the annual requirements of external peer-reviewed funding.

Fortunately, a very special opportunity arose at this time to co-lead, with Nancy Edwards, the evaluation of the emerging Nursing Best Practice Guidelines Program of the Registered Nurses' Association of Ontario. The guidelines include a synthesis of the available research evidence developed by expert panels on priority topics, such as fall prevention, pressure ulcers, asthma control, breastfeeding, and support for families.

Subsequently, over the next eight years, Nancy and I, along with many others, have conducted studies of implementation interventions, surveys of nurses' attitudes, qualitative interviews of barriers and facilitators, observations of teaching tools, and chart audits of nursing practice and client outcomes. The mandate of our nursing best practice research unit is to bring the best knowledge to nursing and health care, enhance practice, and improve health and system outcomes. The goal is to promote best nursing knowledge everywhere.

Currently, my research on best practice addresses sustainability factors, interprofessional collaboration, and system changes. I am also supervising master's and Ph.D. students and postdoctoral fellows who are working on such important elements as leadership and policy integration for evidence-based practice.

Some academics criticize the notion of best practice, commenting on the harms of a hierarchy of evidence that unduly glorifies the randomized controlled trial as the gold standard of research methodology. My view is that a randomized controlled trial is the preferred research design to determine whether one treatment is more effective than another treatment. However, health has multiple determinants, and health care is provided in a complex environment by many types of health care professionals. Thus, it is equally important to conduct qualitative research studies to better understand the factors influencing the promotion of health for all.

Finally, I offer a few words about values, preferences, and best practice. At the core of best practice is the notion that decisions and interventions need to be client centred. Assessing preferences, clarifying values, and informing clients and their families about the risks and benefits of options are essential. Early in my research career, while doing my M.Sc.N. thesis on factors influencing the decisions of

women of advanced maternal age to have genetic amniocentesis, I discovered that women perceived the same risk of "1 in 100" very differently. Each woman, each spouse, and the genetic nurse counsellor had their own and sometimes conflicting perspectives. Conducting this genetic research has heightened my awareness of variances in client and provider values and the need for thoughtful reflection about clients and my own values regarding what constitutes best practice.

In conclusion, although best practice is an admirable goal, I now question whether anyone can ever achieve such a state. Nevertheless, the quest to achieve excellence in nursing practice still drives my research journey. What drives your work in practice, education, or research? What type of evidence counts for you? What does "best practice" mean to you?

Barbara Davies
RN, PhD
Associate Professor,
   Nursing
University of Ottawa
Premiers Research
   Excellence Award
Co-Director Nursing Best
   Practice Research Unit
Ottawa, Ontario

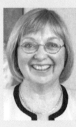

Marita G. Titler
Cherylyn Cameron

CHAPTER 20

Use of Research in Practice

LEARNING OUTCOMES

After reading this chapter, the student should be able to do the following:

- Differentiate among the conduct of nursing research, research utilization, and evidence-based practice (EBP).
- Describe the steps of evidence-based practice.
- Identify three barriers to evidence-based practice and strategies to address each barrier.
- List three sources for finding evidence.
- Describe strategies for implementing evidence-based practice changes.
- Identify steps for evaluating an evidence-based change in practice.
- Use research findings and other forms of evidence to improve the quality of care.

KEY TERMS

conduct of research
Delphi technique
diffusion of innovations
dissemination
evidence-based practice (EBP) guidelines
evidence-based practice (EBP)
integrative review
knowledge-focused triggers
opinion leaders
problem-focused triggers
research utilization
translation science

STUDY RESOURCES

evolve Go to Evolve at
http://evolve.elsevier.com/Canada/LoBiondo/Research/
for Weblinks, content updates, and additional
research articles for practice in reviewing
and critiquing.

The conduct of research is only the first step in improving practice through the use of research (Titler & Everett, 2001). Because of the gap between the discovery and the use of knowledge in practice (Farquhar, Stryer, & Slutsky, 2002; Feldman & Kane, 2003; Lavis, Robertson, Woodside, McLeod, & Abelson, 2003), concentrated efforts must focus on methods to speed the translation of research findings into practice. Development and dissemination of evidence-based practice (EBP) guidelines are essential steps but alone do little to promote knowledge uptake by direct care providers. Promoting the use of evidence in practice is an active process that is facilitated, in part, by modelling and imitation of others who have successfully adopted the innovation, an organizational culture that values and supports the use of evidence, and localization of the evidence for use in a specific health care setting (Berwick, 2003; Gillbody, Whitty, Grimshaw, & Thomas, 2003; Rogers, 2003). The Canadian Nurses Association (2002) has indicated that

> *professional associations, regulatory bodies for nurses, specialty groups for nurses[,] individual nurses, schools of nursing, organizations employing nurses, accreditation councils, governments, health information agencies and nurse researchers share the responsibility of facilitating evidence-based decision-making and evidence-based practice. These responsibilities extend to identifying the barriers and enhancing the factors within organizational structures that facilitate and promote evidence-based practice. (p. 2)*

Translation of research into practice is a multifaceted, systemic process of promoting adoption of EBPs in the delivery of health care services that goes beyond dissemination of evidence-based (EB) guidelines (Farquhar, Stryer, & Slutsky, 2002). Dissemination activities take many forms, including publications, conferences, consultations, and training programs, but promoting knowledge uptake and changing practitioner behaviours require active interchange with those in direct care.

This chapter presents an overview of EBP—the process of implementing evidence into practice to improve client outcomes—and a description of translation science.

OVERVIEW OF EVIDENCE-BASED PRACTICE

The relationships among conduct, dissemination, and utilization of research are illustrated in Figure 20–1. **Conduct of research** is the analysis of data collected from a homogeneous group of subjects who meet study inclusion and exclusion criteria for the purpose of answering specific research questions or testing specified hypotheses. Research design, methods, and statistical analyses are guided by the state of the science in the area of investigation. Traditionally, conduct of research has included **dissemination** of findings via research reports in journals and at scientific conferences. In comparison, **research utilization** is the process of using *research findings* to improve client care. Research utilization encompasses dissemination of scientific knowledge; critique of studies; synthesis of research findings; determination of the applicability of findings for practice; development of an evidence-based standard or guideline; implementation of the standard; and evaluation of the practice change with respect to staff, clients, and cost or resource utilization (Titler et al., 2001).

Evidence-based practice (EBP) has been defined by some experts as the synthesis and use of scientific findings from randomized clinical trials only (Estabrooks, 2004), whereas others define EBP more broadly to include use of empirical evidence from other scientific methods (e.g., descriptive studies) and use of information from case reports and expert opinion (Cook, 1998; DiCenso, Guyatt, & Ciliska, 2005; Sackett, Straus, Richardson, Rosenberg, & Haynes, 2005). The definition used in this book is offered by DiCenso et al. (2005), who defined EBP as "the integration of best research evidence with clinical expertise and patient values to facilitate clinical decision making" (p. 4). As illustrated in the knowledge generation and use cycle (see Figure 20–1), application of research findings in practice may not only improve quality care but also may create new and exciting questions to be addressed via the conduct of research.

The terms *research utilization* and *evidence-based practice* are sometimes used interchangeably. Although these two terms are related, they are not synonymous. EBP is the conscious and judicious use of the current "best" evidence in the care of clients and delivery of health care services, whereas research utilization is a subset of EBP that focuses on the application of research findings. EBP is a broader term that not only encompasses research utilization but also includes the use of case reports and expert opinion in deciding the practices to be used in health care. When sufficient research is available, health care professionals are generally recommended to base their evidence-based practice on the research. In some cases, a sufficient body of research may not be available, and the health care professional may need to supplement research findings with other types of evidence, such as expert opinion and case reports, when developing an EBP guideline. As more research is done in a

specific area, the research evidence can be used to update and refine the guideline.

Evidence-Based Practice Tip

Remember that Registered Nurses (R.N.s) are expected to access, appraise, and incorporate research evidence into their professional judgement and decision making, as well as consider the preferences and values of their client population.

Use of Evidence in Practice

Nursing has a rich history of using research in practice, pioneered by Florence Nightingale, who used data to change practices that contributed to high mortality rates in hospitals and communities (Nightingale, 1858, 1859, 1863a, 1863b). Although during the early and mid-1900s, few nurses built on the solid foundation of research utilization exemplified by Nightingale, the nursing profession has provided major leadership for improving care through the application of research findings in practice (Kirchhoff, 2004). Today, nurses are being prepared as scientists in nursing and are leading

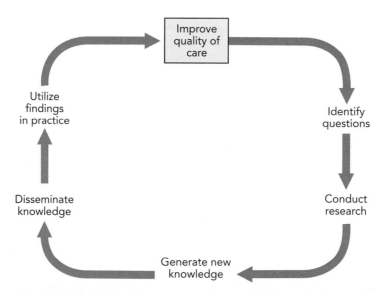

Figure 20–1 The model of the relationship among conduct, dissemination, and use of research

Redrawn from Weiler, K., Buckwalter, K., & Titler, M. (1994). Debate: Is nursing research used in practice? In J. McCloskey & H. Grace (Eds.), *Current issues in nursing* (4th ed.). St. Louis, MO: Mosby.

the way in translation science; as a result, the scientific body of nursing knowledge is growing. It is now every nurse's responsibility to facilitate the use of nursing knowledge in practice.

Cronenwett (1995), Estabrooks (2004), and others have described two forms of using research evidence in practice: conceptual and decision driven. Conceptually driven forms influence the thinking of the health care professional but not necessarily the action. Exposure to new scientific knowledge occurs, but the new knowledge may not be used to change or guide practice. An **integrative review** of the literature, formulation of a new theory, or generation of new hypotheses may be the result. Use of knowledge in this way is referred to as knowledge creep or cognitive application. Knowledge creep is often used by individuals who read and incorporate research into their critical thinking. Decision-driven forms of using evidence in practice encompass application of scientific knowledge as part of a new practice, policy, procedure, or intervention. In this type of application of research findings, a critical decision to change or endorse current practice is based on review and critique of studies applicable to that practice. Examples of decision-driven models of using research in practice are the Iowa Model of Evidence-Based Practice to Promote Quality Care (Titler et al., 2001), the Promoting Action on Research Implementation in Health Services (PAR-IHS) model (Rycroft-Malone et al., 2002), and the Conduct and Utilization of Research in Nursing (CURN) model (Haller, Reynolds, & Horsley, 1979; Horsley, Crane, Crabtree, & Wood, 1983).

Multifaceted active dissemination strategies are needed to promote the use of research evidence in clinical and administrative health care decision making, and they need to address *both* the individual practitioners and the organization. When nurses decide individually what evidence to use in practice, considerable variability in practice patterns results, potentially resulting in adverse client outcomes. For example, a solely "individual" perspective of EBP would leave the decision about the use of evidence-based endotracheal suctioning techniques to each nurse. Some nurses may be familiar with the research findings for endotracheal suctioning, whereas others may not. This situation is likely to result in different and conflicting practices being used because nurses change shifts every 8 to 12 hours. From an organizational perspective, policies and procedures are written that are based on research, and then adoption of these practices by nurses is systematically promoted in the organization.

Models of Evidence-Based Practice

Multiple models of EBP and translation science are available (Berwick, 2003; Dufault, 2004; Olade, 2004; Rosswurm & Larrabee, 1999; Rycroft-Malone et al., 2002; Soukup, 2000; Stetler, 2003; Titler & Everett, 2001; Titler et al., 2001; Wagner et al., 2001). The common elements of these models are syntheses of the evidence, implementation of the evidence, evaluation of the impact on client care, and consideration of the context or setting in which the evidence is implemented.

Evidence-Based Practice Tip

After you have chosen an EBP model to guide your EBP projects think about whether it focuses on individual or organizational change.

THE IOWA MODEL OF EVIDENCE-BASED PRACTICE

The Iowa Model of Evidence-Based Practice is offered here as an example of an EBP *practice* model (see Figure 20–2). This model has been widely disseminated and adopted in academic and clinical settings (Titler et al., 2001). Since the original publication of this model in 1994 (Titler, Moss, et al., 1994), the authors have received 152 written requests to use the model for publications, presentations, graduate and undergraduate research courses, and clinical research programs, and the social sciences citation indicates that by 2003 the model was cited 44 times in nursing journal articles (Social Science Citation Index, 2003). This organizational, collaborative model incorporates conduct of research, use of research evidence, and other types of evidence

**The Iowa Model of
Evidence-Based Practice to Promote Quality Care**

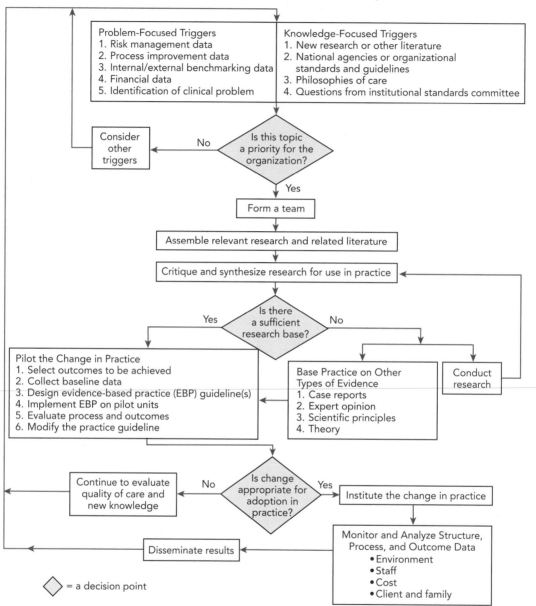

Figure 20–2 The Iowa Model of Evidence-Based Practice to Promote Quality Care

Redrawn from Titler, M. G., Kleiber, C., Steelman, V. J., Rakel, B. A., Budreau, G., Buckwalter, K. C., et al. (2001). The Iowa Model of Evidence-Based Practice to Promote Quality Care. *Critical Care Nursing Clinics of North America, 13*(4), 587–604.
EBP: evidence-based practice.

(Titler et al., 2001). The authors of the Iowa model adopted the definition of EBP as the conscientious and judicious use of current best evidence to guide health care decisions (Sackett, Rosenberg, Gray, Haynes, & Richardson, 1996). Levels of evidence range from meta-analysis and randomized clinical trials to case reports and expert opinion. In this model, knowledge-focused and problem-focused "trigger(s)" lead staff members to question current nursing practice and whether client care can be improved through the use of research findings.

If, through the process of literature review and critique of studies, nurses find that an insufficient number of scientifically sound studies exist to use as a base for practice, consideration is often given to conducting a study. Nurses in practice can collaborate with scientists in nursing and other disciplines to conduct clinical research that addresses practice problems encountered in the care of clients. The findings from such studies are then combined with the findings from existing scientific knowledge to develop and implement these practices. If insufficient research exists to guide practice, and conducting a study is not feasible, other types of evidence (e.g., case reports, expert opinion, scientific principles, theory) are used or combined with available research evidence to guide practice. Priority is given to projects in which a high proportion of practice is guided by research evidence. Practice guidelines usually reflect research and nonresearch evidence and therefore are called EBP guidelines.

Evidence-Based Practice Tip

Knowledge-focused and problem-focused triggers that represent information needs from clinical practice are converted into focused, structured clinical questions.

Several steps are involved in developing an EBP guideline. First, based on the relevant evidence, the recommended practices are compared with current practices, and health care professionals decide whether a practice change is warranted. If a decision is made to proceed with a practice change, the changes are implemented through a process of planned change. The practice is first implemented with a small group of patients, and an evaluation is carried out. Based on this evaluation, the EBP is refined, and the revised practice is implemented with a second client population. Health care professionals monitor the practice's fiscal implications and its impacts on clients, their families, and staff.

Successful use of evidence in care delivery relies on both organizational and administrative supports.

Two Canadian examples of models for EBP are discussed by Ross-Kerr and Wood (2003, pp. 153–154):

The Registered Nurses Association of British Columbia (RNABC) developed a model based on the work of Stetler (1985). The following four phases of the model were identified:

1. *Articulation or definition of the problem and location of research reports*
2. *Evaluation or critical review of research findings for scientific merit and clinical significance*
3. *Comparison of findings to the practice setting*
4. *Application or definition of the contribution to practice and evaluation if implemented*

Application of this framework requires partnerships among nurses with clinical expertise, research experience, and administrative responsibilities. Each phase requires particular nurses to be involved, decisions to be made, and resources to be accessed. The framework can be modified and explained in greater detail by individual agencies, thus making it relevant to both staff needs and the organizational structure.

As an example of this framework's usefulness, one health-care agency in British Columbia has used it as a strategy to promote research-based nursing practice. The nursing research committee—with staff, administrative, and educator representation—worked on explicating the objectives of and responsibilities for each phase, changing terminology to fit the agency's mission, and setting and identifying resources required for each phase. The committee's work has been discussed at general nursing council meetings and with staff. Refinements based on their input have resulted in an agency-specific research-utilization framework that maintains the integrity of the original and addresses the needs of the agency. The intent is to decentralize further work with the framework to areas of practice where it will be used and evaluated against the process of recommending and adopting research-based nursing practices.

Another example can be found in Alberta, where nurses at the Cross Cancer Institute (CCI) in Edmonton tackled the problem of incorporating research findings into their practice using the CURN model as their framework (Alberta Association of Registered Nurses [AARN], 1997). They created an office of nursing research staffed by a full-time clinical nurse researcher. She was responsible for reviewing existing research and for setting up the systems for facilitating the use of research in clinical practice. Communication was aided by providing copies of the contents of nursing journals on all nursing units and providing copies of articles as requested by the staff. CCI also created a quarterly newsletter, which reviewed a major article in each issue. Athabasca University provided evening courses at CCI on research design and statistics. Pilot testing was done on the criteria for reviewing research studies as part of the CURN project. Dr. Joanne Horsley, director of the CURN Project, served as a consultant to the staff as they implemented their research-utilization project.

From these two examples, it is evident that using a framework to guide the process should be part of any research-utilization project (see Table 20–1). Regardless of the research-utilization framework used, the importance of the strategy is that it fosters an inquiring, curious attitude and results in problem identification and resolution. In the long run, this will facilitate adoption of innovations into research-based nursing practice.

Logan and Graham (1998) developed a model for interdisciplinary health care research use called the Ottawa Model of Research Use (OMRU). The framework was created to "be used by policy-makers seeking to increase the use of health research by practitioners, as well as by researchers interested in studying the process by which research becomes integrated into practice" (p. 228). They identified the following six components of research utilization: (1) the practice environment, (2) potential adopters, (3) the evidence-based innovation, (4) transfer strategies, (5) adoption, and (6) health-related and other outcomes (see Figure 20–3). Constant assessment, monitoring, and evaluation parallel the progression through the components. As barriers are identified, strategies are developed to surmount them and to enhance supports.

The previous models described to guide research utilization all have a common linear design; in other words, each describes a series of steps that, if followed, will result in change. However, Kitson, Harvey, and McCormack's (1998) conceptualization of research dissemination

---

TABLE 20–1 Principles of Research Utilization

1. Research utilization depends on the interest, commitment, and expertise of nurses in all areas and cannot be achieved by any one individual working in isolation.
2. The success of research utilization requires that it be proactive, deliberate, and systematic, addressing the process of adopting innovation.
3. Research utilization frameworks provide guides for nursing practice, research, and educational and administrative systems.
4. Relevant research utilization frameworks include phases aimed at identifying the problem, critically reviewing the literature, translating findings to practice, implementing the new practice, and evaluating the outcome.

From Ross-Kerr, J., & Wood, M. (2003). *Canadian nursing: Issues and perspectives* (p. 154). Toronto: Mosby.

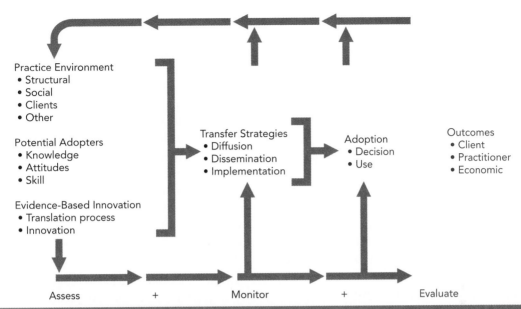

Figure 20–3 The Ottawa Model of Health Care Research Use

Adapted from Logan, J., & Graham, I. (1998). Toward a comprehensive interdisciplinary model of health care research use. *Science Communication,* 20(2), 229.

recognized the often-nonlinear processes involved. A formula—SI = f(E,C,F), or **S**uccessful **I**mplementation is a function of **E**vidence, **C**ontext, and **F**acilitation—is applied to a facilitation approach. Each of the elements (evidence, context, and facilitation) is assessed on a continuum. The research findings are more likely to be accepted and put into practice because each of the elements is rated on the high end of the continuum. To enable the implementation of the research, the elements that are rated as being low must be moved along the continuum.

STEPS OF EVIDENCE-BASED PRACTICE

The Iowa Model of Evidence-Based Practice to Promote Quality Care (Titler et al., 2001) (see Figure 20–2) and Rogers's diffusion of innovations model (Rogers, 1995, 2003; Titler & Everett, 2001) provide guiding steps for actualizing EBP. A team approach is most helpful in fostering a specific EBP, with one person in the group providing the leadership for the project.

Selection of a Topic

The first step in carrying out an EBP project is to select a topic. Ideas for EBP come from several sources, categorized as problem- and knowledge-focused triggers. **Problem-focused triggers** are those identified by staff through quality improvement, risk surveillance, benchmarking data, financial data, or recurrent clinical problems. An example of a problem-focused trigger is increased incidence of deep venous thrombosis and pulmonary emboli in trauma and neurosurgical clients (Blondin & Titler, 1996; Stenger, 1994). **Knowledge-focused triggers** are ideas generated when staff read research, listen to scientific papers at research conferences, or encounter EBP guidelines published by federal agencies or specialty organizations. Examples initiated from knowledge-focused triggers include pain management, prevention of skin breakdown, assessing placement of nasogastric and nasointestinal tubes, and use of saline to maintain the patency of arterial lines. Sometimes, topics arise from a combination of problem- and knowledge-focused triggers, such as the length of bedrest time after femoral artery catheterization. In selecting a topic, nurses must consider how the topic fits with organization, department, and unit priorities to garner support from leaders within the organization and the necessary resources to successfully complete the project.

Individuals should work collectively to achieve consensus in topic selection. Working in groups to review performance improvement data, brainstorm about ideas, and achieve consensus about the final selection is helpful. For example, a unit staff meeting may be used to discuss ideas for EBP; quality improvement committees may identify three to four practice areas in need of attention based on quality improvement data (e.g., for elderly clients, practice concerns would include urinary tract infections, reducing the use of restraints, and preventing constipation); an EBP task force may be appointed to select and address a clinical practice issue (e.g., pain management), or a **Delphi survey technique** may be used to prioritize areas for EBP.

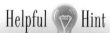

Helpful Hint

Regardless of the method used to select an EBP topic, the staff members who will implement the potential practice changes need to be involved in selecting the topic. They also need to view the study as contributing significantly to the quality of care and client outcomes (Cole & Gawlinksi, 1995).

Forming a Team

A team is responsible for the development, implementation, and evaluation of the EBP. The team or group may be an existing committee, such as the quality improvement committee, the practice council, or the research committee. A task force approach also may be used, in which a group is appointed to address a specific practice issue and use research findings or other evidence to resolve the issue or improve practice. The composition of the team is directed by the topic selected and should include stakeholders interested in the delivery of care. For example, a team working on EBP pain management should be interdisciplinary and include pharmacists, nurses, physicians, and psychologists. In contrast, a team working on the EBP of bathing might include a nurse expert in skin care, staff nurses, and the nurse clinician or educator. In addition to forming a team, key stakeholders who can facilitate the EBP project or put up barriers against successful implementation should be identified. A key stakeholder is an individual or a group of individuals who will be directly or indirectly affected by the implementation of the EBP. Some of these stakeholders are likely to be members of your team. Others may not be team members but are key individuals within the organization or unit who can adversely or positively influence the adoption of the EBP. Questions to consider in the identification of key stakeholders include the following:

- How are decisions made in the practice areas in which the EBP will be implemented?
- What types of system changes will be needed?
- Who is involved in decision making?
- Who is likely to lead and champion implementation of the EBP?
- Who can influence the decision to proceed with implementation of an EBP?
- What type of cooperation do you need from which stakeholders to be successful?

Failure to involve or keep supportive stakeholders informed may place the success of the EBP project at risk because the stakeholders are unable to anticipate or defend the rationale for changing practice, particularly with resistors (nonsupportive stakeholders) who may have a great deal of influence among their peer group.

An important early task for the EBP team is to formulate the EBP question, which helps set boundaries around the project and assists in retrieval of the evidence. A clearly defined question should specify the types of people or clients, interventions or exposures, outcomes, and relevant study designs (Alderson, Green, & Higgins, 2003). For types of people, the EBP team should specify the diseases or conditions of interest, the client population (e.g., age, gender, educational status), and the setting. For example, if the topic for the EBP project is pain, the group needs to specify the type of pain (e.g., acute, persistent, cancer), the age of the population (e.g., children, neonates, adults, older adults), and the setting (e.g., inpatient, outpatient, ambulatory care, home care, primary care). For intervention, specify the types of interventions of interest to the project and the comparison interventions (e.g., standard care, alternative treatments). For the pain example, the interventions of interest might include pharmacological treatment, analgesic administration methods (e.g., client-controlled analgesia, epidural, intravenous), pain assessment, nonpharmacological treatment, and client and family education regarding self-care pain management. For outcomes, select those outcomes of primary importance and consider the type of outcome data that will be needed for decision making (e.g., benefits, harm, cost). Avoid including outcomes that may be interesting but of little importance to the project. Finally, consider the types of study designs that are likely to provide reliable data to answer the question and search for the highest level of evidence available. A similar type of approach to formulating the practice question is PICO: *Patient, population, or problem; Intervention/treatment;*

Comparison *intervention/treatment,* and *Outcome(s)* (University of Illinois at Chicago, 2003). This approach is illustrated in Table 20–2.

Evidence-Based   Practice Tip

The PICO approach is very helpful in formulating the clinical question. PICO is also a helpful format to use when organizing written documentation of the findings related to your EBP project.

Evidence Retrieval

Once a topic is selected, relevant research and related literature need to be retrieved and should include clinical studies, meta-analyses, integrative literature reviews, and existing EBP guidelines. Use the rating systems in Table 20–3 to help you think about the level of evidence provided by the relevant research and related literature. Because more evidence is available to guide practice, professional organizations and federal agencies are developing and making EBP guidelines available. It is important that these guidelines are accessed as part of the literature retrieval process.

TABLE 20–2 Using PICO to Formulate the EBP Question

	Patient/ Population/ Problem	Intervention/ Treatment	Comparison Intervention	Outcome(s)
Tips for building the question	How would we describe a group of clients similar to ours?	Which main intervention are we considering?	What is the main alternative to compare with the intervention?	What can we hope to accomplish?
Example 1	Pain management for elders admitted to hospital with a hip fracture	Pain assessment or pain tool; client-controlled analgesia	Standard of care Nurse-administered analgesic	Regular (e.g., every 4 hr) pain assessment Less pain intensity Earlier mobility Decreased LOS
Example 2	Pain assessment of elderly clients with cognitive impairment	Pain assessment tool designed for assessing pain in elderly clients with cognitive impairment in a long-term care setting	No pain assessment Yes or no question	Regular pain assessment with treatment of pain Fewer residents in pain

Adapted from University of Illinois at Chicago. *P.I.C.O. model for clinical questions.* Retrieved March, 2004, from http://www.uic.edu/depts./lib/lhsp/resources/pico.shtml
LOS: length of stay.

For example, in 1999, the Registered Nurses' Association of Ontario (RNAO) initiated the Nursing Best Practice Guidelines Project to develop practice guidelines for nurses providing client care. The project has published 32 completed guidelines as of October 2008, and additional guidelines are under development. Each Best Practice Guideline (BPG) is developed in phases: planning, development, implementation, evaluation, and dissemination. The BPGs range from smoking cessation to screening for delirium, dementia, and depression in older adults.

The plan for dissemination of the guidelines is three-fold. First, the RNAO requested proposals from interested and eligible health care organizations to work in collaboration to plan, implement, and evaluate nursing BPGs and disseminate knowledge from demonstrated experiences with guidelines. Second, the Best Practice Champions Network was established to prepare nurses to disseminate the BPG in their practices throughout Ontario. Third, the RNAO sponsored 10 demonstration projects for colleges and universities to integrate BPG into nursing curricula.

The guidelines program has now extended to include the offering of an annual doctoral fellowship of $25,000 to eligible candidates. Additionally, advanced clinical/practice fellowships are offered to provide R.N.s with a "focused self-directed learning experience to develop clinical, leadership or best practice guideline implementation knowledge and skills, with support from a mentor(s), the organization where the RN is employed, and the RNAO. This initiative is aimed at developing and promoting nursing knowledge and expertise, and improving client care and outcomes in Ontario" (RNAO, 2007, p. 1).

In the United States, the Agency for Healthcare Research and Quality (AHRQ) funds Evidence-Based Practice Centers (see Box 20–1) that develop evidence reports on selected clinical topics. Canadian centres include McMaster University, University of Alberta, and University of Ottawa. The AHRQ also sponsors a National Guideline Clearinghouse, where abstracts of EBP guidelines are published on a Web site (http://www.guideline.gov). Other professional organizations with EBP guidelines available are the RNAO (http://www.rnao.org); the American Pain Society (http://www.ampainsoc.org); the Oncology Nursing Society (http://www.ons.org); the American Association of Critical-Care Nurses (http://www.aacn.org); the Association for Women's Health, Obstetrics, and Neonatal Nursing (http://www.awhonn.org); the Gerontological Nursing Interventions Research Center (http://www.nursing.uiowa.edu/excellence/nursing_interventions/index.htm); and the American Thoracic Society (http://www.thoracic.org). Current best evidence from specific studies of clinical problems can be found in an increasing number of electronic databases, such as the Cochrane Library (http://www.update-software.com/publications/cochrane; http://www.updateusa.com), the Canadian Cochrane Network and Centre (http://www.ccnc.cochrane.org), the Center for Health Evidence (http://www.cche.net), and the Center for Best Evidence (http://www.acponline.org; see Clinical Information). Another electronic database, Evidence-Based Medicine Reviews (EBMR) from Ovid Technologies (http://www.ovid.com) combines several electronic databases, including the Cochrane Database of Systematic Reviews, Best Evidence, Evidence-Based Mental Health, Evidence-Based Nursing, CancerLit, HealthSTAR, AIDSLINE, BIOETHICSLINE, and MEDLINE, plus links to over 200 full-text journals. EBMR links these databases to one another; if a study on a topic of interest is found on MEDLINE and also has been included in a systematic review in the Cochrane Library, then the review can also be readily and easily accessed. In using these sources, it is important to identify key search terms and to use the expertise of health science librarians in locating publications relevant to the project. Additional information about locating the evidence is in Chapter 5.

Once the literature has been located, it is helpful to classify the articles as clinical (nonresearch),

BOX 20–1	Agency for Healthcare Research and Quality Evidence-Based Practice Centers

- Blue Cross and Blue Shield Association, Technology Evaluation Center
- Duke University
- Evidence–Based Practice Center
- Johns Hopkins University
- McMaster University
- Oregon Evidence–Based Practice Center
- RTI International—University of North Carolina
- Southern California
- Stanford University–University of California, San Francisco
- Tufts-New England Medical Center
- University of Alberta
- University of Connecticut
- University of Minnesota
- University of Ottawa
- Vanderbilt University

From Agency for Healthcare Research and Quality. (2007). Evidence-based practice centers. Retrieved November 5, 2007, from http://www.ahrq.gov/clinic/epc/

integrative reviews, theory articles, research articles, and EBP guidelines. Before reading and critiquing the research, nurses will find it useful to read theoretical and clinical articles to get an overview of the nature of the topic and related concepts and then to review existing EBP guidelines. Ideally, articles should be read in the following order:

1. Clinical articles, to understand the state of the practice
2. Theory articles, to understand the various theoretical perspectives and concepts that may be encountered in critiquing studies
3. Systematic review articles, to understand the state of the science (e.g., meta-analyses and other nonquantitative systematic reviews)
4. EBP guidelines and evidence reports
5. Research articles (e.g., individual randomized clinical trials

Evidence-Based Practice Tip

The focused clinical question is used as a basis for searching the literature to identify relevant external evidence from research.

Schemas for Grading the Evidence

No consensus exists among professional organizations or across health care disciplines regarding the best system to use for denoting the type and quality of evidence or the grading schemas to denote the strength of the body of evidence (West et al., 2002). As illustrated in Table 20–3, for example, the joint American College of Chest Physicians/American Association of Cardiovascular and Pulmonary Rehabilitation ACCP/AACVPR Pulmonary Rehabilitation guidelines panel (1997) used an A, B, C rating scale to reflect the quality of the studies, including study designs and the consistency of the results of the scientific evidence.

In comparison, the US Preventative Services Task Force classifies the hierarchy of research design, grades the quality of each study on a three-point scale (good, fair, poor), and then grades recommendations using one of five classifications (A, B, C, D, or E) reflecting the strength of the evidence and the magnitude of net benefit (Harris et al., 2001). Table 20–3 presents the hierarchy of evidence models used throughout this book for rating evidence.

In "grading the evidence," two important areas are essential to address: (1) the quality of the individual research and (2) the strength of the body of evidence. The important domains and elements to include in grading the strength of the evidence are defined in Table 20–4.

Before critiquing research articles, reading relevant literature, and reviewing EBP guidelines, the organization or group responsible for the review need to agree on methods for noting the type of research, rating the quality of individual articles, and grading the strength of the body of evidence. Users need to evaluate which systems are most appropriate for the task being undertaken, the

TABLE 20-3 Summary of Evidence-Based Practice Rating Systems

Guideline for Management of Acute and Chronic Pain in Sickle Cell Disease	ACCP/AACVPR Pulmonary Rehabilitation Guideline Panel	US Preventative Services Task Force
Type of Evidence	Strength of Evidence	Quality of Evidence
I. Meta-analysis of multiple well-designed controlled studies II. At least one well-designed experimental study III. Well-designed, quasiexperimental studies, such as nonrandomized controlled, single-group pre/post, cohort, time series, or matched-case controlled studies IV. Well-designed nonexperimental studies such as comparative and correlational descriptive and case studies V. Case reports and clinical examples	A. Scientific evidence provided by well-designed, well-conducted, controlled trials (randomized and nonrandomized) with statistically significant results that consistently support the guideline recommendation B. Scientific evidence provided by observational studies or by controlled trials with less consistent results to support the guideline recommendation C. Expert opinion that supports the guideline recommendation because available scientific evidence did not present consistent results or because controlled trials were lacking	I. Evidence obtained from at least one properly randomized controlled trial II-1. Evidence obtained from well-designed controlled trials without randomization II-2. Evidence obtained from well-designed cohort or case-control analytical studies, preferably from more than one centre or research group II-3. Evidence obtained from multiple time series with or without intervention; dramatic results in uncontrolled experiments (such as the results of the introduction of penicillin treatment in the 1940s) also could be regarded as this type of evidence III. Opinions of respected authorities, based on clinical experience, descriptive studies and case reports, or reports of expert committees

TABLE 20-3 Summary of Evidence-Based Practice Rating Systems—cont'd

Guideline for Management of Acute and Chronic Pain in Sickle Cell Disease	ACCP/AACVPR Pulmonary Rehabilitation Guideline Panel	US Preventative Services Task Force
Strengths and Consistency of Evidence	Type of Evidence	Category Rating Validity of Each Study
A. Evidence of type I or consistent findings from multiple studies of type II, III, or IV B. Evidence of type II, III, or IV and generally consistent findings C. Evidence of type II, III, or IV but inconsistent findings D. Little or no evidence or type V evidence only	I. Evidence from a systematic review or meta-analysis of all relevant randomized controlled trials (RCTs) or EBP clinical practice guidelines based on systematic reviews or RCTs II. Evidence from at least one well-designed RCT III. Evidence from well-designed controlled trials without randomization IV. Evidence from well-designed case-control and cohort studies V. Evidence from systematic reviews of descriptive and qualitative studies VI. Evidence from a single descriptive or qualitative study VII. Evidence from the opinion of authorities or reports of expert committees (Melnyk & Fineout-Overholt, 2005)	Good = meets all criteria for this study design Fair = does not meet all criteria for this study design but has no fatal flaws that invalidate the results Poor = study contains a fatal flaw **Recommendation Grades** A. Strongly recommends that clinicians routinely provide [the service] to eligible clients (found good evidence that [the service] improves important health outcomes and concludes that the benefits substantially outweigh the harms) B. Recommends that clinicians routinely provide [the service] to eligible clients (found at least fair evidence that [the service] improves important health outcomes and concludes that the benefits outweigh the harms) C. Makes no recommendation for or against routine provision of [the service] (found at least fair evidence that [the service] can improve health outcomes but concludes that the balance of benefits and harms is too close to justify a general recommendation) D. Recommends against routinely providing [the service] to asymptomatic clients (found at least fair evidence that [the service] is ineffective or that the harms outweigh the benefits) E. Concludes that evidence is insufficient to recommend for or against routinely providing [the service] (evidence that [the service] is effective is lacking, of poor quality, or conflicted and the balance of benefits and harms cannot be determined)

The data in column 1 are from American Pain Society. (1999). *Guideline for the management of acute and chronic pain in sickle cell disease.* Glenview, IL: American Pain Society. The data in column 2 are from American College of Chest Physicians/American Association of Cardiovascular and Pulmonary Rehabilitation (ACCP/AACVPR). (1997). Special report: Pulmonary rehabilitation: Joint ACCP/AACVPR evidence-based guidelines. *Chest, 112,* 1363–1396. The data in column 3 are adapted from Harris et al., (2001). Current methods of the US Preventative Services Task Force: A review of the process. *American Journal of Preventative Medicine, 20(3S),* 21–35.

ACCP/AACVPR: American College of Chest Physicians/American Association of Cardiovascular and Pulmonary Rehabilitation; EBP: evidence-based practice.

length of time to complete each instrument, and its ease of use (West et al., 2002). They will also need to decide how the strength of the evidence will be reflected in the guideline.

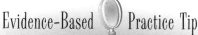

Evidence-Based Practice Tip

Research evidence from both systematic reviews and individual research studies is critically appraised for strength, quality, and consistency, which will influence the validity and generalizability of the studies.

Critique of Evidence-Based Practice Guidelines

As the number of EBP guidelines proliferates, it becomes increasingly important that nurses critique these guidelines, including the methods used for formulating them, and consider how they might be used in their institution (RNAO, 2002). Critical areas that should be assessed when critiquing EBP guidelines include the following:

1. Date of publication or release
2. Authors of the guideline
3. Endorsement of the guideline
4. Clear indication of what the guideline covers and client groups for which it was designed
5. Types of evidence (research, nonresearch) used in formulating the guideline
6. Types of research included in formulating the guideline (e.g., "We considered only randomized and other prospective controlled trials in determining efficacy of therapeutic interventions . . .")

7. Description of the methods used in grading the evidence
8. Search terms and retrieval methods used to acquire research and nonresearch evidence used in the guideline
9. Well-referenced statements regarding practice
10. Comprehensive reference list
11. Review of the guideline by experts
12. Indication as to whether the guideline has been used or tested in practice and, if so, with what types of clients and in what types of settings

Evidence-based (EB) guidelines that are formulated using rigorous methods provide a useful starting point for nurses to understand the evidence base of certain practices. However, more research may have become available since the publication of the guideline, and refinements may be needed. Although information in well-developed national EB guidelines is a helpful reference, nurses usually find it necessary to localize the guideline using institution-specific evidence-based policies, procedures, or standards before application within a specific setting. A useful tool for critiquing guidelines is the AGREE tool available at http://www.agreecollaboration.org/. This tool evaluates six areas: scope and purpose, stakeholder involvement, rigour of development, clarity and presentation, applicability, and editorial independence. The instrument recommends that four to six people with expertise in the area complete the ratings.

Some professional organizations, such as the RNAO, have appraised guidelines using a systematic and rigorous process. However, incorporating

TABLE 20–4	**Important Domains and Elements for Systems to Grade the Strength of Evidence**
Quality	Aggregate of quality ratings for individual studies, predicated on the extent to which bias was minimized
Quantity	Magnitude of the effect, numbers of studies, and sample size or power
Consistency	For any given topic, the extent to which similar findings are reported using similar and different study designs

Adapted from Agency for Healthcare Research and Quality. (2002). *Systems to rate the strength of scientific evidence. Evidence Report/Technology Assessment No. 47* (AHRQ Publication No. 02-E016). Rockville, MD: Agency for Healthcare Research and Quality, US Department of Health and Human Services.

EB guidelines into an organization requires more than a rating or assessment of the guideline itself: stakeholders must be consulted, an analysis of the impact on financial resources must be initiated, policies and procedures must be updated, and a procedure for the introduction, support, and implementation must be planned. The RNAO has published a comprehensive toolkit designed to assist health care agencies to implement EB guidelines (available at http://www.rnao.org).

Critique of Research

The critique of each study should use the same methodology, and the critiquing process should be a shared responsibility. It is helpful, however, to have one individual provide leadership for the project and design strategies for completing critiques. A group approach to critiques is recommended because it distributes the workload, helps those responsible for implementing the changes to understand the scientific basis for the change in practice, arms nurses with citations and research-based facts to use in effecting practice changes with peers and other disciplines, and provides novices with an environment in which to learn how to critique and apply research findings. Methods to make critiquing fun and interesting include the following:

- Using a journal club to discuss critiques done by each member of the group
- Pairing a novice and an expert to do critiques
- Eliciting assistance from students who may be interested in the topic and want experience doing critiques
- Assigning the critique to graduate students interested in the topic
- Making a class project of critique and synthesis of research for a given topic

Resources available to assist with the critique include the following:

- *Reading Research: A User-Friendly Guide for Nurses and Other Health Professionals* (Davies & Logan, 2008)

- *Evidence-Based Nursing: A Guide to Clinical Practice* (DiCenso et al., 2005)
- *The Evidence-Based Practice Manual for Nurses* (Craig & Smyth, 2007)
- *Evidence-Based Medicine: How to Practice and Teach EBM* and accompanying compact disc (Sackett et al., 2005)

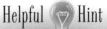
Helpful Hint
Keep critiquing simple and encourage participation by staff members who are providing direct client care.

Synthesis of Research Findings

After the studies have been critiqued, the group can decide which studies should be included in the synthesis of research studies to be used for application to clinical practice. When considering the inclusion of a study in the synthesis of findings, factors to be considered include the overall scientific merit of the study, the type of subjects enrolled in the study (e.g., age, gender, pathology) and their similarity to the client population to which the findings will be applied, and the relevance of the study to the topic in question. For example, if the practice area is prevention of deep venous thrombosis in postoperative clients, a descriptive study using a heterogeneous population of medical clients is not appropriate for inclusion in the synthesis of findings.

To synthesize the findings from research critiques, it is helpful to use a summary table in which critical information from studies can be documented. Essential to include in such summaries are the following:

- The study purpose
- Research questions or hypotheses
- The variables studied
- A description of the study sample and setting
- The type of research design
- The methods used to measure each variable

TABLE 20–5 Example of a Summary Table for Research Critiques												
Citation	Purpose and Research Question	Research Design*	Sample	Independent Variables and Measures	Dependent Variables and Measures	Statistical Tests	Results	Implications	General Strengths	General Weaknesses	Overall Quality of Study†	Summary Statements for Practice

*Identify the level of evidence provided by the design using a consistent hierarchy of evidence model (e.g., Table 3–3 or Table 20–3).
†Use a consistent rating system (e.g., good, fair, poor).

- A detailed description of the independent variable or intervention tested
- The study findings

An example of a summary form is illustrated in Table 20–5. The summary form should be modified for qualitative research.

Helpful Hint

Use of a summary form helps identify commonalities across several studies with regard to study findings and the types of clients to whom study findings can be applied.

Evidence-Based Practice Tip

The written synthesis of the evidence highlights the strengths and weaknesses of the available evidence, which will guide you in making a decision about its applicability to practice for your client population.

Setting Forth Evidence-Based Practice Recommendations

Based on the critique of EBP guidelines and synthesis of research, recommendations for practice are set forth. The type and strength of evidence used to support the practice need to be clearly delineated. Box 20–2 is a useful tool to assist with this activity. The following are examples of practice recommendation statements:

- "Small, informal group health education classes, delivered in the antenatal period, have a better impact on breastfeeding initiation rates than breastfeeding literature alone or combined with formal, non-interactive methods of teaching" (strength of recommendation = B) (RNAO, 2003, p. 46).
- Older people who have recurrent falls should be offered long-term exercise and balance training (strength of recommendation = B) (American Geriatrics Society, British Geriatrics Society, American Academy of

Orthopaedic Surgeons, and Panel on Falls Prevention, 2001, p. 668).

- Every client should be screened to identify those most likely to be affected by asthma. As part of the basic respiratory assessment, nurses should ask every client two questions:
  1. Have you ever been told by a physician that you have asthma?

BOX 20–2	**Consistency of Evidence from Critiqued Research, Appraisals of Evidence-Based Practice Guidelines, Critiqued Systematic Reviews, and Nonresearch Literature**

1. Is there replication of studies with consistent results?
2. Are the studies well designed?
3. Are recommendations consistent among systematic reviews, EBP guidelines, and critiqued research?
4. Are there identified risks to the client by applying EBP recommendations?
5. Are there identified benefits to the client?
6. Have cost analysis studies been conducted on the recommended action, intervention, or treatment?
7. Have recommendations about assessments, actions, and interventions or treatments from the research, systematic reviews, and EB guidelines been summarized with an assigned evidence grade?

ONE EXAMPLE OF GRADING THE EVIDENCE

A. Evidence from well-designed meta-analyses or other systematic reviews
B. Evidence from well-designed controlled trials, both randomized and nonrandomized, with results that consistently support a specific action (e.g., assessment, intervention, or treatment)
C. Evidence from observational studies (e.g., correlational descriptive studies) or controlled trials with inconsistent results
D. Evidence from expert opinion or multiple case studies

Adapted from Titler, M. G. (2002). *Toolkit for promoting evidence-based practice.* Iowa City, IA: Department of Nursing Services and Patient Care, University of Iowa Hospitals and Clinics.

---

2. Have your ever used a puffer or inhaler or asthma medication for breathing problems? (strength of recommendation = D) (RNAO, 2004, p. 30).

Decision to Change Practice

After studies are critiqued and synthesized and EBPs are set forth, the next step is to decide whether the findings are appropriate for use in practice. Criteria to consider in making these decisions include the following:

- Relevance of research findings for practice
- Consistency in findings across studies or guidelines
- Studies with sample characteristics similar to the population being considered for a change in practice
- Consistency among evidence from research and other nonresearch evidence
- Feasibility for use in practice
- Risk-to-benefit ratio (risk of harm; potential benefit for the client)

It is recommended that practice changes be based on knowledge or evidence derived from several sources (e.g., several research studies) that demonstrate consistent findings.

A synthesis of study findings and other evidence may lead to support for current practice, minor practice modifications, major practice changes, or development of a new area of practice. For example, a project on gauze versus transparent dressings did not result in a practice change because the studies that were reviewed substantiated current practice (Pettit & Kraus, 1995). In comparison, a guideline for assessing the return of bowel motility after abdominal surgery used a combination of research findings and expert consultation and resulted in a change in practice for assessing bowel motility in this adult inpatient population (Madsen et al., 2005). This project resulted in (1) deleting bowel sound assessment as a marker of return of gastrointestinal motility and (2) using the return of flatus, the first bowel movement, and the absence of abdominal distention as primary indicators of return of bowel motility following abdominal surgery in adults.

Development of Evidence-Based Practice

The next step is to put in writing the evidence base of the practice (Haber et al., 1994) using the agreed-upon grading schema. When the results of the critique and synthesis of evidence support current practice or suggest a change in practice, a written EBP protocol is warranted.

A written EBP protocol (e.g., standard, policy, procedure) is necessary so that individuals know (1) that the practices are based on evidence and (2) the type of evidence (e.g., randomized clinical trial, expert opinion) used in developing the protocol. Several different formats can be used to document EBP changes. The format chosen is influenced by what the document will be used for and how. Written EBPs should be part of the organizational policy and procedure manual and should include detailed references to the parts of the policy and procedure that are based on research and other types of evidence.

For example, two staff nurses participating in a pilot EBP program to develop unit-based Research Resource Nurses (R.R.N.s) formulated a clinical question related to the "best practice for management of an inwelling urinary catheter in hospitalized adults 65 years and older." The format used at their medical centre was a process standard that is equivalent to an EBP policy or protocol.

Clinicians (e.g., nurses, physicians, pharmacists) who adopt EBPs are influenced by the perceived participation they have had in developing and reviewing the protocol (Titler, 2004). Once the EBP standard is written, key stakeholders must have an opportunity to review it and provide feedback to the individual(s) responsible for writing it.

In the example above, initially, the standard for management of indwelling urinary catheters was presented at the Nursing Practice Council and then to another important stakeholder, the Infection Control Committee, followed by the Medical Products Committee (for cost/benefit analysis), and, finally, the Information Systems Committee for modification of the electronic client record to include a three-day post–urinary catheter insertion prompt for nurses and physicians to evaluate discontinuation of the catheter (Haber, personal communication, 2005).

The use of focus groups is a practical way to provide discussion about the evidence-based standard and to identify key areas that may be potentially troublesome during the implementation phase. Box 20–3 lists key questions that can be used in the focus groups.

Evidence-Based Practice Tip

Use a consistent approach to writing EBP standards and referencing the research and related literature.

Implementing the Practice Change

If a practice change is warranted, the next steps are to implement the EB changes in practice. This process goes beyond writing a policy or procedure that is evidence based; implementing a practice change requires interaction among direct care providers to champion and foster evidence

---

BOX 20–3   Key Questions for Focus Groups

1. What do nurses and physicians need to know to use the protocol with clients in a specific area of practice (i.e., paediatrics)?

2. In your opinion, how will this protocol improve client care in your unit or practice?

3. What modifications would you suggest in the evidence-based protocol before using it in your practice?

4. What content in the protocol is unclear or needs revision?

5. What would you change about the format of the protocol?

6. What part of this protocol or practice change do you view as being the most challenging?

7. Do you have any other suggestions?

adoption, leadership support, and system changes. Rogers's seminal work on **diffusion of innovations** (Rogers, 1995) is extremely useful in facilitating adoption of EBPs. Other investigators describing barriers to and strategies for adoption of EBPs have used Rogers's (2003) model (Sackett et al., 2005). According to this model, diffusion of an innovation (e.g., an EBP) is influenced by the nature of the innovation and the manner in which it is communicated (communication process) to members (health care professionals) of a social system (e.g., acute care hospital, nursing unit) (Rogers, 1995). Strategies for promoting adoption of EBPs must address these four areas within a context of participative, planned change (see Figure 20–4).

NATURE OF THE INNOVATION OR EBP

When implementation processes encourage health care professionals to adapt or reinvent the guidelines for use in their local agency, adherence to the guidelines increases (Schoenbaum et al., 1995a, 1995b; Titler & Everett, 2001). Studies funded by the AHRQ (Farquhar et al., 2002) and others suggested that a positive effect on aligning practices with the evidence can be achieved when clinical systems, computerized decision support, and prompts support practice (e.g., decision-making algorithms) (Oxman, Thomson, Davis, & Haynes, 1995). To move evidence from the "book to the bedside," information from EBPs must have perceived benefits for clients, nurses, physicians, and administrators; be "reinvented" and integrated into daily client care processes; impart evidence in a readily available format; and make evidence-based practices observable for practitioners (Berwick, 2003; Rogers, 2003). Those responsible for implementing the EBP standard need to consider the use of practice prompts, decision support systems, and quick reference guides as part of the implementation process. An example of a quick reference guide is shown in Figure 20–5.

Evidence-Based Practice Tip

When marketing a proposed EBP change to key stakeholders in your organization remember the importance of effective communication.

METHODS OF COMMUNICATION

Methods of communicating the EBP standard to those delivering care affects adoption of the practice (Funk, Tornquist, & Champagne, 1995; Rogers, 1995). Essential components of the implementation process include education of staff; use of opinion leaders, change champions, and core groups; and consultation with experts in the content area (e.g., advanced practice nurses). Continuing education alone does little to change practice behaviour (Mazmanian, Daffron, Johnson, Davis, & Kantrowitz, 1998; Oxman et al., 1995; Schneider

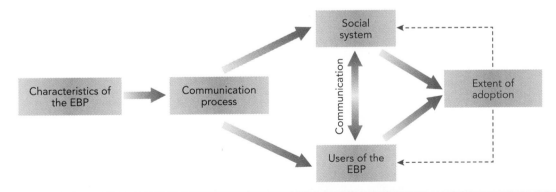

Figure 20–4 Implementation model

Redrawn from Rogers, E. (1995). *Diffusion of innovations.* New York: The Free Press; and Titler, M. G., & Everett, L. Q. (2001). Translating research into practice: Considerations for critical care investigators. *Critical Care Nursing Clinics of North America, 13,* 587–604.
EBP: evidence-based practice.

Use this quick reference guide to help in the assessment of pain:
• Before clients undergo medical procedures or surgeries that can cause pain
• When clients are experiencing pain from recent surgeries, medical procedures, trauma, or other acute illness

General principles for assessing pain in older adults:
• Verify sensory ability (Can the person see you? Hear you?).
• Allow time to respond.
• Repeat questions/instructions as necessary.
• Use printed materials with large type and dark lines.

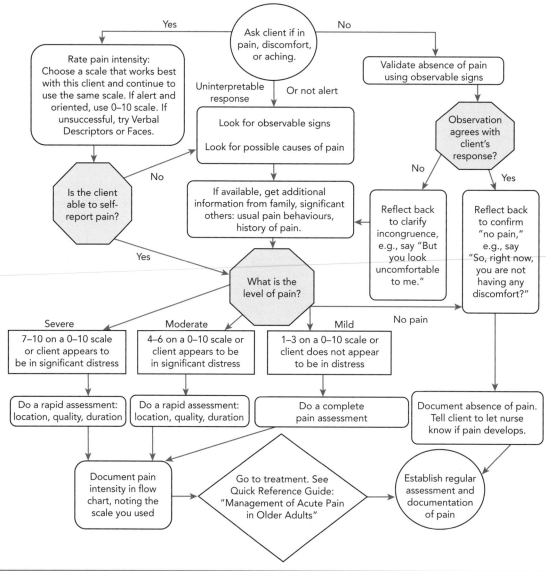

Figure 20–5   Quick reference guide: assessment of acute pain in older adults

Redrawn from Herr, K., Titler, M., Sorofman, B., Ardery, G., Schmitt, M., & Young, D. (2000). Evidence-based guideline: Acute pain management in the elderly. In L. Grant (Ed.), *From book to bedside: Acute pain management in the elderly* (Written for Agency for Healthcare Research and Quality: 1 R01 HS10482-01). Iowa City, IA: University of Iowa.

and Eisenberg, 1998). Interactive education and didactic education, used in combination with other practice-reinforcing strategies, have more positive effects than education alone (Bookbinder et al., 1996; Oxman et al., 1995; Schneider & Eisenberg, 1998).

It is important that staff know the scientific basis for the changes in practice and the improvements in quality of care anticipated by the change. Disseminating this information to staff needs to be done creatively, using various educational strategies. In-service training sessions may not be the most effective method and may not reach the majority of the staff. Although it is unrealistic for all staff to have participated in the critique or to have read all studies used to develop the EBP, staff need to know the myths and realities of the practice. Education of staff also must include ensuring that they are competent in the skills needed to carry out the new practice. For example, if pH is to be used to check placement of nasogastric and nasointestinal tubes rather than auscultation, staff knowledge and skill in obtaining aspirate from small-bore feeding tubes are essential (Rakel et al., 1994).

One method of communicating information to staff is through the use of colourful posters that identify myths and realities or describe the essence of the change in practice (Titler, Moss, et al., 1994). Visibly identifying those who have learned the information and are using the EBP (e.g., with buttons, ribbons, pins) stimulates interest in others who may not have internalized the change. As a result, the "new" learner may ask questions about the practice and be more open to learning the EBP. Other educational strategies, such as train-the-trainer programs, computer-assisted instruction, and competency testing, are helpful in educating staff.

Several studies have demonstrated that opinion leaders are effective in changing the behaviours of health care practitioners (Berner et al., 2003; Cullen, 2005; Locock, Dopson, Chambers, & Gabbay, 2001a, 2001b; Oxman et al., 1995; Thomson O'Brien et al., 2002). **Opinion leaders** are individulas from the local peer group who are viewed as a respected source of influence, are considered by associates to be technically competent, and are trusted to judge the fit between the EBP and the local situation. The key characteristic of an opinion leader is that he or she is trusted to evaluate new information in the context of group norms. Thus, an opinion leader must be considered by associates to be technically competent and a full and dedicated member of the local group (Oxman et al., 1995; Rogers, 2003). Social interactions such as "hallway chats," one-on-one discussions, and addressing questions are important but often overlooked components of translation (Berwick, 2003; Rogers, 2003).

Change champions are also necessary for implementing EBP changes in practice (Rogers, 2003; Titler, 2004). They are practitioners within the local group who are expert clinicians, passionate about the clinical topic, committed to improving quality of care, and have a positive working relationship with other health care professionals (Harvey et al., 2002; Rogers, 2003). They circulate information, encourage peers to align their practice with the best evidence, arrange demonstrations, and orient staff to the EBP (Shively et al., 1997; Titler, 2004). The change champion believes in an idea, will not take "no" for an answer, is undaunted by insults and rebuffs, and, above all, persists. For potential research-based changes in practice to reach the bedside, it is imperative that one or two "change champions" be identified for each client care unit or service where the change is being made (Titler, 2003). Staff nurses are some of the best change champions for EBP.

Using a "core group" in conjunction with change champions is another helpful strategy for implementing the practice change (Titler et al., 2001). A core group is a select group of practitioners with the mutual goal of disseminating information regarding a practice change and facilitating the change in practice by other staff in their unit or peer group. The success of the core group approach requires that core group members work well with the change champion and represent various shifts, days of the week, and tenure in the practice setting. Core group members become knowledgeable about the scientific basis for the practice, assist with disseminating the evidence-based information to other staff, and reinforce the practice change on a daily basis. The change champion educates the core group members and assists them in changing their practices. Each member of the core group, in turn, takes responsibility for effecting the change in two to three of their peers. Core group members provide positive feedback to their assigned staff who are changing their practices and encourage those reluctant to change to try the new practice. Core group members also are able to assist the change champion in identifying the best way to teach staff about the practice change and to proactively solve issues that arise (Titler et al., 2001). Using a core group approach in conjunction with a change champion results in a critical mass of practitioners promoting adoption of the EBP (Rogers, 2003).

Outreach and consultation by an expert in the practice have been shown to promote positive changes in the practice behaviours of nurses and physicians (Thomson O'Brien et al., 2003b). *Outreach (academic detailing)* is done by an expert who meets one-on-one with practitioners in their setting to provide information about the EBP and to give feedback on provider performance; outreach can be accomplished either alone or in combination with others and results in positive changes in health care practices (Thomson O'Brien et al., 2003a, 2003b). Nurse clinicians can provide one-on-one consultation to staff regarding the use of the EBP with specific clients, assist staff in troubleshooting issues in application of the practice, and provide feedback on provider performance regarding use of the EBP. Studies have demonstrated that the use of nurse clinicians as facilitators of change promotes adherence to the EBP (Bauchner & Simpson, 1998; Hendryx et al., 1998).

Evidence-Based ⬤ Practice Tip

Opinion leaders and change champions are essential to the success of implementing an EBP change. They are often found among the informal leaders of an organization.

USERS OF THE INNOVATION OR EBP

Members of a social system influence how quickly and widely EBPs are adopted (Rogers, 2003). The strategies of audit and feedback, performance gap assessment (PGA), and use of the EBP have been tested (Lomas et al., 1991; Rogers, 2003; Titler, Kleiber, et al., 1994; Titler et al., 2001). PGA and audit and feedback have consistently shown a positive effect with regard to changing the practice behaviour of health care professionals (Fiore et al., 1996; Lomas et al., 1991; Thomson O'Brien et al., 2003a). PGA (performance gap assessment or baseline practice performance) informs members, at the *beginning* of change, about a practice performance and opportunities for improvement. Specific practice indicators selected for PGA are related to the practices that are the focus of change, such as pain assessment every four hours for acute pain management.

The strategy of audit and feedback involves an ongoing audit of performance indicators (e.g., pain assessment every four hours) throughout the implementation process and discussion of the findings with practitioners *during* the practice change (Jamtvedt, Young, Kristofferson, Thomson O'Brien, Oxman, 2004; Titler, 2004). This strategy helps staff see how their efforts to improve care and client outcomes are progressing throughout the implementation process. Audit and feedback should be done at regular intervals throughout the implementation process (e.g., every 4 to 6 weeks) (Jamtvedt et al., 2004; Thomson O'Brien et al., 2003a). Performance gap assessment and audit and feedback data can be provided in run charts, statistical process control charts, or bar graphs (Carey, 2002) (see Figure 20–6).

The characteristics of the users, such as educational preparation, practice specialty, and views on innovativeness, influence adoption of an innovation (Rogers, 2003; Schneider & Eisenberg, 1998). Users of an innovation usually try it for a period of time before adopting it in their practice (Meyer & Goes, 1988; Rogers, 2003). When "trying an EBP" (piloting the change) is incorporated as part of the implementation process, users have an opportunity to try it for a period of time, provide feedback to those in charge of implementation, and modify

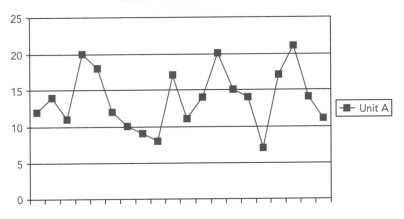

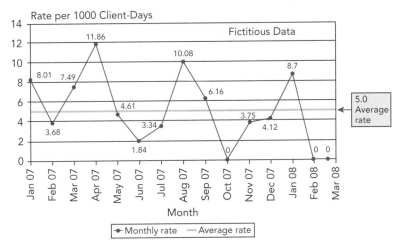

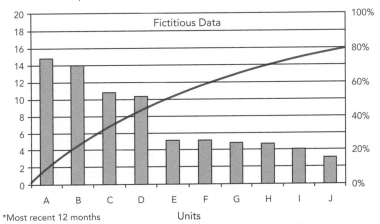

*Most recent 12 months

Figure 20–6 Examples of audit and feedback data

the practice if necessary. Piloting the EBP as part of implementation has a positive influence on the extent of adoption of the new practice (Rogers, 2003; Titler, 2003; Titler et al., 2001).

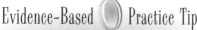

Evidence-Based Practice Tip

Collecting baseline data before implementation of a new EBP, and at specified intervals thereafter, provides staff members with a concrete picture of how this evidence-based change in practice is contributing to improving client outcomes.

SOCIAL SYSTEM

The social system (context) has a high degree of influence on adoption of an innovation (Foxcroft, Cole, Fulbrook, Johnston, & Stevens, 2002; Fraser, 2004a, 2004b; Institute of Medicine, 2001; Rogers, 2003; Thompson, 2001). Leadership support is critical for promoting the use of EBPs (Baggs & Mick, 2000; Berwick, 2003; Carr & Schott, 2002; Nagy, Lumby, McKinley, & Macfarlane, 2001; Retsas, 2000; Stetler, 2003) and is expressed by providing the necessary resources, materials, and time to fulfill assigned responsibilities. Additional organizational variables that influence adoption include the following: (1) access to inventors or researchers; (2) authority to change practice; and (3) support from and collaboration with peers, other disciplines, and administrators to align practice with EBPs (Bach, 1995; Funk et al., 1995; Nutley and Davies, 2000; Thomson O'Brien et al., 2002; Tranmer, Coulson, Holtom, Lively, & Maloney, 1998; Walshe and Rundall, 2001). It is important that organizational and unit practice standards, as well as documentation systems, support the use of the EBPs (Titler, 2004).

The role of the nurse manager is critical in making EBP changes a reality for staff at the bedside. Nurse managers must expect that staff will participate in EBP activities, role-model the change in their practice, and provide written and verbal support for the practice change. When selecting a potential topic, the nurse manager must value the idea and support the potential changes.

Clinical nurse specialists are critical to helping staff retrieve and critique the studies and other evidence on the selected topic. Although staff nurses are often willing to participate, the nurse clinician provides significant leadership in the process by facilitating synthesis of the research and other evidence, critically analyzing which practices should be changed, assisting staff in communicating these changes to their peers, and role-modelling changes in practice.

As part of the work of implementing the change, the social system—unit, service line, or clinic—must ensure that policies, procedures, standards, clinical pathways, and documentation systems support the use of the EBPs. Documentation forms or clinical information systems may need revision to support changes in practice; documentation systems that fail to readily support the new practice impede change. For example, if staff members are expected to reassess and document pain intensity within 30 minutes following administration of an analgesic agent, then documentation forms must reflect this practice standard. The role of upper- and middle-level leadership is to ensure that organizational documents and systems are flexible and supportive of the EBPs.

Thus, making an evidence-based change in practice involves a series of steps and a process that is often nonlinear. Implementing the change will take several weeks to months, depending on the nature of the practice change. Those leading the project must be aware of change as a process and continue to encourage and teach peers about the change in practice. Moreover, the new practice must be continually reinforced and sustained or the practice change will be intermittent and soon fade, allowing more traditional methods of care to return.

Evaluation

Evaluation provides an opportunity to collect and analyze data with regard to use of a new EBP and then to modify the practice as necessary. The evidence-based change needs to be evaluated in both the pilot area and, when the practice is changed, additional client care areas. The importance of the evaluation

Evidence-Based Practice Tip

Obtaining support from nurse managers is essential since they need to support the staff nurses working on the EBP project. Support includes arranging for release time and coverage from client care responsibilities to provide time to think about and formulate the clinical question, search the literature, appraise the evidence, and develop the EBP product (e.g., policy, standard, protocol), as well as present and market the innovation to the appropriate organization. stakeholders.

BOX 20–4   Steps of Evaluation for Evidence-Based Projects

1. Identify process and outcome variables of interest.
   Example: Process variable: clients >65 years of age will have a Braden scale completed upon admission
   Outcome variable: presence or absence of a nosocomial pressure ulcer; if present—identify stage (I, II, III, or IV)

2. Determine methods and frequency of data collection.
   Example: Process variable: chart audit of all clients >65 years old, 1 day a month
   Outcome variable: client assessment of all clients >65 years old, 1 day a month

3. Determine baseline and follow-up sample sizes.

4. Design data collection forms.
   Example: Process chart audit abstraction form
   Outcome variable: pressure ulcer assessment form

5. Establish the content validity of data collection forms.

6. Train data collectors.

7. Assess interrater reliability of data collectors.

8. Collect data at specified intervals.

9. Provide "on-site" feedback to staff regarding the progress in achieving the practice change.

10. Assist feedback of analyzed data to staff.

11. Use data to assist staff in modifying or integrating the EBP change.

---

cannot be overemphasized: it provides information for PGA, audit, and feedback for determining whether the EBP should be retained, modified, or eliminated.

A desired outcome achieved in a more controlled environment, when a researcher is implementing a study protocol to a homogeneous group of clients (conduct of research), may not result in the same outcome when the practice is implemented in the natural clinical setting by several caregivers to a more heterogeneous client population. The steps in the evaluation process are summarized in Box 20–4.

Evaluation should include both process and outcome measures (Lepper & Titler, 1999; Rosswurm & Larrabee, 1999). The process component focuses on how the EBP change is being implemented. It is important to know whether staff are using the practice in care delivery and whether they are implementing the practice as noted in the written EBP standard. Evaluation of the process also should note (1) barriers that staff encounter in carrying out the practice (e.g., lack of information, skills, or necessary equipment), (2) differences in opinion among health care professionals, and (3) difficulty in carrying out the steps of the practice as originally designed (e.g., shutting off tube feedings one hour before aspirating the contents to check for the placement of nasointestinal tubes). Process data can be collected from staff and client self-reports, medical record audits, or observation of clinical practice.

Outcome data are an equally important part of evaluation. The purpose of outcome evaluation is

to assess whether the client, staff, and fiscal outcomes expected are achieved. Therefore, baseline data needs to be used for a pre/post comparison (Cullen, 2005; Titler et al., 2001). The outcome variables measured should be those that are projected to change as a result of changing practice (Rosswurm & Larrabee, 1999; Soukup, 2000). For example, research demonstrates that less restricted family visiting practices in critical care units result in improved satisfaction with care. Thus, client and family member satisfaction should be an outcome measure that is evaluated as part of changing visiting practices in adult critical care units. Outcome measures should be measured before the change in practice is implemented, after implementation, and every six to 12 months thereafter. The findings must be provided to clinicians to reinforce the impact of the change in practice and to ensure that the changes are incorporated into quality improvement programs.

The evaluation process should include feedback to staff who are making the change. This feedback needs to include verbal or written appreciation for the work and visual demonstration of both the progress in implementation and the improvement in client outcomes. The key to effective evaluation is to ensure that the evidence-based change in practice is warranted (e.g., will improve the quality of care) and that the intervention does not harm the clients (Lepper & Titler, 1999). For example, when instituting a change in practice for assessing the return of bowel motility following abdominal surgery in adults, an important step was informing staff that using other markers for return of bowel motility, rather than bowel sound assessment, did not result in increased paralytic ileus or bowel obstruction (Madsen et al., 2005).

Helpful Hint

Include client outcome measures (e.g., pressure ulcer prevalence) and cost (e.g., cost savings, cost avoidance) in your evaluation of a new evidence-based practice.

BARRIERS TO RESEARCH UTILIZATION

Ross-Kerr and Wood (2003, pp. 144–145) described barriers to research utilization as follows:

> Barriers to research utilization closely follow the concepts in Rogers's model. Communication has been cited as a major barrier (Bock, 1990; Chambers, 1989; King, Barnard, & Hoehn, 1981; Repko, 1990). Clinical nurses have difficulty finding relevant studies (Funk, Champagne, Wiese, & Tornquist, 1991; Haughey, 1988;

> Pank, Rostron, & Stenhouse, 1984). They find that much of the literature includes findings with little relevance to the clinical situation, or if relevant, studies are presented in an unusable form (Pank et al., 1984). Researchers often present findings in tentative terms in response to hypothetical inquiries and discuss results as they relate to theory and the need for further inquiry. They may use standard research jargon and emphasize methodological or statistical issues instead of implications for practice. While sometimes appropriate among researchers, this style of communication provides little on which practitioners can base their care (Funk, Tornquist, & Champagne, 1989). To overcome this barrier, it is suggested that researchers make the practice setting the focus of their scientific inquiry and disseminate their findings in a comprehensible and relevant manner to practitioners.

> Other barriers to research utilization include cost and time constraints, negative attitudes toward research, the quality and relevance of the research, time to read and implement research, and a variety of organizational and workplace limitations.

> A survey of all clinical agencies (hospitals, public health units, and home-care departments) in British Columbia found very few with supportive infrastructure in place, particularly in public health units and home-care departments (Registered Nurses Association of British Columbia [RNABC], 1993). If research-based nursing practice was part of the nursing department's philosophy and goals, the most common and often the only form of infrastructure support was an nursing research committee (NRC). To date, little attention has been paid to nurses' job descriptions and responsibilities for research-based nursing practice; however, most of the

health-care agencies expected staff nurses to question practice and use research findings. This suggests that even though nurses might be involved in research activities and might change practice based on research findings, it is unlikely that they will receive support or recognition for such in their performance appraisals.

Carole Estabrooks, an associate professor from the University of Alberta, has built a research program based on knowledge utilization and translating research into practice. She believes that the importance of the role of organizations and nursing service administrators has been underestimated in developing a practice environment conducive to a culture of evidence-based decision making. Estabrooks (2003) hypothesized the following:

- "Without the right climate, individual factors promoting research utilization may not be realized"
- "Personal experience and interactions are not given due recognition as sources of knowledge in the scientific and academic communities"
- "Clinicians and students are both users and producers of knowledge"
- "Knowledge is produced and travels readily within communities of practice." (p. 62)

Administrators who develop appropriate cultures that foster and build on communities of practice, where knowledge is produced and shared by bedside nurses, will facilitate the increased use of research in clinical practice (Estabrooks, 2003).

Another barrier to use of research in practice identified by Estabrooks, O'Leary, Ricker, and Humphrey (2003) is the lag in use of the Internet for sources of knowledge. In a culture in which nurses are rewarded for client care activity, accessing the Internet is considered nonproductive. Nurses do not typically engage in intellectual work or research at the bedside; they do bedside nursing care. Additionally, the infrastructure does not support strategically located and accessible computers for nurses.

TRANSLATION SCIENCE

Although a myriad of initiatives aimed at increasing use of evidence in practice exist, little systematic evidence is available of the effectiveness of these initiatives (Nutley, Davies, & Walter, 2003; Thompson, Estabrooks, Scott-Findlay, Moore, & Wallin, 2007). **Translation science** is the investigation of methods, interventions, and variables that influence adoption of EBPs by individuals and organizations to improve clinical and operational decision making in health care (Kovner, Elton, & Billings, 2000; Titler & Everett, 2001; Walshe & Rundall, 2001). This investigation includes testing the effect of interventions on *promoting* and *sustaining* adoption of EBPs. Examples of translation studies include describing facilitators and barriers to knowledge uptake and use, organizational predictors of adherence to ambulatory care guidelines, and attitudes toward EBPs and defining the structure of the scientific field (Dykes, 2003; Estabrooks, 2004; Kirchhoff, 2004; Titler, 2004).

FUTURE DIRECTIONS

Use of research across health care systems for improving the quality of care is essential. As the profession continues to understand the science of nursing and synthesize this science for application in practice, it will become increasingly necessary that we test and understand how to best promote the use of this science in daily practice.

Ross-Kerr and Wood (2003, p. 155) detailed some of the challenges in the future of the research process:

Facilitating research utilization in nursing practice is not an easy task, but neither is it an impossible dream. Some activities that might facilitate the research process include the following:

- *Funding key research positions*
- *Creating institutional infrastructures*
- *Encouraging and assisting nurses to attend practice-based research workshops and conferences*

- *Providing continuing education courses to assist nurses in critiquing research*
- *Creating a reward system within the agency for research utilization in practice*
- *Promoting collaborative efforts between agency personnel and other health-care agencies or educational institutions*
- *Establishing a means for nurses to access research reports relevant to their practice*
- *Promoting demonstration projects that illustrate the cost-effectiveness of changing from a traditional, intuitively based practice to one that is research-based*
- *Ensuring that research utilization is a role expectation for all nursing positions (management, educational, and clinical) and that it is reinforced in job descriptions, agency policy, and the institution's philosophy of nursing.*

Diagnosing barriers, and planning and implementing strategies to overcome them, are challenges. The first challenge is to demonstrate the cost-effectiveness of nursing research and to justify the allocation of resources and personnel to create the necessary infrastructures. The second challenge is to reduce the time gap between when knowledge is developed and when it is used. The third challenge is to create agency infrastructures that will support the transformation of nursing practice from a ritual base to a research base. Efforts to address these challenges require partnerships among practitioners, researchers, administrators, and disciplines.

Education of nurses must include knowledge and skills in the use of research evidence in practice. Nurses are increasingly being held accountable for practices based on scientific evidence. Thus, we must communicate and integrate into our profession the expectation that all nurses have a professional responsibility to read and use research in their practice and to communicate with nurse scientists the many and varied clinical problems for which we do not yet have a scientific base.

Critical Thinking Challenges

- Discuss the difference between nursing research, research utilization, and EBP. Support your discussion with examples.
- Why would it be important to use an EBP model, such as the Iowa Model of Evidence-Based Practice, to guide a practice project? In what part of this model can a consumer of research participate effectively? Justify your response.
- Discuss the role of technology that can be used to implement the steps of an EBP model. Include in your discussion the contributions that can be made by computer electronic databases and support your position with examples.
- You are a graduate nurse assigned to an adult cardiac unit. Many of your nursing colleagues do not understand EBP. How would you implement EBP in your new clinical setting?
- What barriers do you see in applying EBP in the clinical setting? Discuss strategies to use to overcome these barriers.

KEY POINTS

- *Evidence-based practice (EBP)* is a broad term that encompasses use of the best research evidence with clinical expertise and client values or preferences in deciding the evidence for practice.
- Two forms of research evidence are used: conceptual and decision driven.
- Several models of EBP exist. A key feature of all models is the judicious review and synthesis of research regarding a nursing practice to develop an EBP standard.
- The steps of EBP using the Iowa Model of Evidence-Based Practice are selection of a topic, formation of a team, literature retrieval, schemas for grading the evidence, critique of EBP guidelines, critique of research articles, synthesis of research findings, development of an EBP, and implementation of the change.
- Adoption of EBP standards requires education and dissemination to staff and use of change strategies, such as the use of opinion leaders, change champions, a core group, and consultants.

- Overall, EBP change involves unfreezing old behaviours or attitudes, adopting new behaviours or practices, and integrating the change into the work role or practice setting.
- Evaluating the change is important. Evaluation provides information for PGA, audit, and feedback and for determining whether the practice should be retained.
- Evaluation includes both process and outcome measures.
- Organizations must create a culture of EBP. The creation of this culture requires an interactive process. Organizations need to provide access to information, access to individuals who have the skills necessary for EBP, and written and verbal commitments to EBP in the organization's operations.

REFERENCES

Agency for Healthcare Research and Quality. (2002). *Systems to rate the strength of scientific evidence. Evidence Report/Technology Assessment No. 47* (AHRQ Publication No. 02-E016). Rockville, MD: Agency for Healthcare Research and Quality, US Department of Health and Human Services.

Agency for Healthcare Research and Quality. (2007). *Evidence-based practice centers.* Retrieved November 5, 2007, from http://www.ahrq.gov/clinic/epc/

Alberta Association of Registered Nurses. (1997). *Nursing research dissemination and utilization.* Retrieved May 6, 2004, from http://nurses.ab.ca/publications/papers.html#Research

Alderson, P., Green, S., & Higgins, J. P. T. (2003). *Cochrane reviewers' handbook* 4.2.1. Retrieved March 30, 2004, from http://www.cochrane.org/resources/handbook/handbook.pdf

American College of Chest Physicians/American Association of Cardiovascular and Pulmonary Rehabilitation (ACCP/AACVPR). (1997). Special report: Pulmonary rehabilitation: Joint ACCP/AACVPR evidence-based guidelines. *Chest, 112,* 1363–1396.

American Geriatrics Society, British Geriatrics Society, American Academy of Orthopaedic Surgeons, and Panel on Falls Prevention. (2001). Guideline for the prevention of falls in older persons. *Journal of the American Geriatrics Society, 49,* 664–672.

American Pain Society. (1999). *Guideline for the management of acute and chronic pain in sickle cell disease.* Glenview, IL: American Pain Society.

Bach, D. M. (Ed.). (1995). *Implementation of the Agency for Health Care Policy and Research postoperative pain management guideline,* Vol. 30. Philadelphia: WB Saunders.

Baggs, J. G., & Mick, D. J. (2000). Collaboration: A tool addressing ethical issues for elderly patients near the end of life in intensive care units. *Journal of Gerontological Nursing, 26*(9), 41–47.

Bauchner, H., & Simpson, L. (1998). Specific issues related to developing, disseminating, and implementing pediatric practice guidelines for physicians, patients, families, and other stakeholders. *Health Services Research, 33,* 1161–1177.

Berner, E. S., Baker, C. S., Funkhouser, E., Heudebert, G. R., Allison, J. J., Fargason, C. A., et al. (2003). Do local opinion leaders augment hospital quality improvement efforts? A randomized trial to promote adherence to unstable angina guideline. *Medical Care, 41,* 420–431.

Berwick, D. M. (2003). Disseminating innovations in health care. *Journal of the American Medical Association, 289,* 1969–1975.

Blondin, M. M., & Titler, M. G. (1996). Deep vein thrombosis and pulmonary embolism prevention: What roles do nurses play? *Medsurg Nursing, 5,* 205–208.

Bock, L. (1990). From research to utilization: Bridging the gap. *Nursing Management, 21*(3), 50–51.

Bookbinder, M., Coyle, N., Kiss, M., Goldstein, M. L., Holritz, K., Thaler, H., et al. (1996). Implementing national standards for cancer pain management: Program model and evaluation. *Journal of Pain & Symptom Management, 12,* 334–347.

Canadian Nurses Association. (2002). *Position statement: Evidence-based decision-making and nursing practice.* Retrieved on October 27, 2007, from http://www.cna-nurses.ca/CNA/documents/pdf/publications/PS63_Evidence_based_Decision_making_Nursing_Practice_e.pdf

Carey, R. A. (2002). *Improving healthcare with control charts: Basic and advanced SPC methods and case studies.* Milwaukee, WI: American Society for Quality.

Carr, C. A., & Schott, A. (2002). Differences in evidence-based care in midwifery practice and education. *Journal of Nursing Scholarship, 34,* 153–158.

Chambers, C. (1989). Barriers to the dissemination and use of research in nursing practice. *NRIG Newsletter, 8*(2), 2–3.

Cole, K. M., & Gawlinski, A. (1995). Animal-assisted therapy in the intensive care unit. *Nursing Clinics of North America, 30,* 529–537.

Cook, D. (1998). Evidence-based critical care medicine: A potential tool for change. *New Horizons, 6*(1), 20–25.

Craig, J. V., & Smyth, R. L. (2007). *The evidence-based practice manual for nurses* (2nd ed.). London: Churchill Livingstone.

Cronenwett, L. R. (1995). Effective methods for disseminating research findings to nurses in practice. *Nursing Clinics of North America, 30,* 429–438.

Cullen, L. (2005). Evidence-based practice: Strategies for nursing leaders. In Huber, D. (Ed.), *Leadership and nursing care management* (3rd ed., pp. 461–478). Philadelphia: Elsevier.

Davies, B., & Logan, J. (2008). *Reading research: A user-friendly guide for nurses and other health professionals* (4th ed.). Toronto: Mosby.

DiCenso, A., Guyatt, G., & Ciliska, D. (2005) *Evidence-based nursing: A guide to clinical practice.* St. Louis, MO: Elsevier.

Dufault, M. A. (2004). Testing a collaborative research utilization model to translate best practices in pain management. *Worldviews on Evidence-Based Nursing, 1*(Suppl. 1), S26–S32.

Dykes, P. C. (2003). Practice guidelines and measurement: State-of-the-science. *Nursing Outlook, 51,* 65–69.

Estabrooks, C. A. (2003). Translating research into practice: Implications for organizations and administrators. *Canadian Journal of Nursing Research, 35,* 53–68.

Estabrooks, C. A. (2004). Thoughts on evidence-based nursing and its science: A Canadian perspective. *Worldviews on Evidence-Based Nursing, 1,* 88–91.

Estabrooks, C. A., O'Leary, K., Ricker, K., & Humphrey, C. (2003). The Internet and access to evidence: How are nurses positioned? *Journal of Advanced Nursing, 42,* 73–81.

Farquhar, C. M., Stryer, D., & Slutsky, J. (2002). Translating research into practice: The future ahead. *International Journal of Quality Health Care, 14,* 233–249.

Feldman, P. H., & Kane, R. L. (2003). Strengthening research to improve the practice and management of long-term care. *Milbank Quarterly, 81,* 179–220.

Fiore, M. C., Bailey, W. C., Cohen, S. J., Dorfman, S. F., Goldstein, M., Gritz, E. R., et al. (1996, April). *Smoking cessation: information for specialists* (AHCPR Publication No. 96-0694). Rockville, MD: US Department of Health and Human Services, Public Health Service, Agency for Health Care Policy and Research and Centers for Disease Control and Prevention.

Foxcroft, D. R., Cole, N., Fulbrook, P., Johnston, L., & Stevens, K. (2002). Organisational infrastructures to promote evidence based nursing practice (protocol for a Cochrane Review). *Cochrane Library* 2.

Fraser, I. (2004a). Organizational research with impact: Working backwards. *Worldviews on Evidence-Based Nursing, 1*(Suppl. 1), S52–S59.

Fraser, I. (2004b). Translation research: Where do we go from here. *Worldviews on Evidence-Based Nursing, 1*(Suppl. 1), S78–S83.

Funk, S. G., Champagne, M. T., Wiese, R. A., & Tornquist, E. M. (1991). Barriers: The barriers to research utilization scales. *Applied Nursing Research, 4*(1), 39–45.

Funk, S. G., Tornquist, E. M., & Champagne, M. T. (1989). Application and evaluation of the dissemination model. *Western Journal of Nursing Research, 11,* 486–491.

Funk, S. G., Tornquist, E. M., & Champagne, M. T. (1995). Barriers and facilitators of research utilization: An integrative review. *Nursing Clinics of North America, 30,* 395–408.

Gillbody, S., Whitty, P., Grimshaw, J., & Thomas, R. (2003). Educational and organizational interventions to improve the management of depression in primary care (A systematic review). *Journal of the American Medical Association, 289,* 3145–3151.

Haber, J., Feldman, H., Penney, N., Carter, E., Bidwell-Cerone. S., & Rose Hott, J. (1994). Shaping nursing practice through research-based protocols. *Journal of the New York State Nurses Association, 25*(3), 3–8.

Haller, K. B., Reynolds, M. A., & Horsley, J. O. (1979). Developing research-based innovation protocols: Process, criteria, and issues. *Research in Nursing & Health, 2*(2), 45–51.

Harris, R. P., Helfan, M., Woolf, S. H., Lohr, K. N., Mulrow, C. D., Teutsch, S. M., et al. (2001). Current methods of the US Preventive Services Task Force: A review of the process. *American Journal of Preventative Medicine, 20*(3S), 21–35.

Harvey, G., Loftus-Hills, A., Rycroft-Malone, J., Titchen, A., Kitson, A., McCormack, B., et al. (2002). Getting evidence into practice: The role and function of facilitation. *Journal of Advanced Nursing, 37,* 577–588.

Haughey, B. (1988). Utilizing research findings in nursing. *Clinical Nurse Specialist, 2,* 184.

Hendryx, M. S., Fieselmann, J. F., Bock, M. J., Wakefield, D. S., Helms, C. M., & Bentler, S. E. (1998). Outreach education to improve quality of rural ICU care: Results of a randomized trial. *American Journal Respiratory and Critical Care Medicine, 158,* 418–423.

Herr, K., Titler, M., Sorofman, B., Ardery, G., Schmitt, M., & Young, D. (2000). Evidence-based guideline: Acute pain management in the elderly. In L. Grant (Ed.), *From book to bedside: Acute pain management in the elderly* (Written for Agency for Healthcare Research and Quality: 1 R01 HS10482-01). Iowa City, IA: University of Iowa.

Horsley, J., Crane, J., Crabtree, M. K., & Wood, D. J. (1983). *Using research to improve nursing practice: A guide.* Philadelphia: W.B. Saunders.

Institute of Medicine. (2001). *Crossing the quality chasm: A new health system for the 21st century.* Washington, DC: National Academy Press.

Jamtvedt, G., Young, J. M., Kristoffersen, D. T., Thomson O'Brien, M. A., & Oxman, A. D. (2004). Audit and feedback: Effects on professional practice and health care outcomes (Cochrane Review). *The Cochrane Library, Issue 1.* Chichester, UK: John Wiley and Sons, Ltd.

King, D., Barnard, K., & Hoehn, R. (1981). Disseminating the results of nursing research. *Nursing Outlook, 29,* 164–169.

Kirchhoff, K. T. (2004). State of the science of translational research: From demonstration projects to intervention testing. *Worldviews on Evidence-Based Nursing, 1*(Suppl. 1), S6–S12.

Kitson, A., Harvey, G., & McCormack, B. (1998). Enabling the implementation of evidence based practice: A conceptual framework. *Quality in Health Care, 7,* 149–158.

Kovner, A. R., Elton, J. J., & Billings, J. (2000). Evidence-based management. *Frontline Health Services Management, 16*(4), 3–24.

Lavis, J. N., Robertson, D., Woodside, J. M., McLeod, C. B., & Abelson, J. (2003). Knowledge Transfer Study Group: How can research organizations more effectively transfer research knowledge to decision makers? *Milbank Quarterly, 81,* 221–248.

Lepper, H. S., & Titler, M. G. (1999). Program evaluation. In M. A. Mateo & K. T. Kirchhoff (Eds.), *Using and conducting nursing research in the clinical setting* (2nd ed., pp. 90–104). Philadelphia: W.B. Saunders.

Locock, L., Dopson, S., Chambers, D., & Gabbay, J. (2001a). Implementation of evidence-based medicine: Evaluation of the Promoting Action on Clinical Effectiveness program. *Journal of Health Services Research Policy, 6,* 23–31.

Locock, L., Dopson, S., Chambers, D., & Gabbay, J. (2001b). Understanding the role of opinion leaders in improving clinical effectiveness. *Social Science & Medicine, 53,* 745–757.

Logan, J., & Graham, I. (1998). Toward a comprehensive interdisciplinary model of health care research use. *Science Communication, 20,* 227–246.

Lomas, J., Enkin, M., Anderson, G. M., Hannah, W. J., Vayda, E., & Singer, J. (1991). Opinion leaders vs. audit and feedback to implement practice guidelines: Delivery after previous cesarean section. *Journal of the American Medical Association, 265,* 2202–2207.

Madsen, D., Sebolt, T., Cullen, L., Folkedahl, B., Mueller, T., Richardson, C., et al. (2005). Why listen to bowel sounds? Report of an evidence-based practice project. *American Journal of Nursing, 105,* 40–49.

Mazmanian, P. E., Daffron, S. R., Johnson, R. E., Davis, D. A., & Kantrowitz, M. P. (1998). Information about barriers to planned change: A randomized controlled trial involving continuing medical education lectures and commitment to change. *Academic Medicine, 73,* 882–886.

Melnyk, B. M., & Fineout-Melnyk, E. (2005). *Evidence-based practice in nursing and healthcare.* Philadelphia: Lippincott.

Meyer, A. D., & Goes, J. B. (1988). Organizational assimilation of innovations: A multilevel contextual analysis. *Academy of Management Journal, 31,* 897–923.

Nagy, S., Lumby, J., McKinley, S., & Macfarlane, C. (2001). Nurses' beliefs about the conditions that hinder or support evidence-based nursing. *International Journal of Nursing Practice, 7,* 314–321.

Nightingale, F. (1858). *Notes on matters affecting the health, efficiency, and hospital administration of the British Army.* London: Harrison and Sons.

Nightingale, F. (1859). *A contribution to the sanitary history of the British Army during the late war with Russia.* London: John W. Parker and Sons.

Nightingale, F. (1863a). *Notes on hospitals.* London: Longman, Green, Roberts, and Green.

Nightingale, F. (1863b). *Observation on the evidence contained in the statistical reports submitted by her to the Royal Commission on the Sanitary State of the Army in India.* London: Edward Stanford.

Nutley, S., & Davies, H. T. O. (2000). Making a reality of evidence-based practice: Some lessons from the diffusion of innovations. *Public Money & Management, 20*(4), 35–42.

Nutley, S., Davies, H., & Walter, I. (2003). *Evidence based policy and practice: Cross sector lessons from the UK.* Wellington, NZ: Keynote paper for the Social Policy Research and Evaluation Conference.

Olade, R. A. (2004). Evidence-based practice and research utilization activities among rural nurses. *Journal of Nursing Scholarship, 36*(3), 220–225.

Oxman, A. D., Thomson, M. A., Davis, D. A., & Haynes, R. B. (1995). No magic bullets: A systematic review of 102 trials of interventions to improve professional practice. *Canadian Medical Association Journal, 153,* 1423–1431.

Pank, P., Rostron, W., & Stenhouse, M. (1984). Using research in nursing. *Nursing Times, 80*(11), 44–45.

Pettit, D. M., & Kraus, V. (1995). The use of gauze versus transparent dressing for peripheral intravenous catheter sites. *Nursing Clinics of North America, 30,* 495–506.

Rakel, B. A., Titler, M., Goode, C., Barry-Walker, J., Budreau, G., & Buckwalter, K. C. (1994). Nasogastric and nasointestinal feeding tube placement: An integrative review of research. *AACN Clinical Issues in Critical Care Nursing, 5,* 194–206.

Registered Nurses Association of British Columbia. (1993). *Nursing and research in clinical agencies: A.B.C. survey.* Vancouver: Author.

Registered Nurses' Association of Ontario. (2002). *Toolkit: Implementation of clinical practice guidelines.* Toronto: Author.

Registered Nurses' Association of Ontario. (2003). *Breastfeeding Best Practice Guidelines for nurses.* Toronto: Author.

Registered Nurses' Association of Ontario. (2004). *Adult asthma care guidelines for nurses: Promoting control of asthma.* Toronto: Author.

Registered Nurses' Association of Ontario. (2007). *Best Practice Guidelines.* Retrieved August 2007 from http://www.rnao.org

Repko, L. (1990). Turn research reports into an assessment challenge. *RN, 53*(8), 56–61.

Retsas, A. (2000). Barriers to using research evidence in nursing practice. *Journal of Advanced Nursing, 31,* 599–606.

Rogers, E. (1995). *Diffusion of innovations.* New York: The Free Press.

Rogers, E. M. (2003). *Diffusion of innovations* (5th ed.). New York: The Free Press.

Ross-Kerr, J., & Wood, M. (2003). *Canadian nursing: Issues and perspectives.* Toronto: Mosby.

Rosswurm, M. A., & Larrabee, J. H. (1999). A model for change to evidence-based practice. *Image, 31,* 317–322.

Rycroft-Malone, J., Kitson, A., Harvey, G., McCormack, B., Seers, K., Titchen, A., et al. (2002). Ingredients for change: Revisiting a conceptual framework. *Quality Safety Health Care, 11,* 174–180.

Sackett, D. L., Rosenberg, W. M. C., Gray, J. A. M., Haynes, R. B., & Richardson, W. S. (1996). Evidence based medicine: What it is and what it isn't. *British Medical Journal, 312,* 71–72.

Sackett, D. L., Straus, S. E., Richardson, W. S., Rosenberg, W., & Haynes, R. B. (2005). *Evidence-based medicine: How to practice and teach EBM* (2nd ed.). London: Churchill Livingstone.

Schneider, E. C., & Eisenberg, J. M. (1998). Strategies and methods for aligning current and best medical practices: The role of information technologies. *Western Journal of Medicine, 168,* 311–318.

Schoenbaum, S. C., Sundwall, D. N., Bergman, D., Buckle, J. M., Chernov, A., George, J., et al. (1995a). *Using clinical practice guidelines to evaluate quality of care, Volume 1: Issues* (AHCPR Publication No. 95-0045). Rockville, MD: US Department of Health and Human Services, Public Health Service, Agency for Health Care Policy and Research.

Schoenbaum, S. C., Sundwall, D. N., Bergman, D., Buckle, J. M., Chernov, A., George, J., et al. (1995b). *Using clinical practice guidelines to evaluate quality of care, Volume 2: Methods.* Rockville, MD: U.S. Department of Health and Human Services, Public Health Service, Agency for Health Care Policy and Research.

Shively, M., Riegel, B., Waterhouse, D., Burns, D., Templin, K., & Thomason, T. (1997). Testing a community level research utilization intervention. *Applied Nursing Research, 10,* 121–127.

Soukup, S. M. (2000). The center for advanced nursing practice evidence-based practice model. *Nursing Clinics of North America, 35,* 301–309.

Stenger, K. (1994). Putting research to good use. *American Journal of Nursing, 94*(Suppl.), 30–38.

Stetler, C. (1985). Research utilization: Defining the concept. *Image, 17,* 40–44.

Stetler, C. B. (2003). Role of the organization in translating research into evidence-based practice. *Outcomes Management, 7,* 97–105.

Thompson, C. J. (2001). The meaning of research utilization: A preliminary typology. *Critical Care Nursing Clinics of North America, 13,* 475–485.

Thompson, D. S., Estabrooks, C. A., Scott-Findlay, S., Moore, K., & Wallin, L. (2007). Interventions aimed at increasing research use in nursing: A systematic review. *Implementation Science, 2:*15. Retrieved October, 2007, from http://www.implementation-science.com/content/2/1/15

Thomson O'Brien, M. A., Oxman, A. D., Davis, D. A., Haynes, R. B., Freemantle, N., & Harvey, E. L. (2003a). Audit and feedback versus alternative strategies: Effects on professional practice and health care outcomes. *The Cochrane Library,* Issue 2. Oxford: Update Software.

Thomson O'Brien, M. A., Oxman, A. D., Davis, D. A., Haynes, R. B., Freemantle, N., & Harvey, E. L. (2003b). Educational outreach visits: Effects on professional practice and health care outcomes. *The Cochrane Library,* Issue 2. Oxford: Update Software.

Thomson O'Brien, M. A., Oxman, A. D., Haynes, R. B., Davis, D. A., Freemantle, N., & Harvey, E. L. (2002). Local opinion leaders: Effects of professional practice and health care outcomes (Cochrane Review). *The Cochrane Library,* Issue 2. Oxford: Update software.

Titler, M. G. (2002). *Toolkit for promoting evidence-based practice.* Iowa City, IA: Department of Nursing Services and Patient Care, University of Iowa Hospitals and Clinics.

Titler, M. (2003). *TRIP intervention saves healthcare dollars and improves quality of care (abstract/poster),* July 22–24. Paper presented at the Translating Research Into Practice: What's Working? What's Missing? What's Next?, Sponsored by the Agency for Healthcare Research and Quality, Washington, DC.

Titler, M. G. (2004). Methods in translation science. *Worldviews on Evidence-Based Nursing, 1*, 38–48.

Titler, M. G., & Everett, L. Q. (2001). Translating research into practice: Considerations for critical care investigators. *Critical Care Nursing Clinics of North America, 13*, 587–604.

Titler, M. G., Kleiber, C., Steelman, V., Goode, C., Rakel, B., Barry-Walker, J., et al. (1994). Infusing research into practice to promote quality care. *Nursing Research, 43*, 307–313.

Titler, M. G., Kleiber, C., Steelman, V. J., Rakel, B. A., Budreau, G., Buckwalter, K. C., et al. (2001). The Iowa Model of Evidence-Based Practice to Promote Quality Care. *Critical Care Nursing Clinics of North America, 13*, 497–509.

Titler, M. G., Moss, L., Greiner, J., Alpen, M., Jones, G., Olson, K., et al. (1994). Research utilization in critical care: An exemplar. *AACN Clinical Issues in Critical Care, 5*, 124–132.

Tramner, J. E., Coulson, K., Holtom, D., Lively, T., & Maloney, R. (1998). The emergence of a culture that promotes evidence based clinical decision making within an acute care setting. *Canadian Journal of Nursing Administration, 11*(2), 36–58.

University of Illinois at Chicago. (2003). *Evidence based medicine. Finding the best literature.* Retrieved March 2004 from http://www.uic.edu/depts/lib/lhsp/resources/pico.shtml

Wagner, E. H., Austin, B. T., Davis, C., Hindmarsh, M., Schaefer, J., & Bonomi, A. (2001). Improving chronic illness care: Translating evidence into action. *Health Affairs (Millwood), 20*, 64–78.

Walshe, K., & Rundall, T. G. (2001). Evidence-based management: From theory to practice in health care. *Milbank Quarterly, 79*, 429–457.

Weiler, K., Buckwalter, K., & Titler, M. (1994). Debate: Is nursing research used in practice? In J. McCloskey & H. Grace (Eds.), *Current issues in nursing* (4th ed., pp. 61–75). St. Louis, MO: Mosby.

West, S., King, V., Carey, T. S., Lohr, K. N., McKoy, N., Sutton, S. F., et al. (2002). *Systems to rate the strength of scientific evidence.* (Evidence Report/Technology Assessment No. 47, prepared by the Research Triangle Institute-University of North Carolina Evidence-Based Practice Center under Contract No. 290-97-0011, AHRQ Publication No. 02-E016). Rockville, MD: Agency for Healthcare Research and Quality.

APPENDIX A

From the *Journal of Psychiatric and Mental Health Nursing*, 2005;12:556–564. © 2005 Blackwell Publishing Ltd.

Therapeutic Relationships: From Psychiatric Hospital to Community

C. Forchuk, RN, PhD
Professor/Scientist
School of Nursing, University of Western
    Ontario/Lawson Health Research Institute
London, Ontario

M.-L. Martin, RN, MEd, MScN
Clinical Nurse Specialist/Associate Clinical Professor
St. Joseph's Health Care Hamilton, School of Nursing
Hamilton, Ontario

Y.L. Chan, PhD, CMA
Associate Professor
DeGroote School of Business, McMaster University
Hamilton, Ontario

E. Jensen, RN, PhD
Scientist
Lawson Health Research Institute
London, Ontario
Assistant Professor
School of Nursing, York University
Toronto, Ontario

KEYWORDS

health system research
mental illness
overlapping staff
peer support
Peplau
transitional discharge model

The objective of this study was to determine the cost and effectiveness of a transitional discharge model (TDM) of care with clients who have a chronic mental illness. The model was tested in a randomized clinical trial using a cluster design. This model consisted of: (1) Peer support for 1 year and (2) Ongoing support from hospital staff until a therapeutic relationship was established with the community care provider. Participants (n = 390) were interviewed at discharge, 1 month post-discharge, 6 months post-discharge and 1 year post-discharge. Data collected included demographics, quality of life, health care utilization, levels of functioning and the degree of intervention received. The intervention group post-discharge costs and quality of life were not significantly improved compared with the control group. Although not predicted a priori, intervention subjects were discharged an average of 116 days earlier per person. Based on the hospital per diem rate this would be equivalent to $12M CDN hospital costs. Both under-implementation among implementation wards and contamination in control wards were found. This study demonstrates some of the multiple challenges in health system research.

THERAPEUTIC RELATIONSHIPS:
From Hospital to Community

The mental health care system is in the midst of continued change and reform in the province of Ontario, Canada. The number of psychiatric hospital beds is being dramatically reduced and the emphasis is on service provision in the community. This pattern is similar to other jurisdictions. For example, it is reported that in the USA the number of long-stay occupied beds decreased by 50% between 1991 and 1997 (Desai & Rosenheck, 2003). The transition from hospital to community is complex and can be challenging for individual clients. A recent study of 85 long-term patients showed that 25% met the criterion for relocation trauma when moved from hospital to community (Farhall *et al.* 2003). In order to successfully move the focus of care to the community, effective models of care are required.

Transitional Discharge Model (TDM)

From 1993 to 1996, a pilot project called 'Bridge to Discharge' took place on a tertiary care ward in which care was provided to individuals diagnosed with schizophrenia who had been hospitalized for a minimum of 5 years. Prior to the implementation of the pilot, few clients were successfully returned to the community. Data provided from the clinical records' department of the hospital revealed that in 5 years prior to the pilot, discharges ranged from one to four patients annually. The average census increased from 30 to 38 clients over this five-year period (1988–1993). The pilot study involved clients, staff, a community mental health program, a consumer-survivor group and researchers in the process of developing strategies for successful transition to the community. A Transitional Discharge Model (TDM) was developed based on a safety net of professional and peer relationships (Forchuk *et al.* 1998a). The TDM builds on Peplau's interpersonal theory of nursing (Peplau, 1991). It assumes that the quality of interpersonal relationships has an influence and impact on quality of life and that a supportive social network will promote less need for expensive interventions such as hospitalization. This TDM had two components that included: (1) in-patient staff continued to care for discharged clients until therapeutic relationships were established with the community care providers; and (2) a friendship model of peer support (Schofield *et al.* 1997; Forchuk *et al.* 1998a, b).

The pilot was successful in improving the discharge rate; there were 11 clients discharged the initial year with only two brief re-admissions. Quality of life improved significantly for those discharged as well as those who remained on the ward (Forchuk *et al.* 1998c). The differences in costs of this approach compared with those of continued hospitalization were just under $0.5 million CDN (Forchuk *et al.* 1998c). The pilot became the ongoing model of care and all 38 clients originally on the ward were discharged by 1999 and since 1997 the average length of stay has been around 10 months with an average of 38 discharges per year. The ward census has been reduced to 30 clients. Many clients went on to independent living in apartments and competitive gainful employment (Schofield *et al.* 1997).

Although the pilot study findings were positive, there was no comparison group and no randomization. The client population was not typical since the length of hospital stay had been so prolonged. A recent pilot study on acute admission wards in Scotland replicated the results of the Bridge to Discharge pilot study. Clients from three acute admission wards were randomized on the day of discharge to either TDM or usual follow-up care. The TDM was offered by a group of transitional nurses and trained peer volunteers. Fewer symptoms, fewer re-admissions and better functioning were noted among clients randomized to the TDM group (Reynolds *et al.* 2004). Although these initial studies were promising, a test with a wider range of psychiatric wards was needed to determine if the model would be useful across a range of psychiatric wards.

Peer Support

The provision of peer support has been shown to improve several areas of quality of life, such as satisfaction with living situation, personal safety and financial management (Felton *et al.* 1995; Forchuk *et al.* 1998c). Better communications between case managers and clients and increased client engagement with the program as a result of peer involvement have been reported (Forchuk *et al.* 1998c).

Solomon & Draine (1996) describe the use of consumers as case managers in mental health. The consumer case managers were no more likely than non-consumer case managers to use alternative, non-mental health services for their clients. Consumer case managers were more likely to interact daily with clients. There were no differences in client outcomes based on the type of case manager. The sample was very small, with seven members in each of the two teams.

Davidson *et al.* (1999) conducted a review of the literature on peer support in mental illness. They describe three types of peer support and include: (1) naturally occurring mutual support, (2) consumer run services, and (3) mental health consumers as providers within clinical and rehabilitative settings. Mutual support has been studied, generally using self-reports and descriptive methods. Only one controlled outcome study was included in the review. Mutual support is one potential way to improve social reintegration. The authors conclude mutual support alone and in its current form, is not a sufficient strategy; and they recommend controlled prospective studies are needed. Consumer run services were originally established as an alternative to the formal mental health system but have evolved and are entering a phase of partnership and collaboration with the system. Six studies of consumer run services were located, of which only one used random assignment and assessed outcomes. This one study found no difference on employment variables between a consumer-run employment centre and traditional vocational services. The use of consumers as service providers is the third form of peer support. The authors also located six studies, of which only two used random assignment and only one of those examined client outcomes. They did conclude that this last group of studies support that consumers can be adequately trained to take on roles other than that of 'patient'. They also offer a cautionary note. When consumers are part of the mental health system as peer supporters, there is a tendency for the prevailing clinical culture to co-opt them into providing therapy services, at the expense of the provision of peer support. The preliminary research reported in this paper supports the role of peer support, however, there is a need for more and better designed studies with larger samples to address the many questions that are as yet unanswered.

A research review by Simpson & House (2002) related to the involvement of consumers in the delivery and evaluation of mental health services included five randomized trials and seven other comparative studies. The roles of consumers varied with these studies and included being employees of mental health services, trainers and researchers. The authors concluded that involving consumers in mental health service delivery did not have any detrimental effects on clients, their symptoms, functioning or quality of life. Rather, clients experienced improved quality of life and had fewer and shorter hospital re-admissions with longer periods between admissions. A survey of 311 clients of mental health services (Hodges *et al.* 2003) found that the use of self-help groups was associated with greater satisfaction with professional mental health services.

Davidson *et al.* (2004) describe the results of a clinical trial testing three different models of supported socialization with a group of 260 people with psychiatric disabilities. All participants receive a stipend of $28 per month to cover the expenses of engaging in social activities. One group was given only the stipend. The second group was assigned a volunteer partner who had a history of mental illness and the third group were partnered with volunteers who did not have a history of mental illness. The only two groups to show significant improvements over the 9 month follow-up were the people assigned peer support who did not meet with the volunteers and the people assigned a non-peer volunteer who did meet. The researchers drew on data from the qualitative data collected to try to make sense of the quantitative results. They suggest that both of these scenarios may indicate that moving away from the mental health system supports recovery and that internalized stigma may have played a role. They conclude that recovery is a heterogeneous process with wide variation from one person to the next. The authors also recommended using both qualitative and quantitative methods concurrently in order to improve interpretability of results.

Overlapping Professional Care and Continuity of Care

A further strategy to assist in the transition to community is planning for an overlap of services provided by the inpatient and outpatient professionals during the discharge period. Olfson *et al.* (1998) studied 104 subjects with schizophrenia or schizo-affective disorders, half of whom had contact with the outpatient therapist prior to hospital discharge. This approach improved the control of symptoms and the likelihood of following through on outpatient care (Olfson *et al.* 1998). One study found that individuals moving to a community location from a long-stay ward had fewer adverse effects when there were six or more visits to the new site over a period of 4 months or more (Farhall *et al.* 2003).

Adair *et al.* (2003) reviewed the general concept of continuity of care and its associations with clinical outcomes. They concluded after reviewing eight studies that there was limited support for the concept that continuity of care improves outcomes, primarily owing to the underdevelopment of appropriate measures. Greenberg & Rosenheck (2005) examined three forms of continuity of care, including continuity across organizational boundaries, in a large American nationwide study. They found several significant associations between continuity measures and improved clinical measures such as the global assessment of functioning. Interestingly, these relationships were primarily noted in continuity for the transitional period between hospital care and initial out-patient care.

Brooten's transitional model of care of early hospital discharge and transitional community care has been reported to improve client outcomes and reduce health care costs in diverse non-psychiatric settings (Brooten *et al.* 1988; Naylor *et al.* 1994; Brooten & Duffin, 1999). Continuity of care, communication among hospital and community care providers and a multidisciplinary approach have been identified as the most important factors of transitional services (Brooten & Duffin, 1999).

As the mental health care system strives to contain costs and move care into the community, the call for care and treatment to be evidence-based is becoming more paramount (Drake *et al.* 2001). Outcomes, particularly community tenure, quality of life and functional status of the client are becoming the measures by which the worth of interventions is being judged (Brooten & Duffin, 1999).

OBJECTIVES AND HYPOTHESES

The overall objective of this study was to assist individuals hospitalized with a persistent mental illness in successful community living. Specific objectives were to determine the cost and effectiveness of a TDM of care and compare the results to those of a standard model of discharge care. Outcome measures included quality of life and costs. It was hypothesized that in the year following discharge from a psychiatric hospital, individuals participating in the TDM would: (1) have an improved quality of life and (2) incur fewer health and social services costs compared with individuals receiving standard discharge care. The specific health and social costs to be addressed in this analysis were hospital admissions, emergency room use, and jail/incarceration.

METHODS

The study employed a cluster-randomised design (Donner & Klar, 1994). Clusters, or units of randomization, were 26 wards located in four provincial psychiatric hospitals in Ontario, Canada. Units of analysis were the clients discharged from wards. This design eliminated the logistical problems and risk of increased contamination posed by treating selected clients differently on the same ward. A total of 26 wards from four hospital sites located in Southern Ontario were paired and then randomized to either the experimental group using the new TDM, or to the control group, receiving usual care. The number of participating wards at each site ranged from five to eight.

Pairing of wards was based on similarity of length of stay, staffing levels, current discharge practice, and the general focus of the ward (e.g., admission, forensic, specialized diagnostic groups such as schizophrenia, mood disorders, or developmental disability). An additional six wards agreed to participate but were unable to do so as there were no appropriate matches. The paired matching ensured similarity between the intervention and control groups. It was anticipated that the pair matching would be broken for analysis purposes, given the likelihood that matching would only be slightly to moderately effective (Diehr *et al.* 1995).

Sample Size Calculation

To detect differences between groups, *t*-tests with a power of 0.80 and a significance level of 0.05 (one-tailed) were used. Based on Cohen (1988) and previous score results from the Lehman QOLI-Brief Version (Lehman *et al.* 1994) and the anticipation of a medium effect size required a minimum sample size of 64 per group, when randomization of individuals is used. Similar calculations using other outcome measures yield smaller sample requirements. To account for the cluster randomization, the method recommended by Donner *et al.* (1981) was used to adjust the initial calculation. This brought the minimum sample to 125 per group. This was further inflated by 30% to adjust for drop-outs and 20% for possible contamination between intervention and control groups. Thus, the minimum sample was set at 188 per group (or 376 total).

Blinding Randomization

The three research assistants and six student assistants who conducted the data collection were blind to the ward assignment in the study. To determine if blinding was maintained, staff were asked to guess which wards were intervention wards and which were controls after the study was underway for a year. Only 60% of the staff guesses were accurate. This may indicate that over time the research assistants began to determine which wards were providing the TDM.

Implementation of TDM

The TDM consisted of the same two components as found successful in the pilot: (1) overlap of in-patient and community staff in which the in-patient staff continued their relationship with clients, until the clients had a working relationship with a community care provider; and (2) peer support was available to the client for a minimum of 1 year.

Overlap of Staff

In order to implement the new model, each staff person on the intervention wards was given 12 h of training. The staff were to continue with the client until the community care provider was in the working phase of a therapeutic relationship. The working phase of the relationship started when the client was comfortable identifying problems to be worked on within the context of their therapeutic relationship. A consensus between hospital staff, community staff and the consumer was used to determine this. The decision was assisted by the use of the Relationship Form (Forchuk & Brown, 1989). The time for this varied from 0 weeks to 12 months, but the median of the bridging relations between the ward staff and the client was 3 months. Weekly ward-staff contact included home visits, telephone contact and/or meeting at an agreed location. The community care provider might also be present at these meetings. The focus of these meetings was to support the development of the therapeutic relationship with the community care provider. If the client was returning to a former community care provider it was determined whether or not there was already a therapeutic relationship with that community care provider by reviewing the relationship form with the client. If a working therapeutic relationship existed the ward staff did not need to continue seeing the client after discharge.

Peer Support

Former consumers of the mental health care system who had been in the community for at least a year and had completed a peer-training program provided by one of the 17 participating consumer-survivor groups provided the peer support. Peer volunteers promoted friendship, provided understanding, taught community living skills and encouraged current clients in making the transition from psychiatric hospital to community. Common activities included having a coffee together, visiting free community events or having a telephone conversation. Peer support volunteers were screened, trained and provided with ongoing support from part time volunteer coordinators within the consumer/survivor organizations. Eleven of the groups received funds from The Trillium Foundation (Government of Ontario) which was primarily used to fund peer support volunteer coordinators. The average cost for each peer support coordinator was $24 000 CDN for a 0.6 full time equivalent. Although the coordinators were paid, the peer supporters were volunteers. Over 300 volunteers were trained.

Ethics Review

Ethical approval was obtained from the research ethics boards at University of Western Ontario as well as the hospital sites. Participation in both the study and the intervention (if in intervention group) was voluntary.

Sample and Data Collection

After randomization, staff training occurred on the intervention wards and partnerships were formed between intervention wards and consumer

organizations involved in the provision of peer support. Sequential patients discharged from the study wards were invited to participate in the study. Inclusion criteria for selection included patients with a minimum 2 week admission, proficiency in English to the degree necessary to complete the interview and that the discharge was planned (i.e. not a discharge against medical advice). Exclusion criteria included organic brain problems and language difficulties. Wards had different discharge rates and therefore accrued study subjects at different rates. The maximum number recruited from each ward was capped at 20 and a minimum of 10 was recruited from each ward. The average number of subjects from each ward was 15.

A total of 390 clients were enrolled in the study. Interviews took place at the point of discharge, 1 month post-discharge, 6 months post-discharge and 1 year post-discharge. At 1 year post-discharge, 249 individuals remained in the sample (a 36% drop-out rate). The sample size calculation had assumed a dropout rate of 30%, which was slightly less than what occurred. The high drop-out rate was related to difficulty in tracking people who moved after discharge.

Instruments

Data were collected from individual participants using a demographic questionnaire, the Lehman Quality of Life-Brief Version [QOLI-Brief] (Lehman, 1988; Lehman et al. 1994), a modified form of the Utilization of Health & Social Services [UHSS] (Browne et al. 1990), the Discharge/Process of Follow-up Questionnaire [DPFQ] and the Criteria for Degree of Treatment Implementation Form [CDTIF]. Investigators developed the demographic instrument and the last two instruments specifically for this study. In addition, wards and consumer groups sent monthly reports summarizing any unusual events, issues, or concerns.

The Quality of Life-Brief Version (Lehman, 1988; Lehman et al. 1994) was derived from the QOLI-Full Version and measures both objective quality of life (what people do and experience) and subjective quality of life (what people feel about these experiences). It consists of 45 items, measuring eight domains: living situation, daily activities and functioning, family relations, social relations, finances, work and school, legal and safety issues and health. Internal consistency with people with chronic mental illness ranges from 0.56 to 0.87 (Lehman 1988). Internal consistency on the various sub-scales in this study ranged from 0.50 to 0.90 and the overall life satisfaction alpha was 0.72.

The Utilization of Health and Social Services (UHSS) was designed to measure self-reported direct and indirect costs of health and social services in Ontario (Browne *et al.* 1990). The form contains 30 items that ask about the use of services such as physician visits, medication use, re-admissions, use of emergency room services, involvement with legal services and income support programs. The questions refer to use of services within the past month. To calculate annual costs, the monthly rates were extrapolated to 12 months. Researchers (Browne *et al.* 1990) have validated a portion of the form by having 141 cardiac patients' reports on laboratory tests compared to clinical records. Observed agreement ranged from 0.72 to 0.99 and when adjusted for chance agreement, the kappa statistic ranged from 0.48 to 0.89.

The Discharge Process of Follow-up Questionnaire (DPFQ) consisted of six open-ended questions that explore the experience of discharge, description of activities/issues that help or hinder the process, co-interventions and validation of the experimental vs. control discharge process. The qualitative responses to these questions were used to generate a numeric score that measured the degree of implementation of the intervention, as experienced by the study participant, on the Criteria for Degree of Treatment Implementation Form (CDTIF). For example, participants were asked whether they received any support from former consumers of the mental health system and how often this took place. If so, this was described to determine if it was formal peer support or informal friendships and the frequency of the support. Similar questions were asked about continuing contact with hospital staff. This was a fidelity scale for measuring the degree of implementation of the transitional discharge intervention. Reliability (Cronbach's Alpha) for the CDTIF was 0.79.

Analysis

Descriptive analysis was completed on all variables. *T*-tests were used to test the hypotheses comparing intervention and control groups. The level of statistical significance was set at 0.05 and the tests were unidirectional as the hypotheses were unidirectional. According to Chow (1996) the decision to conduct unidirectional tests requires the hypotheses to be unidirectional a priori, as was done in this study. If the stated hypotheses had been non-directional, convention would require all tests to be two-tailed.

RESULTS

Characteristics of Participants

The characteristics of the participants who were enrolled in the study are summarized in Table A1-1. The intervention and control participants appeared similar at enrolment and therefore additional variables were not controlled for during the analysis. As the study did not include any medical record review, the diagnoses were self-reported and may not be fully accurate. A significant difference between the two groups was length of stay after the intervention had been put in place and patient enrolment began. The average length of stay for the control ward participants was 333.5 days, while the average length of stay for the intervention ward participants was 217.5 days. The baseline data of wards (prior to randomization) average length of stay had been less than 1 day's difference between intervention and control wards.

Degree of Implementation/Contamination

The degree of implementation/contamination was evaluated at individual interviews with each data collection interview. All discharged clients were

TABLE A1-1 Participant Demographic and Baseline Characteristics by Group

Characteristics	Control (n = 189)	Intervention (n = 201)
Female	87 (46%)	103 (51.2%)
Male	102 (54%)	98 (48.8%)
Age-mean years (SD)	39.5 (10.7)	43.4 (11.3)
Age-range	18–83	18–70
Age of onset of illness	20.8	21.9
Total lifetime psychiatric hospitalization (years)	2.5	2.1
Length of admission (days)	333.5 (1068.5)	217.5 (498.5)
Mean (SD)		
Primary diagnosis (self reported)	n = 185*	n = 199*
Schizophrenia	98 (53.0%)	82 (41.2%)
Mood disorder	64 (34.6%)	91 (45.7%)
Substance related	0 (0.0%)	1 (0.5%)
Personality disorder	4 (2.2%)	8 (4.0%)
Anxiety disorder	2 (1.1%)	3 (1.5%)
Developmental delay	4 (2.2%)	6 (3.0%)
Organic disorder	3 (1.6%)	0 (0.0%)
Schizo-affective disorder	1 (0.5%)	2 (1.0%)
Other	9 (4.9%)	6 (3.0%)

*includes those who knew a diagnosis only.

asked questions to determine if they were receiving peer support and ongoing contact with hospital staff. At all times the intervention group received more of the intervention than the control group. The degree of implementation achieved was 38% overall in the intervention group and 26.6% in the control group. Implementing the peer support was done only 22% of the time on the intervention wards and 17% on the control wards. Overlapping the services from hospital to community was implemented 54% of the time on the intervention wards and 37.7% of the time on the control wards. As the study progressed past the initial 9 months, control wards started to increasingly implement the intervention. Issues related to information about implementation were gathered qualitatively through ward and consumer group data and will be described in a different report.

HYPOTHESES

Hypothesis 1 stated that within 1 year, the participants who received the intervention would have a better quality of life. The intervention group did not have a significant improvement in global quality of life (control group mean of 4.65, SD = 1.31; intervention mean = 4.78, SD = 1.31, $F(1,22) = 0.38$, $P = 0.27$). Similarly the sub-scales were not significantly improved. The exception was that quality of life related to social relations where the specific area targeted by the intervention was improved significantly [$F(1,22) = 6.99$, $P = 0.015$].

Hypothesis 2 stated that individuals participating in the TDM would incur fewer health and social services costs after discharge compared to individuals receiving standard care. Key indicators of consumption of health and social services were examined. The use of hospital and emergency room services were selected for analysis since they are the most costly services likely to be accessed. In the first year after discharge, the intervention group consumed $4400 CDN less hospital and emergency room services, per person, than the control group. However, this was not statistically significant ($P = 0.09$). Jail and legal event costs were to be compared but they occurred too infrequently for any meaningful analysis. Specifically, only one participant had 1 day in jail for the year after discharge.

DISCUSSION

The hypotheses related to post-discharge hospital costs and quality of life were not supported by this trial. However, the length of stay was significantly less for participants enrolled on the intervention wards, despite no difference between length of stay on intervention and control wards prior to the implementation of the intervention. The reduced length of stay on the intervention wards was not predicted a priori but may well have contributed to the difficulty in detecting differences after discharge. Although the pilot study had resulted in shorter lengths of stay, hospital partners in this trial were emphatic that due to recent cutbacks and bed closures, further reductions in length of stay were not realistic. Monthly reports from all wards revealed the only ward level change between intervention and control wards had been the introduction of the TDM being tested by the study. Hospital staff first alerted the researchers to the shortening length of stay through monthly ward and reports and feedback from the staff training. Feedback from two intervention wards at two different hospitals made the observation that with the TDM change in practice that 'People are leaving in 6 weeks instead of 6 months'. Staff reported that with the support that the TDM provided, they felt comfortable discharging clients earlier. At a rate of $632.30 CDN per day cost for a bed in a psychiatric hospital, the people in the intervention group consumed $12 212 242 CDN less in hospital services than the control group, prior to discharge. Despite this shorter length of stay (average 116 fewer days per person), the intervention group did not access more hospital services after discharge. It is recommended that future study of similar interventions include an examination of length of stay.

Both under-implementation by some intervention wards and contamination (i.e. the control wards using the intervention) were issues. The training strategies used may have been inadequate to promote this change. In a separate evaluation of the training, staff indicate that although 66.7% felt more able to successfully bridge clients to the community after the training, only 34.8% reported actually doing this (Martin *et al.* 2002). It was noted that some staff were never chosen to bridge with clients although they had received the training. Some reasons given for this included part time hours, lack of therapeutic relationship, sickness and working very few day shifts. This could also reflect the difficulty in changing individual and hospital system practice. As well, some clients on the control wards sought out peer support after discharge. Towards the end of the enrollment process two control wards contacted two different consumer groups in an effort to establish a relationship and systematic method of referral, despite an agreement that they would not do so. In both cases, the consumer groups requested the wards wait until the end of the study. However, individual clients seeking peer help from the consumer groups, even if from control wards, were not turned down. Shortly after the study sample was enrolled (but not completely followed-up), one hospital implemented a peer support program based on a belief that this was making a difference to the client discharge experience and re-admission. All of these issues related to contamination and under-implementation reduce the effect size. There was far less difference in practice between implementation and control wards than anticipated. These issues illustrate the 'messiness' of systems research compared with, for example, a classic drug trial. Vingilis & Pederson (2001) describe some of the multiple reasons that findings of intervention failure may be misleading (Vingilis & Pederson, 2001). These reasons include inadequate implementation, inadequate strength of intervention, and measurement that is not sufficiently sensitive. The first two reasons were clearly factors in this study.

CONCLUSION

With the reduction of psychiatric hospital beds there is a demand for quality mental health services to be provided within the community. This study compared a TDM to usual discharge practices with clients who have a chronic mental illness. The TDM included peer support and bridging from hospital staff until a working therapeutic relationship was established with the community care provider. This model was to assist individuals hospitalized with a chronic mental illness to achieve successful community living. Hypotheses related to improved quality of life and fewer post discharge costs for the intervention group were unsupported. The participants on the intervention wards were discharged 116 days earlier than the control wards. Although this was not predicted *a priori*, it is clinically significant. Both under-implementation on intervention wards and contamination on control wards occurred and reduced the potential effect size. This study is an example of some of the challenges encountered in health systems research, where the use of the intervention cannot be rigorously controlled.

ACKNOWLEDGMENTS

This research was supported by grants from the Canadian Health Services Research Foundation, the Lawson Health Research Institute and the Donner Canadian Foundation and by in-kind support from: Mountain Centre for Health Services, St. Joseph's Healthcare Hamilton (formerly Hamilton Psychiatric Hospital), Regional Mental Health Care, St. Joseph's Healthcare, London/St. Thomas (formerly London/St. Thomas Psychiatric Hospital), Whitby Mental Health Centre. Support for the peer support program was received from the Trillium Foundation. We would like to thank the psychiatric consumer survivors who participated, throughout the project.

REFERENCES

Adair, C., McDougall, M., Beckie, A., Joyce, A., Mitton, C., Wild, C., Gordon, A., & Costigan, N. (2003). History and measurement of continuity of care in mental health services and evidence of its role in outcomes. *Psychiatric Services, 54,* 1351–1356.

Brooten, D., Brown, L. P., Munro, B. H., York, R., Cohen, S. M., Roncoli, M., & Hollingsworth, A. (1988). Early discharge and specialist transitional care. *IMAGE. Journal of Nursing Scholarship, 20,* 64–68.

Brooten, D., & Duffin, N. M. (1999). Transitional environments. In: A. S. Hinshaw, S. L. Feetham, & J. L. F. Shaver (Eds.), *Handbook of clinical nursing research* (pp. 641–653). Thousand Oaks, CA: Sage.

Browne, G., Arpin, K., Corey, P., Fitch, M., & Gafni, A. (1990). Individual correlates of health services utilization and the cost of poor adjustment to chronic illness. *Medical Care, 28,* 43–58.

Chow, S. L. (1996). *Statistical significance.* London: Sage.

Cohen, J. (1988). *Statistical power analysis for the behavioral sciences* (2nd ed.). Hillsdale, NJ: Lawrence Erlbaum Associates.

Davidson, L., Chinman, M., Kloos, B., Weingarten, R., Stayner, D., & Tebes, J. K. (1999). Peer support among individuals with severe mental illness: A review of the evidence. *Clinical Psychology: Science and Practice, 6,* 165–187.

Davidson, L., Shahar, G., Strayner, D. A., Chinman, M., Rakfeldt, J., & Tebes, J. K. (2004). Supported socialization for people with psychiatric disabilities: Lessons from a randomized controlled trial. *Journal of Community Psychology, 32,* 453–477.

Desai, M., & Rosenheck, R. (2003). Trend in discharge disposition, mortality and service use among long-stay psychiatric patients in the 1990s. *Psychiatric Services, 54,* 542–548.

Diehr, P., Martin, D. C., Koepell, T., & Cheadle, A. (1995). Breaking the matches in a paired *t*-test for community interventions when the number of pairs is small. *Statistics in Medicine, 14,* 1491–1504.

Donner, A., Birkett, N., & Buck, C. (1981). Randomization by cluster: Sample size requirements and analysis. *American Journal of Epidemiology, 114,* 906–914.

Donner, A., & Klar, N. (1994). Cluster randomization trials in epidemiology: Theory and application. *Journal of Statistical Planning and Inference, 42,* 37–56.

Drake, R. E., Goldman, H. H., Leff, H. S., Lehman, A. F., Dixon, L., Mueser, K. T., & Torrey, W. C. (2001). Implementing evidence-based practices in routing mental health service settings. *Psychiatric Services, 52,* 79–182.

Farhall, J., Trauer, T., Newton, R., & Cheung, P. (2003). Minimizing adverse effects on patients of involuntary relation from long-stay wards to community residences. *Psychiatric Services, 54,* 1022–1027.

Felton, C. J., Stastny, P., Shern, D. L., Blanch, A., Donahue, S. A., Knight, E., & Brown, C. (1995). Consumers as peer specialists on intensive case management teams: Impact on client outcomes. *Psychiatric Services, 46,* 1037–1040.

Forchuk, C., & Brown, B. (1989). Establishing a nurse-client relationship. *Journal of Psychosocial Nursing, 27,* 30–34.

Forchuk, C., Jewell, J., Schofield, R., Sicelj, M., & Valledor, T. (1998a). From hospital to community: Bridging therapeutic relationships. *Journal of Psychiatric and Mental Health Nursing, 5,* 197–202.

Forchuk, C., Schofield, R., Martin, M. L., Sircelj, M., Woodcox, V., Jewell, J., Valledov, T., Overby, B., & Chan, L. (1998b). Process: Staff and client experiences over time. *Journal of the American Psychiatric Nurses Association, 4,* 128–133.

Forchuk, C., Chan, L., Schofield, R, Sircelj, M., Woodcox, V., Jewell, J., Valledor, T., & Overby, B. (1998c). Bridging the discharge process. *Canadian Nurse, 94,* 22–26.

Greenberg, G., & Rosenheck, R. (2005). Special section on the GAF: Continuity of care and clinical outcomes in a national health system. *Psychiatric Services, 56,* 427–433.

Hodges, J., Markward, M., Keele, C., & Evans, C. J. (2003). Use of self-help services and consumer satisfaction with professional mental health services. *Psychiatric Services, 54,* 1161–1163.

Lehman, A. (1988). A quality of life interview for the chronically mentally ill. *Evaluation and Program Planning, 111,* 51–62.

Lehman, A., Kernan, E., & Postrado, L. (1994). *Toolkit for evaluating quality of life for persons with severe mental illness.* Cambridge, MA: The Evaluation Centre.

Martin, M. L., Forchuk, C., Coatsworth-Puspoky, R., Lysiak-Globe, T., Ricci, A., Jensen, E., Sloan, K., & Holbert, S. (2002). Staff education to support research. *Therapeutic Relationships: From Hospital to Community.* [Dissemination Conference.] London, May 15.

Naylor, M., Brooten, D., Jones, R., Lavizzo-Mourey, R., Mezey, M., & Pauly, M. (1994). Comprehensive discharge planning for the hospitalized elderly. *American College of Physicians, 120,* 990–1006.

Olfson, M., Mechanic, D., Boyer, C. A., & Hansell, S. (1998). Linking inpatients with schizophrenia to outpatient care. *Psychiatric Services, 49,* 911–916.

Peplau, H. E. (1991). *Interpersonal relations in nursing: A conceptual framework of reference for psychodynamic nursing.* New York: Springer.

Reynolds, W., Lauder, W., Sharkey, S., Maciver, S., Veitch, T., & Cameron, D. (2004). The effect of transitional discharge model for psychiatric patients. *Journal of Psychiatric and Mental Health Nursing, 11,* 82–88.

Schofield, R., Valledor, T., Sircelj, M., Forchuk, C., Jewell, J., & Woodcox, V. (1997). Evaluation of bridging institution and housing: A joint consumer-care provider initiative. *Journal of Psychosocial Nursing, 35,* 9–14.

Simpson, E. L., & House, A. O. (2002). Involving users in the delivery and evaluation of mental health services: Systematic review. *British Medical Journal, 325,* 1265.

Solomon, P., & Draine, J. (1996). Perspectives concerning consumers as case managers. *Community Mental Health Journal, 32,* 41–46.

Vingilis, E., & Pederson, L. (2001). Using the right tools to answer the right questions: The importance of evaluative research techniques of health services evaluation in the 21st century. *Canadian Journal of Program Evaluation, 16,* 1–26.

APPENDIX B

From *Advances in Nursing Science*, 2006;29(2):E27–E44. © 2006 Lippincott Williams & Wilkins, Inc.

Bringing Safety and Responsiveness into the Forefront of Care for Pregnant and Parenting Aboriginal People

Dawn Smith, PhD, RN
School of Nursing
University of Ottawa
Ottawa, Ontario

Nancy Edwards, PhD, RN
School of Nursing and Department of
    Community Health and Epidemiology
University of Ottawa
Ottawa, Ontario

Colleen Varcoe, PhD, RN
School of Nursing
University of British Columbia
Vancouver, BC

Patricia J. Martens, PhD, IBCLC
Department of Community Health Sciences,
Faculty of Medicine
University of Manitoba
Winnipeg, Manitoba

Barbara Davies, PhD, RN
School of Nursing
University of Ottawa
Ottawa, Ontario

Poor access to prenatal care for Aboriginal people is well documented, and is explicated as an unethical barrier to care resulting from colonial and neocolonial values, attitudes, and practices. A postcolonial standpoint, participatory research principles, and a case study design were used to investigate 2 Aboriginal organizations' experiences improving care for pregnant and parenting Aboriginal people. Data were collected through exploratory interviews and small-group discussions with purposefully selected community leaders, providers, and community members. The study found that safety in healthcare relationships and settings, and responsiveness to individuals' and families' unique experiences and capacities must be brought into the forefront of care. Results suggest that the intention of care must be situated within a broader view of colonizing relations to improve early access to, and relevance of, care during pregnancy and parenting for Aboriginal people.

KEYWORDS

ethical practice and policy
Indigenous peoples
maternal/child healthcare
participatory research
postcolonial
pregnancy and parenting
responsiveness
safety

Providing care that is safe and competent is a minimum moral obligation for nursing. This long-standing obligation is enshrined in Codes of Ethics, with safety being a key feature of codes such as those developed by the International Council of Nurses (ICN) and the American Nurses Association (ANA).[1] Increasingly, nurses have recognized that all forms of marginalization and discrimination are ethical issues.[2,3] Codes of Ethics explicitly directs nurses to attend to such issues in the provision of safe and competent care. For example, the ICN Code of Ethics directs nurses to "initiate and support action ... particularly for vulnerable populations."[4(p2)] The Canadian Nurses Association specifies that nurses "must not discriminate ... based on a person's race, ethnicity, culture, spiritual beliefs, marital or social status, sex, sexual orientation, age, health status, life style, mental or physical ability and/or ability to pay,"[5(p15)] further directing that nurses should advocate for fair and inclusive practices, policies, and resource allocation.

As in most Western countries, Aboriginal* people in Canada have not fared well under colonialism, with poor health being but one consequence. Late or no access and poor use of prenatal care, as well as poor pregnancy outcomes among Indigenous[†] women globally[6–10] demonstrate the problems and lost benefits incurred by colonial-style healthcare delivery systems. In Canada, many healthcare programs and practices continue to reflect the oppressive values and attitudes that underlie colonization[11] and create demeaning, disrespectful, or dismissive environments and interactions between providers and Aboriginal people.[12–14] The often taken-for-granted, problematic legacy and enduring presence of colonial values, ideologies, and structures serve to disenfranchise Aboriginal people in the context of healthcare interactions and relationships. This has created a dynamic in healthcare in which Aboriginal[‡] people may avoid healthcare services or use services only at the point of crisis. Although these dynamics may be unintended, they nevertheless contribute to unethical barriers to care. As a result, individuals and populations lose the benefits of preventive interventions during pregnancy and parenting. Thus fostering safe and competent care for Aboriginal people is a priority ethical concern for nursing and for healthcare more generally.

The purpose of this study was to describe community-based stakeholders' perspectives on their experience improving care for pregnant and parenting Aboriginal women and families. "Community-based stakeholders" were defined as Aboriginal people, providers, and organizations mandated to provide care tailored to the needs of the Aboriginal people. Results are being reported in a series of papers.[†] In an earlier article,[15] we described Aboriginal parents' views of the importance of pregnancy and parenting. Focusing on perspectives of Aboriginal parents in the study sample, findings suggested that pregnancy and parenting must be understood on the one hand relative to Aboriginal peoples' unique individual and family life experiences, and on the other within a broad understanding of the intergenerational impact of residential schools as an instrument of collective violence. The results highlighted the need to recognize colonizing policies as one of the root causes of inequities in health and access to services experienced by Aboriginal people. Participants' views that healthcare interventions

---

*The term Aboriginal "refers to organic political and cultural entities that stem historically from the original Peoples in North America, rather than collections of individuals united by so-called 'racial' characteristics" (Royal Commission on Aboriginal Peoples, 1996). These include the First Nations, Inuit, and Métis Peoples of Canada.

[†] The term Indigenous is a globally inclusive term, while the term Aboriginal is used primarily in Canadian contexts. Both terms are used in this paper, depending on the context to which we are referring.

[‡] A final set of papers will report on results for the final 3 research questions: (1) How does safe and responsive care developed by innovative Aboriginal organizations make a difference to Aboriginal women and families; (2) What was the process of transforming care for pregnant and parenting Aboriginal people; and (3) What was the influence of context on Aboriginal communities' experience of innovating care for pregnant and parenting Aboriginal people?

must flow from the perspective and values of the people they serve set the context for answering the remaining research questions.

In this article we report on results for the research question, "What are community-based stakeholders' views on care during pregnancy and parenting?" Results extend current use of the concept of safety in healthcare, and describe how experiences of safe and responsive care may improve early access to and relevance of care during pregnancy and parenting for Aboriginal people. The importance of *safe* care is understood within a socio-historically situated understanding of unsafe healthcare encounters resulting from systemic disenfranchisement or "othering" of Aboriginal people. Imposed models of healthcare intervention based on racialized explanations and prescriptive solutions for health concerns experienced by Aboriginal people create an unethical paradox of care. At best, imposed models of care incongruent with clients' values, beliefs, and personal strengths and resource diminish the relevance of care. At worst, imposed models of care violate human rights and create unethical race-based barriers to effective care.[16] In contrast, *responsive* care and practice begins with understanding of the fundamental right to practice one's cultural beliefs and values, and respect and appreciation for the strengths each person develops through their unique life experiences. Implications for extending current use of the concept of patient safety, and improving responsiveness in healthcare, are considered. Importantly, this analysis supports and understanding of safety as reflected in nursing codes of ethics—a broad ethical mandate that extends well beyond narrow concerns with physical safety—and emphasizes the emotional and cultural dimensions of safety.

BACKGROUND

Aboriginal women and families need more culturally appropriate maternal/child healthcare that is relevant to their needs and strengths.[17–20] Some evidence for intervention suggests that culturally appropriate perinatal services improved Indigenous women's satisfaction with care and early initiation of care, and increased rates of breastfeeding initiation and duration, although interventions deemed to be culturally appropriate varied. Research programs[21,22] and evaluation studies[23,24] with Indigenous communities have found that community involvement in program design, implementation, and evaluation improved participant satisfaction, promoted early access and participation in care, enhanced women's health behaviors, resulting in improved nutrition and decreased tobacco and alcohol consumption; and engendered feelings of mastery about infant care. These findings support the argument that "until the effects on the healthcare system of inequalities in power between groups in society are addressed,"[25(p453)] significant improvement in healthcare for Aboriginal people is unlikely.[26] Racism-driven inequities in health between populations, exacerbated by institutionalized inequities in access to safe care, are ethical issues for nurses, organizations, and societies.

Impact of Colonization on Healthcare for Aboriginal People

About 3.33% (approximately 1,000,000) of Canada's total population self-identify as First Nations, Métis, or Inuit. Delivery of healthcare to Aboriginal people in Canada crosses provincial and federal jurisdictional responsibilities for healthcare. However, colonization of Aboriginal people in Canada has resulted in complex arrangements for jurisdiction, administration, and governance over healthcare, which in turn fostered inequities in health and social conditions and inconsistencies in design and capacity to deliver maternal/child healthcare. Since the Indian Act of 1876,[27] the federal government has had jurisdiction over primary healthcare services for those in First Nations' and Inuit communities.* About 30% of the Aboriginal people live in 602 communities under federal jurisdiction for provision

*Métis peoples were not included in the Indian Act. However, growing awareness of Métis issues, improvements in recognition of Métis rights, and better enumeration has brought recognition of Métis needs for appropriate healthcare.

of health services. Responsibility for providing healthcare to the majority (70%) of Aboriginal peoples is a provincial responsibility south of the 55th parallel, and a territorial responsibility north of it.[†][28,29] Many Aboriginal communities are geographically isolated, having either no road access or access for only part of the year.

In federal jurisdictions, the First Nations and Inuit Health Branch [FNIHB] delivers health services to First Nations communities either directly, or through transfer agreements with First Nations–controlled health authorities. Health transfer has enabled First Nations to exert more control over health priorities and solutions, and has assisted the federal government to meet its fiduciary responsibilities. As of September 2005, 80% of eligible First Nations communities were involved in the transfer of some level of health services to First Nations control (FNIHB, 2005). Poor participation in and outcomes of healthcare have been attributed to inequities in access to services, an imposed biomedical rather than holistic approach to interventions, lack of responsiveness to differences in cultures and community realities, and federal government rather than Aboriginal authority and community control over health systems.[30–32]

Inequities in health and social conditions between Aboriginal and mainstream Canadian populations have been well documented.[33,34] For example, 46% of the people in First Nations communities live in inadequate housing,[35] compared to 20% of non-Aboriginal people in rental accommodation. Poverty is widespread, with 60% of all Aboriginal children from birth to 6 years of age living in low-income families (compared to 25% in the Canadian population).[36] Forty-four percent of people residing in Aboriginal communities live below the low-income cut-off point (compared to 20% in the Canadian population).[36] Aboriginal people experience significant perinatal and infant health challenges such as teen pregnancy (9% of Aboriginal children live with teenage mothers compared to 1%

in the non-Aboriginal population), Fetal Alcohol Spectrum Disorder (estimates of prevalence among Aboriginal people range from 2.8 to 9.1/1000 live births, vs 0.3/1000 in the Canadian population)[37] and infant mortality from injuries (4 times the rate in non-Aboriginal populations).[38] A growing body of evidence suggests that these inequitable health and social conditions have their root in the "othering" of Aboriginal peoples that began with colonization, which directly challenges discriminatory and socially unjust racialized explanations that have underpinned many health intervention programs for Aboriginal people.[39]

Design and Delivery of Maternal/Child Healthcare

The FNIHB's maternal/child health program comprises prenatal and postnatal care, including evacuation from rural and remote settings to provincial tertiary care facilities for birth.[40] Prenatal and postnatal programs are delivered primarily by registered nurses who work with community health representatives [CHRs*],[41] and alongside several related programs such as the Canada Prenatal Nutrition Program, the Fetal Alcohol Syndrome/Fetal Alcohol Effects Prevention Program, and the Aboriginal Head Start on Reserve Program. Nursing services across the regions are predominated by individualistic, biomedically oriented tertiary interventions. However, single regions have adopted particular emphases such as evidence-based prevention and population health approaches, prenatal screening, or family-centered care. The presence, size, and scope of the related programs also vary among the 602 First Nations communities since small geographically isolated communities often do not have the population, resources, or capacity to support infrastructure or staffing for full program delivery. The result

---

[†]Health care for populations living north of 55 was outside the focus of this study.

*CHRs are lay health workers with variable amounts of formal and/or informal education who assist individuals, families, and groups of people in the community to take responsibility for their own health; to work with other healthcare teams to improve and maintain the spiritual, physical, intellectual, social, and emotional well-being of the individuals, families, and community.

is a collection of maternal/child health services with disparate administrative, governance, and implementation systems. Furthermore, service continuity and depth of care over the childbearing continuum are disrupted by evacuation for birth, geographical barriers to delivery of care, and high rates of staff turnover. These shortcomings and challenges contribute to the inequities in access to relevant and responsive maternal/child health services for Aboriginal people[42] set up by colonization.

Over the last decade, some improvements have been noted, such as greater congruence between healthcare services and local values and beliefs; increased emphasis on the role of family, culture, and prevention; and more effective integration between traditional and Western approaches.[43,44] However, the process and characteristics of the innovations have not been systematically documented or disseminated. Furthermore, models addressing social determinants of health and each community's unique cultural, social, economic, and political circumstances have yet to be described.

METHODS

A critical postcolonial stance and participatory research principles[45,46] shaped the study methods. Postcolonial and participatory research perspectives are inclusive of different value systems and sensitive to differences, view all forms of knowledge as valuable, and seek to generate knowledge that is relevant to stakeholders and useful for solving practical problems.

Postcolonialism is concerned with "the unequal relations of power that are the legacy of the colonial past and neocolonial present, and the ways in which the cultures of dominant groups have redefined local meanings, and dictated social structures, including healthcare delivery systems."[47(p197)] Postcolonial scholarship aims to expose, describe, and change ideological and social structures that maintain inequities between Aboriginal and non-Aboriginal populations. A critical postcolonial perspective recognizes Aboriginal people as central agents of this change, and moves beyond us-them ways of thinking,

toward recognition and valuing of the strengths made available through integrating diverse ways of knowing, doing, and being.[48,49]

Participatory research methodologies acknowledge and aim to redress the troubled history of research *on* Aboriginal people. "Many Aboriginal people have been the subjects of research that they had little say in or no control over, that misrepresented or misinterpreted their experiences, and failed to create knowledge that was useful to the community."[50(p4)] Participatory research views all forms of knowledge as valuable, and maintains that knowledge should be useful for solving practical problems and be relevant to stakeholders. Participatory research is particularly suited to exploring the potentially disparate knowledge, values, and worldviews of stakeholders (eg, community members, providers, and policy makers) for the purpose of acquiring the practical knowledge needed to improve care for pregnant and parenting Aboriginal people.

A 2-phase case study design enabled collection of in-depth contextual data to understand the determinants and processes of individual and organizational participants' experiences improving care for pregnant and parenting Aboriginal people in each setting.[51]

Phase 1

The study was set in the province of British Columbia, Canada. The study setting was chosen on the basis of the following: (*a*) the goal of learning from Aboriginal organizations with successful approaches to prenatal care; (*b*) the goal of exploring the interplay between complex jurisdictional, administrative, and governance arrangements for healthcare for Aboriginal people; and (*c*) recognizing that the depth of data collection and analysis would depend on development of partnerships with organizations and trusting relationships with participants. The researcher had preexisting professional relationships with several Aboriginal organizations in this setting, expediting the initial steps of identification, recruitment, and development of agreements with the organizations and communities in phase 2.

Concurrent data collection and analysis for phase 1 began in February of 2004 following approval from the University of Ottawa Health and Social Sciences ethics review board. Sixteen key informants working in policy, leadership, and provider positions in maternal/child health within the province of British Columbia were purposefully selected using network sampling techniques.[52] Policy makers and providers who worked in early childhood services, infant development programs, nursing, and pregnancy support were included. Leaders were from policy organizations, First Nations communities, and Aboriginal health service organizations. During either telephone or face-to-face interviews, key informants share their perspectives about issues and influences on Aboriginal women's and families' pregnancy experiences, and identified healthcare delivery organizations with a reputation for high rates of early access and participation in prenatal care by Aboriginal women. Consequently, several communities from both provincial and federal jurisdictions were identified and approached regarding their interest in participating in phase 2.

Phase 2

One urban and one rural Aboriginal healthcare delivery organization geographically located in one health region agreed to participate in the community-based case study in phase 2. The 2 sites represented complementary jurisdictional, geographical, and program development characteristics. Ethical approval for phase 2 was obtained from the University of Ottawa Health and Social Sciences ethics review board, the ethical review committee of the participating Tribal Council, and Chief and Council of the participating communities. Fieldwork was conducted from June to September of 2004 in the 2 settings. Participants in each setting were purposefully selected using network sampling techniques to obtain a variety of perspectives from community members, providers, and leaders. Sampling decisions were made to juxtapose stakeholder group perspectives (eg, leaders, providers, and community members) on the research questions. Data were collected by the first author using one-to-one exploratory interviews and small-group discussions according to the preference of each participant. Interviews lasted from 45 to 120 minutes depending on the communication style and the stories and perspectives the participant wished to share. Time was taken at the beginning of the interview to create a safe, trusting, respectful environment and dynamic in the researcher-participant relationship and to emphasize the importance of many ways of knowing, particularly feelings or embodied knowledge.[53,54] Many participants held multiple stakeholder positions, such as parent, provider, and community leader, so a longer period of time was required to discuss their related experiences. Interviews were taped with participants' consent* and transcribed. Supplementary documents and field notes were also included in the data set.

Documents reviewed reflected both the program design and the process of health system change. Examples of documents reflecting the process of health system change included the following: government reports; proceedings from community meetings; memoranda of understanding; strategic policy documents; organizations' mission and mandate, and terms of reference for tribal councils, boards, and advisory committees; newspaper articles; and annual reports. Documents capturing program design and/or innovation included consultant and pilot project reports, program descriptions, utilization statistics, staff job descriptions, and reports of audits and external evaluations.

Criteria for enhancing methodological rigor included critical reflexivity, maintaining integrity of participants' voices in context, taking direct action on the research problem,[55] confirmability, credibility, and fittingness.[56] Peer debriefing, member checking, prioritizing trust and relationship building in research encounters, reflective writing, and engagement were used to enact these criteria.

---

* Three participants preferred to have notes taken during the interview.

Critical reflexivity is a process of deliberately noticing, recording, and reflecting on the research process and experience, and the nature of knowledge being constructed. It is a method for observing, making explicit, and continuously revising the influence of the researcher as the primary instrument in research, and records influence of the researcher's voice and perspectives vis-à-vis those of participants.[57] Critical reflexive strategies included regular reflective writing and peer debriefing as a way of "mining" the subjective experience of doing the research for potential problematic situations, perceptions, values, and attitudes. Integrity of participants' voices was facilitated through giving control of time, place, and format of interviews to participants; making time and space to develop a comfortable and safe interaction; member checking during analysis to deepen understanding of themes and subthemes; and privileging verbatim quotes in presentation of results. For example, participants chose to do interviews alone or with a trusted peer or colleague. Hard copies of preliminary results were distributed to participants in the study sites, and workshops and luncheons were hosted by the researcher (first author of this article) to discuss and critique themes and subthemes and their presentation.

Data were analyzed by the first author using an interpretive descriptive method[58] supported by NVIVO software during a prolonged period of immersion in the data. Analysis proceeded from a wholly inductive approach, and became increasingly deductive as important themes were identified. Analysis included iterative cycles of coding, collapsing, and reorganizing coding structure, and consideration of thematic patterns across different sites and different participant groups (eg, community member, providers, and leaders). Once preliminary results were drafted, all participants were invited to discuss them in 3-hour workshops held in the study communities in April of 2005.

RESULTS

A total of 73 key informants and community-based leaders, providers, and community members participated. Table B-1 shows a profile of participants in each phase of the study. Over 60% of the sample self-identified as Aboriginal and 90% were women. Nearly half of phase 2 participants were providers ($n = 25$); and 20 of these had more than 10 years ($n = 20$) of experience working in an Aboriginal health service delivery organization. Providers included registered nurses ($n = 9$); lay providers ($n = 7$) such as nutrition counselors, community health representatives, or family support workers; and other health and social service professionals ($n = 9$) such as nutritionists, social workers, and professional counselors. The remainder were community members, including mothers, fathers, grandparents, and

TABLE B-1 Sample Composition by Phase, Aboriginal Identity and Gender				
Study Phase and Setting	Sample Subgroup	Total*	Aboriginal Identity No. (%)	Female No. (%)
Phase 1		16	8 (50)	15 (93.7)
Phase 2		57	36 (63)	51 (89.5)
Case A: remote setting		29	21 (72.4)	25 (86.2)
	Leaders	8	7 (87.5)	6 (75)
	Providers	10	2 (20)	9 (90)
	Community members	11	11 (100)	9 (81.8)
Case B: urban setting		28	15 (53.6)	26 (92.9)
	Leaders	9	4 (44.4)	9 (100)
	Providers	15	7 (46.7)	14 (93.3)
	Community members	4	4 (100)	3 (75)
Study Totals		73	44 (60.3)	66 (90.4)

*Although many participants fit into more than 1 category, they are only counted once in this profile.

elders; and leaders such as band administrators, chief and council members, health center administrators, and advisory committee members. Participants were assigned to the group according to the criterion by which they were chosen to participate. However, most Aboriginal participants held multiple stakeholder positions: for example, participants may have been both a leader and a provider, or both a parent and a provider, or both a leader and a parent (as well as other family roles), and in some cases held all 3 roles (leader, provider, parent). Many of these participants brought critically reflexive understandings gained through multiple roles, thus enriching the insights into the research questions.

Table B-2 shows the themes and subthemes resulting from our analysis. Each of these themes and subthemes are described below, followed by discussion of implications for policy, practice, and education of health providers.

Pregnancy as an Opportunity for Change

"Successful" intervention approaches were described by participants as acknowledging individual and collective history, and responding to pregnancy and parenting as a significant opportunity to facilitate and support Aboriginal peoples' efforts to create a better future for their children. Respondents described pregnancy as a powerful opportunity to support and facilitate people to choose a healing path. Participants indicated that pregnancy was often a time when prospective parents examined the influence of the intergenerational impact of residential schools on their values, beliefs, and capacity for healthy parenting. Speaking from her experience as a parent, this provider explains:

> I've found having children really makes you question the spiritual, your spirituality.... So if you're ambiguous before, you weren't sure what you believed, it's pretty hard to talk about that with you kids.... I think questioning as you become a parent is a normal part of becoming a parent, but there probably are a lot more conflicting issues I think, if you have the residential school issues. Even if you weren't there yourself, but a child of someone who went to residential school because it's passed down for sure. But they were never taught how to be a parent. They were never parented. (Provider P2-A3)

TABLE B-2 Themes and Subthemes in Results	
Themes	**Subthemes**
Pregnancy as an opportunity for change	• Wanting children to have the gifts but not the pain of the intergenerational impact of residential schools • Children are highly valued • Parents are highly motivated to heal past hurts, and reconnect with self, family, and culture
Safe healthcare places and relationships	• Nonjudgmental • Respectful • Strengths-based • Facilitating healing and trusting relationships
Responsive care	• Holistic • Client-directed • Integrating multiple ways of knowing, with greater emphasis on experiential and cultural knowledge
Making intervention safe and responsive	• Reaching out—being visible • Empowerment education • Including fathers and family • Feeding body, mind, and soul

As well as revisiting a painful childhood, becoming a parent represented a time of significant hope for a better future for their children.

> I was abused. I was neglected, I was physically abused by my parents, by my friends. This is something I don't want to happen to the next generation of children. I want things to be different for my kids. I want them to succeed—I can see they are going to succeed. They are doing well in school and they are going to have a chance. (Community member P2-A10)

Participants described high value placed on children by families, culture, and community as an "enormous" motivator for parents to make and sustain healthier choices.

> The real cultural belief is that all children are a gift from God. So no matter what the circumstances . . . if the woman is drinking, if she's doing drugs . . . it doesn't matter [to the importance placed on the child], that child is a gift. And that has an enormous influence on the women. (Provider P2-A2)

Safe and Responsive Care

Safety and *responsiveness* were seen by participants as central to an approach to care that fundamentally changed the nature of their relationships with healthcare organizations and providers. They saw attention to safety and responsiveness as enabling healthcare to facilitate Aboriginal peoples' efforts to "turn around" the intergenerational impact of residential schools. The subthemes involved in design, implementation, and evaluation of safe and responsive care for pregnant and parenting Aboriginal people are described below.

Safe Places and Safe Relationships

Safe places and relationships were described as essential to support Aboriginal parents in their efforts to turn around the intergenerational impact of residential schools. Safe places are important from multiple perspectives. Participants described how mainstream healthcare environments were often perceived and experienced as unsafe. Speaking about experiences in mainstream healthcare setting, one leader said:

> Lots of time they don't feel comfortable [at the mainstream health agency]. It's not a culturally acceptable place. The rules are very rigid. You have to come at a certain time. They [agency staff] don't understand the difficulty of getting rides, they don't understand how appointments can be missed . . . and also they [Aboriginal parents] feel they're being judged on the way the baby looks, or how they talk or . . . health nurses assume they're stupid or they're slow and they can't read, or, you know, these sorts of things. (Leader P2-B1b)

Participants described how the risks associated with past care-seeking experiences have made safe places and safe people in the Aboriginal health organization critical. Safe places require a non-judgmental attitude on the part of the whole program and organization.

> It took a long time for trust to be established. That this was a safe place and that it had benefits versus the risks of coming into this place. I think we have to acknowledge for people who have been marginalized, the risks need to be weighed out versus those benefits. And you know, some of the risks might be that it puts on the table that you are using a substance that could cause harm to the fetus or if you have other children at home and you identify that you are using a drug of some sort . . ., I mean just coming out of the closet and telling people that you have a problem has its own risks. And that's where the trust factor comes in. You know if, if the way that that problem solving is handled is respectful, effective, and client focused, then that's why people will come. The word of mouth is going to put it out there that it's okay to take that risk. (Leader P2-B6)

Participants described the characteristics of a safe place, emphasizing the importance of the energy, or the feeling, of a place:

> It's also the environment, the place; it's warm, friendly and caring and we have time for people. There is a different energy in programs built from an Aboriginal perspective . . . the pace is different . . . the environment is more relaxed, friendly, casual . . . it is a comfortable place to be with couches and the coffee room. There is a mix of staff that is similar to the mix of participants [including some] First Nations staff. We dress differently. . . . I don't dress up to see participants. . . . We are people-friendly, not appointment book–friendly . . . it feels like home here. (Provider P1-16)

Aboriginal parents said that to heal, you have to face up to the pain, to the weaknesses and the problems, which can be very difficult. Therefore, you need supportive relationships with people who will not judge you, but will walk beside you, who will listen and acknowledge your pain and your strengths along with the mistakes you may have committed as a human being. Respect in everything that is said and done, whether consciously or unconsciously, influenced people's feelings of emotional safety.

> But I think the more First Nation's groups I know, the more I know just to treat everyone like individuals. It truly is. You know, you make these assumptions based on what they should be culturally and then you get challenged and told that's wrong. So, I find it's always best to work with them as individuals and say . . . and treat them as people, with respect, and then you get amazing results. (Provider P2-B1a)

The client-provider relationship was seen as an opportunity to build understanding and capacity for healthy relationships. Participants emphasized facilitating healthy reconnection and relationships with self, significant others, and family, rather than creating dependencies on providers.

> You have to have, I feel, for me to even connect with them and to be open and honest so that we can work with that, is to say, "What has life shown you?" "What's your biggest issue, what's your biggest concern?" And when it's coming from them, then probably 95% of the time, people come out and say what their issue is . . . and [ultimately] they wanted a healthy relationship and they wanted to treat each other respectfully so that their children could come into a world where they were treated respectfully. (Provider P2-A22)

Safe relationships meant providers being open, and seeking to understand and acknowledge, rather than to judge. Along with acknowledging the pain and struggles people have experienced, participants thought it critical to recognize the gifts and assets that people have developed through their struggles.

> That's all people want, is that acknowledgement. I think we all want that as people, trust that I can make my own decision and trust that I will do the best that I can with the skill set that I have. And when you give me that credit . . . then I'm going to aspire for more. (Provider P2-A22)

Connecting with people at a "heart" or "spirit" level through developing safe, trusting relationships was described by all groups of participants (eg, leaders, providers, community members) as the most important difference between the approach developed by Aboriginal health organizations compared to conventional care. This became increasingly clear as the interviews progressed, so the question was posed, "What happens if you don't connect with people at a heart level?" Responses to this question ranged from "You might as well pack your bags and head home," to "Nothing. Absolutely nothing happens." One participant put it like this:

> If [connecting at heart/spirit level] isn't there, they're not there. That's what happens. People just don't feel comfortable. My take . . . is that they're not going to come

> *back, because that's the feedback that I have got from people . . . when they feel respected and when they feel accepted, when they feel that you care and they'll test you out . . . and they know . . . they've been through an experience for so long that they know from their teachings and also from their experience and all the kinds of painful things that have happened what works and what doesn't. (Leader P2-B7)*

Responsiveness

Responsiveness of care is a fundamental shift by providers and organizations. Rather than entering into care relationships with unexamined and often unconscious worldviews, values, and priorities for health-related experiences, care is offered in a way that seeks to understand, respect, and respond to those of communities' and clients'. Responsiveness encompasses being holistic, being client-directed, and integrating ways of knowing into relationships and care. Participants in this study described *holistic* as

> *There is that kind of spiritual dimension in everything that takes place . . . the spiritual, mental, emotional, physical aspects of life all need to be considered and in balance for us to really be able to participate fully in who we are and in our families and in our communities. And that's a juggling act. Anybody who has tried to become balanced knows that. But, so we need all kinds of support to do that . . . we need understanding, we need encouragement. (Leader P2-B7)*

Client-directed care was differentiated from client-centered care and was described as the client setting the agenda, making the decisions and taking responsibility for living with the consequences. For example,

> *Most of it, I truly believe, if I look back over the years . . . it's about 50 to 60% emotional support. I might have an agenda that I'd like to talk about breastfeeding today, but*

> *that might be the last thing on their agenda, so if we can't do what's on their mind and their focus, then how can we really reach what we need to do. (Provider P2-A22)*

Responsiveness means that many ways of knowing are respected and integrated into care. Ways of knowing included the traditional knowledge, experiential knowledge, "heart knowledge," and clinical knowledge from both clients and providers. However, there was a consistent emphasis on bringing traditional and experiential knowledge, and "heart knowledge," into the forefront of care. Participants explained why:

> *We're trying to work with women to invite them to explore some of the traditional practices, like before they give birth, and try to incorporate it into a birth plan. And even through the pregnancy, to try to use some of those belief systems and have that guidance instead of white society telling you what you should and shouldn't do. (Provider P2-A3)*

An emphasis on personal and cultural knowledge reverses the pattern of care, from imposing and shaming based on mainstream knowledge and practices, to connecting with clients, and acknowledging and affirming their cultural knowledge and identity:

> *Well I think that to be strong on the culture is such a good tool to try to turn it around because, you know I talked to a lot of women and there's a lot of anger, there's a lot of being made to feel ashamed of yourself that sort of results in sex and abuse issues. And I think going back to the traditional ways of giving pride and food can help to undo some of that. I see that as the answer. And I think it will come. It's going to be slow. But I think that's the answer, going back to the traditional teachings and beliefs. (Provider P2-B16)*

The importance of an approach that incorporates many ways of knowing is evident in descriptions of experiences of moving back and forth between living in small isolated First Nations communities and larger mainstream communities. The difficulties of trying to fit into the values and lifestyle of mainstream society heightened some participants' awareness of their unique way of being and knowing as an Aboriginal person:

> It was like two collisions . . . this world with that world . . . and it took many years to realize . . . how do I fit into this society? How do I adjust to this society? How do I meet up to their standards, their education, their lifestyle, their raising of their children was so different from the way . . . we were raised as children . . . and ah, it was hard. It took me many years to adjust. (Community member P2-B3)

Providers, leaders, and community members were clear that up-to-date scientific and expert clinical knowledge is important, and integrated as needed. Providers indicated that deciding how and when to use different ways of knowing comes from reflective engagement with their own emotional wisdom, as well as being emotionally "tuned-in" and respectful of the choice and priorities of the people with whom they are working.

Making Intervention Strategies Safe and Responsive

Safe and responsive care meant that providers and organizations reoriented their role and relationship with the community and clients. Paramount was understanding and embracing the local cultural values, norms, and practices as an organizing framework for engaging with clients and community, with other ways of knowing such as professional nursing standards, evidence-based knowledge or expert clinical knowledge being woven in. This is in direct contrast to clients' and providers' experience of working within an imposed model of care:

> In the past, the emphasis had always been on perceived rigid rules and regulations coming from the outside. [Though] we wanted to honor our professional code (eg,

nursing standards for practice), we also wanted to honor the cultural codes and protocols of the [local] people. We needed to understand the [local cultural] code, to respect it, to abide by it, and to be guided by it. So that the cultural code was the main code, and the professional code was the add-on piece, rather than the other way round. (Provider P2-A4)

Safe and responsive care for Aboriginal parents during pregnancy and parenting involved a collection of innovative strategies that are qualitatively different from conventional care. These strategies were identified as critically important by all 3 groups of participants in both communities (ie, community members, providers, and leaders). Examples illustrating this difference include reaching out and being visible, empowerment education, inclusion of fathers and families, and an emphasis on the role of food. Examples highlighted below demonstrate how the imperatives of safety and responsiveness shaped providers' practice.

REACHING OUT AND BEING VISIBLE

Reaching out acknowledges the barriers that the history of unsafe environments, people and relationships may have on care seeking. Reaching out was also seen as indication of being with people because you genuinely cared about them. Reaching out was an example of following the local cultural codes, rather than imposing or limiting care to the norms of mainstream society. Reaching out was the "way we do things around here—it's our way." For example,

> There is, I think, very positive support with [the community health nurse], who is able to get out into the homes and do a one-on-one, and that's what really works. There is a very big weakness, in a sense, with people and their safety and their issues to walk into the health clinic. They don't feel safe. They don't feel that they can trust the staff [who] work there. They don't feel trust in, not just the people, but in the whole entire

government structure. . . . Fear is a big thing—fear to talk to somebody about sex and sexual education [for example]. (Provider P2-A9)

Being visible went hand in hand with reaching out.

To me, one of the most important things is being visible. I found that being visible in the community, consistently . . . I'll see Elders, I'll work with the mothers, I'll go to the school, I'll do baby shots . . . a lot of stuff, where people come in and they're looking for something or they want some screening done, and then I'll talk to them about that . . . about anything. I found that the women come much earlier. (Provider P2-A2)

EMPOWERMENT EDUCATION

In contrast to the straight information-giving approach of conventional and less well-received programs, an empowering approach to education was a distinct aspect of supportive programs. Providers described a one-to-one responsive style of teaching and learning that was noticeably different than simply providing people with verbal or written information. They described an ongoing dialogue with clients that integrated client's knowledge of themselves, and their goals and constraints, with provider's knowledge of such things as bodily functioning, the healthcare system, and client's rights.

Now they're thinking about it. They know that if they want to get pregnant they want to be healthy. They want to have healthy babies . . . I teach them [about their menstrual cycle]. . . . Pretty much all those women know when they are ovulating now. And we all should. I tell them, don't feel bad if you don't know, 80% of the population doesn't. I mean, it's the truth. So, they all know. To me, that's empowering them. They are empowering themselves with that awareness of when they need to . . . not have sex when . . . you know, if they are

going out for the weekend, there is more planning involved than I have ever seen before. (Provider P2-A22)

INCLUDING FATHERS AND FAMILY

Safe and responsive care recognized the disconnections resulting from the intergenerational impact of residential schools, and seized the positive opportunity presented by pregnancy and parenting to encourage families to develop stronger connections and build healthy relationships. Providers encouraged family members to participate directly in care. For example,

When [the nurse] is doing the prenatal, she welcomes them. . . . I don't think I've seen a dad come through here that wasn't just beaming when he left after the prenatal session. I think that even that early involvement and that early education about what's happening with the wife's body is an important step for, for men to have, for all people to have. And it's teamwork, it's not just all mom's job because the baby's in mom . . . you need that support. (Provider 14)

Participants also described how clients were encouraged to reach out to family members to explore how the tasks and issues of pregnancy and childbearing, such as dietary habits and naming have been managed in previous generations. This served to reconnect family members over a positive common interest that often provided an opening for healing past hurts.

FEEDING THE BODY, MIND, AND SOUL

Food was described as a positive, culturally based method of connecting, building relationships, and passing on knowledge and a traditional way of imparting knowledge.

Culturally our way is to, when you feed someone, what you're feeding them is, you're feeding them information once you're feeding them nutritionally also. You know, what I mean, is you're feeding their mind. You're feeding their body and you're feeding their soul when you're giving them the respect. And you're giving them the honor that they deserve. Everybody needs to be well-respected when they walk in that door regardless of who they are. That's the way I envision it. Feed the mind. Feed the body. Feed the soul. (Provider 15)

However, food security and food literacy were also described as urgent concerns for pregnant and parenting families. Food insecurity was identified as a consequence of poverty, and a gap in knowledge and skills resulting from the loss of traditional food sources and the consequences of the intergenerational impact of residential schools.

We also have to recognize that the parents of today's pregnant women may have been in residential schools. And so they didn't learn how to cook. Therefore, they didn't do what you're doing with your family. They didn't make from scratch or teach their children what is a balanced meal. So we've got some [food] illiteracy. (Leader P2-B6)

In summary, the stakeholders in this study saw pregnancy as an important opportunity for change. However they emphasized that in order for such change to be realized, healthcare organizations and relationships must be safe and responsive. Safety and responsiveness require taking history and inequities into account, and working partnership among all stakeholders.

DISCUSSION

These results expand notions of safety as currently used in healthcare. Patient safety broadens the concepts of medical or physical safety as criteria for quality in healthcare.[59] Patient safety, defined most broadly, supports the argument that a "major objective of any healthcare system should be the safe progress of consumers through all parts of the system. Harm from their care, by omission or commission, as well as from the environment in which it is carried out, must be avoided and risk minimized in care delivery processes."[60(p2)] This understanding of safety includes the concept of harm due to negligent or intentional action or inaction.[61] However, the risk of *emotional* harm in healthcare settings and interactions is rarely discussed as a patient safety issue. Indeed, Storch has pointed out that current narrow interpretations of patient safety may distort and obscure broader needs such as those for emotional safety.[62] Results of this current study suggest that emotional safety is an important dimension of patient safety for Aboriginal people in healthcare interactions and settings and warrants further attention.

Results identified the emotional dimension of safety as having a crucial influence on **access** to prenatal care. That is, experiences of unsafe care can deter access. Emotional safety has been discussed in the context of mental healthcare, and as an issue in care and healing from interpersonal and collective violence, rather than as an issue of patient safety that is central to all healthcare encounters. The extent to which one feels safe in healthcare encounters is affected by past experiences with safety or lack of safety. One's willingness to engage in healthcare encounters is also influenced by peer and social network views about how likely organizations and providers are to be safe and caring. This community-level influence is also a reflection of the influence of past experiences with unsafe healthcare interactions or institutions.[63] Further research is needed to understand the influence of emotional safety on both access to and experience of healthcare interactions and settings.

As described in the cultural safety literature, some healthcare settings and interactions are routinely unsafe for Aboriginal people.[64] Unexamined, demeaning, and disrespectful attitudes, values, and beliefs of healthcare providers and organizations of colonized societies have fostered behaviors that are hurtful for Aboriginal people.[65] Transforming this systemic impact of collective violence on Aboriginal peoples' experiences of both internal and external safety in healthcare has been termed *culturally safe care* and is described as "actions which recognize, respect and nurture the unique cultural identity of [Aboriginal people], and safely meet their needs, expectations and rights."[66] Identifying safety as an important influence on early access and use of care during pregnancy and parenting is an important finding, and complements the emerging body of evidence on cultural safety.

Results suggest that Aboriginal people are working on understanding, healing, and transforming their sense of safety and well-being in interpersonal relationships, including relationships in the context of healthcare. Participants described the approach taken by both providers and organizations to work *in partnership* with Aboriginal people to create relationships, places, and interactions that feel safe. Furthermore, healthcare organizations and providers must develop the skills and understanding to assess the extent to which they *are* providing safe care. The extent to which institutions responsible for the basic preparation of health professionals, such as undergraduate schools of nursing, are equipping graduates with the skills to understand and develop safe care must be examined. Research and education could build on the work of nursing organizations and educational institutions in New Zealand to develop competencies and organizational support for culturally safe practice.[68]

Findings highlight the importance of responsiveness to the diversity of individual and families' lived experiences, and the need to provide care that respects these differences. Responsiveness is qualitatively different from "sensitivity," particularly as it is used in relation to culture, in at least 2 ways. First, responsiveness is more active than "sensitivity" and places responsibility on healthcare providers to act. Second, responsiveness implies particular individuals and situations rather than sensitivity to groups based on generalized assumptions and stereotypes. Third, responsiveness is an ethical alternative to imposing a dominant model that dictates the rightness of a particular set of healthcare issues and priorities

on the basis of a taken-for-granted worldview (Western) and values, priorities, and actions (eg, biomedicine). In contrast, responsiveness positions healthcare organizations and providers as responsible to (*a*) recognize their own positions, (*b*) seek to understand that of others, and (*c*) ethically make the resources and support available to address their priorities rather than judging difference as somehow wrong or inferior. Furthermore, a strengths-based orientation to responsive intervention seems critical to improve real access to care and to facilitate women's choices related to family planning and timing of pregnancies. These results illustrate how safe, trusting relationships are prerequisite to understanding individual circumstances and needs for basic determinants of health such as housing, food, advocacy with mainstream health and social systems, and encouragement to start and sustain further education. Results exemplify *how* the approach to care can enhance Aboriginal peoples' feelings of safety and relevance, thereby increasing early access, participation, and outcomes of care.

Finally, this study adds to awareness of discrimination, inequity, and safety as ethical concerns. Importantly, as Applebaum has argued, racism is a particularly serious ethical issue.[68,69] Furthermore, the findings suggest links among ethical concepts such as justice, competence, autonomy, and respect. Safety is a minimum ethical standard for nursing practice. A broader conceptualization of safety suggests that to practice ethically and competently, inequities and discrimination must be addressed in both individual and organizational practices.

CONCLUSION

This qualitative community-based study of the innovations developed by Aboriginal organizations in 2 unique geographical, jurisdictional, and demographic contexts explored perspectives of providers, leaders, and community members to describe their views of care during pregnancy and parenting. Although several strategies were used to capture the richness of their experience, and differentiate research and participant voice and interpretation, these results represent only a beginning understanding of community-based perspectives. Further research is needed across a greater number and diversity of settings to confirm or add to our understanding of salient aspects of approaches to and evaluation of care during pregnancy and parenting for Aboriginal people. Adequate time and resources are required to enable community-based participants with long-standing, trusting relationships to take a more active role in research design and implementation, thus enabling Aboriginal perspectives to guide and inform knowledge, policy, and practice development.

Pregnancy and parenting represent a culturally and developmentally significant opportunity for Aboriginal people to heal from and resist the ongoing impacts of colonialism. Results highlight the critical importance of building successful programs on an understanding of the history of colonization, and its impacts on Aboriginal people's relationships and experiences in healthcare. Results describe how the approach to care positions providers and organizations to work in partnership with Aboriginal people toward their vision to transform both the impact of this history and the nature of relationships. Situating care within a wider historical timeframe profoundly influences the goals, roles and relationships, resources, and expected outcomes of care. This study also underscores the importance of planning programs to recognize and respond to the unique experiences of individuals, families, and communities. These results warrant further exploration of the notion of safety in healthcare, particularly how experiences of emotionally safe care may improve early access to, and relevance of, care during pregnancy and parenting for Aboriginal people. We conclude that ethically, healthcare providers and organizations must work in closer harmony with Aboriginal people toward their vision, rather than reinforcing the colonizing relations that are a legacy of our past and often an ongoing feature of daily practices.

REFERENCES

1. American Nurses Association. (2001). *Code of ethics.* Retrieved December 18, 2005, from http://www.nursingworld.org/ethics/ecode.htm

2. Peternelj-Taylor, C. (2005). An exploration of othering in forensic psychiatric and correctional nursing. *Canadian Journal of Nursing Research, 36,* 130–147.

3. Varcoe, C. (2004). Widening the scope of ethical theory, practice and policy: Violence against women as an illustration. In J. Storch, P. Rodney, & R. Starzomski (Eds.), *Toward a moral horizon: Nursing ethics for leadership and practice* (pp. 414–432). Toronto: Pearson.

4. International Council of Nurses. (2000). *Code of ethics.* Geneva, Switzerland: Author.

5. Canadian Nurses Association. (2002). *Code of ethics.* Ottawa: Author.

6. De Costa, C., & Child, A. (1996). Pregnancy outcomes in urban Aboriginal women. *Medical Journal of Australia, 164,* 523–526.

7. Goldman, N., & Glei, D. (2003). Evaluation of midwifery care: Results from a survey in rural Guatemala. *Social Science & Medicine, 56,* 685–700.

8. Hoyert, D., Freedman, M., Strobino, D., & Guyer, B. (2001). Annual summary of vital statistics: 2000. *Pediatrics, 108,* 1241–1255.

9. Humphrey, M., & Holzheimer, D. (2000). A prospective study of gestation and birthweight in Aboriginal pregnancies in far north Queensland. *The Australian & New Zealand Journal of Obstetrics and Gynaecology, 40,* 326–330.

10. Luo, Z., Kierans, W., Wilkins, R., Liston, R., Uh, S., & Kramer, M. (2004). Infant mortality among First Nations versus non-First Nations in British Columbia: Temporal trends in rural versus urban areas, 1981–2000. *International Journal of Epidemiology, 33,* 1252–1259.

11. Royal Commission on Aboriginal People. (1996). *Gathering strength,* Vol. 3 (pp. 223–224). Ottawa: Author. Retrieved May 6, 2003, from http://www.ainc-inac.gc.ca/ch/rcap/rpt/index_e.html

12. Browne, A., & Smye, V. (2002). A postcolonial analysis of health care disclosures addressing Aboriginal women. *Nurse Researcher, 9*(3), 28–41.

13. Browne, A. (2005). Discourses influencing nurses' perceptions of First Nations patients. *Canadian Journal of Nursing Research, 37*(4), 62–87.

14. Browne, A. & Fiske, J. (2001). First Nations women's encounters with mainstream health care services. *Western Journal of Nursing Research, 23,* 126–147.

15. Smith, D., Varcoe, C., & Edwards, N. (2005). Turning around the intergenerational impact of residential schools on Aboriginal people: Implications for health

policy and practice. *Canadian Journal of Nursing Research, 37*(4), 38–61.

16. Krieger, N., & Gruskin, S. (2001). Frameworks matter: Eco-social and health and human rights perspectives on disparities in women's health—the case of tuberculosis. *Journal of the American Medical Women's Association, 56,* 137–142.

17. Long, C., & Curry, M. (1998). Living in two worlds: Native American women and prenatal care. *Health Care for Women International, 19,* 205–215.

18. Powell, J., & Dugdale, A. (1999). Obstetric outcomes in an Aboriginal community: A comparison with the surrounding rural area. *Australian Journal of Rural Health, 7*(1), 13–17.

19. Sokolowski, E. (1995). Canadian First Nations women's beliefs about pregnancy and prenatal care. *Canadian Journal of Nursing Research, 27*(1), 89–100.

20. Westenberg, L., van der Klis, K., Chan, A., Dekker, G., & Keane, R. (2002). Aboriginal teenage pregnancies compared with non-Aboriginal in South Australia, 1995–1999. *The Australian & New Zealand Journal of Obstetrics and Gynaecology, 42,* 187–192.

21. Affonso, D., Mayberry, L., Inaba, A., Matsuno, R., & Robinson, E. (1996). Hawaiian-style "Talkstory": Psychosocial assessment and intervention during and after pregnancy. *Journal of Obstetric, Gynecologic & Neonatal Nursing, 25,* 737–742.

22. Martens, P. (2002). Increasing breastfeeding initiation and duration at a community level: An evaluation of Sagkeeng First Nation's community health nurse and peer counsellor programs. *Journal of Human Lactation, 18,* 236–246.

23. Bucharski, D., Brockman, I., & Lambert, D. (1999). Developing culturally appropriate prenatal care models for Aboriginal women. *Canadian Journal of Human Sexuality, 34,* 151–154.

24. Fisher, P., & Ball, T. (2002). The Indian family wellness project: An application of the tribal participatory research model. *Prevention Science, 3,* 235–240.

25. Polashek, N. (1998). Cultural safety: A new concept in nursing people with different ethnicities. *Journal of Advanced Nursing, 27,* 452–457.

26. Smye, V., & Browne, A. (2002). 'Cultural safety' and the analysis of health policy affecting Aboriginal people. *Nurse Researcher, 9*(3), 42–51.

27. Government of Canada. (1985). *Indian Act.* Retrieved June 6, 2005, from http://laws.justice.gc.ca/en/I-5/text.html

28. Indian and Northern Affairs Canada. (2004). *Basic departmental data—2003.* Ottawa: First Nations and Northern Statistics Section, Corporate Information Management Directorate, Information Management Branch. Retrieved June 6, 2005, from http://www.ainc-inac.gc.ca/pr/sts/bdd03/bdd03_e.html

29. Statistics Canada. (2003). *Aboriginal Peoples survey.* Ottawa: Author.

30. Romanow, R. (2002). A new approach to Aboriginal health. In: *Building on values: The future of health care in Canada.* Ottawa: Commission on the Future of Health Care in Canada. Retrieved March 14, 2003, from http://www.hc-hc.gc.ca/english/care/romanow/hcc0086.html.

31. Jasen, P. (1997). Race, culture, and the colonization of childbirth in northern Canada. *Social History of Medicine, 10,* 383–400.

32. O'Neil, J. (1995). Issues in health policy for Indigenous peoples in Canada. *Australian Journal of Public Health, 19,* 559–566.

33. Federal/Territorial/Provincial Advisory Committee on Population Health. (1999). *Second report on the health of Canadians.* Ottawa: Author.

34. First Nations and Inuit Regional Health Survey National Steering Committee. (1999). *First Nations and Inuit regional health survey, national report.* Akwesasne Mohawk Territory, St. Regis, QC: Author.

35. Indian and Northern Affairs Canada. (2002). *Basic departmental data—2001.* Ottawa: First Nations and Northern Statistics Section, Information Management Directorate. Retrieved October 10, 2003, from http://www.ainc-inac.gc.ca/pr/sts/bdd01/bdd01_e.html

36. Federal/Territorial/Provincial Advisory Committee on Population Health. (1999). *Second report on the health of Canadians.* Ottawa: Author.

37. Canadian Pediatric Society. (2002). Fetal alcohol syndrome. Position statement (II 2002-01). *Pediatrics & Child Health, 7,* 161–174.

38. Assembly of First Nations. (1999). *Aboriginal and Inuit regional health surveys.* Ottawa: First Nations and Inuit Regional Health Surveys Steering Committee, Assembly of First Nations.

39. Adelson, N. (2004). *Reducing health disparities and promoting equity for Aboriginal populations in Canada: Synthesis paper.* Toronto: Department of Anthropology, York University.

40. Kornelsen, J., & Grzybowski, S. (2005). The costs of separation: The birth experiences of women in isolated and remote communities in British Columbia. *Canadian Women's Studies, 24*(1), 75–80.

41. McCulla, K. (2004). *A comparative review of community health representatives scope of practice in international indigenous communities.* Prepared for the National Indian and Inuit Community Health Representatives Organization, Kahnawake, Quebec. Retrieved September 5, 2005, from http://www.niichro.com/2004/pdf/international-chr-study.pdf

42. Dion-Stout, M., & Kipling, G. (1999). *Emerging priorities for health of First Nations and Inuit children and youth.* Ottawa: Program Policy Transfer

Secretariat and Planning Directorate, First Nations and Inuit Health Branch, Health Canada.

43. Royal Commission on Aboriginal People. (1996). *Highlights from the Report of the Royal Commission on Aboriginal Peoples—People to people, nation to nation.* Ottawa: Author. Retrieved July 21, 2003, from http://www.ainc-inac.gc.ca/ch/rcap/rpt/index_e.html

44. Smylie, J. (2000). A guide for health professionals working with Aboriginal peoples. Aboriginal health resources. *Journal of the Society of Obstetricians and Gynaecologists of Canada, 23,* 255–270.

45. Fletcher, C. (2002). Community-based participatory research relationships with Aboriginal communities in Canada: An overview of context and process. *Pimatziwin, 1*(1), 29–61.

46. Macaulay, A., Delormier, T., McComber, A., et al. (1998). Participatory research with native community of Kahnawake creates innovative code of research ethics. *Canadian Journal of Public Health, 89,* 105–108.

47. Anderson, J., Perry, J., Blue, C., et al. (2003). Rewriting cultural safety within the postcolonial and postnational feminist project toward new epistemologies of healing. *Advances in Nursing Science, 26,* 196–214.

48. Battiste, M. (Ed.). (2000). *Reclaiming indigenous voice and vision.* Vancouver: UBC Press.

49. Reimer-Kirkham, S., & Anderson, J. (2002). Postcolonial nursing scholarship: From epistemology to method. *Advances in Nursing Science, 25*(1), 1–17.

50. National Aboriginal Health Organization. (2003). *Ways of knowing: A framework for health research.* Ottawa: Author. Retrieved January 17, 2004, from http://www.naho.ca/english/pdf/research_waysof.pdf

51. Abelson, J. (2001). Understanding the role of contextual influences on local health-care decision making: Case study results from Ontario, Canada. *Social Science & Medicine, 53,* 777–793.

52. Burns, N., & Grove, S. (2005). *The practice of nursing research: Conduct, critique, and utilization.* St. Louis. MO: Elsevier/Saunders.

53. Jaggar, A. (1989). Love and knowledge: Emotion in feminist epistemology. In A. M. Jaggar & S. R. Bordo (Eds.), *Gender/body/knowledge: Feminist reconstructions of being and knowing* (pp. 145–171). New Brunswick, NJ: Rutgers University Press.

54. Kleinman, S., & Kopp, M. (1993). *Emotions and fieldwork—Qualitative research methods* (Vol. 28). Newbury Park, CA: Sage.

55. Fontana, J. (2004). A methodology for critical science in nursing. *Advances in Nursing Science, 27,* 93–101.

56. Erlandson, D., Harris, E., Skipper, B., & Allen, S. (2003). *Doing naturalistic inquiry: A guide to methods.* Newbury Park, CA: Sage.

57. Thorne, S., & Varcoe, C. (1998). The tyranny of feminist methodology in women's health research. *Health Care for Women International, 19,* 481–493.

58. Thorne, S., Reimer-Kirkham, S., & Flynn-Magee, K. (2004). The analytic challenge in interpretive description. *International Journal of Qualitative Methods, 3*(1), article 1. Retrieved April 10, 2004, from http://www.ualberta.ca/~iiqm/backissues/3_1/htm/thorneetal.html

59. Gardner, J., Baker, G., Norton, P., & Brown, A. (2002). *Governments and patient safety in Australia, the United Kingdom and the United States: A review of policies, institutional and funding frameworks, and current initiatives.* Prepared for the Advisory Committee on Health Services Working Group on Quality of Health Care Services. Retrieved June 4, 2005, from http://www.hc-sc.gc.ca/english/care/patient_safety.html#2_1

60. New South Wales Health. (2001). *A framework for managing the quality of health services in NSW.* Sydney, NSW, Australia: New South Wales Health.

61. The Canadian Patient Safety Initiative. (2003). *The Canadian patient safety dictionary* [online]. Retrieved July 10, 2005, from http://rcpsc.medical.org/publications/PatientSafetyDictionary_e.pdf

62. Storch, P. (2005). Patient safety: Is it just another bandwagon? *Canadian Journal of Nursing Leadership, 18*(2), 39–55.

63. Moffitt, P. (2004). Colonization: A health determinant for pregnant Dogrib women. *Journal of Transcultural Nursing, 15,* 323–330.

64. Browne, A. (2005). Discourses influencing nurses' perceptions of First Nations patients. *Canadian Journal of Nursing Research, 37*(4), 62–88.

65. Browne, A. (2001). First Nations women's encounters with mainstream health care services. *Western Journal of Nursing Research, 23,* 126–147.

66. Wood, P., & Schwass, M. (1993). Cultural safety: A framework for changing attitudes. *Nursing Praxis in New Zealand, 8*(1), 4–15.

67. Nursing Council of New Zealand. (2005). *Nursing Council of New Zealand 2005 Guidelines for Cultural Safety, the Treaty of Waitangi and Maori Health in Nursing Education and Practice.* Wellington, New Zealand: Author. Retrieved from June 19, 2005, http://www.nursingcouncil.org.nz/Cultural%20Safety.pdf

68. Applebaum, B. (1997). Good liberal intentions are not enough! Racism, intentions and moral responsibility. *Journal of Moral Education, 26,* 409–411.

69. Applebaum, B. (2005). In the name of morality: Moral responsibility, whiteness and social justice education. *Journal of Moral Education, 34,* 277–290.

APPENDIX C

From *Canadian Journal of Nursing Research*, 2006;38(1):58–80. © McGill University School of Nursing.

Relationship among Employment Status, Stressful Life Events, and Depression in Single Mothers

Joan Samuels-Dennis, RN, PhD (c)
School of Nursing, University of Western Ontario
London, Ontario

KEYWORDS

determinants of health
depression
stress
single mothers
welfare

The purpose of this study was to extend our understanding of employment status as a social determinant of psychological distress among single mothers. A cross-sectional survey assessing stressful life events and depression was completed with 96 single mothers (48 employed and 48 social assistance [SA] recipients) between November 2003 and March 2004. The prevalence of depressive symptoms was significantly higher for the SA recipients. Mild, moderate, and severe depressive symptoms were reported by 2%, 23%, and 67%, respectively, of SA recipients. Total stressful events were markedly greater for SA recipients. In addition, SA recipients reported larger numbers of housing, health, social, and financial stressors. Regression analysis indicated that 40.6% of the variation in depressive symptoms among single mothers was explained by their employment status and stressful events. The findings suggest that women's employment status significantly impacts on their psychological well-being. Implications for nursing practice, policy development, and future research are identified and discussed.

INTRODUCTION

Among the many social and economic factors that influence and shape the health of Canadians, income has been identified as the single most important determinant of health (Raphael, 2004). For the 12.7% of Canadian families headed by single mothers (Statistics Canada, 2001), poverty is a particular challenge to psychological well-being (Avison, 2002). Single mothers, when compared to the general population, have almost double the 12-month prevalence rates of depression (15.4% vs. 7.9–8.6%) (Cairney, Thorpe, Rietschlin, & Avison, 1999).

Single mothers receiving social assistance (SA) are at particularly high risk for psychological distress because of established relationships between mental illness and family structure (Avison, 2002), poverty (Belle, 1990; Bryne & Brown, 1998; Gyamfi, Brooks-Gunn, & Jackson, 2001), and life adversities (Davies, Avison, & MacAlpine, 1997; Ford-Gilhoe, Berman, Laschinger, & Laforet-Fliesser, 2000; Tolman & Rosen, 2001). The chronic strains that accompany single motherhood, including economic hardship, parental stress, and role strain, have been credited with much of the responsibility for the disproportionate burden of mental illness experienced by this population (Avison).

Having identified single-parent families as vulnerable to increased risk for poor health, the National Children's Agenda has, over the past three decades, launched national and provincial health promotion programs (i.e., Healthy Babies Healthy Children, Ontario Early Years Initiatives, and Community Action for Children) directed at improving the health status of at-risk families with children under 6 years of age (Ministry of Health and Long-Term Care, 2002; National Children's Agenda, 2005). Historically, nursing interventions offered by such programs have focused on enhancing the social competencies or personal resilience of single parents and have often failed to address the socio-economic factors that contribute to the heightened risk for health disparities among single-parent families.

This article highlights the findings of an exploratory study examining the influence of the socio-economic context of single mothers' lives on their psychological well-being. A premise of the study was that family structure alone is not a risk factor for poor health. It is acknowledged, however, that single mothers are a heterogeneous group with significant differences in level of education, employment and socio-economic status, access to resources, and life experiences (Ford-Gilhoe et al., 2000). Given that these differences may affect one's vulnerability to psychological distress, it is essential for the development of group-specific nursing interventions that nurse researchers identify those subgroups of single mothers in which mental health disparities are most pronounced.

LITERATURE REVIEW

The Stress Process Model (Pearlin, 1989, 1999, 2002) provided the theoretical framework for the study. According to this model, stress is a dynamic and evolving process that incorporates three core elements: stressors, stress moderators, and stress outcomes.

Stressors

In general, stressors are tension-producing stimuli or forces — problems, hardships, or threats — whose reduced impact requires the mobilization of cognitive and behavioural efforts (Pearlin, 1999, 2002; Wheaton, 1999). Pearlin (1999, 2002) and Wheaton identify three primary categories of social stressor: life events, chronic stressors, and trauma. Life events are significant life changes that are discrete and observable, have a relatively clear onset, and have a well-defined set of sub-events that progress from stressor initiation to stressor termination. In contrast to life events, chronic stressors or strains arise insidiously and may either surface repeatedly or maintain a presence over a considerable period of time. Chronic stressors represent the enduring problems, conflicts, and threats that individuals face in their daily lives and that may arise from systems of inequality such as class, institutionalized social roles, social networks, neighbourhoods and communities, or households (Pearlin, 1999, 2002; Wheaton). Traumatic events are typically more severe than normal stressful events; they occur both as isolated events and as long-term chronic events, and, because of their level of severity, their impact is long-lasting (Pearlin, 1999, 2002; Wheaton). Traumas include a potentially wide range of severe situations and events, including war, natural disasters, sexual abuse during childhood or adulthood, and physical violence and abuse.

A key feature of the Stress Process Model is what Pearlin (2002) calls *stress proliferation*. This refers to the human reality that individuals are frequently exposed to multiple stressors that may negatively impact on their well-being (Pearlin, 2002). According to the Stress Process Model, exposure to one set of stressors eventually leads to other stressors (Pearlin, 2002). Job loss, for example, is a precursor to chronic financial strain, which increases single mothers' risk for insufficient food, housing insecurity, and psychological distress or depression.

In addition to socio-economic disadvantages, a wide range of life adversities in both early and adult life have been identified as significant contributors to higher rates of psychological distress among single mothers (Avison, 2002; Davies et al., 1997; Ford-Gilboe et al., 2000). McLanahan (1983) examined the relationship between family headship (single-mother and two-parent families) and three types of stressor: chronic life strains (demographic characteristics — race, income, age); major life strains (events that lead to a disruption of social networks or life patterns); and the absence of social and psychological support. That study revealed that single-mother families were more likely than other families to experience chronic strains commonly associated with poverty, being black, and being less educated. Income change, change in household composition, and residence change were identified as the major life events most frequently experienced by single mothers. In other studies (Scarini, Ames, & Brantley, 1999; Wagner & Menke, 1991) with low-income single mothers, the most common stressful life events reported were related to

intra-family strains, finance, work-family transitions, health status of individuals and family, and change in social activities.

An important life adversity endemic to single-parent families, particularly those receiving SA, is intimate partner violence (IPV). Tolman and Rosen (2001) used data from a random sample of women from welfare caseloads in Michigan County, in the United States, to investigate the prevalence of domestic violence and its association with mental health, physical health, and economic well-being. They found 12-month and lifetime prevalence rates of IPV to be 25% and 62.8%, respectively. Ford-Gilboe et al. (2000), in a community sample of 236 mothers, found that 86%, 78%, 65%, and 52% had experienced emotional, verbal, physical, and sexual abuse, respectively, during their lifetime. Compared to women who had never experienced intimate partner abuse, recent victims had markedly higher rates of five psychiatric disorders: depression, generalized anxiety disorder, post-traumatic stress disorder, drug dependence, and alcohol dependence (Tolman & Rosen). In addition, chronic strains most frequently reported by IPV survivors include financial strain, homelessness, eviction, discontinuation of utility services, food insufficiencies, physical and mental illness, and harassment (Campbell, 2002; Ford-Gilboe et al.; Tolman & Rosen).

Stress Moderators

Early research relevant to stressful life events was based on the assumption that all life events (positive or negative) are potentially stressful, with the degree of stressfulness varying with the magnitude of readjustment required by the specific event (Holmes & Rahe, 1967). Research has since revealed that stressor impact (beneficial or detrimental) is determined by five factors: the time-frame in which the stressor occurs, the past and present mental and physical health status of the individual, the nature and intensity of the stressor, the amount of energy required by the individual to adjust, and, most important, the moderating resources available to the individual (Davies et al., 1997; Pearlin, 2002; Wheaton, 1999).

Moderators, including the individual's coping repertoire, level of social support, and mastery (sense of control over one's life), represent the social and personal resources that individuals and families mobilize to contain, regulate, or otherwise ameliorate the effects of stressors (Pearlin, 2002). Moderating resources help us to understand why individuals exposed to the same stressors experience an array of different outcomes. Moderators serve a protective function that can be exercised in three ways: by acting proactively to preclude or prevent the occurrence of a stressor, by modifying or minimizing the harmful impact of stressful conditions, and by perceptually controlling the meaning of the stressor in ways that reduce their threat and potential painful consequences. From the few studies that have examined the coping repertoire of single mothers, it is evident that this population uses an array of strategies to manage chronic and traumatic stress, including active and passive strategies such as obtaining social support, seeking spiritual guidance, engaging in active problem-solving, and using passive appraisal or avoidant coping (Felsten, 1998; Hall, Gurley, Sachs, & Kryscio, 1991; Wagner & Menke, 1991). For further exploration of coping as a moderator of stress, see Pearlin (1989, 1999, 2002) and Pearlin and Johnson (1977).

Stressor Outcomes

The final major component of the Stress Process Model is the outcome (Pearlin, 2002). Outcome refers to physiological and psychological manifestations of "organismic" stress (Pearlin, 1989). Studies looking at stress and health outcomes among single mothers often compare single-parent families with two-parent families and have consistently documented greater psychological distress among separated and divorced parents than among two-parent families (Avison, 2002; Cairney et al., 1999; Davies et al., 1997; Lipman, Offord, & Boyle, 1997). The authors of these studies suggest that dissolution of a marital or common-law relationship is often accompanied by increased levels of stress or chronic strain (for example, economic hardship, parenting difficulties, and child-care demands) that continue long after the divorce or separation and, consequently, increase single mothers' risk of experiencing psychological distress or depression (Avison). Consistent with the Stress Process Model, much of this work has purposely attempted to uncover the ways in which single mothers' response to stress differs not only by family structure but also by social and economic status (Pearlin, 1999, 2002). Pearlin (1999, 2002) proposes that the stress process occurs within a social context whereby life events and/or chronic strains largely arise from, and are influenced by, social structures and people's location within them. Finding its roots in critical social theory, the model suggests that systemic embodiment of unequal distribution of resources and opportunities inevitably results in stressful conditions for those with the lowest status (Pearlin, 1999, 2002).

Researchers examining the association between childhood adversity and mental health suggest that childhood maltreatment (physical, emotional, and sexual abuse) creates early vulnerability to psychiatric difficulties that is activated by periods of interpersonal stress in later life (Davies et al., 1997; Lipman et al., 1997). Davies et al. used data from a case-comparison longitudinal survey of single and married mothers in London, Ontario, to examine the relationship between early-life adversities, depressive episodes, and family structure. Higher rates of depression among single mothers were related to greater exposure to stressors (i.e., low maternal attachment, parental depression, parental substance abuse, and child abuse/neglect) in the woman's family of origin that, in turn, increased the likelihood of early-onset depression and subsequent depressive episodes.

The association between poverty and psychological distress among single mothers is well documented (Avison, 2002; Bryne & Brown, 1998; Gyamfi et al., 2001; Lennon, Blome, & English, 2001). Among single mothers with the lowest incomes, the 12-month prevalence rate of major depressive disorder ranges from 12% to 36% (Lennon et al.). Bryne and Brown's assessment of depression levels among single mothers receiving SA revealed that 32.5%, 10.4%, and 2.5% reported symptoms consistent with major depression, dysthmia (moderate chronic depression), and double depression (major depression and dysthmia), respectively.

Employment, regardless of income, offers some protection against depressive episodes (Belle, 1990). Hall, Williams, and Greenberg (1985) examined the relationship between social support, everyday stressors, and mental health in a sample of low-income single mothers. They report that mothers who had extremely low incomes or were unemployed were more likely to report severe depressive symptoms (48%). More recently, Gyamfi et al. (2001) investigated the association between financial strain and maternal depressive affect among single mothers who were formerly ($n = 95$) and currently ($n = 95$) receiving SA. Employed mothers reported fewer symptoms of depression and stress than non-employed mothers. However, for those women transitioning from welfare to work, being employed did not reduce financial strain. The authors suggest that the lack of change in financial strain reflects the fact that a majority of single mothers transitioned from welfare to low-paying jobs without benefits. They also note that while employed mothers continued to experience financial strain, the strain no longer affected the level of depression. Among the unemployed, however, financial strain was positively correlated with depression. The authors surmise that employment and a resultant increase in levels of perceived self-efficacy may mediate depressive symptoms.

Low-income women are the target of many social programs, ranging from welfare and workfare programs to interventions designed to prevent problems in pregnancy and to enhance maternal competence. While research has identified factors that may cause psychological distress in single mothers, few studies have specifically examined variations in stressful events and psychological distress among single mothers caused by differences in employment status or access to income. A greater understanding of the factors that contribute to health disparities among subgroups of single mothers is essential for the development of effective public health nursing interventions.

PURPOSE AND HYPOTHESES

The purpose of this study was to assess the association between employment status or access to income, stressful life events, and depression among single mothers. Three hypotheses were formulated: Hypothesis 1: *SA recipients will report greater stressful events than employed single mothers.* Hypothesis 2: *SA recipients will report greater depressive symptoms than employed single mothers.* Hypothesis 3: *Employment status and stressful events will predict depression among single mothers.*

METHOD

Design

This cross-sectional, descriptive correlational study used survey data to assess predictors of depression in two groups of single mothers, those employed and those receiving SA, as part of a larger study examining the association between employment status, stressful events, coping repertoire, and psychological distress (Samuels-Dennis, 2004).

Participants

A convenience sample of 96 single mothers (48 employed and 48 receiving SA) was recruited from community agencies in a large city in the Canadian province of Ontario. Power analysis determined that a sample of 91 single mothers was needed based on $\alpha = .05$, multiple regression with five independent variables, and a medium effect size (Cohen, 1992). Women were asked to participate in the study if they met the following criteria: (a) 18 years or older; (b) self-identified as a separate, divorced, widowed, or never-married woman who was the primary caregiver of at least one child 4 to 18 years old; (c) employed or receiving SA; and (d) fluent in English.

Women were recruited using: (a) contacts in health and social agencies that provide services to single mothers and their children; (b) a list of active SA recipients generated by Ontario Works, the provincial welfare provider; and (c) referral of other single mothers by the study participants. Twenty-one potential Ontario Works participants could not be reached because of cancelled telephone service. Of the 74 SA recipients contacted, 70 agreed to participate and 48 returned completed questionnaires, for a response rate of 68%. Of the 75 employed single mothers contacted, 73 agreed to participate and 48 returned completed questionnaires, for a response rate of 65.8%. The combined response rate across the two groups was 67%.

Instruments

Exposure to stressful life events was captured using the Social Readjustment Rating Scale (SRRS) (Holmes & Rahe, 1967). The SRRS was developed to identify the incidence of recent life changes and to measure the intensity of anticipated readjustment to 43 specific life events. It is a short survey in checklist form that assesses participant exposure to stressors such as divorce, physical illness, and financial difficulties. Life Change Units (LCUs), assigned to the various life events, allow researchers to determine the cumulative amount of stress an individual has experienced over a 24-month period. The SRRS was adapted to assess single mothers' exposure to chronic strains, daily hassles, and traumatic stressors. The LCU component of the scale was excluded and eight stressors relevant to woman abuse, mental illness, and homelessness that were not previously captured using the SRRS were added to the checklist. Single mothers were asked to indicate if they had encountered specific events in the past 24 months by checking the appropriate box. The total number of life events experienced was computed by summing the number of checked boxes. Possible scores ranged from 0 to 51, with higher scores indicating more stressful events. Face validity of the revised SRRS was determined by a panel of three experts. Test-retest scores for the unaltered SRRS range from .72 to .91 and internal consistency ranges from .59 to .83 (Holmes & Rahe). In this study, Cronbach's alpha reliability coefficient was .69.

The BDI-II is a self-report instrument designed to measure the severity of depression in adults and adolescents aged 13 years and older (Beck, Brown, & Steer, 1996). It contains 21 items and was developed to assess symptoms corresponding to the criteria for diagnosing depressive disorders listed in the American Psychiatric Association's *Diagnostic and Statistical Manual of Mental Disorders, 4th edition* (DSM-IV) (Beck et al.). Participants were asked to indicate the extent to which they had experienced each symptom on a four-point Likert scale (0 = I do not feel sad; 3 = I am so sad or unhappy that I can't stand it). A total score is computed by summing the ratings of all 21 items and reflects the following clinical interpretation: 0 to 13, minimal depression (representing normal ups and downs of everyday living); 14 to 19, mild depression; 20 to 28, moderate depression; 29 to 63, severe depression (Beck et al.). Internal consistency and 1-week test-retest values range from .92 to .93. In the present study, Cronbach's alpha reliability coefficient was .93.

Data Collection

After ethical approval had been obtained, a questionnaire was delivered or mailed to the homes of women who had consented to participate. No incentives were offered for participation in the study. A return envelope with prepaid postage was included with each questionnaire. Participants completed and returned the questionnaire by mail. Follow-up phone calls were made to those single mothers who had not returned the questionnaire after 3 months.

Data Analysis

Data were analyzed using SPSS Version 12. Descriptive statistics appropriate to the level of measurement were generated for all study variables. *T* tests were used to test hypotheses 1 and 2, while multiple regression analysis was used to examine the extent to which employment status and stressful life events contributed to variations in depressive symptoms among the single mothers. The significance level for all analyses was $\alpha = .05$.

RESULTS AND DISCUSSION

Demographic comparisons between employed mothers and mothers receiving SA are presented in Table C-1. Comparative analysis revealed that the two groups were similar in age ($\bar{x}_E = 38.60$, $SD = 7.203$, $\bar{x}_{SA} = 40.0$, $SD = 6.425$, $t = -.990$, $p = .325$). However, SA recipients had a significantly larger number of children currently in their care ($\bar{x}_E = 1.92$, $SD = .942$, $\bar{x}_{SA} = 2.42$, $SD = 1.048$, $t = -2.458$, $p = .016$). Chi-square analysis indicated marked differences in racial makeup of the groups ($\chi^2 = 19.337$, $p = .001$) and the highest level of education reached ($\chi^2 = 26.736$, $p = .001$).

Hypothesis 1

The first hypothesis was that SA recipients would report more stressful events than their employed counterparts. As predicted, SA recipients encountered a larger number of stressful life events than employed mothers ($X_E = 6.94$, $X_{SA} = 8.81$, $t = -2.233$, $p = 0.28$: see Table C-2). Financial strain was more pronounced among SA recipients (50% vs. 18.8%), as this group reported that their financial status was much worse than usual, experienced greater difficulty paying their rent or mortgage (56.3% vs. 16.7%), and were more frequently evicted from their homes (8.3% vs. 0%). Employed

TABLE C-1 Sociodemographic Characteristics of Single Mothers, by Employment Status

	Employment (n = 48)		Social Assistance (n = 48)	
	n	%	*n*	%
Race				
Caucasian	14	29.2	21	43.8
Afro-Canadian	27	56.3	11	22.9
Native	1	2.1	1	2.1
South Asian	1	2.1	9	18.8
Asian	4	8.3	1	2.1
Latino	1	2.1	3	6.3
Arabic	0	0.0	1	2.1
Other	0	0.0	1	2.1
Number of Children				
1	18	37.5	9	18.8
2	20	41.7	19	39.6
3	7	14.6	13	27.1
4	2	4.2	5	10.4
5 or more	1	2.1	2	4.2
Annual Income				
$0–19,999	4	8.5	47	97.9
$20,000–39,999	23	48.9	1	2.1
$40,000–59,999	10	21.3	0	0.0
$60,000–79,999	9	19.1	0	0.0
$80,000 and above	1	2.1	0	0.0
Marital Status				
Single	22	45.8	20	41.7
Separated	14	29.2	7	14.6
Divorced	12	25.0	19	39.6
Widowed	0	0.0	2	4.2
Level of Education				
Grade school	0	0.0	5	10.4
High school	9	18.8	27	56.3
College/university	27	56.3	15	31.3
Graduate/professional	12	25.0	1	2.1

TABLE C-2 Comparison of Stressful Events According to Employment Status						
	Employment (n = 48)			Social Assistance (n = 48)		
Stressful Event	%	$\bar{x}$	SD	%	$\bar{x}$	SD	t
Started/changed school	14.6	.15	.357	20.8	.21	.410	-0.796
Graduated from school	22.9	.23	.425	12.5	.13	.334	1.335
Problems in school	4.2	.04	.202	8.3	.08	.279	-0.838
Failed school	2.1	.02	.144	0	.00	.000	1.000
Got married	2.1	.02	.144	0	.00	.000	1.000
Marital separation	12.5	.13	.334	8.3	.08	.279	0.663
Divorce	10.4	.10	.309	14.6	.15	.357	-0.612
Reconciled relationship	10.4	.10	.309	6.3	.06	.245	0.733
Increased arguments with partner	20.8	.21	.410	8.3	.08	.279	1.744
Improved relations with partner	10.4	.10	.309	8.3	.08	.279	0.347
Emotionally abused by partner	20.8	.21	.410	22.9	.23	.425	-0.244
Physically abused by partner	2.1	.02	.144	4.2	.04	.202	-0.581
Sexually abused by partner	0	.00	.000	2.1	.02	.144	-1.000
Change in residence	41.7	.42	.498	39.6	.40	.494	0.206
Repeated difficulty paying rent or mortgage	16.7	.17	.377	56.3	.58	.539	-4.374*
Eviction from home	0	.00	.000	8.3	.08	.279	-2.067*
Mortgage or loan for a major purchase	31.3	.31	.468	0	.00	.000	4.622*
Foreclosure of mortgage or loan	0	.00	.000	0	.00	.000	–
Pregnancy	8.3	.08	.279	8.3	.08	.279	0.000
Abortion	2.1	.02	.144	8.3	.46	.504	-1.377
Gained new family member	6.3	.31	.468	2.1	.02	.144	1.016
Son or daughter left home	6.3	.06	.245	22.9	.23	.425	-2.356*
Change in amount of contact with family members	31.3	.06	.245	45.8	.08	.279	-1.469*
Trouble with in-laws	14.6	.46	.504	4.2	.65	.483	1.761
Change in amount and type of recreation	45.8	.15	.357	64.6	.04	.202	-1.861
Change in church activities	33.3	.33	.476	54.2	.54	.504	-2.082*
Change in social activities	47.9	.48	.505	68.8	.69	.468	-2.096*
Physical or mental illness	22.9	.23	.425	79.2	.79	.410	-6.598*
Personal injury or accident	8.3	.08	.279	25.0	.25	.438	-2.224*
Death of a close friend	8.3	.08	.279	14.6	.15	.357	-0.956
Death of a close family member	20.8	.27	.676	31.3	.38	.703	-1.159
Death of a pet	2.1	.02	.144	10.4	.10	.309	-1.694
Change in health of family member	20.8	.21	.410	20.8	.21	.410	0.000
Frequent minor illness	31.3	.31	.468	54.2	.54	.504	-2.309*
Minor violation of the law	6.3	.06	.245	6.3	.06	.245	0.000
Jail time served	0	.00	.000	0	.00	.000	–
Loss, robbery, or damage of personal property	10.4	.10	.309	20.8	.21	.410	-1.405
Vacation	39.6	.40	.494	6.3	.06	.245	4.188
Spouse started/stopped work	4.2	.04	.202	0	.00	.000	1.430
Started work for the first time	14.6	.15	.357	22.9	.23	.425	-1.041
Promotion	8.3	.08	.279	4.2	.04	.202	0.838
Demotion	0	.00	.000	0	.00	.000	–
Laid off from work	10.4	.10	.309	14.6	.15	.357	-0.612
Fired from work	2.1	.02	.144	6.3	.06	.245	-1.016
Trouble with boss or co-workers	18.8	.19	.394	6.3	8.81	3.595	1.866
Major improvement in financial status	20.8	.21	.410	0	.00	.000	3.517*
Financial status a lot worse than usual	18.8	.19	.394	50.0	.50	.505	-3.378*
Total Stressors	–	6.94	4.573	–	8.81	3.595	-2.233*

*p < .05; t value not calculated due to non-occurrence.

mothers reported significantly greater improvements in their financial status (20.8% vs. 0%) and a greater amount of the financial stability required to obtain a loan for a major purchase such as a car or mortgage (33.3% vs. 0%).

The results prove the hypothesis that employment does offer protection against poor health. SA recipients reported significantly greater health problems (physical, mental, and social). In the 2 years prior to completion of the questionnaire, 79.2% of SA recipients, compared to 22.9% of employed mothers, experienced a serious physical or mental illness; in addition, they reported a considerably larger number of personal injuries or accidents (25.0% vs. 8.3%) and more frequent minor illnesses (54.2% vs 31.3%).

Social interaction evident in changes to church and social activities was significantly greater among SA recipients (54.2% vs. 33.3% and 68.8% vs. 47.9%, respectively). In addition, change in family composition (a son or daughter leaving home) was reported more frequently by SA recipients (22.9% vs. 6.3%). These results speak not only to the limited amount of social interaction available to single mothers receiving SA, but also to the poor quality of social interaction and the social exclusion that is endemic to this population (Nezlek, Hampton, & Shean, 2000; Raphael, 2004).

Hypothesis 2

The second hypothesis was that single mothers receiving SA experience higher levels of depressive symptoms than employed single mothers. SA recipients were found to experience significantly higher levels of depressive symptoms than their employed counterparts ($t = -7.634$, $p < .000$). Mean BDI-II scores for the employed and SA groups were 13.85 ($SD = 9.694$) and 30.79 ($SD = 11.907$), respectively. This finding is alarming when compared to Bryne and Brown's (1998) finding of 32.5% of SA recipients experiencing major depression and 10.4% moderate depression. As expected, a disproportionate burden of illness is carried by SA recipients. Among SA recipients, 66.7% and 22.9% reported symptoms

consistent with severe and moderate depression, respectively, while for the employed group the figures were 14.6% and 25.0%. In a broader context, employed mothers experienced depression at twice the rate for the general population, while SA recipients experienced depression at 11 times the rate for the general population (Health Canada, 2002).

Hypothesis 3

Hierarchical multiple regression analysis was used to examine the extent to which employment status and stressful events predict depression among single mothers (Table C-3). Prior to analysis, employment status was dummy coded in the following way: 1 = employed full time or part time; 2 = SA. Demographic variables, including employment status, age, and number of children, were entered at step 1 of the analysis, while the number of stressful events was entered at step 2. At step 1, mother's age, number of children, and employment status predicted 37.7% of the variance in mother's depression [$F (3.89) = 17.951$, $p = .000$]. At step 2, the addition of stressful events contributed an additional 2.9% to the explained variance of depressive symptoms, and this change was significant [$F (4.88) = 4.290$, $p = .041$]. The final model (age, number of children, employment status, and stressful events) explained 40.6% of the variance in depressive symptoms, with employment status being the primary contributor ($\beta = .591$, $p = .000$).

There are two explanations for the patterned association between socio-economic status (SES) and mental illness (Yu & Williams, 1999). The social-selection hypothesis suggests that mental illness keeps individuals from obtaining or retaining jobs that would preserve their SES status or enhance their social mobility. Within this perspective, it may be argued that the presence of mental illness, perhaps in childhood or early adolescence, leads to lower socio-economic status by interfering with the single mother's ability to advance her education or acquire appropriate job skills (see Gyamfi et al., 2001). In contrast, the social-causation hypothesis argues that socio-economic adversities linked

Step	R	R Square	Adjusted R Square	Standard Error of the Estimate
TABLE C-3 Predictors of Depression among Single Mothers			
1	.614[a]	.377	.356	10.831
2	.637[b]	.406	.379	10.636

Final variables in the equation

Steps		Standardized Coefficients			Correlations	
		Beta	t	Sig.	Partial	Part
1	Age	-.043	-.514	.608	-.054	-.043
	Number of children	-.112	-1.292	.200	-.136	-.108
	Employment status	.637	7.309	.000	.612	.611
2	Age	-.014	-.166	.868	-.018	-.014
	Number of children	-.100	-1.166	.247	-.123	-.096
	Employment status	.591	6.687	.000	.580	.549
	Total stressful life events	.178	2.071	.041	.216	.170

Tolerance = .919.
[a] Predictors: employment status, age, number of children.
[b] Predictors: employment status, age, number of children, total stressful life events.

to low-SES positions cause or exacerbate mental health problems among single mothers (Yu & Williams). The Stress Process Model represents a social-causation hypothesis, and the findings of this study illustrate that single mothers in the lowest socio-economic positions do indeed experience higher rates of psychological distress and functional impairment. While employment or access to income does not explain single mothers' depression entirely, the socio-economic context of women's lives accounts for a considerable portion of single mothers' psychological well-being; 98% of SA recipients, compared to 8.5% of employed mothers, had incomes below $20,000, a finding that has fundamental implications for access to the social and material resources (e.g., food, shelter, transportation, and social activities) needed to promote one's health (Raphael, 2004).

DISCUSSION AND IMPLICATIONS

The purpose of this study was to examine the factors that contribute to health disparities among subgroups of single mothers. Specifically, the study explored the association between employment status, stressful experiences, and depressive symptoms. The findings present us with some significant health promotion challenges and opportunities. Health promotion represents a comprehensive social and

political process that embraces not only actions directed at strengthening the skills and capabilities of individuals, but also actions directed at changing social, environmental, and economic conditions so as to reduce their negative impact on individual health (World Health Organization, 1986). The findings of this study present a number of health promotion challenges and opportunities for both SA programs such as Ontario Works and public health nursing. They suggest that, first, workfare programs intended to address the mental health concerns of single mothers could achieve greater success in ensuring the mothers' ability to obtain and sustain employment; second, the prevalence and severity of depression among single mothers indicate the need for reorientation of health services towards a multidisciplinary approach to mental health promotion; and third, the need to ensure that the basic necessity of single-parent families for food and secure housing is met through the development of healthy public policies.

In recent years, federal and provincial governments in Canada have invested extensive resources in the reform of SA and welfare programs. Ontario Works currently provides temporary financial assistance to those individuals who are determined to be most in need while they satisfy obligations to find and retain employment (Ministry of Community and Social Services, 2001). Implicit to welfare reform is the assumption that SA recipients are similar, in status and function, to the general population. However, the findings of this study suggest that mental health concerns pose a strong barrier to employment. Ecologically sound workfare strategies are needed to address the many factors that affect women's employment status, including physical and mental illness and lack of employment training, child care, and social support (Youngblut, Brady, Brooten, & Thomas, 2000). When the Bough Breaks (Browne et al., 2001) is one ecologically sound intervention program that has proved effective in reducing levels of dysthmia, enhancing social adjustment, and increasing single mothers' success in obtaining and sustaining employment. It speaks to the social and economic feasibility of providing single mothers receiving SA with services such as health promotion and case management, recreation and skill development for children, employment retraining, and child care.

The pervasive functional impairments that accompany depression require a multidisciplinary approach whereby mental health professionals (i.e., nurses, general practitioners, psychologists, psychiatrists, and lay practitioners) use a number of strategies to enhance the social functioning, coping capacity, and health promoting behaviours of single mothers. The findings of this study suggest that single mothers who experience psychological distress would be most effectively served by health and service providers who use an array of mental health promotion strategies appropriate to the multiple problems that single mothers may experience over their lifetime — for example, IPV, homelessness, and economic hardship. Nurses with advanced knowledge and understanding of mental illness, including its assessment, diagnosis, and management, have an essential role to play in helping single mothers to manage and overcome psychological distress. An intervention study conducted by Beeber, Holditch-Davis, Belyea, and Funk (2004) demonstrated the feasibility of master's-prepared nurses positively impacting on not only single mothers' mental health status but also their success in managing depressive symptoms, improving

problematic life issues, accessing social support, and parenting effectively while symptomatic. It is important to note, however, that enhanced expertise must be accompanied by a conscious and systematic effort to understand the context and culture of single mothers' lives. Likewise, nursing interventions for single mothers must be innovative and tailored to their personal needs and life goals (Beeber et al.; Cauce et al., 2000).

Public health nurses are ideally positioned to influence the development of public policies designed to reduce chronic and daily stressors that may exacerbate psychological distress among single mothers. The findings of this study suggest that housing insecurity is an important stressor for single mothers, particularly those receiving SA. Adequate living allowance and rent geared to income programs would significantly reduce this problem. While the average rent for a two-bedroom apartment in Ontario is $1,165, a single mother with two children currently receives SA of $1,215 monthly (Canadian Council on Social Development, 2003). The socio-economic conditions under which single mothers live increase their risk for homelessness. Risk for homelessness and its negative impact on the psychological well-being of single mothers cannot be underestimated (Bogard, Trillo, Schwartz, & Gerstel, 2001). Bassuk, Browne, and Bucker (1996) identify three factors that greatly affect the ability of a poor single mother to retain housing: lack of education ensures that single mothers have the lowest-paying jobs and will likely live below the poverty line even when employed full time; frequently, one quarter of a single mother's monthly income goes to child care; and pervasive physical, emotional, and sexual violence, in both childhood and adulthood, decreases single mothers' physical, emotional, and social well-being and, in turn, their ability to work outside the home. As posited by the Stress Process Model, the present findings suggest that the health of single mothers is determined by the structural social inequality that predominates in Canadian society (Avison, 2002; Davies et al., 1997; Pearlin, 1989; Tolman & Rosen, 2001). The involvement of public health nurses in developing public policies designed to address the structural inequalities that impede single mothers' access to food and secure housing is essential to promoting the mental health of those mothers.

This study has several limitations. The cultural diversity of the sample (Caucasian 36.8%, Afro-Canadian 40%, Aboriginal 1.1%, South Asian 10.5%, Asian 5.3%, Latino 4.2%, Arabic 1.1%) may limit the generalization of its findings to less culturally diverse populations. Second, a substantial number of women ($N = 21$) who were eligible for participation in the study were not included because their telephones had been disconnected. This group might have presented data different from those presented by women who were able to maintain their telephone subscriptions and consequently participated in the study. Third, the modified SRRS was not pretested and was by no means exhaustive of the types of stressor frequently encountered by single mothers. Fourth, the small sample size precluded an examination of whether depressive symptoms were similar for those single mothers who were employed but whose incomes resembled those of SA recipients. A larger sample, including single mothers from three socio-economic groups — those employed with middle and high incomes, those employed with low incomes, and those receiving SA — would allow researchers to examine this issue more thoroughly. Additionally, comparable studies may employ a qualitative or mixed-method (quantitative and qualitative) approach to exploring the incidence of stressful events not captured by the SRRS, as well as the perceived positive or negative impact of those stressors. Another essential area for further investigation is the prevalence of comorbid conditions — more than one mental illness such as post-traumatic stress disorder, anxiety disorders, and bipolar disorders — and its impact on employment status.

CONCLUSION

This study used the Stress Process Model to examine trajectories of depression among single mothers in the context of socio-economic status.

Analyses of variations in patterns of stressful events and depression by employment status (employment or SA) revealed that single mothers receiving SA reported a larger number of stressful events specific to housing instability, social isolation, family composition, physical and mental illness, and financial instability than employed single mothers. The prevalence of depressive symptoms in this sample of single mothers was extremely high, with more than 65% of participants reporting symptoms consistent with moderate or severe depression. However, much of the burden of illness fell on participants with the lowest socio-economic status. Fifteen percent of employed parents reported symptoms consistent with severe depression, compared to 67% of SA recipients. Results of multiple regression analysis revealed that 41.5% of the variation in depressive symptoms among single mothers was explained by employment status and stressful events, with employment status contributing most of the variance.

REFERENCES

Avison, W. R. (2002). Family structure and mental health. In A. Maney & J. Ramos (Eds.), *Socioeconomic conditions, stress and mental disorders: Toward a new synthesis of research and public policy* (pp. 1–38). Bethesda, MD: NIH Office of Behavioral and Social Research.

Bassuk, E., Browne, A., & Bucker, J. C. (1996). Single mothers and welfare. *Scientific American, 275*(4), 60–67.

Beck, A. T., Brown, G. K., & Steer, R. A. (1996). *BDI-II, Beck Depression Inventory: Manual* (2nd ed.). San Antonio,TX: Psychological Corporation.

Beeber, L. S., Holditch-Davis, D., Belyea, M. J., & Funk, S. G. (2004). In-home intervention for depressive symptoms with low-income mothers of infants and toddlers in the United States. *Health Care for Women International, 25,* 561–580.

Belle, D. (1990). Poverty and women's mental health. *American Psychologist, 45,* 385–389.

Bogard, C. J., Trillo, A., Schwartz, M., & Gerstel, N. (2001). Future employment among homeless single mothers: The effects of full-time work experience and depressive symptomatology. *Welfare Work and Well-Being, 32*(1/2), 137–157.

Browne, G., Bryne, C., Roberts, J., Gafni, A., Watt, S., Ewart, B., et al. (1998, June). *When the Bough Breaks: Provider-initiated comprehensive care is more effective and less expensive for sole-support parents on social assistance.*

Hamilton, ON: Ontario Ministry of Health. Retrieved December 1, 2004, from http://www.fhs.mcmaster.ca/slru/paper/GWA4yrf.pdf

Bryne, C., & Browne, G. (1998). Surviving social assistance: 12-month prevalence of depression in sole-support parents receiving social assistance. *Canadian Medical Association Journal, 158*, 881–894.

Cairney, J., Thorpe, C., Rietschlin, J., & Avison, W. R. (1999). 12-month prevalence of depression among single and married mothers in the 1994 National Population Health Survey. *Canadian Journal of Public Health, 90*, 320–324.

Campbell, J. (2002). Health consequences of intimate partner violence. *Lancet, 359,* 1331–1336.

Canadian Council on Social Development. (2003, May). *Estimated 2002 annual basic social assistance income by type of household.* Retrieved June 2, 2005, from http://www.ccsd.ca/factsheets/basicsa02.htm

Cauce, A. M., Paradise, M., Ginzler, J. A., Embry, L., Morgan, C. J., & Lohr, Y. (2000). The characteristics and mental health of homeless adolescents: Age and gender differences. *Journal of Emotional and Behavioural Disorders, 8*, 230–239.

Cohen, J. (1992). A power primer. *Psychological Bulletin, 112*, 155–159.

Davies, L., Avison, W. R., & MacAlpine, D. D. (1997, May). Significant life experiences and depression among single and married mothers. *Journal of Marriage and the Family, 59*, 294–308.

Felsten, G. (1998). Gender and coping: Use of distinct strategies and associations with stress and depression. *Anxiety, Stress and Coping, 11,* 289–309.

Ford-Gilboe, M., Berman, H., Laschinger, H., & Laforet-Fliesser, Y. (2000). T*esting a causal model of family health promotion behaviour in mother-headed single families (final report).* London, ON: University of Western Ontario.

Gyamfi, P., Brooks-Gunn, J., & Jackson, A. P. (2001). Association between employment and financial and parental stress in low-income single black mothers. *Women and Health, 32*(1/2), 119–135.

Hall, L. A., Gurley, D. N., Sachs, B., & Kryscio, R. J. (1991). Psychological predictors of maternal depressive symptoms, parenting attitudes, and child behavior in single-parent families. *Nursing Research, 40*, 214–220.

Hall, L. A., Williams, C. A., & Greenberg, R. S. (1985). Supports, stressors, and depressive symptoms in low-income mothers and young children. *American Journal of Public Health, 75*, 518–522.

Health Canada. (2002). *A report on mental illnesses in Canada.* Ottawa, ON: Health Canada. Retrieved November 15, 2002, from http://www.hc-sc.gc.ca

Holmes, T. H., & Rahe, R. H. (1967). The Social Readjustment Rating Scale. *Journal of Psychosomatic Research, 11*, 213–218.

Lennon, M. C., Blome, J., & English, K. (2001, March). *Depression and low-income women: Challenges of TANF and welfare to work policies and programs.* Retrieved November 30, 2002, from http://www.researchforum.org

Lipman, E. L., Offord, D. R., & Boyle, M. H. (1997). Single mothers in Ontario: Sociodemographic, physical and mental health characteristics. *Canadian Medical Association Journal, 156*, 639–645.

McLanahan, S. S. (1983). Family structure and stress: A longitudinal comparison of two-parent and female-headed families. *Journal of Marriage and the Family, 45*, 317–357.

Ministry of Community and Social Services. (2001, May). *Ontario Works Program overview.* Toronto: Author.

Ministry of Health and Long-Term Care. (2002). *Children's health.* Retrieved February 12, 2003, from http://www.health.gov.on.ca/english/public/program/child/child_mn.html

National Children's Agenda. (2005). *Supporting families and children: Government of Canada initiatives.* Retrieved December 3, 2005, from http://www.socialunion.gc.ca/nca/supporting_e.html

Nezlek, J. B., Hampton, C. P., & Shean, G. D. (2000). Clinical depression and day-to-day social interaction in a community sample. *Journal of Abnormal Psychology, 109*(1), 11–19.

Pearlin, L. I. (1989). The sociological study of stress. *Journal of Health and Social Behaviour, 30,* 241–256.

Pearlin, L. I. (2002). Some conceptual perspectives on the origins and prevention of social stress. In A. Maney & J. Ramos (Eds.), *Socioeconomic conditions, stress and mental disorders: Toward a new synthesis of research and public policy* (pp. 1–35). Bethesda, MD: NIH Office of Behavioral and Social Research. Retrieved May 2, 2002, from http://www.mhsip.org/pdfs/pearlin.pdf

Pearlin, L. I., & Johnson, J. S. (1977). Marital status, life strains, and depression. *American Sociological Review, 42*, 704–715.

Raphael, D. (2004). Introduction to the social determinants of health. In D. Raphael (Ed.), *Social determinants of health: Canadian perspective* (pp. 1–18). Toronto: Canadian Scholars' Press.

Samuels-Dennis, J. (2004). *Assessing stressful life events, psychological well-being and coping styles in sole-support parents.* Unpublished master's thesis, D'Youville College, Buffalo, NY.

Scarini, I. C., Ames, S. C., & Brantley, P. J. (1999). Chronic minor stressors and major life events experienced by low-income patients attending primary care clinics: A longitudinal examination. *Journal of Behavioural Medicine, 22*, 143–156.

Statistics Canada. (2001). *Population attributes*. Retrieved June 17, 2005, from http:www.statcan.ca/english/freepub/82-221-XIE/00604/community/community1.htm

Tolman, R. M., & Rosen, D. (2001). Domestic violence in the lives of women receiving welfare. *Violence Against Women, 7,* 141–158.

Wagner, J., & Menke, E. (1991). Stressors and coping behaviours of homeless, poor, and low-income mothers. *Journal of Community Health Nursing, 8*(2), 75–84.

Wheaton, B. (1999). Social stress. In C. S. Aneshensel & J. C. Phelan (Eds.), *Handbook of the sociology of mental health* (pp. 277–297). New York: Kluwer Academic/Plenum.

World Health Organization. (1986). *Ottawa Charter for Health Promotion.* Geneva: Author.

Youngblut, J. M., Brady, N., Brooten, D., & Thomas, D. J. (2000). Factors influencing single mothers'employment status. *Health Care for Women International,* 21, 125–136.

Yu, Y., & Williams, D. R. (1999). Socioeconomic status and mental health. In C. S. Aneshensel & J. C. Phelan (Eds.), *Handbook of the sociology of mental health* (pp. 151–163). New York: Kluwer Academic/Plenum.

AUTHORS' NOTE

Sincere thanks are extended to Marilyn Ford-Gilboe and Richard Dennis for reading and commenting on earlier drafts of this paper. I am particularly grateful to Dr. Ford-Gilboe for her insightful comments and encouragement as I embarked on the journey to complete this manuscript and evolve in my thinking about the mental health of single mothers.

Comments or queries may be directed to Joan Samuels-Dennis, School of Nursing, Health Sciences Addition H3A, University of Western Ontario, 1151 Richmond Street, London, Ontario, N6A 5C1 Canada. E-mail: jsamuel4@uwo.ca

APPENDIX D

From *Canadian Journal of Nursing Research*, 2004;36(1):22–39. © McGill University School of Nursing.

Adolescent Constructions of Nicotine Addiction

Joan L. Bottorff, PhD, RN, FCAHS
Professor, Distinguished University Scholar,
  and CIHR Investigator
School of Nursing, UBC Okanagan
Kelowna, British Columbia

Joy L. Johnson, PhD, RN
Professor and CIHR Investigator
School of Nursing, University of British Columbia
Vancouver, British Columbia

Barbara Moffat, MSN, RN
Project Coordinator
School of Nursing, University of British Columbia
Vancouver, British Columbia

Jeevan Grewal, BSc
Research Assistant
School of Nursing, University of British Columbia
Vancouver, British Columbia

Pamela A. Ratner, PhD, RN
Associate Professor and CIHR Health Research Scholar
School of Nursing, University of British Columbia
Vancouver, British Columbia

Cecilia Kalaw, MA
Project Coordinator
School of Nursing, University of British Columbia
Vancouver, British Columbia

The purpose of this qualitative study was to extend our understanding of how adolescents view nicotine addiction. This secondary analysis included 80 open-ended interviews with adolescents with a variety of smoking histories. The transcribed interviews were systematically analyzed to identify salient explanations of nicotine addiction. These explanations presuppose causal pathways of nicotine exposure leading to addiction and include repeated use, the brain and body "getting used to" nicotine, personal weakness, and family influences. A further explanation is that some youths pretend to be addicted to project a "cool" image. These explanations illustrate that some youths see themselves as passive players in the formation of nicotine addiction. The findings can be used in the development of programs to raise youth awareness about nicotine addiction.

KEYWORDS

adolescents
smoking
nicotine addiction
nicotine dependence
tobacco

Nicotine dependence in adolescents is usually classified at about half the rate observed in adults; however, the majority of adolescent smokers consider themselves to be addicted and find it difficult to stop smoking (Colby, Tiffany, Shiffman, & Niaura, 2000a). Although youth smoking has been linked to social factors, some researchers have observed that the reasons for smoking most frequently cited by adolescents are pleasure and addiction (Eiser, 1985; Sarason, Mankowski, Peterson, & Dinh, 1992). Daughton, Daughton, and Patil (1997) found that 52% of high-school smokers were already "hooked" on cigarettes or believe they had a good chance of becoming addicted within 5 years. However, although some adolescent smokers recognize their susceptibility to nicotine addiction, a significant proportion do not. Applying risk-perception theory, Virgili, Owen, and Sverson (1991) concluded that adolescent smokers perceive less personal risk of addiction than "experimenters" (i.e., occasional smokers), former smokers, and those who have never smoked.

Researchers acknowledge the need for more work focusing on nicotine addiction in adolescents (Colby, Tiffany, Shiffman, & Niaura, 2000b; Kassel, 2000; Moffat & Johnson, 2001; Shadel, Shiffman, Niaura, Nichter, & Abrams, 2000). Developments in social science underscore the need for professionals to understand the lay knowledge that underpins health beliefs and practices (Popay & Williams, 1996). In addition, theories of health behaviour suggest that the way in which one views a health risk has implications for decision-making and lifestyle choices (Montano, Kasprzyk, & Taplin, 1997; Strecher & Rosenstock, 1997). It is well known that most addicted adults started smoking in adolescence. If we are to reduce nicotine addiction, we need a better grasp of how teenagers understand and explain nicotine addiction. The view of 10- and 11-year-old children on smoking and addiction indicate that they are vulnerable to taking up smoking and becoming addicted (Rugkasa, Knox, et al., 2001). Adolescent girls' experiences of nicotine addiction include resistance to a smoking identity, failure to view addiction as a

consequence of their smoking, and surprise at how quickly they could become addicted (Moffat & Johnson, 2001). Ongoing close attention to adolescents' views could inform health promotion interventions to better address nicotine addiction among youths.

Several explanatory models of nicotine addiction have been proposed to delineate the causal factors. Genetic researchers have proposed that genetic and environmental factors influence smoking initiation and continuation (Koopmans, Slutske, Heath, Neale, & Boomsma, 1999; True et al., 1997) and that specific genes play a role in determining smoking behaviour (Mah, Tang, Liauw, Nagel, & Schneider, 1998; Marubio & Changeux, 2000; Rosecrans, 1989). Others have proposed a "sensitivity" model in which an individual's initial sensitivity to nicotine determines the development of tolerance for, and thus dependence on, nicotine (Pomerleau, 1995; Pomerleau, Collins, Shiffman, & Pomerleau, 1993). Physiological models also have been proposed to explain the action of nicotine on nicotinic receptors in the brain (Mah et al.; Marubio & Changeux; Lueders et al., 1999, Rosecrans). An additional source of exposure to nicotine is environmental tobacco smoke (ETS). While cotinine levels reveal that many youths are exposed to nicotine via ETS (Ashley et al., 1998), there is no evidence that this exposure increases their risk of addiction. Psychological models focus on affective and emotional factors that predispose a person to nicotine dependence. For example, the self-medication model (Gilbert & Gilbert, 1995) describes how individuals cope with difficult situations by smoking and may explain the addictive potential of nicotine in persons with depression (Balfour, 2000; Benowitz, 1999).

Although influenced directly by emerging scientific and medical evidence, societal explanations of addiction are culturally bound and have shifted over time with changes in dominant social and moral values. Researchers have described the social constructions of addiction to drugs and alcohol, highlighting the common-sense understandings of various publics and how they function as paradigms for constructing the world and give meaning to experience (Heim, Davies, Cheyne, & Smallwood, 2001; Nichter, 2003; Peele, 1985). These constructions are multidimensional and sometimes contradictory. For example, Heim et al. suggest that the concept of addiction is used to remove blame for unfavourable behaviour and simultaneously to stigmatize morally. With the increasing public attention on tobacco control, scientific theories of nicotine addiction are entering public discourse and influencing the ways in which society views nicotine addiction.

Constructivists argue that constructions and reconstructions of reality are experientially based and dependent for their form and content on consensus among individuals or groups (Guba, 1990). Adolescents are exposed to education on the adverse effects of smoking through school programs, television, and the guidance of parents and health professionals. However, little is known about how youths view nicotine addiction in the context of health education, their personal experiences with smoking, and other factors such as policies aimed at limiting youth access to tobacco. The purpose of this qualitative study was to examine dialogues with teenagers about tobacco use and to describe their views on nicotine addiction, no matter how partial or implausible.

METHODS

In this qualitative study (Lincoln & Guba, 1985), we carried out a secondary analysis of interviews with youths conducted as part of several research projects focused on teenagers' experiences with tobacco use. Adolescents with a variety of smoking histories were recruited. They included regular smokers, occasional or social smokers, and those who considered themselves to be former smokers. The open-ended interviews were based on techniques described by Kvale (1996) and focused on gaining in-depth accounts of adolescents' experiences with tobacco. The interviews covered a wide range of topics, including personal experiences with cigarettes and smoking, observations of others' smoking behaviour, and views on addiction. The interviews lasted from 45 to 60 minutes and were audiotaped and transcribed. All youths provided informed consent prior to participating in the interviews.

We began by analyzing a set of 47 individual interviews and one focus group interview that were available for secondary analysis. Six youths who were recruited for a pilot study participated in a focus group exploring issues of tobacco use. The majority of the individual interviews ($n = 35$) were collected as part of a qualitative study examining the transition from experimentation to regular tobacco use among adolescents (Johnson et al., 2003). We recruited youths who self-identified as casual, regular, or former smokers, as well as a few who had only experimented with smoking. Another 12 interviews were conducted with adolescent female smokers in a study to explore the meaning of nicotine addiction (Moffat & Johnson, 2001). Using NVivo, a computer program that facilitates qualitative analysis, we searched the data set for segments of text that included explanations of dependence, addiction, lack of control over smoking, and experiences associated with cessation. These sections of data were then subjected to detailed thematic analysis that compared and contrasted explanations to identify unique explanations of addiction and the strategies used to construct them.

The research team discussed the analyses and interpretation at regular intervals. Questions were raised on the basis of the data reviewed, and directions for additional search and analytic strategies were set. After the initial phase of data analysis, preliminary findings were verified and refined through an additional secondary analysis with a second set of open-ended interviews ($n = 19$) from an ongoing study of dimensions of adolescent tobacco dependence (Johnson et al., 2002). These interviews also focused on adolescents' experiences with tobacco and included individuals with a variety of smoking histories. Finally, eight primary interviews were conducted with selected adolescents. Some of these interviews were conducted with individuals who had been interviewed previously, because they were good informants. The questions in these final interviews focused specifically on adolescents' understanding of how nicotine addiction arises and provided an opportunity to validate the findings.

RESULTS

In total, interviews with 80 adolescents were analyzed in this study. Slightly more males than females participated and the average age was 16 years (see Table D-1). On average, participants tried their first cigarette at age 13 (range 9 to 17 years) and smoked for 3 years (range 1 to 7 years). Adolescents with a variety of smoking histories were included in the data sets used in this study: 41 defined themselves as regular or daily smokers, 21 as occasional or social smokers, and 18 as former smokers.

Adolescent Constructions of Nicotine Addiction

The participants constructed their understanding of nicotine addiction in the context of their observations of smokers, integrating what they heard from peers, family members, educators, and the media with their own experiences with cigarettes. Some youths began by admitting that they had "no clue" about addiction and indicated that they had never thought about what made them want cigarettes. The interview represented the first time they

had reflected on or discussed the development of nicotine addiction. Many of the participants puzzled over nicotine addiction, stating that they did not know much about it. For example, one youth who indicated that she was aware of the health effects of smoking said she did not know how long it takes before one becomes so addicted that it is difficult to abstain [15-year-old female, daily smoker, 3–4 quit attempts]. Others had well-formed opinions and explanations. Nonetheless, when probed, all the participants attempted to understand nicotine addiction. For example, one youth said: "I don't know if your lungs become dependent on the smoke you inhale. It seems kind of silly, because of course they don't want the smoke, so why would they?" [16-year-old male, occasional smoker]

The adolescents tended to use several strategies to distance themselves from nicotine addiction. Few admitted to being addicted or even to being vulnerable to nicotine addiction. They drew on their observations of other smokers (who they thought were addicted) instead of exploring their own addiction. Others talked about nicotine addiction in a depersonalized way — for example, by describing the effects of nicotine on "the body" and "the brain," effectively separating addiction from their subjective and embodied experiences with smoking. Yet others focused on factors beyond one's control (e.g., the actions of others, personality traits), and in so doing presented some teenagers as passive, vulnerable, and powerless in the face of addiction.

Our analysis of adolescents' constructions of nicotine addiction revealed four broad explanations. These presuppose causal pathways of nicotine exposure leading to addiction. Some concentrate on the phenomenon of addiction itself, others on the factors or circumstances that lead to it. A possible fifth explanation is that some youths pretend to be addicted in order to project a "cool" image. While the data support five predominant constructions, some teenagers drew on several concurrently in an attempt to provide a full account of nicotine addiction. Each of the five explanations is described below.

TABLE D-1	Demographic Information for All Participants (n = 80)	
Characteristics	**N**	**%**
Gender		
Male	45	56
Female	35	44
Smoking status		
Occasional/social	21	26
Regular/daily	41	51
Former	18	23
	Mean Years (SD)	**Range in Years**
Age at time of interview	16 (1.3)	13–19
Age at first whole cigarette	13 (1.5)	9–17
Duration of smoking	3 (1.7)	< 1–7

NICOTINE ADDICTION AS REPEATED USE

Some adolescents explained that addiction occurs with sustained smoking, arguing that nicotine "adds up over the years." This was perhaps the simplest and most obvious explanation; the more one smokes, the greater one's chances of becoming addicted. At times, the tone used by adolescents in offering this explanation suggested that the cause of nicotine addiction is self-evident. For example, one youth stated, "It's not like someone with red hair becomes addicted; it's just who becomes addicted to it smokes enough and starts to need it" [14-year-old female, daily smoker, 2 quit attempts]. The informants further emphasized that addiction is associated with lengthy periods of smoking, daily smoking, excessive smoking, or "overdoing smoking."

Some adolescents explained why they believed that repeated use leads to addiction. Three postulations were provided, one focusing on the accumulation of nicotine, another on the development of a "taste" for or enjoyment of smoking, and the third on the development of a smoking habit.

According to the first postulation, nicotine "builds up" in the body and creates a need for more nicotine. One adolescent described the process of nicotine addiction as follows: "You start off with a little bit and you just build up and build up… That's the way their addiction forms. They just need a little bit and then they need more and then they need more" [16-year-old female, occasional smoker]. Others tried to formulate a more sophisticated response but admitted that they did not know how this "build-up" of nicotine leads to addiction: "I guess it's just tolerance. I don't know if there's a certain tolerance that your body has for addiction… I actually don't know the basis of addiction. I don't know if it's a mental aspect or biological" [18-year-old female, occasional smoker].

The second postulation is that "repeated use" leads to greater enjoyment. This explanation implies that addiction occurs as one acquires a taste for or appreciation of smoking: "You start to like it more, and so the more you like it, the more often you want it. So I think the more that somebody smokes for a while, the greater the chance of them getting addicted" [16-year-old female, daily smoker, 1 quit attempt].

In her effort to understand the phenomenon of "enjoying" an addictive substance, one girl compared nicotine addiction to "addiction to a job," associating addiction with enjoyment of a chosen activity: "Addiction means mostly, like, you get addicted because you enjoy it…. Say you like a certain job, and you like it a lot, and you start getting addicted to it. That's how it goes" [15-year-old female, daily smoker].

The third way some adolescents believed repeated use leads to addiction is through habituation, or "getting used to" smoking. One adolescent explained how smoking had become part of her everyday life:

> When you're a smoker you get used to smoking at different points in the day. Like, it's weird to think, but certain times, like before I go to bed, I have to have a cigarette. As soon as I wake up and have my coffee I have a cigarette…. There's certain times where…when I'm driving I have to have a cigarette…I smoke a lot more when I'm driving just because it's what I do, like, I drive and I smoke. It's natural to me now. [17-year-old female, daily smoker]

Some adolescents, it was suggested, become attached to smoking routines and used to the actions involved in smoking (e.g., holding a cigarette), the implication being that addiction occurs because smoking is associated with certain events, activities, and feelings, and as a result people "just keep on doing it."

Many of the participants who believed that nicotine addiction is related to repeated use introduced the idea of degrees of addiction — light, moderate, and heavy. Some speculated that "heavy addiction" occurs among older people who have smoked for extended periods. One youth explained: "I think that for someone who has been smoking for maybe 60 years…their addiction is going to be a lot stronger and a lot harder to break, as opposed to someone who is only smoking for 6 months" [16-year-old female, daily smoker, no quit attempts]. These adolescents reasoned that those who smoke relatively little or who have smoked for a short period experience less addiction: "Our friend who just took up smoking is lightly addicted because he doesn't smoke very much. I'm moderately addicted because I will feel the need for a cigarette every so often" [16-year-old male, occasional smoker]. One adolescent who described her smoking as a "habit" did not believe she had reached the point of being addicted because she had not yet started "craving" cigarettes. Nevertheless, because of her concerns about addiction she remained vigilant for signs of craving so she could stop smoking before passing "the point of no return" [16-year-old female, daily smoker, no quit attempts].

The teenagers drew on observations of people they knew who were addicted to support their conclusions: "My God, Mom…smokes a lot and she's…always, like, 'Oh, I need one, I can't concentrate…' I think that's just because she has been smoking her whole life and she just smokes really a lot of cigarettes" [16-year-old female, daily smoker, no quit attempts].

NICOTINE ADDICTION AS THE BODY AND BRAIN "GETTING USED TO IT"

Some adolescents suggested that addiction occurs when the body and the brain "get used to" nicotine, thereby creating a continuous need for nicotine to "function normally." Without nicotine, an addicted individual experiences cravings: "Your body says you need one at that time; you just can't ignore what your body says." Some focused on the sensations or effects that the body experiences in the absence of nicotine: "My understanding is that addiction is when…the body can't function without it, when the body goes, like, nauseous, gets all stressed out and, you know, just doesn't function, just like your whole mind doesn't think right or anything" [17-year-old female, daily smoker].

Thus, nicotine addiction was conceptualized by these youths as beyond one's control and was equated by some with the body's need for food. Others focused on the role of the brain in nicotine addiction: "The brain forces you to think you need a cigarette." Although some of the adolescents used the terms "brain" and "body" interchangeably, others were adamant that addiction is caused by one or the other, and still others referred to the combined roles of the brain and the body.

The descriptions of the mechanisms by which the brain and body "get used to it" varied in sophistication and detail. Some of the adolescents were unable to specify the addictive component(s) of cigarettes: "…tar or something in the cigarette." They pointed to a vague bodily process that causes people to lose the ability to control their smoking: "You're not wanting it, really wanting it [a cigarette]….but, inside, something's just, like, needing it…. It's like the person inside you is wanting just to have one" [18-year-old make, daily smoker, 2 quit attempts].

Others were more specific about the mechanisms by which the brain and body "get used to it." They suggested that as people smoke more frequently their nicotine "levels go up" and as their body becomes "more tolerant" there is a greater need for nicotine: "That's the way their addiction forms. They just need a little bit and then they need more and then they need more." Some of these youths spoke of nicotine in the way one speaks of drugs such as heroin, using terms such as "dose," "levels," and "withdrawal." Others used the concept of "refuelling" to explain the need for nicotine—stating, for example, that smokers lose nicotine through sweating, creating a need to "refuel" the body by smoking to top up their nicotine level. They postulated that this explains why smokers crave cigarettes after exercise and sexual activity.

Finally, some of the adolescents offered more sophisticated explanations, reasoning that it is the "cells" that become addicted. They theorized that certain people become addicted to nicotine because their bodies lack a chemical or lack a protective gene. Others maintained that the body stops producing naturally occurring chemicals with prolonged smoking:

Just like Chapstick [lip balm], it stops your body from producing the stuff that makes your lips moist. Like, nicotine is replacing a chemical that makes you calm when you are stressed out. And so, when you take away your cigarette, your body doesn't know how to produce the chemical any more, and your body gets all freaked out. [17-year-old male, daily smoker, 3 quit attempts]

These adolescents spoke of the consequences of not acquiring sufficient nicotine. The short-term consequences, they believed, include irritability and cravings.

NICOTINE ADDICTION AS PERSONAL WEAKNESS

A third explanation of nicotine addiction was based on the premise that it develops because of "weakness" or vulnerability due to "personal problems." The youths explained that this weakness is reflected in smokers' admission that they had not really wanted to start smoking, as well as their inability to cut down or quit. One youth maintained that adolescents often take up smoking when they feel vulnerable in certain situations and have a cigarette whenever they experience this feeling. Another suggested that smokers typically have low self-esteem and smoke to "prove they are better" or to "look cool." It was argued that not all teenagers who smoke become addicted, that the development of addiction "depends on what kind of person they are." Thus, addiction was viewed by some as a result of "mental weakness" or "weak-mindedness" rather than as a physical condition.

In these explanations of nicotine addiction as a personal weakness, a moral tone was evident in the language used and the adolescents tended to distance themselves from addicted smokers by disclosing their own perceived character strengths. For example, some maintained that the weak become addicted while those who are "in control" of their lives and their smoking do not: "I've been so comfortable with smoking and I'm not really getting addicted because I know I'm so much in control of my life… If people had more control of their lives, perhaps they [would] know when enough is enough" [16-year-old female, occasional smoker]; "Very few young people are lucky enough to be strong enough to not get addicted" [16-year-old female, daily smoker, 3 quit attempts]; "It shows that they are weak if they are addicted because they don't have the willpower to quit" [15-year-old female, daily smoker, 3–4 quit attempts].

Some adolescents associated personal weakness with a particular kind of "addictive" personality characterized by lack of confidence, inability to resist peer pressure, and lack of personal conviction. One boy reasoned that immaturity is a factor in susceptibility to addiction: "When you are younger you have…a more addictive personality" [17-year-old male, occasional smoker]. Because of the focus on willpower and mental control of smoking, some adolescents suggested that nicotine addiction is not a true addiction, like heroin addiction, and referred to the need to smoke cigarettes as a "so-called addiction." Although they admitted that some youths need to smoke, they believed that smoking cigarettes "is not really an addiction if you can control it."

NICOTINE ADDICTION AS FAMILY INFLUENCE

Some of the adolescents explained that nicotine addiction occurs because of the influence of both immediate and extended family members. Instead of viewing nicotine addiction as stemming from personal characteristics or choices, they believed that people become *passively* addicted. Many of the participants who held this position were regular smokers and had several relatives who smoked. Three central arguments were used to support this position: the availability of cigarettes in the home, exposure to smoking and ETS, and an inherited predisposition to addiction.

If family members smoke, reasoned some youths, cigarettes are readily available and the likelihood of their becoming addicted increases: "If they can get their hands on them, chances are they'll become addicted" [15-year-old female, daily smoker, no quit attempts]. These youths suggested that they have no choice but to smoke when cigarettes are available: "I might as well smoke it if I have it" [18-year-old male, daily smoker, 2 quit attempts].

Many of the adolescents maintained that seeing others smoke and being exposed to ETS, particularly in the home, creates an addiction to nicotine. They reasoned that when family members smoke, children "get used" to smoking and ETS and hence view it as "normal." They explained that even the smell of smoke becomes a part of everyday life and is associated with the home:

> *If your parents smoke, you have so much more chance of becoming [addicted]. For one [thing], you've had it in your system, like second-hand smoke, as long as your parents have smoked. And then it's just…second nature. It doesn't smell like stale cigarettes. It smells like home [laughs] or like…the living room. [17-year-old male, occasional smoker]*

These teenagers expressed a belief that continued exposure to smoking creates a disposition to smoke and to become addicted. One youth said that after her parents divorced she was no longer exposed to cigarette smoke because her father, a regular smoker, had left the home. She started to have feelings of panic and reasoned that she was experiencing nicotine withdrawal even though she was a non-smoker at the time. She maintained that this prompted her to take up smoking and to become a regular smoker [15-year-old female, daily smoker].

One boy reasoned that daily exposure in the home leads to "smoke being in your system." Another adolescent offered a detailed account of how children's exposure to smoke sensitizes them to cigarettes and puts them at risk for addiction:

> *When you're younger and there's smoke around you…there's potential for being addicted to it just from the clouds of smoke that go onto children's faces. And so they [parents] might already be creating this addiction that they are not even aware of. And so when they [the children] have that first cigarette, it'll be sort of a re-enactment of when they were younger with all the smoke around them. [17-year-old female, former smoker, 3–4 quit attempts]*

This girl attributed sensitization to the subconscious acceptance of smoking that occurs when everyone smokes: "And if they're smoking it gives you this idea, in your head, that…what those kinds of people do is okay… I think subconsciously, somewhere in my brain, it is still…okay, everyone does this."

A third attribution of addiction to family influences was based on the proposition that if one's relatives smoke or have other addictions there might be a hereditary component to nicotine addiction. When asked why some people are more prone to addiction than others, one girl stated, "I don't know if it's hereditary, but both my mother and [I] smoke" [16-year-old female, occasional smoker, 1 quit attempt]. Others traced the smoking patterns in their family: "My mom and my auntie and my uncles, they all smoke. And my cousins smoke. And even my dad's side smoke, his sister and all my cousins. So maybe it's in your family or something. When they smoke, then you smoke" [16-year-old male, daily smoker, approximately 10 quit attempts]. Some were convinced they were susceptible to addiction because of a family predisposition. One youth who was a daily smoker stated:

> *I have an addictive personality because people in my family have been addicted to…certain drugs and…alcohol and stuff like that. My dad had a drug addiction and people…my grandparents and…in the family, like, genes, kind of. My dad always tells me I have to be careful with everything. Because of him I can get addicted easily to more stuff, because of him having the addiction. [16-year-old female, daily smoker]*

NICOTINE ADDICTION AS "IMAGE"

Most of the youths described nicotine addiction as something they recognized in others. A few theorized that there is no such thing as nicotine addiction, particularly among teenagers, because people can stop smoking if they really want to. They further suggested that youths who claim they are addicted are simply pretending to be addicted, arguing that smoking "doesn't seem to come naturally to them" and that they do not look like "real smokers." They referred to this phenomenon as "false" or "made-up" addiction, explaining that teenagers smoke to impress and to project a "cool" image:

> You get that person who has, like, one smoke a month and "Oh, I am so addicted, I am so addicted, blah, blah, blah." And they just blurt out things they have heard before. They are trying to make it sound like they smoke all the time. [16-year-old male, daily smoker, 7–8 quit attempts]

The adolescents who subscribed to the notion of addiction as image suggested that teenagers who pretend to be addicted are more dependent on the image than on nicotine. Acting addicted was said to offer certain advantages. For example, one youth admitted to "acting addicted" in order to "hang out" with a certain group [14-year-old female, occasional smoker]. Another suggested that people who want to be "known as smokers" act addicted because it is "cool" [16-year-old male, daily smoker].

DISCUSSION

Other researchers have described children's ideas concerning nicotine addiction (Rugkasa, Kennedy, et al., 2001; Rugkasa, Knox, et al., 2001) and adolescent girls' experiences of it (Moffat & Johnson, 2001). However, this is the first study to focus specifically on adolescent constructions of nicotine addiction. Compared to the ideas of children, which focus almost exclusively on the dangers and costs of addiction, those of adolescents are more complex and include less dramatic and harmful images of nicotine addiction. We also noticed a tendency for adolescents to recognize and focus on nicotine addiction in others rather than in themselves, and to implicate other smokers in youths' vulnerability to nicotine addiction. These perspectives on nicotine addiction extend our understanding of the profound influence of parents who smoke on the smoking behaviour of children, beyond that suggested by social modelling theories. Echoing the findings of Moffat and Johnson, the participants in this study downplayed the link between individual behaviour and the development of addiction; a number of them saw themselves as immune to addiction even though they smoked.

Why do teenagers minimize their role in nicotine addiction? It is possible that they are simply resisting the warnings of authority figures about addiction. It is also possible that these findings reflect a tendency to distance oneself from the label of addiction because in social discourse addiction is often associated with lack of control and immorality and is viewed as distasteful. Some might suggest that the findings reflect theories of a heightened egocentrism during adolescence that contributes to perceived invulnerability to natural hazards and behaviour-linked risks. Nevertheless, there is a growing body of research challenging commonly held views related to adolescent competence in judging risk and uncovering the multidimensional components of risk judgements (Millstein & Halpern-Felsher, 2002).

The constructions of nicotine addiction provided by these adolescents reflect elements of different models of addiction that have had credence in public discourse, such as genetic, exposure, and adaptation theories (Peele, 1985). In general, however, the youths ascribed far less importance to scientific "facts" than to personal experiences and observations, hunches, and, sometimes, misinformation as they struggled to understand the mechanisms involved in nicotine addiction. Other studies have also found that lay conceptualizations of addiction reflect personal knowledge of addictive substances and morals, rather than facts about the addicted state (Heim et al., 2001).

Teenagers clearly draw on various sources of information regarding addiction (and addicts). The challenge for nurses engaged in health education is to be aware of how adolescents position themselves in relation to "addiction" and to be mindful of how education campaigns around tobacco and other drugs impact the social climate for disclosure and dialogue with regard to substance use. By removing some of the moral censure that accompanies "addiction," and by facilitating meaningful dialogue with youths about tobacco use and addiction, we will be able to provide a foundation for introducing a scientific understanding of nicotine addiction. Our knowledge of nicotine addiction is evolving rapidly, with new discoveries being made related to genetics (Li, 2003; Yoshimasu & Kiyohara, 2003) and the influence of sex and gender on addiction (Benowitz & Hatsukami, 1998). In addition, there is new evidence suggesting that some teenagers develop nicotine addiction more rapidly than previously theorized (DiFranza, Savageau, Fletcher, et al., 2002; DiFranza, Savageau, Rigotti, et al., 2002). Many of these discoveries have received media attention and inevitably inform adolescents' views on tobacco use. It is important for nurses to keep up to date with new discoveries and incorporate relevant findings into health education programs focusing on tobacco.

Lay theories of health and illness are embedded in causal schemas that are grounded in life experiences (Stein, Roeser, & Markus, 1998). The realities described by the participants in the present study pose considerable challenges for nurses and health educators. How can we provide support for adolescents who do not want to smoke yet belong to families in which smoking is "normal" and in which encouragement to quit is non-existent? Furthermore, as suggested by Stein et al., lay theories may not be easily replaced because the behaviours these causal schemas support become enmeshed in individuals' self-concepts.

The youths interviewed were interested in the topic of nicotine addiction and puzzled over it, but questions remain. What notions of nicotine addiction should be cultivated among youths, and to what end? Tobacco-reduction programs for children and adolescents have concentrated on smoking bans on school premises (Northrup, Ashley, & Ferrence, 1998; Pickett, Northrup, & Ashley, 1999) as well as on prevention regarding the long-term, often delayed, adverse health effects of smoking and strategies for resisting smoking (BC Ministry of Education & BC Ministry of Health, 2000). The limited attention given to nicotine and its immediate effects is perhaps reflected in the views expressed by the participants in the present study.

The findings of this study suggest some priorities for nurses involved in youth tobacco control, including the fostering of accessible and accurate health education related to the action of nicotine. Although information about nicotine addiction will likely be insufficient to deter adolescents from smoking, knowledge that responds to their social contexts and experiences is key to empowering them to make decisions about their health.

REFERENCES

Ashley, M. J., Cohen, J., Ferrence, R., Bull, S., Bondy, S., Poland, B., et al. (1998). Smoking in the home: Changing attitudes and current practices. *American Journal of Public Health, 88,* 797–800.

Balfour, D. J. (2000). The effects of nicotine on neural pathways implicated in depression: A factor in nicotine addiction? *Pharmacology, Biochemistry and Behavior, 66,* 79–85.

BC Ministry of Education & BC Ministry of Health. (2000). *bc.tobaccofacts: A tobacco prevention resource for teachers.* Retrieved January 20, 2004, from http://www.prevention.alphabet.ca

Benowitz, N. L. (1999). Nicotine addiction. *Primary Care, 26,* 611–631.

Benowitz, N. L., & Hatsukami, D. (1998). Gender differences in the pharmacology of nicotine addiction. *Addiction Biology, 3,* 383–404.

Colby, S. M., Tiffany, S. T., Shiffman, S., & Niaura, R. S. (2000a). Are adolescent smokers dependent on nicotine? A review of the evidence. *Drug and Alcohol Dependence, 59,* S83–S95.

Colby, S. M., Tiffany, S. T., Shiffman, S., & Niaura, R. S. (2000b). Measuring nicotine dependence among youth: A review of available approaches and instruments. *Drug and Alcohol Dependence, 59,* S23–239.

Daughton, J. M., Daughton, D. M., & Patil, K. D. (1997). Self-recognition of alcohol and cigarette dependency among high school seniors. *Perceptual and Motor Skills, 85,* 115–120.

DiFranza, J. R., Savageau, J. A., Fletcher, K., Ockene, J. K., Rigotti, N. A., McNeill, A. D., et al. (2002). Measuring the loss of autonomy over nicotine use in adolescents: The DANDY (Development and Assessment of Nicotine Dependence in Youths) study. *Archives of Pediatrics and Adolescent Medicine, 156,* 397–403.

DiFranza, J. R., Savageau, J. A., Rigotti, N. A., Fletcher, K., Ockene, J. K., McNeill, A. D., et al. (2002). Development of symptoms of tobacco dependence in youths: 30-month follow-up data from the DANDY study. *Tobacco Control, 11,* 228–235.

Eiser, J. R. (1985). Smoking: The social learning of an addiction. *Journal of Social and Clinical Psychology, 3,* 446–457.

Gilbert, D. G., & Gilbert, B. O. (1995). Personality, psychopathology, and nicotine response as mediators of the genetics of smoking. *Behavior Genetics, 25,* 133–147.

Guba, E. G. (1990). The alternative paradigm dialogue. In E. G. Guba (Ed.), *The paradigm dialogue* (pp. 17–27). Newbury Park, CA: Sage.

Heim, D., Davies, J., Cheyne, B., & Smallwood, J. (2001). Addiction as a functional representation. *Journal of Community and Applied Social Psychology, 11,* 57–62.

Johnson, J. L., Bottorff, J. L., Moffat, B., Ratner, P. A., Shoveller, J. A., & Lovato, C. Y. (2002). Tobacco dependence: Adolescents' perspectives on the need to smoke. *Social Science and Medicine, 56,* 1481–1492.

Johnson, J. L., Lovato, C. Y., Maggi, S., Ratner, P. A., Shoveller, J. A., Baillie, L., et al. (2003). Smoking and adolescence: Narratives of identity. *Research in Nursing and Health, 26,* 387–397.

Kassel, J. D. (2000). Are adolescent smokers addicted to nicotine? The suitability of the nicotine dependence construct as applied to adolescents. *Journal of Child and Adolescent Substance Abuse, 9,* 27–49.

Koopmans, J. R., Slutske, W. S., Heath, A. C., Neale, M. C., & Boomsma, D. I. (1999). The genetics of smoking initiation and quantity smoked in Dutch adolescent and young adult twins. *Behavior Genetics, 29,* 383–393.

Kvale, S. (1996). *InterViews: An introduction to qualitative research interviewing.* Thousand Oaks, CA: Sage.

Li, M. D. (2003). The genetics of smoking related behavior: A brief review. *American Journal of Medical Science, 326,* 168–173.

Lincoln, Y. S., & Guba, E. G. (1985). *Naturalistic inquiry.* Newbury Park, CA: Sage.

Lueders, K. K., Elliott, R. W., Marenholz, I., Mischke, D., DuPree, M., & Hamer, D. (1999). Genomic organization and mapping of the human and mouse neuronal beta$_2$-nicotinic acetylcholine receptor genes. *Mammalian Genome, 10,* 900–905.

Mah, S. J., Tang, Y., Liauw, P. E., Nagel, J. E., & Schneider, A. S. (1998). Ibogaine acts at the nicotinic acetylcholine receptor to inhibit catecholamine release. *Brain Research, 797,* 173–180.

Marubio, L. M., & Changeux, J. (2000). Nicotinic acetylcholine receptor knockout mice as animal models for studying receptor function. *European Journal of Pharmacology, 393,* 113–121.

Millstein, S., & Halpern-Felsher, B. (2002). Judgments about risk and perceived invulnerability in adolescents and young adults. *Journal of Research on Adolescence, 12,* 399–422.

Moffat, B. M., & Johnson, J. L. (2001). Through the haze of cigarettes: Teenage girls' stories about cigarette addiction. *Qualitative Health Research, 11,* 668–681.

Montano, D. E., Kasprzyk, D., & Taplin, S. H. (1997). The theory of reasoned action and the theory of planned behavior. In K. Glanz, F. Marcus Lewis, & B. K. Rimer (Eds.), *Health behavior and health education: Theory, research and practice* (pp. 85–112). San Francisco: Jossey-Bass.

Nichter, M. (2003). Smoking: What does culture have to do with it? *Addiction, 98,* 139–145.

Northrup, D. A., Ashley, M. J., & Ferrence, R. (1998). The Ontario ban on smoking on school property: Perceived impact on smoking. *Canadian Journal of Public Health, 89,* 224–228.

Peele, S. (1985). *The meaning of addiction — Compulsive experience and its interpretation.* Toronto: Lexington.

Pickett, W., Northrup, D. A., & Ashley, M. J. (1999). Factors influencing implementation of the legislated smoking ban on school property in Ontario. *Preventive Medicine, 29,* 157–164.

Pomerleau, O. F. (1995). Individual differences in sensitivity to nicotine: Implications for genetic research on nicotine dependence. *Behavior Genetics, 25,* 161–177.

Pomerleau, O. F., Collins, A. C., Shiffman, S., & Pomerleau, C. S. (1993). Why some people smoke and others do not: New perspectives. *Journal of Consulting and Clinical Psychology, 61,* 723–731.

Popay, J., & Williams, G. (1996). Public health research and lay knowledge. *Social Science and Medicine, 42,* 759–768.

Rosecrans, J. A. (1980). Nicotine as a discriminative stimulus: A neurobehavioral approach to studying central cholinergic mechanisms. *Journal of Substance Abuse, 1,* 287–300.

Rugkasa, J., Kennedy, O., Barton, M., Abaunza, P. S., Treacy, M. P., & Knox, B. (2001). Smoking and symbolism: Children, communication and cigarettes. *Health Education Research, 16,* 131–142.

Rugkasa, J., Knox, B., Sittlington, J., Kennedy, O., Treacy, M. P., & Abaunza, P. S. (2001). Anxious adults vs. cool children: Children's views on smoking and addiction. *Social Science and Medicine, 53,* 593–602.

Sarason, I. G., Mankowski, E. S., Peterson, A. J., & Dinh, K. T. (1992). Adolescents' reasons for smoking. *Journal of School Health, 62,* 185–190.

Shadel, W. G., Shiffman, S., Niaura, R., Nichter, M., & Abrams, & D. B. (2000). Current models of nicotine dependence: What is known and what is needed to advance understanding of tobacco etiology among youth. *Drug and Alcohol Dependence, 59,* S9–S22.

Stein, K. F., Roeser, R., & Markus, H. R. (1998). Self-schemas and possible selves as predictors and outcomes of risky behaviors in adolescents. *Nursing Research, 47,* 96–106.

Strecher, V. J., & Rosenstock, I. M. (1997). The health belief model. In K. Glanz, F. Marcus Lewis, & B. K. Rimer (Eds.), Health behavior and health education: Theory, research and practice (pp. 41–59). San Francisco: Jossey-Bass.

True, W. R., Heath, A. C., Scherrer, J. F., Waterman, B., Goldberg, J., Lin, N., et al. (1997). Genetic and environmental contributions to smoking. *Addiction, 92,* 1277–1287.

Virgili, M., Owen, N., & Sverson, H. H. (1991). Adolescents' smoking behavior and risk perceptions. *Journal of Substance Abuse, 3,* 315–324.

Yoshimasu, K., & Kiyohara, C. (2003). Genetic influences on smoking behavior and nicotine dependence: A review. *Journal of Epidemiology, 13,* 183–192.

AUTHORS' NOTE

This research was supported by grants from the British Columbia Medical Services Foundation and the National Cancer Institute of Canada, and through career awards from the Canadian Institutes of Health Research (CIHR) to Drs. Bottorff, Johnson, and Ratner.

Comments or inquiries may be directed to Dr. Joan L. Bottorff, Nursing and Health Behaviour Research Unit, School of Nursing, T201-2211 Wesbrook Mall, Vancouver, British Columbia V6T 2B5 Canada. Telephone: 604-822-7438. Fax: 604-822-7466. E-mail: bottorff@nursing.ubc.ca

Glossary

a priori From Latin, meaning "the former," that is, before the study or analysis.

abstract A brief, comprehensive summary of a study.

accessible population A population that meets the population criteria and is available.

accuracy The characteristic of all aspects of a study systematically and logically following from the research problem.

after-only design An experimental design with two randomly assigned groups: a treatment group and a control group. This design differs from the true experiment in that both groups are measured only after the experimental treatment; also known as *post-test-only control group design.*

after-only nonequivalent control group design A quasiexperimental design similar to the after-only experimental design, but subjects are not randomly assigned to the treatment group or the control group.

aims of inquiry The goals of the research, which vary with the *paradigm.*

alpha Considered a prior probability because it is set before the data are collected; the alpha is a conditional probability because the null hypothesis is assumed to be true.

alpha coefficient See *reliability coefficient.*

alternate form reliability A reliability measure in which two or more alternate forms of a measure are administered to the same subjects at different times. The scores of the two tests determine the degree of relationship between the measures.

analysis The division of the content into parts to understand each aspect of the study.

analysis of covariance (ANCOVA) A statistic that measures differences among group means and uses a statistical technique to equate the groups under study in relation to an important variable.

analysis of variance (ANOVA) A statistic that tests whether group means differ from each other; instead of testing each pair of means separately, ANOVA considers the variation among all groups.

animal rights Guidelines used to protect the rights of animals in the conduct of research.

anonymity A research participant's protection in a study so that no one, not even the researcher, can link the subject with the information given.

antecedent variable A variable that affects the dependent variable but occurs before the introduction of the independent variable.

assent An aspect of informed consent that pertains to protecting the rights of children as research subjects.

assumptions Accepted truths, key concepts and ideas, reasons and justifications, supporting examples, parallel experiences, implications and consequences, and any other structural features of the written text used to interpret and assess it accurately and fairly.

auditability The researcher's development of the research process in a qualitative study that allows a researcher or reader to follow the thinking or conclusions of the researcher.

behavioural/materialist perspective In ethnographical studies, the perspective that sees culture as observed through a group's patterns of behaviour and customs, their way of life, and what they produce.

beneficence An obligation to do no harm and to maximize possible benefits.

benefits Potential positive outcomes of participation in a research study.

bias A distortion in the data analysis results.

biological measurement Use of specialized equipment to determine the biological status of subjects.

bracketing A process by which the researcher identifies personal biases about the phenomenon of interest to clarify how personal experience and beliefs may colour what is heard and reported. The term comes from the mathematical metaphor of putting "brackets" around our beliefs so they can be put aside.

case study The study of a selected phenomenon that provides an in-depth description of its dimensions and processes.

case study method The study of a selected contemporary phenomenon over time to provide an in-depth description of the essential dimensions and processes of the phenomenon.

chance error An error attributable to fluctuations in subject characteristics that occur at a specific point in time and are often beyond the awareness and control of the examiner; also called *random error*.

chi-square (χ^2) A nonparametric statistic used to determine whether the frequency found in each category is different from the frequency that would be expected by chance.

close-ended item A question that the respondent may answer with only one of a fixed number of choices.

cluster sampling A probability sampling strategy that involves successive random sampling of units. The units sampled progress from large to small; also known as *multistage sampling*.

codes Tags or labels that are assigned to themes in a qualitative study.

coding The progressive marking, sorting, resorting, and defining and redefining of the collected data.

cognitive perspective In ethnographical studies, the perspective that culture consists of beliefs, knowledge, and ideas people use as they live.

cohort The subjects of a specific group that are being studied.

community-based participatory research A method that systematically accesses the voice of a community to plan context-appropriate action.

computer database A database that can be accessed online or on CD-ROM.

concealment An observational method that refers to whether the subjects know that they are being observed.

concept An image or symbolic representation of an abstract idea.

conceptual definition The general meaning of a concept.

conceptual framework A structure of concepts, theories, or both pulled together as a map for the study.

conceptual literature Published and unpublished non–data-based material, such as reports of theories, concepts, synthesis of research on concepts, or professional issues, some of which underlie reported research, as well as other nonresearch material; also called *theoretical literature*.

concurrent validity The degree of correlation between two measures of the same concept that are administered at the same time.

conduct of research The analysis of data collected from a homogeneous group of subjects who meet study inclusion and exclusion criteria for the purpose of answering specific research questions or testing specified hypotheses.

confidence interval An estimated range of values, which is likely to include an unknown population parameter calculated from a given set of sample data.

confidentiality Assurance that a research participant's identity cannot be linked to the information that was provided to the researcher.

consent See *informed consent*.

consistency   An aspect of the data collection process that requires that data be collected from each subject in the study in exactly the same way or as close to the same way as possible.

constancy   An aspect of control in data collection that ensures that methods and procedures of data collection are the same for all subjects.

constant comparative method   In the grounded theory method, a process of continuously comparing data as they are acquired during research.

constant error   See *systematic error*.

construct   An abstraction that is adapted for scientific purpose.

construct validity   The extent to which an instrument is said to measure a theoretical construct or trait.

constructivism   The basis for *naturalistic* (qualitative) research, which developed from writers such as Immanuel Kant, who sought alternative ways of thinking about the world.

constructivist paradigm   The basis of most qualitative research, which is concerned with the ways in which people construct their worlds.

consumer   An individual who actively uses and applies research findings in nursing practice.

content analysis   A technique for the objective, systematic, and quantitative description of communications and documentary evidence.

content validity   The degree to which the content of the measure represents the universe of content or the domain of a given behaviour.

context   The environment where an event occurs or a phenomenon is based (time, place, cultural beliefs, values, and practices).

contrasted-groups approach   A method used to assess construct validity. A researcher identifies two groups of individuals who are suspected of having either an extremely high or an extremely low score on a characteristic. Scores from the groups are obtained and examined for sensitivity to the differences; also called *known-groups approach*.

control   The measures used to hold uniform or constant the conditions under which an investigation occurs.

control group   The group in an experimental investigation that does not receive an intervention or treatment; the comparison group.

convenience sampling   A nonprobability sampling strategy that uses the most readily accessible persons or objects as subjects in a study.

convergent validity   A strategy for assessing construct validity in which two or more tools that theoretically measure the same construct are administered to subjects. If the measures are positively correlated, convergent validity is said to be supported.

correlation   The degree of association between two variables.

correlational study   A type of nonexperimental research that examines the relationship between two or more variables.

credibility   Steps in qualitative research to ensure the accuracy, validity, and soundness of data.

criterion-related validity   The degree of relationship between performance on the measure and the actual behaviour, either in the present (concurrent) or in the future (predictive).

critical reading   An active interpretation and objective assessment of an article, during which the reader is looking for key concepts, ideas, and justifications.

critical thinking   The rational examination of ideas, inferences, principles, and conclusions.

critique   The process of objectively and critically evaluating the content of a research report for scientific merit and application to practice, theory, or education.

critiquing criteria   The criteria used for objectively and critically evaluating a research article.

Cronbach's alpha   A test of internal consistency that simultaneously compares each item in a scale with all others.

cross-sectional study   Nonexperimental research that looks at data at one point in time, that is, in the immediate present.

culture   The system of knowledge and linguistic expressions used by social groups that allows the researcher to interpret or make sense of the world.

Cumulative Index to Nursing and Allied Health Literature (CINAHL)   A print and computerized database; computerized CINAHL is available on CD-ROM and online.

data   Information systematically collected in the course of a study; the plural of *datum.*

data-based literature   Reports of completed research; also called *empirical literature, research literature,* and *scientific literature.*

data display   Compression and organization of data that promotes understanding and visualization and enables conclusions to be drawn.

data reduction   The process of selecting and transforming the data from field notes or transcriptions.

data saturation   A point when data collection can cease; data saturation occurs when the information being shared with the researcher becomes repetitive. Ideas conveyed by the participant have been shared before by other participants; inclusion of additional participants does not result in new ideas.

debriefing   The opportunity for researchers to discuss the study with the participants and for participants to refuse to have their data included in the study.

deductive reasoning   A logical thought process in which hypotheses are derived from theory; reasoning moves from the general to the particular.

degrees of freedom (*df*)   The number of quantities that are unknown minus the number of independent equations linking these unknowns; a function of the number in the sample.

delimitations   Characteristics that restrict the population to a homogeneous group of subjects.

Delphi technique   The technique of gaining expert opinion on a subject. The Delphi techniqe uses rounds or multiple stages of data collection, with each round using data from the previous round.

dependent variable   In experimental studies, the presumed effect of the independent or experimental variable on the outcome.

descriptive/exploratory survey   A type of nonexperimental research that collects descriptions of existing phenomena for the purpose of using the data to justify or assess current conditions or to make plans for improvement of conditions.

descriptive statistics   Statistical details used to describe and summarize sample data.

design   The plan or blueprint for conduct of a study.

developmental study   A type of nonexperimental research that is concerned not only with the existing status and interrelationships of phenomena but also with changes that take place as a function of time.

diffusion of innovations   The strategy for promoting adoption of evidence-based practices.

directional hypothesis   A hypothesis that specifies the expected direction of the relationship between independent and dependent variables.

dissemination   The communication of research findings.

divergent validity   A strategy for assessing construct validity in which two or more tools that theoretically measure the opposite of the construct are administered to subjects. If the measures correlate negatively, divergent validity is said to be supported.

domains In an ethnographic study, symbolic categories that include smaller categories.

effect size Measurement of the magnitude of a treatment effect.

electronic databases The electronic means by which journal sources (periodicals) of data-based and conceptual articles on a variety of topics (e.g., doctoral dissertations) are produced, as well as the publications of professional organizations and various governmental agencies.

element The most basic unit about which information is collected.

eligibility criteria Those characteristics that restrict the population to a homogeneous group of subjects.

emic view The native's or insider's view of the world.

empirical-analytical A general label for quantitative research approaches that test hypotheses.

empirical factors Those things that can be observed through the senses; the obtaining of evidence or objective data.

empirical literature A synonym for data-based literature; see *data-based literature*.

epidemiological study Examines factors affecting the health and illness of populations in relation to the environment.

epistemology The theory of knowledge; the branch of philosophy concerned with how people know what they know.

equivalence Consistency or agreement among observers using the same measurement tool or agreement among alternate forms of a tool.

error variance The extent to which the variance in test scores is attributable to error rather than to a true measure of behaviours.

ethics The theory or discipline dealing with principles of moral values and moral conduct.

ethnographic method A method that scientifically describes cultural groups. The goal of the ethnographer is to understand the natives' view of their world.

ethnographic research See *ethnography*.

ethnography A qualitative research approach designed to produce cultural theory.

etic view An outsider's view of another's world.

evaluation research The use of scientific research methods and procedures to evaluate a program, treatment, practice, or policy outcomes; the analytical means used to document the worth of an activity.

evidence-based practice (EBP) guidelines Principles that help the researcher better understand the evidence base of certain practices.

evidence-based practice (EBP) The conscious and judicious use of the current "best" evidence in the care of clients and the delivery of health care services.

ex post facto study A type of nonexperimental research that examines the relationships among variables after variations have occurred.

experiment A scientific investigation in which observations are made and data are collected by means of the characteristics of control, randomization, and manipulation.

experimental design A research design that has the following properties: randomization, control, and manipulation.

experimental group The group in an experimental investigation that receives an intervention or treatment.

external criticism A process used to judge the authenticity of historical data.

external validity The degree to which the findings of a study can be generalized to other populations or environments.

extraneous variable   A variable that interferes with the operations of the phenomena being studied; also called *mediating variable*.

face validity   A type of content validity that uses an expert's opinion to judge the accuracy of an instrument.

factor analysis   A strategy for assessing construct validity that uses a statistical procedure for determining the underlying dimensions or components of a variable.

feasibility   The capability of the study to be successfully completed.

findings   The statistical results of a study.

Fisher's exact probability test   An analysis used to compare frequencies when samples are small and expected frequencies are less than six in each cell.

fittingness   An evaluation criterion that involves answering the following questions: Are the findings applicable outside the study situation? Are the results meaningful to the individuals not involved in the research?

formative evaluation   Assessment of a program as it is being implemented, usually focusing on evaluation of the process of a program rather than the outcomes.

frequency distribution   A descriptive statistical method for summarizing the occurrences of events under study.

generalizability (generalize)   Inferences that the data are representative of similar phenomena in a population beyond the studied sample.

grand theory   An all-inclusive conceptual structure that tends to include views on person, health, and environment to create a perspective of nursing.

grounded theory   A research approach that is constructed inductively from a base of observations of the world as it is lived by a selected group of people.

grounded theory method   An inductive approach that uses a systematic set of procedures to arrive at theory about basic social processes.

Hawthorne effect   See *reactivity*.

hermeneutics   A theoretical framework to understand or interpret human phenomena from the study of the interpretation of phenomena.

heterogeneity   Dissimilarities of a sample group, which inhibit the researchers' ability to interpret the findings meaningfully and make generalizations.

hierarchical linear modelling (HLM)   A type of regression analysis that allows for analysis of hierarchically structured data simultaneously at all levels.

historical research method   The systematic compilation of data resulting from evaluation and interpretation of facts regarding people, events, and occurrences of the past.

history   The threat to internal validity that events outside of the experimental setting may affect the dependent variable.

homogeneity   A similarity of conditions; also called *internal consistency*.

homogeneous   Having limited variation in attributes or characteristics.

hypothesis   A prediction about the relationship between two or more variables.

hypothesis-testing approach   A strategy for assessing construct validity in which the theory or concept underlying a measurement instrument's design is used to develop hypotheses that are tested. Inferences are made based on the findings about whether the rationale underlying the instrument's construction is adequate to explain the findings.

incidence The number of cases occurring in a particular period.

independent variable The antecedent or variable that has the presumed effect on the dependent variable.

inductive reasoning A logical thought process in which generalizations are developed from specific observations; reasoning moves from the particular to the general.

inferential statistics Statistical details that combine mathematical processes and logic to test hypotheses about a population with the help of sample data.

information literacy The skills needed to consult the literature and answer a clinical question.

informed consent An ethical principle that requires a researcher to obtain the voluntary participation of subjects after informing them of potential benefits and risks.

instrumental case study Research undertaken to pursue insight into an issue or to challenge a generalization.

instrumentation Changes in the measurement of the variables that may account for changes in the obtained measurement.

integrative review Synthesis review of the literature on a specific concept or topic.

internal consistency The extent to which items within a scale reflect or measure the same concept; also called *homogeneity*.

internal criticism The process of judging the reliability or consistency of information within a historical document.

internal validity The degree to which the experimental treatment, not an uncontrolled condition, resulted in the observed effects.

Internet The global electronic network that links a cadre of participating networks (e.g., commercial, educational, and governmental agencies); see also *World Wide Web*.

interrater reliability The consistency of observations between two or more observers; often expressed as a percentage of agreement between raters or observers or a coefficient of agreement that takes into account the element of chance; generally used with the direct observation method.

intersubjectivity The belief that others share a common world with us; an important tenet in phenomenology.

interval measurement The level of measurement used to show rankings of events or objects on a scale, with equal intervals between numbers but with an arbitrary zero (e.g., Celsius temperature).

intervening variable A variable that occurs during an experimental or quasiexperimental study that affects the dependent variable.

intervention An observational method that deals with whether or not the observer provokes actions from those who are being observed.

intervention fidelity Consistency in data collection.

interview A method of data collection in which a data collector questions a subject verbally. An interview may occur face to face or over the telephone and may consist of open-ended or close-ended questions.

intrinsic case study Research undertaken to gain a better understanding of the essential nature of the case.

item-to-total correlation The relationship between each of the items on a scale and the total scale.

justice The principle that human subjects should be treated fairly.

kappa The level of agreement observed beyond the level that would be expected by chance alone.

key informants   Individuals who have special knowledge, status, or communication skills and who are willing to share their expertise with the ethnographer.

knowledge-focused triggers   Ideas that are generated when staff read research, listen to scientific papers at research conferences, or encounter evidence-based practice guidelines published by federal agencies or specialty organizations.

known-groups approach   See *contrasted-groups approach.*

Kuder–Richardson (KR-20) coefficient   The estimate of homogeneity used for instruments that use a dichotomous response pattern.

kurtosis   The relative peakness or flatness of a distribution.

level of significance (alpha level)   The risk of making a type I error, set by the researcher before the study begins.

level of evidence   A measure of the strength of evidence found in a research study.

levels of measurement   Categorization of the precision with which an event can be measured (nominal, ordinal, interval, and ratio).

life context   The matrix of human–human–environment relationships emerging over the course of one's life.

Likert-type scale   A list of statements on which respondents indicate whether they "strongly agree," "agree," "disagree," or "strongly disagree."

limitations   The weaknesses of a study.

Linear Structural Relationships (LISREL)   A computer program developed to analyze covariance and the testing of complex causal models.

literature   Print and nonprint sources, such as books, chapters of books, journal articles, critique reviews, abstracts published in conference proceedings, professional and governmental reports, and unpublished doctoral dissertations.

lived experience   In phenomenological research, the focus on living through events and circumstances (prelingual) as opposed to thinking about these events and circumstances (conceptualized experience).

logistic regression (or logit analysis)   The analysis of relationships between multiple independent variables and a dependent variable that is binary, ordinal, or polynomial.

longitudinal study   A nonexperimental research design in which a researcher collects data from the same group at different points in time.

manipulation   The provision of some experimental treatment, in varying degrees, to some of the subjects in the study.

matching   A special sampling strategy used to construct an equivalent comparison sample group by filling it with subjects who are similar to each subject in another sample group in terms of pre-established variables, such as age and gender.

maturation   Developmental, biological, or psychological processes that operate within an individual as a function of time and are external to the events of the investigation.

mean (*M*)   A measure of central tendency; the arithmetic average of all scores.

measurement   The assignment of numbers to objects or events according to rules.

measurement effects   Administration of a pretest in a study that affects the generalizability of the findings to other populations.

measures of central tendency   Descriptive statistical techniques that describe the average member of a sample (e.g., mean, median, and mode).

measures of variability   A descriptive statistical procedure that describes the level of dispersion in sample data.

median   A measure of central tendency; the middle score.

mediating variable   A variable that is between or occurs between an independent variable and a dependent variable and can produce an indirect effect of the independent variable on the dependent variable; also called *extraneous variable.*

MEDLINE   The print or computerized database of standard medical literature analysis and retrieval system online; it is also available on CD-ROM.

meta-analysis   A research method that takes the results of multiple studies in a specific area and synthesizes the findings to make conclusions regarding the area of focus.

metaparadigm   A broad philosophical or conceptual framework. Nursing's meta-paradigm includes person, environment, health, and nursing.

metasynthesis   A technique for drawing inferences or synthesizing findings from similar or related studies.

methodological research   The controlled investigation and measurement of the means of gathering and analyzing data.

microrange theory   The linking of concrete concepts into a statement that can be examined in practice and research.

midrange theory   A focused conceptual structure that synthesizes practice–research into ideas central to the discipline.

mixed methods research   Research in which the investigator collects and analyzes data, integrates the findings, and draws inferences using both qualitative and quantitative approaches or methods in a single study or a program of inquiry; one form of triangulation.

modal percentage   A measure of variability; percentage of cases in the mode.

modality   The number of peaks in a frequency distribution.

mode   A measure of central tendency; the most frequent score or result.

model   A symbolic representation of a set of concepts that is created to depict relationships.

mortality   The loss of a subject from time 1 data collection to time 2 data collection.

multiple analysis of variance (MANOVA)   A test used to determine differences in group means when a study has more than one dependent variable.

multiple regression   The measure of the relationship between one interval-level dependent variable and several independent variables. Canonical correlation is used when a study has more than one dependent variable.

multistage sampling   A sampling method that involves successive random sampling of units (clusters) that progresses from large to small and meets sample eligibility criteria; also known as *cluster sampling.*

multitrait–multimethod approach   A type of validity that uses more than one method to assess the accuracy of an instrument (e.g., observation and interview of anxiety).

narrative analysis   A field of hermeneutics that focuses on the lived experience and perceptions of experience, using materials such as in-depth interview transcripts, memoirs, stories, and creative nonfiction.

naturalistic research   A general label for qualitative studies that involve the researcher going to a natural setting where the phenomenon being studied is taking place.

network sampling   A strategy used for finding samples that are difficult to locate. It uses social networks and the fact that friends tend to have characteristics in common; subjects who meet the eligibility criteria are asked for assistance in getting in touch with others who meet the same criteria; also known as *snowball effect sampling.*

nominal measurement The level used to classify objects or events into categories without any relative ranking (e.g., gender, hair colour).

nondirectional hypothesis A hypothesis that indicates the existence of a relationship between the variables but does not specify the anticipated direction of the relationship.

nonequivalent control group design A quasi-experimental design that is similar to the true experiment, but subjects are not randomly assigned to the treatment or the control group.

nonexperimental research design A research design in which an investigator observes a phenomenon without manipulating the independent variable(s).

nonparametric statistics Statistics that are usually used when variables are measured at the nominal or ordinal level because they do not estimate population parameters and involve less restrictive assumptions about the underlying distribution.

nonparametric tests of significance Inferential statistics that make no assumptions about the population distribution.

nonprobability sampling A selection technique in which elements are chosen by nonrandom methods.

normal curve A curve that is unimodal and symmetrical about the mean.

null hypothesis A statement that no relationship exists between the variables and that any relationship observed is a result of chance or fluctuations in sampling; also known as a *statistical hypothesis*.

null value When an experimental value indicates no difference between the treatment and control groups; known as *the value of no effect*.

objective Data that are not influenced by anyone who collects the information.

objectivity The use of facts without distortion by personal feelings or bias.

observed test score The actual score obtained in a measure.

odds ratio The probability of an event, which is calculated by dividing the odds in the treated or exposed group by the odds in the control group.

one-group (pretest–post-test) design A study approach used by researchers when only one group is available for study; subjects act as their own controls, and no randomization occurs, thus enhancing the internal validity of the study.

ontology The study of being, of existence, and its relationship to nonexistence.

open-ended item A question that respondents may answer in their own words.

operational definition The measurements used to observe or measure a variable; delineates the procedures or operations required to measure a concept.

operationalization The process of translating concepts into observable, measurable phenomena.

opinion leaders Individuals from the local peer group who are viewed as respected sources of influence, considered by associates to be technically competent, and trusted to judge the fit between the evidence-based practice and the local situation.

ordinal measurement A level used to show rankings of events or objects; numbers are not equidistant, and zero is arbitrary (class ranking).

orientational qualitative inquiry A qualitative approach in which researchers begin with an ideology or orientation (e.g., feminism, Marxism, critical theory) to direct the inquiry, including the research question, methodology, fieldwork, and analysis of the findings.

p value The conditional probability of obtaining, from the study data, the value of the test statistic that is at least as extreme as that calculated from the data, given that the null hypothesis is true.

paradigm   From the Greek word meaning "pattern," this word has been applied to science to describe the way people in society think about the world.

parallel form reliability   See *alternate form reliability.*

parameter   A characteristic of a population.

parametric statistics   Inferential statistics that involve the estimation of at least one parameter, require measurement at the interval level or higher, and involve assumptions about the variables being studied. These assumptions usually include the fact that the variable is normally distributed.

participatory action research   A form of orientation research that seeks to change society; the researcher studies a particular setting to identify problem areas to improve practice, identify possible solutions, and take action to implement changes.

path analysis   A statistical technique in which the researcher hypothesizes how variables are related and in what order and then tests the strength of those relationships or paths.

Pearson correlation coefficient (Pearson *r*)   A statistic that is calculated to reflect the degree of relationship between two interval level variables; also called *Pearson product moment correlation coefficient.*

peer-reviewed journal   See *refereed journal.*

percentile   A measure of rank; percentage of cases a given score exceeds.

phenomenological method   A process of learning and constructing the meaning of human experience through intensive dialogue with persons who are living the experience.

phenomenological research   Research that is based on phenomenological philosophy and is aimed at obtaining a description of an experience as it is lived to understand the meaning of that experience for those who are going through it.

phenomenology   A qualitative research approach that aims to describe experience as it is lived through, before it is conceptualized.

philosophical beliefs   The system of motivating values, concepts, principles, and the nature of human knowledge of an individual, group, or culture; see also *paradigm* and *worldview.*

physiological measurement   The use of specialized equipment to determine the physical status of subjects.

pilot study   A small, simple study conducted as a prelude to a larger-scale study, which is often called the "parent study".

population   A well-defined set that has certain specified properties.

positivism   The "received view" in quantitative research; a philosophical approach that recognizes only observable data.

post hoc analysis   Comparison of all possible pairs of means after conducting an omnibus ANOVA test to determine where the difference lies.

post-test-only control group design   See *after-only design.*

power   The conditional prior probability of the researcher making a correct decision to reject the null hypothesis when it is actually false, denoted as $1 - b$.

prediction study   A type of nonexperimental research design that attempts to make a forecast or prediction derived from particular phenomena.

predictive validity   The degree of correlation between the measure of the concept and some future measure of the same concept.

prevalence   The number of people affected by a disease or health problem.

primary source   Scholarly literature that is written by a person or persons who developed the theory or conducted the research. Primary sources include eyewitness accounts of historical events provided by original documents, films, letters, diaries, records, artifacts, periodicals, and tapes.

print databases   Indexes, card catalogues, and abstract reviews. Print indexes are used to find journal sources (periodicals) of data-based and conceptual articles on a variety of topics, as well as publications of professional organizations and various governmental agencies.

print indexes   See *print databases.*

probability   The probability of an event is the event's long-run relative frequency in repeated trials under similar conditions.

probability sampling   A selection technique that uses some form of random selection when the sample units are chosen.

problem-focused triggers   Research triggers that are identified by staff through quality improvement, risk surveillance, benchmarking data, financial data, or recurrent clinical problems.

process consent   A request for the respondent's continued participation in a study.

product testing   The testing of medical devices.

propositions   The linkage of concepts that lays a foundation for the development of methods that test relationships.

prospective study   A nonexperimental study that begins with an exploration of assumed causes and then moves forward in time to the presumed effect.

psychometrics   The theory and development of measurement instruments.

purpose   The aim or goal the investigator hopes to achieve with the research.

purposive sampling   A nonprobability sampling strategy in which the researcher selects subjects who are considered to be typical of the population.

qualitative research   The study of research questions about human experiences. Qualitative research is often conducted in natural settings and uses data that are words or text, as opposed to numerical data, to describe the experiences being studied.

quantitative research   The process of testing relationships, differences, and cause-and-effect interactions among and between variables. These processes are tested with hypotheses and research questions.

quasiexperiment   Research in which the researcher initiates an experimental treatment, but some characteristic of a true experiment is lacking.

quasiexperimental design   A research approach in which random assignment is not used, but the independent variable is manipulated and certain mechanisms of control are used.

questionnaire   An instrument designed to gather data from individuals.

quota sampling   A nonprobability sampling strategy that identifies the strata of the population and proportionately represents the strata in the sample.

random error   See *chance error.*

random selection   A selection process in which each element of the population has an equal and independent chance of being included in the sample.

randomization   A sampling selection procedure in which each person or element in a population has an equal chance of being selected to either the experimental group or the control group.

range   A measure of variability; the difference between the highest and the lowest scores in a set of sample data.

ratio measurement   The ranking of the order of events or objects that has equal intervals and an absolute zero (e.g., height, weight).

reactivity   The distortion created when those who are being observed change their behaviour because they know that they are being observed; also known as the *Hawthorne effect*.

recommendation   Application of a study to practice, theory, and future research.

records or available data   Information that is collected from existing materials, such as hospital records, historical documents, and videotapes.

refereed (peer-reviewed) journal   A scholarly journal that has a panel of external and internal reviewers or editors; the panel reviews manuscripts submitted for possible publication. The review panel uses the same set of scholarly criteria to judge whether the manuscripts are worthy of publication.

reflexivity   The situation wherein researchers must monitor whether their own perspectives are affecting their research methods, analyses, or interpretations.

relationship/difference study   A study that traces the relationships or differences between variables that can provide a deeper insight into a phenomenon.

reliability   The consistency or constancy of a measuring instrument.

reliability coefficient   A number between 0 and 1 that expresses the relationship between the error variance, true variance, and the observed score. A 0 correlation indicates no relationship. The closer to 1 the coefficient is, the more reliable is the tool; also called the *alpha coefficient*.

representative sample   A sample whose key characteristics closely approximate those of the population.

research base   The accumulated knowledge gained from several studies that have investigated a similar problem.

research-based practice   Nursing practice that is based on research studies, that is, supported by research findings.

research-based protocols   Practice standards that are formulated from the findings of several studies.

research ethics board (REB)   A board established in agencies to review biomedical and behavioural research involving human subjects within the agency or in programs sponsored by the agency.

research hypothesis   A statement about the expected relationship between the variables; also known as a *scientific hypothesis*.

research literature   A synonym for data-based literature; see *data-based literature*.

research question   A key preliminary step wherein the foundation for a study is developed from the research problem and results in the research hypothesis.

research utilization   A systematic method of implementing sound research-based innovations in clinical practice, evaluating the outcome, and sharing the knowledge through the process of research dissemination.

respect for persons   The idea that people have the right to self-determination and to being treated as autonomous agents; that is, they have the freedom to participate or not participate in research.

retrospective data   Data that have been manifested, such as scores on a standard examination.

retrospective study   A nonexperimental research design that begins with the phenomenon of interest (the dependent variable) in the present and examines its relationship to another variable (the independent variable) in the past.

review of the literature   An extensive, systematic, and critical review of the most important published scholarly literature on a particular topic. In most cases, the literature review is not considered exhaustive.

rigour   The quality, believability, or trustworthiness of study findings.

risk   The potential negative outcome(s) of participation in a research study.

risk–benefit ratio   The extent to which the benefits of the study are maximized and the risks are minimized such that the subjects are protected from harm during the study.

sample   A subset of sampling units from a population.

sampling   A process in which representative units of a population are selected for study in a research investigation.

sampling error   The tendency for statistics to fluctuate from one sample to another.

sampling frame   A list of all units of the population.

sampling interval   The standard distance between the elements chosen for the sample.

sampling unit   The element or set of elements used for selecting the sample.

saturation   See *data saturation.*

scale   A self-report inventory that provides a set of response symbols for each item. A rating or score is assigned to each response.

scatter plot   A visual representation of the strength and magnitude of the relationship between two variables.

scholarly literature   Published and unpublished data-based and conceptual literature material found in print and nonprint forms.

scientific hypothesis   The researcher's expectation about the outcome of a study; also known as the *research hypothesis.*

scientific literature   A synonym for data-based literature; see *data-based literature.*

scientific merit   The degree of validity of a study or group of studies.

scientific observation   The collecting of data about the environment and subjects. Data collection has specific objectives to guide it, is systematically planned and recorded, is checked and controlled, and is related to scientific concepts and theories.

secondary analysis   A form of research in which the researcher takes previously collected and analyzed data from one study and reanalyzes the data for a secondary purpose.

secondary source   Scholarly material written by a person or persons other than the individual who developed the theory or conducted the research. Secondary sources are usually published. Often a secondary source represents a response to or a summary and critique of a theorist's or researcher's work. Examples are documents, films, letters, diaries, records, artifacts, periodicals, and tapes that provide a view of the phenomenon from another's perspective.

selection   The generalizability of the results to other populations.

selection bias   The internal validity threat that arises when pretreatment differences exist between the experimental group and the control group.

semi-interquartile range   See *semiquartile range.*

semiquartile range   A measure of variability; the range of the middle 50% of the scores; also known as *semi-interquartile range.*

simple random sampling   A probability sampling strategy in which the population is defined, a sampling frame is listed, and a subset from which the sample will be chosen is selected; members are randomly selected.

skew   The measure of the asymmetry of a set of scores.

snowball effect sampling   A strategy used for finding samples that are difficult to locate. This strategy uses social networks and the fact that friends tend to have characteristics in common; subjects who meet the eligibility criteria are asked for assistance in getting in touch with others who meet the same criteria; also known as *network sampling.*

social desirability   The tendency of a subject to respond in a manner that he or she believes will please the researcher rather than in an honest manner.

Solomon four-group design   An experimental design with four randomly assigned groups: the pretest–post-test intervention group, the pretest–post-test control group, a treatment or intervention group with only post-test measurement, and a control group with only post-test measurement.

split-half reliability   An index of the comparison between the scores on one half of a test with those on the other half to determine the consistency in response to items that reflect specific content.

stability   An instrument's ability to produce the same results with repeated testing.

standard deviation (SD)   A measure of variability; measure of average deviation of scores from the mean.

standard error of the mean   The standard deviation of a theoretical distribution of sample means. It indicates the average error in the estimation of the population mean.

statistic   A characteristic of a sample.

statistical hypothesis   A statement that no relationship exists between the independent and dependent variables; also known as a *null hypothesis.*

stratified random sampling   A probability sampling strategy in which the population is divided into strata or subgroups. An appropriate number of elements from each subgroup are randomly selected based on their proportion in the population.

summative evaluation   Assessment of the outcomes of a program, conducted after the program's completion.

survey study   A descriptive, exploratory, or comparative study that collects detailed descriptions of existing variables and uses the data to justify and assess current conditions and practices or to make more plans for improving health care practices.

symbolic interactionism   A theoretical perspective that holds that the relationship between self and society is an ongoing process of symbolic communication whereby individuals create a social reality.

symmetry   When the two halves of a distribution are mirror images of one another (i.e., when folded over, they can be superimposed on each other).

systematic   A term used when data collection is carried out in the same manner with all subjects.

systematic error   An error attributable to the lasting characteristics of the subject that do not tend to fluctuate from one time to another; also called *constant error.*

systematic review   A summary of research evidence from several studies.

systematic sampling   A probability sampling strategy that involves the selection of subjects randomly drawn from a population list at fixed intervals.

t **statistic**   The test of whether two groups' means are more different than would be expected by chance. The groups may be related or independent.

target population   A population or group of individuals who meet the sampling criteria.

testability   The concept that the variables of a proposed study lend themselves to observation, measurement, and analysis.

testing   The effect on the scores of a post-test as the result of having taken a pre-test.

test–retest reliability   The administration of the same instrument twice to the same subjects under the same conditions within a prescribed time interval, with a comparison of the paired scores to determine the stability of the measure.

text   Data in a contextual form; that is, narrative or words that were written from recorded interviews and then transcribed.

thematic analysis   The process of recognizing and recovering the emergent themes.

themes   Units of data with structured meaning that occur frequently.

theoretical framework   A structure for concepts that exist in the literature, which may provide theoretical rationale for the development of hypotheses.

theoretical literature   A synonym for conceptual literature; see *conceptual literature*.

theoretical sampling   In the grounded theory method, the sampling method used to select experiences that will help the researcher test ideas and gather complete information about developing concepts.

theory   A set of inter-related concepts, definitions, and propositions that present a systematic view of phenomena for the purpose of explaining and making predictions about those phenomena.

time series design   A quasiexperimental design used to determine trends before and after an experimental treatment. Measurements are taken several times before the introduction of the experimental treatment, the treatment is introduced, and measurements are taken again at specified times afterward.

transferability   The findings from one qualitative research study having meaning to others in similar situations.

translation science   The investigation of methods, interventions, and variables that influence the adoption of evidence-based practices.

triangulation   The expansion of research methods in a single study or multiple studies to enhance diversity, enrich understanding, and accomplish specific goals.

true experiment   A study design in which subjects are randomly assigned to an experimental group or a control group, pretest measurements are performed, an intervention or treatment occurs in the experimental group, and post-test measurements are performed; also known as the *pretest–post-test control group design*.

trustworthiness   An accurate portrayal of the experience of the study's participants.

type I error   The researchers' incorrect decision to reject the null hypothesis.

type II error   As a result of the sample data, the failure to reject the null hypothesis when it is actually false; also known as beta (β).

validation sample   The sample that provides the initial data for determining the reliability and validity of a measurement tool.

validity   The determination of whether a measurement instrument actually measures what it is purported to measure.

variables   A defined concept; properties that take on different values and are studied by quantitative researchers.

Web browser   A software program used to connect to or "read" the World Wide Web (e.g., Internet Explorer).

World Wide Web (www)   A conceptual group of servers on the Internet. The Web is multiple hypertexts linked together in a network that criss-crosses the whole Internet like a spider web.

worldview   The way people in society think about the world; a synonym for *paradigm*.

Z score   A rating used to compare measurements in standard units; an examination of the relative distance of the scores from the mean.

Index

Page number followed by b indicates box; f, figure; t, table.